Review Questions and Answers

for
Veterinary Technicians

Review Questions and Answers

for
Veterinary Technicians

Fourth Edition

Thomas Colville, DVM, MSc
Director, Veterinary Technology Program
North Dakota State University
Fargo, North Dakota

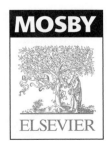
MOSBY
ELSEVIER

MOSBY
ELSEVIER

3251 Riverport Lane
St. Louis, Missouri 63043

Library of Congress Cataloging-in-Publication Data

Review questions and answers for veterinary technicians/[edited by] Thomas Colville.—4th ed.
    p. ; cm.
  Rev. ed. of: Review questions & answers for veterinary technicians / [edited by] Thomas Colville.
3rd ed. 2003.
  ISBN 978-0-323-06801-7 (pbk. : alk. paper)
  1. Animal health technicians—Examinations, questions, etc. 2. Animal health technology—
Examinations, questions, etc. I. Colville, Thomas P. II. Review questions & answers for
veterinary technicians.
  [DNLM: 1. Animal Technicians—Examination Questions. SF 774.4 R454 2010]
  SF774.4.R48 2010
  636.089'076—dc22

                                                                    2009037447

Vice President and Publisher: Linda Duncan
Publisher: Penny Rudolph
Acquisitions Editor: Teri Merchant
Publishing Services Manager: Hemamalini Rajendrababu
Project Manager: Shereen Jameel
Book Designer: Charlie Seibel

Printed in the United States of America

Last digit is the print number: 9 8 7 6 5 4 3 2 1

Contributors

Joann Colville, DVM
Program Director, retired
Veterinary Technology Program
Fargo, North Dakota

Eloyes Hill, BS, MT
Veterinary Technology Program
North Dakota State University
Fargo, North Dakota

Marianne Tear, MS, LVT
Program Director
Veterinary Technology Program
Baker College
Clinton Township, Michigan

Sarah A. Wagner, DVM, PhD, Dipl ACVCP
Assistant Professor of Veterinary Technology
Department of Animal Sciences
North Dakota State University
Fargo, North Dakota

Preface

New editions of books are often more similar to previous editions than different. This fourth edition of *Review Questions and Answers for Veterinary Technicians*, however, departs significantly from previous editions in both form and content.

The content of the book is arranged to allow intuitive review for the Veterinary Technician National Examination (VTNE). The seven main subject areas in the **VTNE Review** section represent the seven "domains" of the VTNE that were in effect when this was written. The subjects included in the **Foundation Knowledge Review** section represent general knowledge that is included in all of the seven VTNE domains.

The 5,000+ questions in this book resulted from a process that began with a rigorous review of each of the questions from the second and third editions. In order to meet the criteria for inclusion in this edition, each question, answer, and rationale had to reflect accurate, contemporary, entry-level veterinary technology knowledge. More than 1,500 of the questions, answers, and explanations are completely new or significantly revised.

The questions in *Review Questions and Answers for Veterinary Technicians* test factual knowledge, reasoning skills, and clinical judgment. To the best of our knowledge, none of the questions in this book has come directly from any current or previous credentialing examination. When properly used, however, the questions can help identify strong and weak subject areas.

Thomas Colville

Acknowledgments

This book is the result of a lot of effort on the part of a knowledgeable and dedicated team. I am honored to have been able to work with these skilled professionals, and I am pleased to acknowledge the vital contributions they made.

I am grateful to Joann Colville, Eloyes Hill, Marianne Tear, and Sarah Wagner, all current or former veterinary technician educators, who took time out of their busy schedules to review, revise, and re-write questions for this book. I know from experience that veterinary technician educators are the "one-armed wallpaper hangers" of the educational world. They (we) are kept very busy filling all the roles necessary to educate veterinary technology students for the complex professional world that awaits them. It is a tribute to the commitment of these individuals that they took the time to prepare such an excellent collection of challenging questions.

I am grateful to Teri Merchant, the project's managing editor at Elsevier, for her patience, perseverance, and perspicacity in bringing our vision of this edition of the book to fruition. The unconventional format of the book, with the complete contents provided in both printed and CD-ROM format, is a testament to Teri's foresight and leadership.

Finally, on behalf of veterinary technician educators everywhere, I would like to acknowledge our students and graduates. They are pioneers in this young profession. Their hard work and devotion to their profession is inspiring and gratifying. It is for them that this book was created, and it is to them that it is dedicated.

Thomas Colville

Credentialing of Veterinary Technicians

In most states and Canadian provinces, individuals who wish to work as veterinary technicians must demonstrate their knowledge and competence by completing a credentialing process that is administered by an appropriate regulatory agency. Successful completion of this credentialing process generally confers the title of Licensed Veterinary Technician (LVT), Certified Veterinary Technician (CVT), or Registered Veterinary Technician (RVT) on the individual, depending on the terminology used in that state.

Nearly all states and provinces that regulate the veterinary technology profession use the Veterinary Technician National Examination (VTNE) as the main component of their credentialing process, although some jurisdictions have additional requirements. Candidates should contact the appropriate regulatory agency in the state or province in which they desire credentialing to obtain information on processes, requirements, and deadlines. Contact information can be found on the website of the American Association of Veterinary State Boards (AAVSB) at http://www.aavsb.org.

The VTNE is offered by the AAVSB under a contractual agreement with the Professional Examination Service (PES). It is designed to evaluate essential job-related knowledge at the entry level, and consists of 225 multiple-choice questions in seven primary subject areas called "domains." The current VTNE domains are:

- Pharmacy and Pharmacology
- Surgical Preparation and Assisting
- Dentistry
- Laboratory Procedures
- Animal Care and Nursing
- Diagnostic Imaging
- Anesthesia and Analgesia

Once the VTNE has been passed in a state or province, the examination score can be transferred to other states or provinces. Information on this process is also available on the AAVSB website.

How to Use This Book

Review Questions and Answers for Veterinary Technicians, Fourth Edition, covers every major aspect of veterinary technology. It contains more than 5,000 questions, answers, and explanations. A CD bound inside each book contains all of the book content in study and quiz modes, and in a 200-question practice test that can be taken in timed examination mode. The questions are divided into two main sections, ***Foundation Knowledge Review*** and ***VTNE Review.***

The subjects covered in the ***Foundation Knowledge Review*** section represent general knowledge that is included in all of the 7 VTNE domains. They are:
- Anatomy and Physiology
- Hospital Procedures
- Medical Calculations
- Medical Terminology

The foundation subjects are particularly important because questions in the second section, *VTNE Review,* are built on the foundational knowledge in the first section. It may be helpful to complete the *Foundation Knowledge Review* section before beginning the *VTNE Review* section.

The subjects covered in the ***VTNE Review*** section correspond to the seven VTNE domains that were in effect when this was written. They are:
- Pharmacology
- Surgical Nursing
- Dentistry
- Clinical Laboratory
- Animal Nursing (consisting of four subsections)
  - Animal Care
  - Emergency Care
  - Pocket Pets/Laboratory Animals
  - Medical Nursing
- Diagnostic Imaging
- Anesthesiology

The primary intent of this book is to help students and graduate veterinary technicians prepare for examinations–either in academic programs or for credentialing purposes. Before beginning a section, review textbooks and course notes pertaining to that subject area, then approach each section as though it were an actual examination.

- *Carefully read each question.* Look for key words such as "most," "best," "least," "always," "never," and "except." Consider only the facts presented in the question. Do not make assumptions and inferences that may not be true.

- *Carefully evaluate each answer choice.* Each question has only one correct answer. The other three choices are incorrect "distractors." If more than one answer choice appears to be correct, closely examine each one for clues that would eliminate it as incorrect.

- *Select an answer for each question.*

- *Compare your answers with the correct answers.* The correct answers are listed at the end of each section. Most are accompanied by an explanation.

- *Identify "weak" areas.* Subject areas with many incorrect answers may indicate the need for further review.

The companion **CD-ROM** is set up in several different modes to better help the student study for the VTNE exam.

The *study mode* includes all of the multiple-choice questions available in the book divided into sections by topic. The student chooses the specific section he or she wishes to study, and he or she can select any number of questions from that section to review. The student receives instant feedback as to whether the question was answered correctly or incorrectly, along with a rationale for the correct answer, where needed.

The *quiz mode* includes all of the multiple-choice questions available in the book, divided into sections by topic. The student chooses a section and selects any number of questions from that section for the quiz. Once the student completes all of the questions the quiz is scored, and the student may review his or her answers and the correct answers in Review mode. The student may also save his or her progress and return to a quiz later. They can bookmark and save questions for future review. Quiz results are archived to allow the student to keep track of his or her progress, and results may be printed.

Exam mode, like the actual VTNE exam, contains 200 questions that are selected randomly from across all section topics. The exam is timed and scored. Once it is completed the student is able to view his or her results in a table that displays the percentage of correct answers from each section to show which sections require further study. The student may then review the exam in its entirety with answers and rationales. As in quiz mode, the student may save progress and return to an exam later, and he or she can bookmark and save questions for future review. Results of the student's performance are archived for comparison with results of exams taken later, and exam results may be printed for reference.

Contents

Part One

FOUNDATION KNOWLEDGE REVIEW

Anatomy and Physiology

Joann Colville

QUESTIONS

1. Where are striated muscles located?
   a. Stomach wall and uterus
   b. Urinary bladder and intestine
   c. Ciliary body of the eye
   d. Heart and skeletal muscles

2. The pressure in the systemic arteries during ventricular contraction is
   a. Diastolic blood pressure
   b. Osmotic pressure
   c. Systolic blood pressure
   d. Low pressure

3. The difference between the systolic and diastolic pressures of the expanding and contracting arterial walls is the
   a. Pulse
   b. Osmotic pressure
   c. End-systolic volume
   d. Stroke volume

4. Input from what system causes vasoconstriction during exercise and therefore an increase in blood pressure?
   a. Sympathetic nervous system
   b. Parasympathetic nervous system
   c. Central nervous system
   d. Peripheral nervous system

5. Cardiac muscle is
   a. Nonstriated involuntary
   b. Striated involuntary
   c. Nonstriated voluntary
   d. Striated voluntary

6. In what order does the impulse for depolarization travel through the heart?
   a. AV node, SA node, bundle of His, Purkinje fibers
   b. SA node, AV node, bundle of His, Purkinje fibers
   c. SA node, AV node, Purkinje fibers, bundle of His
   d. AV node, SA node, Purkinje fibers, bundle of His

7. The wave on an electrocardiogram that is associated with the atrial wall depolarization is the
   a. PR interval
   b. T wave
   c. QRS complex
   d. P wave

8. The SA node is located in the wall of which chamber?
   a. Left atrium
   b. Left ventricle
   c. Right atrium
   d. Right ventricle

9. The muscular sphincter located between the stomach and the duodenum is the
   a. Pylorus
   b. Cardia
   c. Chyme
   d. Rugae

10. The type of cell responsible for the transmission of impulses through the nervous system is the
    a. Neuroglia
    b. Schwann
    c. Neuron
    d. Oligodendrocyte

11. What system is anatomically composed of the brain and spinal cord?
    a. Central nervous system
    b. Peripheral nervous system
    c. Parasympathetic nervous system
    d. Sympathetic nervous system

12. Functions that an animal does not have to consciously control, such as peristalsis in the intestine, are influenced by the
    a. Somatic nervous system
    b. Central nervous system
    c. Peripheral nervous system
    d. Autonomic nervous system

Correct answers are on pages 52-71.

13. The cranial nerves and the spinal nerves are anatomically part of what system?
    a. Central nervous system
    b. Peripheral nervous system
    c. Parasympathetic nervous system
    d. Sympathetic nervous system

14. Sensory nerves are considered
    a. Efferent motor nerves
    b. Motor nerves
    c. Efferent nerves
    d. Afferent nerves

15. An imbalance of what minerals can affect nerve function?
    a. Phosphorus and magnesium
    b. Sodium and potassium
    c. Manganese and chromium
    d. Iron and zinc

16. When a stimulus is strong enough to cause complete depolarization, it has reached
    a. Threshold
    b. Repolarization
    c. Refractory period
    d. Action potential

17. What happens within the neuron that allows local anesthetics to be effective?
    a. Potassium gates open
    b. The charge within the cell becomes positive
    c. The charge within the cell becomes negative
    d. Sodium channels become blocked

18. Smooth muscles can be found in the
    a. Heart
    b. Stomach
    c. Pelvic limb
    d. Diaphragm

19. Which muscle cells have single nuclei?
    a. Skeletal and cardiac
    b. Skeletal and smooth
    c. Smooth and cardiac
    d. Skeletal only

20. Cattle and swine display what type of estrous cycle?
    a. Polyestrous
    b. Seasonally polyestrous
    c. Diestrous
    d. Monoestrous

21. Dogs demonstrate what type of estrous cycle?
    a. Polyestrous
    b. Seasonally polyestrous
    c. Diestrous
    d. Monoestrous

22. What species is an induced ovulator?
    a. Bovine
    b. Equine
    c. Canine
    d. Feline

23. In what stage of the estrous cycle does the corpus luteum develop?
    a. Proestrus
    b. Estrus
    c. Metestrus
    d. Diestrus

24. The hormone produced by a developing ovarian follicle is
    a. Estrogen
    b. Progesterone
    c. Prolactin
    d. Oxytocin

25. What hormone contracts the female reproductive tract to help move spermatozoa into the oviducts?
    a. Estrogen
    b. Progesterone
    c. Prolactin
    d. Oxytocin

26. To achieve a normal pregnancy, the blastocyst attaches to what structure?
    a. Endometrium
    b. Placenta
    c. Oviduct
    d. Cervix

27. Giving birth is known as
    a. Parturition
    b. Gestation
    c. Lactation
    d. Estrous

28. From the estrous cycle to parturition, in what order are the following hormones released?
    a. Estrogen, oxytocin, progesterone
    b. Oxytocin, estrogen, progesterone
    c. Estrogen, progesterone, oxytocin
    d. Progesterone, estrogen, oxytocin

29. Which animal has a cotyledonary placenta?
    a. Cat
    b. Dog
    c. Horse
    d. Sheep

30. In cotyledonary placentation the mother's side of the attachment is called the
    a. Caruncle
    b. Cotyledon
    c. Placentome
    d. Polycyton

31. A pregnant mare has what kind of placentation?
    a. Zonary
    b. Cotyledonary
    c. Diffuse
    d. Discoid

32. A pregnant bitch has what kind of placentation?
    a. Zonary
    b. Cotyledonary
    c. Diffuse
    d. Discoid

33. A pregnant rodent has what kind of placentation?
    a. Zonary
    b. Cotyledonary
    c. Diffuse
    d. Discoid

34. A pregnant queen has what kind of placentation?
    a. Zonary
    b. Cotyledonary
    c. Diffuse
    d. Discoid

35. The canine uterus is shaped like the letter
    a. U
    b. Y
    c. J
    d. V

36. How many mammary glands are typically found on a bitch?
    a. 8–12
    b. 12–14
    c. 4–6
    d. 10–16

37. Which reaction is the result of parasympathetic nervous system stimulation?
    a. Bronchodilation
    b. Pupil dilation
    c. Decreased GI motility
    d. Decreased heart rate

38. Which reaction is the result of sympathetic nervous system stimulation?
    a. Decreased heart rate
    b. Dilated pupils
    c. Increased GI activity
    d. Increased salivation

39. Acetylcholine is released as a neurotransmitter by
    a. Effector organs
    b. Sensory bodies
    c. Postganglionic parasympathetic nerve fibers
    d. Postganglionic sympathetic nerve fibers

40. The neurotransmitter that is most responsible for the "flight or fight" reaction is
    a. Epinephrine
    b. Acetylcholine
    c. Dopamine
    d. Serotonin

41. In the healthy heart, the heartbeat is initiated by the
    a. SA node
    b. Purkinje fibers
    c. Vagus nerve
    d. AV node

42. On an electrocardiogram the T wave is most closely associated with
    a. Atrial depolarization
    b. Atrial repolarization
    c. Ventricular depolarization
    d. Ventricular repolarization

43. On an electrocardiogram the P wave is most closely associated with
    a. Atrial depolarization
    b. Atrial repolarization
    c. Ventricular depolarization
    d. Ventricular repolarization

44. Which of the following conditions is most life threatening?
    a. Atrial fibrillation
    b. Ventricular fibrillation
    c. First–degree heart block
    d. Complete heart block

45. Increasing a neuron's permeability to Na^+ will cause
    a. Hyperexcitability
    b. An increase in the intensity of the stimulus required to generate an action potential
    c. The neuron to become more hyperpolarized
    d. The membrane potential of the neuron to become more negative

Correct answers are on pages 52-71.

46. Atropine works primarily by
    a. Stimulating the sympathetic system
    b. Blocking the sympathetic system
    c. Stimulating the parasympathetic system
    d. Blocking parasympathetic actions

47. The primary constituent of blood responsible for the oncotic (osmotic) pressure of blood is
    a. NaCl
    b. Albumin
    c. Hemoglobin
    d. Red blood cells

48. Edema would mostly likely develop during or after which one of the following conditions?
    a. Salt deficiency
    b. Dehydration
    c. Low blood pressure
    d. Inactivity

49. On inspiration the pressure in the thoracic cavity, as compared with ambient air pressure, is
    a. Negative
    b. Positive
    c. Same as the ambient air pressure
    d. Fluctuating

50. In the healthy, awake cat the primary stimulus in blood for respiration is
    a. Increased CO_2
    b. Decreased O_2
    c. Increased lactic acid
    d. Increased K^+

51. An increased PCV (packed cell volume) could be indicative of
    a. Liver disease
    b. Anemia
    c. Leucocytosis
    d. Dehydration

52. Apnea will cause
    a. Metabolic acidosis
    b. Metabolic alkalosis
    c. Respiratory acidosis
    d. Respiratory alkalosis

53. Dehydration will typically not lead to
    a. Thirst
    b. Urine with a specific gravity greater than 1.015
    c. Increased osmolarity of blood
    d. Polyuria

54. Which of the following nutrients can be used for gluconeogenesis?
    a. Long-chain fatty acids
    b. Amino acids
    c. Vitamin C
    d. Iron

55. Cataracts are due to a problem with transparency of the
    a. Cornea
    b. Vitreous humor
    c. Lens
    d. Aqueous humor

56. A physiologic isotonic solution would contain
    a. 100 mOsm
    b. 200 mOsm
    c. 300 mOsm
    d. 500 mOsm

57. Cholesterol is necessary for
    a. Extracellular transport
    b. Cell membrane production
    c. Urine excretion
    d. Vitamin C metabolism

58. Which is not a function of insulin?
    a. Increased glucose transport into muscle
    b. Lipogenesis
    c. Fatty acid synthesis
    d. Increased blood pressure

59. Insulin resistance is commonly seen in animals that
    a. Are obese
    b. Have high blood pressure
    c. Exercise excessively
    d. Seek warmth

60. Long-term use of glucocorticoids will
    a. Increase lymphocyte production
    b. Increase plasma protein levels
    c. Suppress the immune system
    d. Decrease blood glucose levels

61. Nociceptors are important for detecting
    a. Color
    b. Warmth
    c. Lactic acid
    d. Pain

62. Areas with low sensory sensitivity are characterized by
    a. Nerves with small receptor fields
    b. Overlapping receptor fields
    c. Large numbers of neurons
    d. Lots of convergence

63. The vagus nerve is cranial nerve __.
    a. X
    b. XII
    c. V
    d. VI

64. The cranial nerves originate from the
    a. Cerebellum
    b. Spinal cord
    c. Brainstem
    d. Cerebrum

65. Glaucoma is
    a. Decreased pressure in the posterior chamber of the eye
    b. Increased pressure in the posterior chamber of the eye
    c. Increased pressure in the anterior chamber of the eye
    d. Decreased pressure in the anterior chamber of the eye

66. In a healthy dog, if the right eye is in low light and a light is shown into the left eye, the pupil(s) in
    a. Both eyes would be constricted
    b. Both eyes would be dilated
    c. The right eye would dilate and the pupil in the left eye would constrict
    d. The right eye would constrict and the pupil in the left eye would remain the same

67. Clients should be cautioned against sticking Q-tips in the ears of their pets because they could rupture the
    a. Oval window
    b. Round window
    c. Cochlea
    d. Tympanic membrane

68. Which condition would be typical of hypothyroidism?
    a. Decreased water consumption
    b. Oily hair coat
    c. Very active
    d. Gaining weight

69. In dairy cattle the teats and udder are gently washed before milking to stimulate the release of __, which causes milk let-down.
    a. Adrenalin
    b. Norepinephrine
    c. Dopamine
    d. Oxytocin

70. GnRH will stimulate the release of
    a. FSH
    b. Thyroxine
    c. Cortisol
    d. Insulin

71. ACTH will stimulate the release of
    a. FSH
    b. Thyroxine
    c. Cortisol
    d. Insulin

72. Lymph nodes that are found medial to the caudal part of the jaw are the
    a. Popliteal nodes
    b. Inguinal nodes
    c. Mandibular nodes
    d. Prescapular nodes

73. Lymph nodes found on the caudal aspect of the leg at the level of the patella are the
    a. Popliteal nodes
    b. Inguinal nodes
    c. Mandibular nodes
    d. Prescapular nodes

74. The neurohypophysis is an anatomic section of the __.
    a. Pituitary gland
    b. Hypothalamus
    c. Adrenal gland
    d. Pancreas

75. The portal vein
    a. Carries blood from the spleen to the heart
    b. Delivers blood to the liver
    c. Delivers blood to the kidney
    d. Carries blood from the lungs to the heart

76. To get from a point between the eyes to the tip of a dog's nose, you would move
    a. Rostrally
    b. Cranially
    c. Caudally
    d. Laterally

77. Typically what percentage of an animal's body weight is blood?
    a. 0.1%
    b. 1%
    c. 8%
    d. 30%

78. A dog that weighs 10 kg would have approximately how much blood?
    a. 50 ml
    b. 800 ml
    c. 1.5 L
    d. 2 L

Correct answers are on pages 52-71.

79. Which of the following dissections could be made without cutting through a bone to bone joint?
    a. Forelimb from the body
    b. Hind limb from the body
    c. Head from the neck
    d. Tail from the body

80. If you were to grasp your hands behind your head at the base of your skull, your hands would be over which bone of the skull?
    a. Occipital
    b. Frontal
    c. Temporal
    d. Parietal

81. The initial process of converting glucose into fat is called
    a. Lipogenesis
    b. Gluconeogenesis
    c. Glycogenolysis
    d. Fatty acid synthesis

82. Which of the following is true about anaerobic metabolism?
    a. Fat can be used
    b. Glucose can be used
    c. It takes place in the mitochondria
    d. Oxygen must be present

83. The amount of energy an animal would acquire from burning off adipose tissue would be
    a. 7700 kcal/kg
    b. 4 kcal/g
    c. 4 kcal/kg
    d. 9 kcal/kg

84. Efferent nerves carry nerve impulses
    a. To the body from the central nervous system
    b. To the body from the spinal cord
    c. From the body to the central nervous system
    d. From one part of a limb to another part of the same limb

85. The name for the bile acid–lipid units that carries fat within the gut is
    a. LPL
    b. Micelles
    c. VLDL
    d. Chylomicrons

86. What the lay press calls "good cholesterol" is actually a lipoprotein that is called
    a. Chylomicron
    b. LPL
    c. LDL
    d. HDL

87. Bile acids are important in the digestion of
    a. Carbohydrates
    b. Electrolytes
    c. Fats
    d. Proteins

88. Which of the following lowers blood glucose?
    a. Insulin
    b. Glucagon
    c. Epinephrine
    d. Glucocorticoids

89. What ion is responsible for repolarization of a neuron during an action potential?
    a. Potassium
    b. Calcium
    c. Magnesium
    d. Glucose

90. Insulin stimulates all of the following except
    a. Protein synthesis
    b. Fatty acid synthesis
    c. Glycogen synthesis
    d. Gluconeogenesis

91. The P wave component of a QRS complex usually corresponds to
    a. Atrial contraction
    b. Ventricular contraction
    c. Atrial relaxation
    d. Electrical conduction in Purkinje fibers

92. The islets of Langerhans are found in the
    a. Spleen
    b. Pancreas
    c. Liver
    d. Kidney

93. Renin is secreted by the
    a. Kidney
    b. Hypothalamus
    c. Liver
    d. Adrenal cortex

94. Sympathetic stimulation of the heart increases strength of contractions by
    a. Frank-Starling mechanism
    b. Increasing the firing rate of the SA node
    c. Depolarizing the bundle of His
    d. Increasing permeability of heart muscle to calcium

95. Edema could be caused by
    a. Decreased capillary blood pressure
    b. Increased plasma oncotic pressure
    c. Venous congestion
    d. Dehydration

96. Fat in the lymph would most likely be associated with
    a. HDL cholesterol
    b. Chylomicrons
    c. Chyle
    d. LDL cholesterol

97. Clinical ketosis in dairy cattle is most common in
    a. First-calf heifers
    b. Fat cows
    c. Dairy bulls
    d. Steers

98. Milk fever in dairy cows is typically treated with
    a. IV glucose
    b. IV calcium
    c. Atropine
    d. Antibiotics

99. For an animal that had lost RBCs to a moderate hookworm infection, one would expect the capillary refill time to be
    a. Less than 2 seconds
    b. Greater than 4 seconds
    c. Greater than 2 minutes
    d. Greater than 4 minutes

100. A pulse taken from the inguinal area of a dog would be from the
    a. Femoral artery
    b. Axillary artery
    c. Popliteal artery
    d. Saphenous artery

101. What is called the "knee" in the forelimb of a horse would be called the __ in the human.
    a. Hip joint
    b. Wrist joint
    c. Finger joint
    d. Knee joint

102. The linea alba on a standing cat is __ to the spinal cord.
    a. Ventral
    b. Dorsal
    c. Medial
    d. Contralateral

103. A common sign of a puppy with a cleft palate would be
    a. Inability to breathe
    b. Milk coming out of its nose
    c. Malocclusion of the teeth
    d. Inability to urinate

104. Yellow mucous membranes would suggest
    a. Renal disease
    b. Hepatic disease
    c. Shock
    d. Dehydration

105. A capillary refill time of 2 seconds would suggest
    a. Shock
    b. Anemia
    c. A healthy animal
    d. Dehydration

106. What is the name for the large, flat projection located lateral to the head of the femur?
    a. Lesser trochanter
    b. Greater trochanter
    c. Trochanteric fossa
    d. Tubercle

107. The femur articulates distally with the tibia, forming the
    a. Hip joint
    b. Stifle joint
    c. Tarsal joint
    d. Shoulder joint

108. What is the term for a part closer to a point of attachment or to the trunk?
    a. Distal
    b. Lateral
    c. Proximal
    d. Superficial

109. What is the term used below the carpus for the surface directed caudally or ventrally?
    a. Plantar
    b. Sagittal
    c. Palmar
    d. Longitudinal

110. In growing bone, where does lengthening take place?
    a. Epiphyseal plate
    b. Metaphysis
    c. Diaphysis
    d. Periosteal plane

111. What layer of bone tissue is necessary for attachment of ligaments and tendons?
    a. Periosteum
    b. Endosteum
    c. Cartilage
    d. Meniscus

Correct answers are on pages 52-71.

112. The fibrous covering around the part of the bone NOT covered by articular cartilage is
    a. Endosteum
    b. Ligament
    c. Tendon
    d. Periosteum

113. What two valves comprise the atrioventricular valves?
    a. Mitral valve, pulmonic valve
    b. Aortic valve, pulmonic valve
    c. Mitral valve, tricuspid valve
    d. Pulmonic valve, tricuspid valve

114. What two valves comprise the semilunar valves?
    a. Mitral valve, pulmonic valve
    b. Pulmonic valve, aortic valve
    c. Mitral valve, tricuspid valve
    d. Pulmonic valve, tricuspid valve

115. The normal dentition pattern for an adult cat is
    a. Incisor 3/3, Canine 1/1, Premolar 3/2, Molar 1/1
    b. Incisor 3/3, Canine 1/1, Premolar 4/3, Molar 2/2
    c. Incisor 2/2, Canine 1/1, Premolar 3/2, Molar 2/1
    d. Incisor 2/2, Canine 1/1, Premolar 4/4, Molar 1/1

116. In the avian species, the ventral wall of the esophagus is greatly expanded to form the
    a. Proventriculus
    b. Crop
    c. Gizzard
    d. Duodenum

117. How many air sacs does a chicken have?
    a. 4
    b. 6
    c. 8
    d. 9

118. In birds, the cloaca is
    a. An appendage suspended from the head
    b. A blind sac at the distal end of the jejunum
    c. A cleft in the hard palate
    d. A common passage for fecal, urinary, and reproductive systems

119. In the avian species, the gizzard is also referred to as the
    a. Proventriculus
    b. Ventriculus
    c. Crop
    d. Colon

120. The femoral artery is cranial to what muscle?
    a. Sartorius
    b. Pectineus
    c. Rectus femoris
    d. Tensor fascia lata

121. The uvea consists of the iris, ciliary body, and
    a. Nervous tunic
    b. Fibrous tunic
    c. Anterior chamber
    d. Choroid

122. The shape of the eyeball is maintained by the
    a. Sclera
    b. Vitreous humor
    c. Lens
    d. Fibrous tunic

123. The muscular structure that separates the right and left ventricles is called the interventricular
    a. Sternum
    b. Coronary muscle
    c. Septum
    d. Myocardium

124. The muscular layer that makes up the majority of the heart mass is the
    a. Myocardium
    b. Endocardium
    c. Myometrium
    d. Pericardium

125. The major artery that carries blood out of the left ventricle is the
    a. Subclavian artery
    b. Carotid artery
    c. Pulmonary artery
    d. Aorta

126. All of the following major vessels contribute to blood flowing into the cranial vena cava except for the
    a. Brachiocephalic vein
    b. Thoracic duct
    c. Azygos vein
    d. Femoral vein

127. The structure by which venous blood from the intestines bypasses the liver is the
    a. Ductus arteriosus
    b. Porto-caval shunt
    c. Obturator foramen
    d. Intrahepatic venous plexus

128. The coronary veins empty blood via the coronary sinus into the
   a. Left atrium
   b. Right atrium
   c. Left ventricle
   d. Right ventricle

129. The pulmonary circulation is under
   a. High pressure
   b. Low pressure
   c. Partial pressure
   d. Equilibrium

130. Systemic circulation is under
   a. High pressure
   b. Low pressure
   c. Partial pressure
   d. Equilibrium

131. How many teeth does an adult dog have?
   a. 28
   b. 32
   c. 42
   d. 50

132. Which of these is not a division of the small intestine?
   a. Duodenum
   b. Ilium
   c. Ileum
   d. Jejunum

133. What abdominal organ is absent in the horse and rat?
   a. Right kidney
   b. Gall bladder
   c. Pancreas
   d. Cecum

134. What is unique about the ruminant oral cavity?
   a. Presence of a dental pad
   b. Absence of salivary glands
   c. Absence of molars
   d. Presence of needle teeth

135. What is the average frequency of ruminations for ruminants?
   a. 2/minute
   b. 10/minute
   c. 1/hour
   d. 5/hour

136. What is the most common site of feed impactions in the horse?
   a. Sternal flexure
   b. Diaphragmatic flexure
   c. Stomach
   d. Pelvic flexure

137. Food is moved along the digestive tract by the process known as
   a. Mastication
   b. Prehension
   c. Peristalsis
   d. Reticulation

138. The most distal portion of the monogastric stomach is the
   a. Fundus
   b. Antrum
   c. Cardia
   d. Pylorus

139. All of the following are cells found in the fundus and body of the stomach except
   a. Parietal cells
   b. Chief cells
   c. G cells
   d. Mucous cells

140. Which of the following is not a hormone produced or released by the pituitary gland?
   a. Luteinizing hormone
   b. Oxytocin
   c. Growth hormone
   d. Calcitonin

141. Which of the following is a ductless system?
   a. Exocrine system
   b. Endocrine system
   c. Exogenous system
   d. Lymphatic system

142. The hormone responsible for maintaining pregnancy is
   a. Oxytocin
   b. Luteinizing hormone
   c. Estrogen
   d. Progesterone

143. The structure produced immediately after an ovarian follicle has ruptured and released its ovum is the
   a. Corpus callosum
   b. Corpus luteum
   c. Granulosum
   d. Sertolioma

144. A deficiency in antidiuretic hormone causes
   a. Diabetes insipidus
   b. Diabetes mellitus
   c. Cushings disease
   d. Pancreatic insufficiency

Correct answers are on pages 52-71.

145. What hormone is produced by the kidney?
     a. Antidiuretic hormone
     b. Adrenocorticotropic hormone
     c. Erythropoietin
     d. Adrenal cortex hormone

146. What hormone is produced by the beta cells in the pancreas?
     a. Insulin
     b. Glucagon
     c. Glycogen
     d. Somatostatin

147. The adrenal cortex is made up of all of the following except
     a. Zona glomerulosa
     b. Zona medullata
     c. Zona fasciculata
     d. Zona reticularis

148. The endocrine structure responsible for secreting melatonin is
     a. Pituitary gland
     b. Spleen
     c. Thymus
     d. Pineal gland

149. The lymphatic system is not involved in
     a. Waste material transport
     b. Protein transport
     c. Carbohydrate transport
     d. Fluid transport

150. Which is not a lymphatic structure?
     a. Peyers patches
     b. Haustra
     c. Lacteals
     d. Thoracic duct

151. The lymphatic structure found in the small intestines responsible for the transport of fats and fat-soluble vitamins is
     a. Peyers patches
     b. Lacteals
     c. Popliteal lymph nodes
     d. Spleen

152. Which of the following is a lymphatic structure?
     a. Bile duct
     b. Islets of Langerhans
     c. Thyroid
     d. Tonsil

153. What structure is not found in the brainstem?
     a. Midbrain
     b. Pons
     c. Hypothalamus
     d. Medulla oblongata

154. Which of these is not a catecholamine?
     a. Norepinephrine
     b. Acetylcholine
     c. Epinephrine
     d. Dopamine

155. Which animal does not have a gall bladder?
     a. Goat
     b. Donkey
     c. Cat
     d. Sheep

156. Ruminants have what type of placentation?
     a. Cotyledonary
     b. Zonary
     c. Diffuse
     d. Discoid

157. Which of the following is a posterior pituitary hormone?
     a. Luteinizing hormone
     b. Growth hormone
     c. Oxytocin
     d. Follicle stimulating hormone

158. Sperm cells are produced by the
     a. Seminiferous tubule
     b. Epididymis
     c. Vas deferens
     d. Seminal vesicles

159. What domestic species lacks the bulbourethral gland, also called *Cowpers gland*?
     a. Equine
     b. Feline
     c. Canine
     d. Bovine

160. All of the following are induced ovulators except
     a. Rabbit
     b. Rat
     c. Cat
     d. Ferret

161. The time period from the beginning of one heat cycle to the beginning of the next is called
     a. Estrous
     b. Estrus
     c. Ovulation
     d. The mating cycle

162. What muscle is responsible for pulling the testicles closer to the body?
   a. Retractor penis muscle
   b. Cremaster muscle
   c. Kegel muscle
   d. Retractor testicle muscle

163. When does ovulation occur in the cow?
   a. Midestrus
   b. After estrus
   c. 1 to 2 days after estrus
   d. 12 hours after standing heat

164. What primary ovarian structure is responsible for the release of estrogen?
   a. Follicle
   b. Placenta
   c. Corpus hemorrhagicum
   d. Corpus luteum

165. What hormone is given to prevent pregnancies in dogs that have been unintentionally "mismated"?
   a. Oxytocin
   b. LH
   c. Estrogen
   d. Progesterone

166. The average gestation length in the ferret is
   a. 69 days
   b. 42 days
   c. 151 days
   d. 20 days

167. The condition known as *pseudopregnancy* can result from an exaggerated
   a. Anestrus
   b. Metestrus
   c. Diestrus
   d. Proestrus

168. The thorax is normally under
   a. Partial pressure
   b. Positive pressure
   c. Equilibrium
   d. Negative pressure

169. Skeletal muscles are
   a. Under voluntary control
   b. Nonstriated
   c. Under involuntary control
   d. Found in the walls of hollow organs

170. The two main minerals that make up bone are
   a. Calcium and magnesium
   b. Sodium and potassium
   c. Calcium and phosphorus
   d. Calcium and potassium

171. Basic functions of bones include all of the following except
   a. Protection
   b. Storage
   c. Leverage
   d. Metabolism

172. The hormone primarily responsible for preventing hypocalcemia is
   a. T4
   b. Parathyroid hormone
   c. Calcitonin
   d. Vitamin D

173. The hormone primarily responsible for preventing hypercalcemia is
   a. T4
   b. Parathyroid hormone
   c. Calcitonin
   d. Vitamin D

174. The bone cells responsible for the removal of bone are
   a. Osteoclasts
   b. Osteoblasts
   c. Chondroblasts
   d. Chondroclasts

175. The periosteum
   a. Covers joint cavities
   b. Lines the heart
   c. Lines the marrow cavity of bones
   d. Covers the outer surface of bones

176. Bones come in all of the following shapes except
   a. Flat
   b. Short
   c. Regular
   d. Long

177. The shaft of the bone is also called the
   a. Trunk
   b. Epiphysis
   c. Periosteum
   d. Diaphysis

178. An example of a short bone would be a
   a. Vertebra
   b. Tarsal bone
   c. Scapula
   d. Patella

179. The skull bone that articulates with the first cervical vertebra is the
   a. Parietal bone
   b. Temporal bone
   c. Occipital bone
   d. Frontal bone

Correct answers are on pages 52-71.

180. The bones known collectively as the ossicles include all of the following except the
    a. Sphenoid
    b. Malleus
    c. Stapes
    d. Incus

181. The cat has how many cervical vertebrae?
    a. 13
    b. 7
    c. 3
    d. 10

182. The first cervical vertebra, C1, is referred to as the
    a. Axis
    b. Atlas
    c. Arch
    d. Auricle

183. The breastbone is the
    a. Hyoid
    b. Septum
    c. Tubercle
    d. Sternum

184. The most caudal portion of the sternum is called the
    a. Xiphoid
    b. Coccyx
    c. Manubrium
    d. Costal

185. Claws, hooves, and horns are made up of which type of cell?
    a. Keratinized
    b. Agglutinated
    c. Calcified
    d. Crystallized

186. The average rate of equine hoof growth per month is
    a. 2 inches
    b. 1/2 inch
    c. 1 inch
    d. 1/4 inch

187. Adult cattle have how many upper incisors?
    a. 6
    b. 4
    c. 0
    d. 5

188. The anatomic term for *synovial joints* is
    a. Fibroarthroses
    b. Amphiarthroses
    c. Synarthroses
    d. Diarthroses

189. Which joint is not a synovial joint?
    a. Hinge joint
    b. Gliding joint
    c. Swinging joint
    d. Pivot joint

190. The area of the kidney where blood vessels and nerves enter and leave is called the
    a. Hilus
    b. Medullary rays
    c. Cortex
    d. Collecting ducts

191. In the kidney, the primary site of action of ADH is in the
    a. Loop of Henle
    b. Proximal convoluted tubule
    c. Glomerulus
    d. Collecting ducts

192. The renal corpuscle is located in the
    a. Renal pelvis
    b. Hilus
    c. Medulla
    d. Cortex

193. The renal corpuscle is composed of the
    a. Glomerulus and Bowman capsule
    b. Collecting ducts and proximal convoluted tubule
    c. Descending and ascending loops of Henle
    d. Collecting ducts and afferent arteriole

194. The urinary bladder is not responsible for
    a. Urine storage
    b. Urine filtration
    c. Urine collecting
    d. Urine release

195. The trunk of an animal is defined as
    a. The front half of the animal
    b. The back half of the animal
    c. The thorax of the animal
    d. The thorax and abdomen of the animal

196. The area between the thorax and front leg is called the
    a. Axilla
    b. Inguina
    c. Forearm
    d. Armpit

197. The middle phalanx is located
    a. Lateral to the distal phalanx
    b. Distal to the distal phalanx
    c. Medial to the distal phalanx
    d. Proximal to the distal phalanx

198. The humeroradioulnar joint is located
    a. Lateral to the carpus
    b. Distal to the left of the carpus
    c. Medial to the carpus
    d. Proximal to the carpus

199. The feline liver is normally __ to the kidneys.
    a. Dorsal
    b. Ventral
    c. Caudal
    d. Cranial

200. The leg bone responsible for minimal support is the
    a. Fibula
    b. Femur
    c. Tibia
    d. Humerus

201. The large muscle of the caudal aspect of the canine lower hind leg is the
    a. Tibialis anterior
    b. Gracilis
    c. Semimembranosus
    d. Gastrocnemius

202. Which of the following is not a muscle in the abdominal group?
    a. External oblique
    b. Rectus abdominis
    c. Latissimus dorsi
    d. Internal oblique

203. How many muscle heads are in the canine triceps brachii group?
    a. 4
    b. 3
    c. 2
    d. 1

204. Fascia is described as
    a. The facial muscular surface
    b. A tough sheet of fibrous connective tissue
    c. A broad band of muscle fiber
    d. A lacy network of connective tissue

205. The deltoid muscles allow fine movements of the
    a. Shoulder
    b. Hip
    c. Elbow
    d. Spine

206. Cats have several salivary glands. The gland that is located under the eye above the upper jaw is called the
    a. Interorbital gland
    b. Supraorbital gland
    c. Infraorbital gland
    d. Intraorbital gland

207. The two gastric sphincters of the canine are
    a. Rectal and cecal
    b. Cardiac and pyloric
    c. Cardiac and rectal
    d. Pyloric and rectal

208. The dorsal plane divides the
    a. Upper and lower halves of the body
    b. Front and back halves of the body
    c. Head from the rest of the body
    d. Right and left sides of the body

209. The middle portion of the small intestine is the
    a. Jejunum
    b. Jejunem
    c. Jajunem
    d. Jujunem

210. The __ pleura overlays organs in the body.
    a. Parietal
    b. Viscous
    c. Partial
    d. Visceral

211. The cat larynx is made up of four cartilages. Which one is not one of them?
    a. Arytenoid
    b. Cricoid
    c. Epiglottis
    d. Glottis

212. The muscle that lies along the outer thorax that looks like a fan of fingers or a jagged saw edge is the
    a. Latissimus dorsi
    b. Serratus ventralis
    c. Subscapularis
    d. External intercostals

213. The prepuce is also called the
    a. Foreskin
    b. Flap
    c. Prostate gland
    d. Glans penis

Correct answers are on pages 52-71.

214. The cardiovascular system has four components. Which of the following is not part of the system?
   a. Heart
   b. Blood circulation
   c. Blood vessels
   d. Lungs

215. The appendicular skeleton includes the
   a. Os cordis
   b. Ribs
   c. Pelvic girdle
   d. Clavicles

216. Which animal does not have an os penis?
   a. Dog
   b. Cat
   c. Wolf
   d. Pig

217. Which statement best describes short bones?
   a. Greater size in one dimension than another
   b. Filled with spongy bone and marrow spaces
   c. Thick outer layer of compact bone
   d. Developed along the course of tendons

218. The scapula is an example of a
   a. Long bone
   b. Short bone
   c. Flat bone
   d. Irregular bone

219. An example of an irregular bone is
   a. Cervical vertebra 1
   b. Metacarpal 3
   c. Ulna
   d. Calcaneus

220. Which of the following is not a part of the axial skeleton?
   a. Cervical vertebra 3
   b. Scapula
   c. Skull
   d. Thoracic vertebra 1

221. A cloven-hoofed animal stands on which digits?
   a. 1 and 2
   b. 2 and 3
   c. 3 and 4
   d. 4 and 5

222. A cloven-hoofed animal has how many phalanges on each digit?
   a. 1
   b. 2
   c. 3
   d. 4

223. A common equine disease of the digit in horses is
   a. Navicular disease
   b. EIA
   c. Phalangeal disease
   d. Tripping syndrome

224. A skull suture is an example of what type of joint?
   a. Diarthrosis
   b. Synarthrosis
   c. Amphiarthrosis
   d. Cartilaginous

225. The only true pivot joint in the body is the
   a. Coxofemoral
   b. Tarsal
   c. Carpal
   d. Atlantoaxial

226. Muscles and ligaments attach to structures on bony surfaces. Which of the following is not one of these found in the forelimb?
   a. Trochanter
   b. Tuberosity
   c. Spine
   d. Epicondyle

227. Which structure will not allow blood vessels and nerves to pass through?
   a. Meatus
   b. Sinus
   c. Foramen
   d. Facet

228. The joint between the bony rib and cartilaginous portion of the rib is called the
   a. Cartilaginous junction
   b. Chondrocartilaginous junction
   c. Costochondral junction
   d. Costicartilaginous junction

229. Dogs have how many cervical, thoracic, and lumbar vertebrae?
   a. 7, 13, 6
   b. 7, 12, 7
   c. 6, 13, 7
   d. 7, 13, 7

230. What is the value of X in this cow's dentition chart? I 0/3; C 0/1; PM 3/3–4; M X/3
   a. 4
   b. 3
   c. 2
   d. 1

231. The valves that prevent backflow of blood from the arteries to the ventricles are called the
    a. Tricuspid
    b. Bicuspid
    c. Mitral
    d. Semilunar

232. What structures disseminate electrical impulses across the ventricles?
    a. Perkinje fibers
    b. Purkinje fibers
    c. Purkinge fibers
    d. Perkingi fibers

233. Systole is
    a. Contraction of the atria and ventricles
    b. Relaxation of the atria and ventricles
    c. Contraction of the atria and relaxation of the ventricles
    d. Relaxation of the atria and contraction of the ventricles

234. The aorta leaves the heart from the
    a. Left ventricle
    b. Right ventricle
    c. Left atrium
    d. Right atrium

235. Blood enters the heart from the pulmonary veins in the
    a. Left ventricle
    b. Right ventricle
    c. Left atrium
    d. Right atrium

236. What blood pressure value is not as important in veterinary medicine in comparison to human medicine?
    a. Systolic
    b. Diastolic
    c. Pulse
    d. Vessel

237. Systemic circulation includes
    a. Portal and peripheral circulation
    b. Cardiac and portal circulation
    c. Cardiac and pulmonary circulation
    d. Pulmonary and appendicular circulation

238. The name of the hole between the cardiac atria that closes at birth in the mammal is
    a. Cardiac fossa
    b. Atria foramen
    c. Fossa foramen
    d. Foramen ovale

239. Which of these is not a characteristic of lymph?
    a. Tissue fluids
    b. A large number of neutrophils
    c. Virtually colorless
    d. Part of the circulatory system

240. The tricuspid valve controls the flow of blood
    a. Into the left ventricle
    b. Out of the left ventricle
    c. Into the right ventricle
    d. Out of the right ventricle

241. The thymus
    a. Is another name for the thyroid gland
    b. Produces cells that destroy foreign substances
    c. Is more prominent in adults than in young animals
    d. Is located in the cranial abdomen

242. The eardrum is also called the
    a. Tympanic bulla
    b. Tympanic membrane
    c. Tympanic film
    d. Tympanic ossicle

243. What organ is most commonly associated with the capacity for extramedullary hematopoiesis if necessary?
    a. Spleen
    b. Pancreas
    c. Lung
    d. Prostate

244. Association neurons are part of what system?
    a. Peripheral
    b. Interneuron
    c. Sensory
    d. Extraneuron

245. Efferent neurons are part of what system?
    a. Motor
    b. Interneuron
    c. Sensory
    d. Extraneuron

246. Afferent neurons are part of what system?
    a. Motor
    b. Interneuron
    c. Sensory
    d. Extraneuron

247. The function of the red blood cell is to
    a. Produce antibodies against bacteria and viruses
    b. Act as a phagocyte
    c. Carry oxygen to the tissues
    d. Help increase the osmotic pressure within the vessels

Correct answers are on pages 52-71.

248. What artery carries deoxygenated blood?
    a. Aorta
    b. Pulmonary
    c. Coronary
    d. Carotid

249. Albumin is found in the blood and is a type of
    a. Cell
    b. Phospholipid
    c. Enzyme
    d. Protein

250. Albumin is produced in the
    a. Liver
    b. Red bone marrow
    c. Lymph nodes
    d. Pancreas

251. What blood protein plays a role in hemostasis?
    a. Gamma globulin
    b. Fibrinogen
    c. Beta globulin
    d. Albumin

252. Which chamber of the heart is surrounded by the largest amount of cardiac muscle?
    a. Right atrium
    b. Right ventricle
    c. Left atrium
    d. Left ventricle

253. How does the volume of the right ventricle compare with that of the left ventricle?
    a. The right ventricle has less volume than the left but pumps more blood than the left ventricle
    b. The right ventricle has less volume than the left
    c. The right and left ventricles have the same volume
    d. The right ventricle generally holds more blood than the left but does not pump as much as the left

254. What cells are involved in antibody production?
    a. Erythrocytes
    b. Neutrophils
    c. Lymphocytes
    d. Basophils

255. Which of the following are antibodies?
    a. Gamma globulins
    b. Albumin
    c. Fibrinogen
    d. Thrombocytes

256. The liver receives blood via what two different routes?
    a. Mesenteric arteries and the caudal vena cava
    b. Hepatic artery and the portal veins
    c. Cranial mesenteric artery and the hepatic artery
    d. Hepatic artery and the hepatic vein

257. Red blood cell production is stimulated by
    a. Hypoxia and erythropoietin
    b. Erythropoietin and thrombocytes
    c. Fibrinogen and acetylcholine
    d. Coagulation cascade

258. What structure is the pacemaker of the heart?
    a. Bundle of His
    b. Purkinje fibers
    c. Atrioventricular node
    d. Sinoatrial node

259. What is meant by cardiac output?
    a. Strokes (beats) per minute
    b. Volume of blood pumped per stroke (beat)
    c. Volume of blood pumped per minute
    d. Strokes (beats) per volume

260. When an animal becomes severely dehydrated, it loses both tissue fluid and plasma fluid. What effect would this have on the hematocrit and the PCV?
    a. Increase both values
    b. Decrease both values
    c. Increase the hematocrit but no effect on the PCV
    d. No change in either value

261. In the normal heart ECG, the QRS complex corresponds to what portion of the cardiac cycle?
    a. Atrial systole
    b. Atrial diastole
    c. Ventricular systole
    d. Ventricular diastole

262. What is the function of the blood platelets?
    a. Production of antibodies
    b. Hemostasis
    c. Chemotaxis
    d. Phagocytosis

263. Decreased osmotic pressure in blood would cause
    a. Decreased blood flow
    b. Edema in tissues and/or lungs
    c. Increased hydrostatic pressure
    d. Increased cardiac output

264. Albumin plays a role in
    a. Bladder control
    b. Hydrostatic pressure in the blood
    c. Osmotic pressure in the blood
    d. Nervous stimulation

265. What is the function of erythropoietin?
    a. Stimulates urine production
    b. Stimulates white blood cell production
    c. Stimulates red blood cell production
    d. Stimulates the production of antidiuretic hormone

266. Horses and ruminants gain much of their energy from a product produced by microbes during fermentation. What is this product?
    a. Lipids
    b. Volatile fatty acids
    c. Amylase
    d. Trypsinogen

267. Bile is produced in the
    a. Spleen
    b. Pancreas
    c. Liver
    d. Omasum

268. Bile is needed for the digestion/absorption of
    a. Proteins
    b. Calcium
    c. Lipids
    d. Ash

269. Fermentation in the horse occurs in what two portions of the digestive tract?
    a. Cecum and large colon (ventral and dorsal colons)
    b. Ileum and jejunum
    c. Duodenum and large colon (ventral and dorsal colons)
    d. Cecum and rectum

270. The term for an animal ingesting its own feces is
    a. Corpophagy
    b. Coprophagy
    c. Corpology
    d. Coprology

271. In the bovine, ingesta freely moves back and forth between the rumen and the
    a. Omasum
    b. Abomasum
    c. Reticulum
    d. Duodenum

272. Which of these species does *not* possess a gall bladder?
    a. Pig
    b. Horse
    c. Goat
    d. Dog

273. What hormone stimulates the release of gastric secretions?
    a. Gastrin
    b. Secretin
    c. Calcitonin
    d. Insulin

274. What enzyme breaks down carbohydrates in the digestive tract?
    a. Lipase
    b. Amylase
    c. Protease
    d. Tryptase

275. The lymph vessels that absorb fats within the villi of the small intestine are called
    a. Pylorus
    b. Ileus
    c. Lacteals
    d. Peyers patches

276. What enzyme group breaks down fats within the digestive tract?
    a. Amylase
    b. Lipase
    c. Protease
    d. Secretin

277. What structures in the mucosa of the small intestine increase the surface area?
    a. Fimbria
    b. Cilia
    c. Brush borders
    d. Villi

278. What are the two vitamins produced by the gut bacteria involved in fermentation?
    a. Vitamins C and D
    b. Vitamins B12 and niacin
    c. Vitamins B and K
    d. Vitamins A and E

279. What level of organization in the body is more complex than tissues?
    a. Cells
    b. Organs
    c. Muscles
    d. Organelles

Correct answers are on pages 52-71.

280. Which of the following is isotonic to plasma?
     a. Sterile water
     b. 0.9% saline solution
     c. 7.5% NaCl solution
     d. 0.45% NaCl saline solution

281. Where would you expect to find DNA within the cell?
     a. In the cell membrane
     b. In the ribosomes
     c. In the cytoplasm
     d. In the nucleus

282. Where would you find stratified squamous epithelial tissue in the mammalian body?
     a. In the urinary bladder
     b. In the epidermis
     c. Lining the heart
     d. In the tendons and ligaments

283. Glandular tissue is what type of tissue?
     a. Epithelial
     b. Connective
     c. Nervous
     d. Muscle

284. Hair is
     a. Formed in the dermis where there is no blood supply
     b. Composed of adipose tissue
     c. Produced by glands in the epidermis
     d. Produced at invaginations of epidermis called *follicles*

285. The layer of the integument that contains the blood vessels is the
     a. Epidermis
     b. Stratum corneum
     c. Dermis
     d. Hypodermis

286. What cellular structure is responsible for the production of ATP for energy?
     a. Ribosomes
     b. Mitochondria
     c. Endoplasmic reticulum
     d. RNA

287. What type of epithelial tissue appears to be multilayered, but all cells touch the basement membrane?
     a. Stratified
     b. Simple
     c. Pseudostratified
     d. Columnar

288. What tissue type is responsible for fat storage?
     a. Connective
     b. Adipose
     c. Neural
     d. Glandular

289. Osteons are associated with which of the following?
     a. Stratified epithelial tissue
     b. Fibrous connective tissue
     c. Cartilage
     d. Bone

290. The function of the epiphyseal plate is to
     a. Provide for growth in the thickness of the bone
     b. Provide for growth in the length of the bone
     c. Provide bone for the articular surface within a joint
     d. Provide bone with marrow substance

291. The cells involved in bone destruction are called
     a. Osteoblasts
     b. Osteotomes
     c. Osteons
     d. Osteoclasts

292. What substance provides lubrication to joints and nourishment to articular cartilage cells?
     a. Intra-articular fluid
     b. Plasma
     c. Serum
     d. Synovial fluid

293. The bone type that makes up the diaphysis of long bones is
     a. Cancellous
     b. Spongy
     c. Articular
     d. Compact

294. How many cervical vertebrae do mammals have?
     a. 3
     b. 6
     c. 7
     d. 10

295. Prolonged inactivity causes a decrease in muscle size, which is called
     a. Atrophy
     b. Hypotrophy
     c. Hypertrophy
     d. Inotropy

296. How many bones are found in the normal equine carpus?
  a. 1–2
  b. 3–4
  c. 6–7
  d. 9–10

297. Which of the following is not required for muscular contraction and relaxation?
  a. Calcium
  b. Phosphorus
  c. Sodium
  d. Potassium

298. The function of the muscles making up the quadriceps femoris is
  a. Extension of the elbow
  b. Extension of the stifle
  c. Flexion of the hock
  d. Flexion of the stifle

299. Microscopically, smooth muscle can be differentiated from the other muscle types because
  a. It is striated
  b. It is involuntary
  c. It lacks striations
  d. It possesses Purkinje fibers

300. What substance causes the breakdown of acetylcholine in the synaptic cleft?
  a. Acetylcholinesterase
  b. Choline
  c. Calcium
  d. Actin

301. Toxins that interfere with the function of acetylcholinesterase would have what effect on muscle fibers?
  a. They would prevent contraction completely, so the muscle would be paralyzed
  b. They would cause the muscles to become very weak and flaccid
  c. The muscle fiber would continue to contract, causing tremors and cramping
  d. They would cause rigor mortis

302. The space between the nerve end and the sarcolemma of the muscle is called the
  a. Neurolemma
  b. Synaptic cleft
  c. Nodes of Ranvier
  d. Synaptic knob

303. Aqueous humor is secreted by the
  a. Ciliary body
  b. Sclera
  c. Choroid layer of the retina
  d. Iris

304. The part of the nephron where filtration of the blood takes place is the
  a. Hilus
  b. Ureter
  c. Loop of Henle
  d. Glomerulus

305. A cat presents with a urolith (stone) blocking the urethra. Where is the first place that the urine backs up into?
  a. Renal pelvis
  b. Bladder
  c. Kidney
  d. Ureter

306. The most important function of ADH is to
  a. Decrease water reabsorption by the distal convoluted tubules
  b. Increase water reabsorption by the distal convoluted tubules
  c. Decrease water reabsorption by the glomerulus
  d. Increase water reabsorption by the glomerulus

307. The major factor determining glomerular filtration rate is
  a. Pulse rate
  b. Carbon dioxide saturation of blood
  c. Oxygen saturation of blood
  d. Blood pressure

308. What is a normal function of estrogen?
  a. Inducing estrus
  b. Decreasing blood flow to the uterus
  c. Inducing parturition
  d. Constricting the cervix

309. What two organs have receptors to and thus are responsive to oxytocin?
  a. Ovary and uterus
  b. Ovary and vagina
  c. Uterus and mammary glands
  d. Colon and mammary glands

310. The hormone that regulates sodium reabsorption in the nephron is
  a. ADH
  b. Estrogen
  c. Aldosterone
  d. Calcitonin

311. Osteoclasts are cells involved in bone destruction. Their activity is increased by
  a. Calcitonin
  b. Parathyroid hormone (PTH)
  c. Thyroxine (T4)
  d. Aldosterone

Correct answers are on pages 52-71.

312. The hormone that lowers the level of glucose in the blood by aiding the passage of glucose into cells is
    a. Glucagon
    b. Calcitonin
    c. Growth hormone
    d. Insulin

313. The hormone that is regulated by the rennin-angiotensin system is
    a. Aldosterone
    b. Antidiuretic hormone
    c. Thyroid hormone
    d. Prolactin

314. The hormone that works on a positive-feedback system to cause labor contractions is
    a. Growth hormone
    b. Cortisol
    c. Oxytocin
    d. Epinephrine

315. What type of hormone is bovine somatotropin (BST)?
    a. Estrogen
    b. Growth hormone
    c. Prolactin
    d. Insulin

316. Diabetes insipidus is caused by a lack of what hormone?
    a. Antidiuretic hormone
    b. Aldosterone
    c. Luteinizing hormone
    d. Calcitonin

317. The neuron and all of the muscle fibers it innervates are considered to be a
    a. Neural unit
    b. Motor unit
    c. Nerve fiber
    d. Muscle bundle

318. Cerebrospinal fluid lies within the
    a. Epidural space
    b. Subdural space
    c. Subarachnoid space
    d. Epiarachnoid space

319. The two ions that are actively pumped into and out of cells that result in the polarization of the cells are
    a. Sodium and chloride
    b. Sodium and potassium
    c. Acetylcholine and water
    d. Calcium and chloride

320. Which of the following is not a response of increased stimulation to the parasympathetic division of the autonomic nervous system?
    a. Constriction of the pupils
    b. Dilation of the bronchioles
    c. Decreased heart rate
    d. Increased digestive activity

321. The anterior pituitary hormone that promotes follicular development on the ovary is
    a. LH
    b. Glucagon
    c. FSH
    d. Estrogen

322. What is a normal response to progesterone?
    a. Maintenance of a pregnancy
    b. Inducing estrus
    c. Milk let-down
    d. Initiation of parturition

323. What structure is not part of the "foot" of the horse?
    a. Hoof and corium
    b. Distal end of the proximal phalanx
    c. Distal phalanx
    d. Navicular bone

324. The dermis is also called the
    a. Cutis
    b. Subcutis
    c. Corium
    d. Subcorium

325. What layer of skin contains sebaceous and sweat glands?
    a. Dermis
    b. Epidermis
    c. Subcorium
    d. Hypodermis

326. The oil glands that are responsible for lubricating the skin and hair are called
    a. Anal glands
    b. Mammary glands
    c. Ceruminous glands
    d. Sebaceous glands

327. The glands found in the external ear canal are called
    a. Sebaceous glands
    b. Horn glands
    c. Eccrine sweat glands
    d. Ceruminous glands

328. The glands found on the lips of cats used for marking territory are called
   a. Apocrine sweat glands
   b. Circumoral glands
   c. Horn glands
   d. Anal sacs

329. Dog hair grows
   a. In cycles
   b. Continuously
   c. From specialized glands
   d. In layers

330. What muscle is responsible for "raising the hackles" on a dog's back?
   a. Latissimus dorsi
   b. Subcutis externa
   c. Arrector pili
   d. Epithelia errecti

331. What is the largest organ in the equine body?
   a. Lungs
   b. Liver
   c. Skin
   d. Brain

332. What structure is located most distal on a horse's leg?
   a. Ergot
   b. Elbow joint
   c. Chestnut
   d. Withers

333. Which of the following types of hair make up the undercoat of mammals and are also called *wool hairs?*
   a. Primary
   b. Tactile
   c. Vibrissa
   d. Secondary

334. Where is the sensitive laminae of an equine hoof located?
   a. Frog
   b. Wall
   c. White line
   d. Bars

335. An animal's body temperature is not routinely affected by
   a. Drinking water
   b. Sex of the animal
   c. Exercise
   d. Time of day

336. Evaporation of water from the body results in cooling. Which of the following causes the most common types of evaporated heat loss in animals?
   a. Running, drinking
   b. Drinking, panting
   c. Panting, sweating
   d. Sweating, bathing

337. Inflammation of the mammary glands is termed
   a. Hepatitis
   b. Blepharitis
   c. Mastitis
   d. Enteritis

338. A cat's whiskers are a type of tactile hair that are also called
   a. Vibrissa
   b. Guard hairs
   c. Fimbria
   d. Cilia

339. The absence of normal pigment in the skin is termed
   a. Amelanosis
   b. Albinism
   c. Cyanosis
   d. Keratosis

340. Founder in horses is another name for
   a. Foot rot
   b. Laminitis
   c. Ringbone
   d. Thrush

341. In the equine, what term describes a degenerative condition of the frog associated with filth?
   a. Gravel
   b. Thrush
   c. Toe crack
   d. Corns

342. In the equine, what term describes a drainage tract resulting from a crack in the white line?
   a. Corn
   b. White line disease
   c. Gravel
   d. Seedy toe

343. The shaft or body of a long bone is called the
   a. Epiphysis
   b. Diaphysis
   c. Metaphysis
   d. Tubercle

Correct answers are on pages 52-71.

344. The two enlarged ends of a long bone are called the
   a. Epiphyses
   b. Diaphyses
   c. Metaphyses
   d. Chondrophyses

345. The fibrous layer around bone that is necessary for bone growth, repair, nutrition, and attachment of ligaments and tendons is the
   a. Endosteum
   b. Peritoneum
   c. Periosteum
   d. Mesothelium

346. The innermost part of the shaft of a long bone that contains the bone marrow is called the
   a. Periosteum
   b. Medullary cavity
   c. Compact bone
   d. Cancellous bone

347. What type of joint movement decreases the angle between bones?
   a. Abduction
   b. Adduction
   c. Extension
   d. Flexion

348. The hip joint is classified by which of the following terms?
   a. No joint capsule, ball-and-socket joint, flexion and extension
   b. Synovial joint, hinge joint, freely movable
   c. Synovial joint, ball-and-socket joint, universal movement
   d. No joint capsule, pivot joint, slightly movable

349. The elbow joint is classified by which of the following terms?
   a. Compound hinge joint, synovial joint, flexion and extension
   b. Synovial joint, ball-and-socket joint, universal movement
   c. No joint capsule, pivot joint, rotational movement
   d. Simple hinge joint, contains no joint capsule, universal movement

350. The stifle joint articulates between the
   a. Humerus, radius, and ulna
   b. Tibia, fibula, and tarsal bones
   c. Scapula and humerus
   d. Femur, patella, and tibia

351. The thoracic limb includes the
   a. Pelvis, femur, patella, radius, ulna, tarsals, metatarsals, and phalanges
   b. Scapula, humerus, radius, ulna, carpals, metacarpals, and phalanges
   c. Scapula, femur, tibia, fibula, carpals, metacarpals, and phalanges
   d. Pelvis, humerus, radius, ulna, tarsals, metatarsals, and phalanges

352. The xiphoid process is found on the
   a. Vertebrae
   b. Sacrum
   c. Skull
   d. Sternum

353. The obturator foramen is found
   a. At the base of the skull
   b. In the mandible
   c. In the maxillary bone
   d. In the pelvis

354. During episodes of chronic laminitis, what bone in the equine foot may rotate downward, pressing against the sole causing pain?
   a. Navicular
   b. Coffin
   c. Short pastern
   d. Cannon

355. The anatomic name for the hip joint is the
   a. Temporomandibular joint
   b. Glenohumeral joint
   c. Femorotibial joint
   d. Coxofemoral joint

356. Muscle fibers are held together by connective tissue and are enclosed in a sheet of fibrous membrane called
   a. Tendon
   b. Aponeurosis
   c. Fascia
   d. Ligament

357. A muscle whose movement increases the angle between two bones is known as
   a. Abductor
   b. Adductor
   c. Extensor
   d. Flexor

358. The large, round, lateral cheek muscle used primarily for elevation of the mandible to aid in chewing is the
   a. Sternomastoid
   b. Masseter
   c. Sartorius
   d. Digastric

359. The extensive aponeurosis that covers the lower back to join the superficial muscles in that area is called the
    a. Fascia lata
    b. Cutaneous maximus
    c. Lumbodorsal fascia
    d. Linea alba

360. The muscle that is located on the shoulder, originates on the clavicle, inserts on the ulna, and whose action is to flex the forearm is the
    a. Clavobrachialis
    b. Pectoantebrachialis
    c. Sternomastoid
    d. Latissimus dorsi

361. The opening at the distal end of the simple stomach that allows for emptying of its contents into the duodenum is called the
    a. Fundus
    b. Body
    c. Pylorus
    d. Cardia

362. The gluteal muscles include the gluteus medius, the gluteus maximus, and the
    a. Biceps femoris
    b. Tensor fascia lata
    c. Sartorius
    d. Caudofemoralis

363. Which of the following sequences lists the abdominal muscle layers in order, starting with the most superficial?
    a. External oblique, internal oblique, transverse abdominis
    b. External oblique, internal oblique, rectus abdominis
    c. Internal oblique, external oblique, transverse abdominis
    d. Rectus abdominis, internal oblique, external oblique

364. The muscle that is found in the midventral abdominal area on either side of the linea alba, extending from the pubis to the upper ribs and sternum, is the
    a. Transverse abdominis
    b. Latissimus dorsi
    c. Rectus abdominis
    d. Spinotrapezius

365. Which is a powerful muscle of the head that contributes to the act of chewing by closing the mouth?
    a. Digastricus
    b. Masseter
    c. Mylohyodeus
    d. Platysma

366. What muscle condition would result from lack of use, such as during immobilization of a fractured bone or as a result of nerve damage to a body part?
    a. Myopathy
    b. Atrophy
    c. Hypertrophy
    d. Myalgia

367. What muscle is observed from the medial surface of the thigh?
    a. Gracilis
    b. Gastrocnemius
    c. Biceps femoris
    d. Caudofemoralis

368. The chief action of the quadriceps femoris group is to
    a. Flex the foot
    b. Extend the stifle
    c. Extend the elbow
    d. Abduct the hind leg

369. What is the chief action of the three heads of the triceps brachii?
    a. Extension of the forearm
    b. Flexor of the lower hind limb
    c. Adduction of the shoulder
    d. Flexion of the neck

370. Which of the following is not a function of the muscular system?
    a. Protection
    b. Generation of body heat
    c. Transport of ingesta through intestinal tract
    d. Movement of the skeleton

371. Which one of the following works in opposition to the prime mover, relaxing as the prime mover is contracting?
    a. Fixator
    b. Antagonist
    c. Synergist
    d. Flexor

Correct answers are on pages 52-71.

372. The huge, comma-shaped section of the large intestine of the horse that occupies much of the right side of the abdomen is the
    a. Cecum
    b. Colon
    c. Rectum
    d. Ileum

373. Which of the following lists the sections of the small intestine in order, from anterior to posterior?
    a. Jejunum, ileum, duodenum
    b. Duodenum, colon, jejunum
    c. Ileum, duodenum, cecum
    d. Duodenum, jejunum, ileum

374. In what portion of the ruminant digestive system does most microbial fermentation take place?
    a. Abomasum
    b. Duodenum
    c. Rumen
    d. Omasum

375. In the ruminant animal, the fermentation process produces gas in the rumen, which, if not eliminated, can cause a condition called *bloat*. What instrument can be used to relieve this condition?
    a. Emasculator
    b. Trocar
    c. Burdizzo
    d. Rochester-Carmalt forceps

376. Rumination is a cycle of activity composed of four phases. Which of the following is not included in this process?
    a. Eructation
    b. Remastication
    c. Redeglutition
    d. Reurination

377. Where does fermentation occur in nonruminant herbivores, such as the horse?
    a. Jejunum and ileum
    b. Cecum and colon
    c. Ileum and cecum
    d. Rumen and cecum

378. What organ is located immediately behind the diaphragm in the carnivore?
    a. Liver
    b. Spleen
    c. Pancreas
    d. Kidney

379. Hardware disease is usually associated with ingestion of nails, wire, or other sharp objects. The portion of the digestive tract that collects these objects is the
    a. Reticulum
    b. Omasum
    c. Rumen
    d. Abomasum

380. What animals have a dental pad in place of upper incisors and canines?
    a. Horse, cow
    b. Cow, goat
    c. Dog, sheep
    d. Cat, horse

381. The serosa that covers the organs of the abdominal cavity is called the
    a. Visceral peritoneum
    b. Visceral pleura
    c. Mesentery
    d. Parietal peritoneum

382. The connecting peritoneum that suspends the intestinal tract from the abdominal wall and contains vessels, nerves, and lymphatics that supply their respective organs is the
    a. Mesentery
    b. Omentum
    c. Pleura
    d. Omasum

383. What structure divides the rostral part of the pharynx into the oropharynx and nasopharynx?
    a. Tongue
    b. Hard palate
    c. Epiglottis
    d. Soft palate

384. The nucleus is an essential component of all body cells except for
    a. Liver cells
    b. Immature red blood cells
    c. Kidney cells
    d. Mature red blood cells

385. The cell membrane that surrounds tissue cells is made up of
    a. Two lipid layers that surround a protein layer
    b. Two protein layers that surround a lipid layer
    c. An outer protein layer and an inner lipid layer
    d. An outer lipid layer and an inner protein layer

386. What cell component is primarily responsible for protein synthesis?
    a. Golgi apparatus
    b. Mitochondria
    c. Nucleolus
    d. Granular (rough) endoplasmic reticulum

387. What cell component is primarily responsible for energy supply for various cell processes?
    a. Golgi apparatus
    b. Mitochondria
    c. Nucleolus
    d. Granular (rough) endoplasmic reticulum

388. What cell component is primarily responsible for concentration and packaging of secretory products?
    a. Golgi apparatus
    b. Mitochondria
    c. Nucleolus
    d. Granular (rough) endoplasmic reticulum

389. What cell component is primarily responsible for ribonucleic acid (RNA) production?
    a. Golgi apparatus
    b. Mitochondria
    c. Nucleolus
    d. Granular (rough) endoplasmic reticulum

390. Which of the following functions of the epithelium is indicated when stratified squamous epithelium is highly keratinized?
    a. Absorption
    b. Secretion
    c. Excretion
    d. Protection

391. The lining epithelium of blood vessels is called
    a. Mesothelium
    b. Myoepithelium
    c. Endothelium
    d. Exothelium

392. What type of epithelium lines the upper portion of the respiratory system and plays an important role in the body's defense mechanism?
    a. Pseudostratified ciliated columnar epithelium
    b. Stratified columnar epithelium
    c. Simple ciliated cuboidal epithelium
    d. Stratified squamous epithelium

393. The type of epithelial cell capable of significant variation in shape, depending on changes in the size of the organ that it lines, is called a
    a. Squamous epithelium
    b. Columnar epithelium
    c. Transitional epithelium
    d. Cuboidal epithelium

394. The mineral most important for normal contraction of striated muscle fibers is
    a. Phosphorus
    b. Iron
    c. Calcium
    d. Magnesium

395. Cardiac muscle fibers can be identified by
    a. The presence of cross striations and peripheral nuclei
    b. The absence of cross striations and the presence of central nuclei
    c. The absence of cross striations and the presence of peripheral nuclei
    d. The presence of cross striations and central nuclei

396. The junctions between adjacent cardiac muscle fibers are called
    a. Terminal bars
    b. Intercalated disks
    c. Motor end plates
    d. Synapses

397. Regeneration of cardiac muscle fibers following injury
    a. Is possible when the nucleus and part of the cytoplasm are preserved
    b. Occurs through mitotic division of fibers
    c. Does not occur
    d. Occurs from perivascular connective tissue cells

398. Peritoneum, pleura, and pericardium consist of a flattened arrangement of
    a. Adipose tissue covered by a layer of mesothelium
    b. Hyaline cartilage covered by a layer of endothelium
    c. Loose connective tissue covered by a layer of endothelium
    d. Loose connective tissue covered by a layer of mesothelium

399. The apex of the heart is normally positioned
    a. Caudal and to the left
    b. Caudal and to the right
    c. Cranial and to the left
    d. Cranial and to the right

Correct answers are on pages 52-71.

400. What cardiac chamber receives blood from the systemic veins?
    a. Left atrium
    b. Left ventricle
    c. Right atrium
    d. Right ventricle

401. The valve that prevents blood from flowing back into the left atrium during ventricular systole is the
    a. Aortic
    b. Mitral
    c. Pulmonary
    d. Tricuspid

402. The cardiac chamber that pumps blood into the pulmonary artery is the
    a. Left atrium
    b. Left ventricle
    c. Right atrium
    d. Right ventricle

403. The valve that prevents blood from flowing back into the left ventricle during ventricular diastole is the
    a. Aortic
    b. Mitral
    c. Pulmonary
    d. Tricuspid

404. The second heart sound is produced by
    a. Closure of the aortic and pulmonary valves
    b. Closure of the mitral and tricuspid valves
    c. Closure of the aortic and mitral valves
    d. Closure of the mitral and pulmonary valves

405. What vessel normally carries carbon dioxide–rich blood?
    a. Aorta
    b. Pulmonary vein
    c. Umbilical vein
    d. Vena cava

406. Which of the following organs is not essential to life?
    a. Heart
    b. Liver
    c. Pancreas
    d. Spleen

407. The most numerous type of blood cell is the
    a. Basophil
    b. Monocyte
    c. Neutrophil
    d. Red blood cell

408. Which of the following white blood cells is not a granulocyte?
    a. Basophil
    b. Eosinophil
    c. Monocyte
    d. Neutrophil

409. For what blood cell is phagocytosis the main function?
    a. Basophil
    b. Eosinophil
    c. Monocyte
    d. Red blood cell

410. Chordae tendineae are present on which valve?
    a. Aortic
    b. Lymphatic
    c. Mitral
    d. Pulmonary

411. The mitral valve of the heart is the
    a. Left atrioventricular valve
    b. Left ventricular outflow valve
    c. Right atrioventricular valve
    d. Right ventricular outflow valve

412. The valve that prevents blood from flowing back into the right ventricle at the end of ventricular systole is the
    a. Aortic
    b. Mitral
    c. Pulmonary
    d. Tricuspid

413. What blood vessel normally carries oxygen-rich blood?
    a. Aorta
    b. Pulmonary artery
    c. Umbilical artery
    d. Vena cava

414. What lymphoid organ normally is prominent in young animals only?
    a. Gut-associated lymphatic tissue
    b. Spleen
    c. Thymus
    d. Tonsil

415. The least numerous type of blood cell in circulation is normally the
    a. Basophil
    b. Eosinophil
    c. Lymphocyte
    d. Monocyte

416. Blood vessels that are the site of the transfer of nutrients between the blood and tissues are the
  a. Arteries
  b. Arterioles
  c. Capillaries
  d. Veins

417. The circulatory system is lined by what kind of epithelium?
  a. Simple columnar
  b. Simple squamous
  c. Stratified squamous
  d. Transitional

418. What vessels contain valves?
  a. Arterioles
  b. Capillaries
  c. Lymph capillaries
  d. Medium-sized veins

419. The heart chamber that pumps blood to the lungs is the
  a. Left atrium
  b. Left ventricle
  c. Right atrium
  d. Right ventricle

420. The heart chamber that receives blood from the pulmonary veins is the
  a. Left atrium
  b. Left ventricle
  c. Right atrium
  d. Right ventricle

421. The heart chamber that pumps blood through the aorta is the
  a. Left atrium
  b. Left ventricle
  c. Right atrium
  d. Right ventricle

422. The valve between the right atrium and right ventricle of the heart is the
  a. Aortic
  b. Mitral
  c. Pulmonary
  d. Tricuspid

423. The valve at the outflow tract of the right ventricle is the
  a. Aortic
  b. Mitral
  c. Pulmonary
  d. Tricuspid

424. The left atrioventricular valve is the
  a. Aortic
  b. Mitral
  c. Pulmonary
  d. Tricuspid

425. The left ventricular outflow valve is the
  a. Aortic
  b. Mitral
  c. Pulmonary
  d. Tricuspid

426. The first heart sound is produced by
  a. Closure of the left and right atrioventricular valves
  b. Closure of the pulmonary and aortic valves
  c. Contraction of the left and right atria
  d. Contraction of the left and right ventricles

427. The bundle of His is located in what part of the heart?
  a. Interventricular septum
  b. Left and right ventricular walls
  c. Right atrial wall
  d. Apex of the heart

428. The blood vessel that shunts blood from the pulmonary artery to the aorta in a fetus is the
  a. Ductus arteriosus
  b. Foramen ovale
  c. Umbilicus arteriosus
  d. Umbilicus venosus

429. The main component of the tunica media of muscular arteries is
  a. Cardiac muscle fibers
  b. Elastic fibers
  c. Skeletal muscle fibers
  d. Smooth muscle fibers

430. The pulmonary valve prevents blood from flowing back into the
  a. Left atrium
  b. Right atrium
  c. Left ventricle
  d. Right ventricle

431. The mitral valve prevents blood from flowing back into the
  a. Left atrium
  b. Right atrium
  c. Left ventricle
  d. Right ventricle

Correct answers are on pages 52-71.

432. The aortic valve prevents blood from flowing back into the
    a. Left atrium
    b. Right atrium
    c. Left ventricle
    d. Right ventricle

433. The tricuspid valve prevents blood from flowing back into the
    a. Left Atrium
    b. Right atrium
    c. Left ventricle
    d. Right ventricle

434. Each cardiac cycle in a normal heart results from an impulse that is initiated in the
    a. Atrioventricular node
    b. Bundle of His
    c. Purkinje fibers
    d. Sinoatrial node

435. The ductus arteriosus in a fetus joins the
    a. Aorta and pulmonary artery
    b. Aorta and pulmonary vein
    c. Vena cava and pulmonary artery
    d. Vena cava and pulmonary vein

436. The valve that prevents blood from flowing back into the left ventricle at the end of ventricular systole is the
    a. Aortic
    b. Mitral
    c. Pulmonary
    d. Tricuspid

437. The Purkinje fibers in the heart are located in the
    a. Interventricular septum
    b. Left and right ventricular walls
    c. Right atrial wall
    d. Interatrial septum

438. Blood that has returned to the heart through the cranial and caudal venae cavae first passes through what heart valve?
    a. Aortic
    b. Mitral
    c. Pulmonary
    d. Tricuspid

439. The right atrium receives blood from what blood vessel?
    a. Aorta
    b. Pulmonary artery
    c. Pulmonary vein
    d. Vena cava

440. What heart chamber pumps blood to the systemic circulation?
    a. Left atrium
    b. Left ventricle
    c. Right atrium
    d. Right ventricle

441. The left atrium receives blood from what blood vessel?
    a. Aorta
    b. Pulmonary artery
    c. Pulmonary vein
    d. Vena cava

442. Which structure of the fetal heart largely allows blood to bypass the pulmonary circulation?
    a. Foramen magnum
    b. Foramen ovale
    c. Nutrient foramen
    d. Obturator foramen

443. The large lymphoid organ that stores blood but is not essential to life is the
    a. Kidney
    b. Liver
    c. Pancreas
    d. Spleen

444. What blood component is most important in plugging leaks in damaged blood vessels?
    a. Albumin
    b. Neutrophil
    c. Platelet
    d. Red blood cell

445. Which of the following is not a feature of the right side of the heart?
    a. Atrium
    b. Chordae tendineae
    c. Pulmonary valve
    d. Mitral valve

446. The first cardiac chamber that blood enters after returning from the lungs is the
    a. Left atrium
    b. Left ventricle
    c. Right atrium
    d. Right ventricle

447. What are the effects of parasympathetic nervous system stimulation on the heart?
    a. Decreased rate and decreased force of contractions
    b. Decreased rate and increased force of contractions
    c. Increased rate and decreased force of contractions
    d. Increased rate and increased force of contractions

448. The foramen ovale in the developing fetus allows blood to flow
   a. From the left atrium to the right atrium
   b. From the right atrium to the left atrium
   c. From the left ventricle to the right ventricle
   d. From the right ventricle to the left ventricle

449. What body fluid cannot clot?
   a. Plasma
   b. Serum
   c. Whole blood
   d. Lymph

450. What white blood cell normally contains red-staining granules in its cytoplasm?
   a. Basophil
   b. Eosinophil
   c. Monocyte
   d. Neutrophil

451. What white blood cell is important in immunity production and normally has a single, large nucleus that occupies most of the cell?
   a. Eosinophil
   b. Lymphocyte
   c. Monocyte
   d. Neutrophil

452. Which of the following structures are listed in the order in which they are encountered by a blood cell?
   a. Arteries, veins, capillaries, heart
   b. Capillaries, veins, heart, arteries
   c. Heart, veins, capillaries, arteries
   d. Veins, capillaries, arteries, heart

453. What vessel brings fresh, oxygenated blood from the placenta to a developing fetus?
   a. Ductus arteriosus
   b. Pulmonary vein
   c. Umbilical artery
   d. Umbilical vein

454. What blood cell normally has a multilobed nucleus?
   a. Eosinophil
   b. Lymphocyte
   c. Platelet
   d. Red blood cell

455. Which of the following is not one of the main functions of the digestive system?
   a. Absorption
   b. Digestion
   c. Prehension
   d. Secretion

456. The digestive system of herbivores
   a. Contains an enlarged microbial fermentation vat
   b. Is generally simpler and narrower than that of carnivores
   c. Is made to handle both plant and animal food sources
   d. Relies mainly on enzymatic digestion

457. From the stomach to the anus, the digestive tube is lined by what kind of epithelium?
   a. Simple columnar
   b. Simple squamous
   c. Stratified columnar
   d. Stratified squamous

458. Most of a tooth is made up of what tissue?
   a. Bone
   b. Cementum
   c. Dentin
   d. Enamel

459. The most rostral teeth in the dental arcade are the
   a. Canines
   b. Incisors
   c. Molars
   d. Premolars

460. The smallest ruminant forestomach, and the one most commonly involved in hardware disease, is the
   a. Abomasum
   b. Omasum
   c. Reticulum
   d. Rumen

461. The true stomach of the ruminant is the
   a. Abomasum
   b. Omasum
   c. Reticulum
   d. Rumen

462. The most distal short portion of the small intestine, just before it joins the large intestine, is the
   a. Duodenum
   b. Ileum
   c. Ilium
   d. Jejunum

463. The longest portion of the large intestine is the
   a. Cecum
   b. Colon
   c. Jejunum
   d. Rectum

Correct answers are on pages 52-71.

464. The root of a tooth is normally covered by
    a. Cartilage
    b. Cementum
    c. Dentin
    d. Enamel

465. The most caudal teeth are the
    a. Canines
    b. Incisors
    c. Molars
    d. Premolars

466. The surface area of the small intestinal lining is increased by
    a. Gyri
    b. Papillae
    c. Rugae
    d. Villi

467. The organ that has endocrine functions and also produces many digestive enzymes is the
    a. Liver
    b. Pancreas
    c. Spleen
    d. Thymus

468. The largest ruminant forestomach is the
    a. Abomasum
    b. Omasum
    c. Reticulum
    d. Rumen

469. The crown of a tooth is covered by
    a. Cementum
    b. Dentin
    c. Enamel
    d. Serosa

470. The cranial cheek teeth are the
    a. Canines
    b. Incisors
    c. Molars
    d. Premolars

471. The ruminant forestomach that dehydrates and grinds feed is the
    a. Abomasum
    b. Omasum
    c. Reticulum
    d. Rumen

472. The first short portion of the small intestine that comes off the stomach is the
    a. Cecum
    b. Duodenum
    c. Ileum
    d. Jejunum

473. The longest portion of the small intestine, where most absorption of nutrients occurs, is the
    a. Cecum
    b. Duodenum
    c. Ileum
    d. Jejunum

474. The opening of the esophagus into the stomach is called the
    a. Cardia
    b. Fundus
    c. Pylorus
    d. Ruga

475. The blind-ended sac that is part of the large intestine is the
    a. Cecum
    b. Colon
    c. Duodenum
    d. Rectum

476. The exocrine secretion of the pancreas contains large amounts of
    a. Bile
    b. Digestive enzymes
    c. Hydrochloric acid
    d. Mucus

477. The largest gland in the normal adult animal body is the
    a. Liver
    b. Pancreas
    c. Spleen
    d. Thymus

478. The blood vessel that carries nutrient-rich blood from the intestines to the liver is the
    a. Ductus arteriosus
    b. Portal vein
    c. Pulmonary vein
    d. Vena cava

479. The outermost layer of the digestive tube is the
    a. Mucosa
    b. Muscle layer
    c. Serosa
    d. Submucosa

480. Which of these combinations of digestive structures is lined entirely by simple columnar epithelium?
    a. Anus, duodenum, ileum, stomach
    b. Cecum, colon, jejunum, stomach
    c. Colon, esophagus, ileum, stomach
    d. Duodenum, jejunum, ileum, pancreas

481. Which of the following is not secreted by gastric glands?
a. Acid
b. Chyme
c. Digestive enzymes
d. Mucus

482. The process or structure in a newborn ruminant animal that allows milk to bypass the rumen and reticulum and go directly to the omasum is the
a. Eructation
b. Esophageal groove
c. Reticular folds
d. Rumination

483. What structure is not part of the large intestine?
a. Cecum
b. Colon
c. Ileum
d. Rectum

484. Villi are prominent in the lining of what structure?
a. Esophagus
b. Large intestine
c. Small intestine
d. Stomach

485. Which of the following is not a normal function of the liver in an adult animal?
a. Bile secretion
b. Blood cell formation
c. Destruction of old red blood cells
d. Protein synthesis

486. The correct term for chewing of food is
a. Eructation
b. Mastication
c. Prehension
d. Rumination

487. In which of these animals is microbial fermentation most important in the digestive process?
a. Cat
b. Dog
c. Horse
d. Pig

488. The inner lining of the digestive tube is called the
a. Mucosa
b. Musculorum
c. Serosa
d. Submucosa

489. The teeth that are not present in all common domestic animals are the
a. Canines
b. Incisors
c. Premolars
d. Molars

490. The common passageway of the respiratory and digestive systems is the
a. Esophagus
b. Larynx
c. Pharynx
d. Trachea

491. What fluid contributes least to the process of digestion?
a. Bile
b. Pancreatic juice
c. Saliva
d. Stomach gland secretions

492. In what structure does no significant digestion or absorption take place?
a. Esophagus
b. Large intestine
c. Small intestine
d. Stomach

493. The periodic elimination of excess gas from the ruminant forestomach is termed
a. Eructation
b. Mastication
c. Prehension
d. Rumination

494. The portal vein carries nutrient-rich blood from the intestines to the
a. Liver
b. Pancreas
c. Spleen
d. Stomach

495. What gland is also called the *master gland*?
a. Thyroid
b. Adrenal
c. Pituitary
d. Thymus

496. The anterior pituitary gland secretes
a. Antidiuretic hormone (ADH)
b. Insulin
c. Oxytocin
d. Follicle-stimulating hormone (FSH)

Correct answers are on pages 52-71.

497. The adrenal glands produce
   a. Insulin
   b. Glucocorticoids
   c. Parathormone
   d. Calcitonin

498. The pancreas produces
   a. Thyroxine
   b. Prolactin
   c. Insulin
   d. Progesterone

499. What gland regulates most of the endocrine system?
   a. Thyroid
   b. Pancreas
   c. Thymus
   d. Pituitary

500. What hormones are produced by the thyroid gland?
   a. Thyroxine and insulin
   b. Parathormone and thyroxine
   c. Calcitonin and insulin
   d. Thyroxine and calcitonin

501. What hormone stimulates milk let-down?
   a. Testosterone
   b. Epinephrine
   c. Oxytocin
   d. Relaxin

502. Where is the thyroid gland located?
   a. At the base of the brain
   b. Adjacent to the trachea
   c. Adjacent to the cranial end of each kidney
   d. At the duodenal loop

503. Exocrine glands are
   a. Glands whose secretory products are transported via ducts
   b. Glands whose secretory products enter the bloodstream
   c. Glands whose excretory products are transported via ducts
   d. Glands whose excretory products enter the bloodstream

504. Hypoadrenocorticism is commonly referred to as
   a. Cushings disease
   b. Addisons disease
   c. Bangs disease
   d. Carres disease

505. The adrenal medulla secretes
   a. Thyroxine
   b. Estrogen
   c. Progesterone
   d. Epinephrine

506. What substance is required for production of thyroid hormones?
   a. Insulin
   b. Epinephrine
   c. Iodine
   d. Sodium

507. What clinical sign is associated with hyperthyroidism?
   a. Loss of weight with a normal or increased appetite
   b. Lethargy
   c. Decreased tolerance of cold
   d. Decreased metabolic rate

508. An appreciable enlargement of the thyroid gland is termed
   a. Hypothyroidism
   b. Goiter
   c. Parathyroidism
   d. Lump jaw

509. When one hormone increases the activity of another hormone, the effect is termed
   a. Potentiation
   b. Antagonism
   c. Doubling
   d. Nullification

510. The abbreviation ACTH stands for
   a. Acidic colorotropic hormone
   b. Anterior control trophic hormone
   c. Adrenocorticotropic hormone
   d. Adrenocontrol trophic hormone

511. The most important function of ADH is to
   a. Assist glucose in crossing into body cells
   b. Stimulate parturition
   c. Increase production of thyroid hormone
   d. Help control water loss from the kidneys

512. Following coitus, what hormone that also aids in fetal expulsion is believed to stimulate uterine contraction and thereby aid transport of sperm to the oviducts?
   a. Oxytocin
   b. Progesterone
   c. Testosterone
   d. FSH

513. Where are the adrenal glands located?
    a. Base of the brain
    b. Adjacent to the trachea
    c. Near the kidneys
    d. Caudal to the eyes

514. Parathyroid hormone is one of the major factors controlling the blood level of
    a. Iodine
    b. Magnesium
    c. Chloride
    d. Calcium

515. The number of parathyroid glands in all species is
    a. 2
    b. 4
    c. 10
    d. Variable

516. The disease caused by a lack of insulin or the body's inability to use insulin is
    a. Diabetes mellitus
    b. Diabetes insipidus
    c. Addisons disease
    d. Cushings disease

517. Insulin is produced in the pancreas by the beta cells in the islets of Langerhans. What is produced by the alpha cells?
    a. Thyroxine
    b. Glucagon
    c. Estrogen
    d. Calcium

518. What type of hormone transmission uses interstitial fluid to diffuse the hormone through the body?
    a. Endocrine
    b. Neurocrine
    c. Paracrine
    d. Exocrine

519. What substance is not classified as an endocrine hormone?
    a. Pancreatic juice
    b. Polypeptide (protein)
    c. Steroid
    d. Amine

520. The epithelium of the skin is
    a. Simple squamous, keratinized
    b. Simple squamous, nonkeratinized
    c. Stratified squamous, keratinized
    d. Stratified squamous, nonkeratinized

521. The sweat glands in the skin are
    a. Compound alveolar
    b. Compound tubular
    c. Simple alveolar
    d. Simple tubular

522. The wall of the hoof grows distally from the
    a. Coronary band
    b. Chestnut
    c. Frog
    d. Periople

523. What hoof structure normally has the firmest consistency?
    a. Frog
    b. Periople
    c. Sole
    d. Wall

524. The sebaceous glands of the skin are
    a. Compound alveolar
    b. Compound tubular
    c. Simple alveolar
    d. Simple tubular

525. Which of the following is not a skin gland?
    a. Mammary
    b. Salivary
    c. Sebaceous
    d. Sudoriferous

526. Which statement about the dermis is most accurate?
    a. It contains blood vessels.
    b. Its deepest layer contains pigment cells.
    c. It is composed of stratified squamous epithelium.
    d. Its surface is keratinized.

527. A hair is produced by the
    a. Bulb
    b. Epidermis
    c. Follicle
    d. Root

528. What structure is located most proximal on a horse's leg?
    a. Chestnut
    b. Coronary band
    c. Ergot
    d. Frog

529. Which of the following is not a function of the integument?
    a. Secretion and excretion
    b. Sensation
    c. Synthesis of vitamin E
    d. Temperature regulation

Correct answers are on pages 52-71.

530. The oil glands of the skin are the
    a. Anal glands
    b. Mammary glands
    c. Sebaceous glands
    d. Sudoriferous glands

531. The portion of a hair that is visible above the skin surface is the
    a. Bulb
    b. Follicle
    c. Root
    d. Shaft

532. If a hair is pigmented, the pigment granules are present in what layer?
    a. Cortex
    b. Cuticle
    c. Medulla
    d. Periople

533. The arrector pili muscles are attached to
    a. Guard hairs
    b. Hair beds
    c. Hair clusters
    d. Wool hairs

534. Which of the following is a sweat gland?
    a. Mammary
    b. Salivary
    c. Sebaceous
    d. Sudoriferous

535. Which of these statements about the epidermis is most accurate?
    a. It contains blood vessels.
    b. Its surface layer contains pigment cells.
    c. It is composed of stratified squamous epithelium.
    d. Its surface layer is made up of living cells.

536. Which of these statements about the skin is least accurate?
    a. It is involved in synthesis of vitamin D.
    b. It is the largest organ in the body.
    c. Its underlayer (dermis) consists of epithelial and connective tissues.
    d. The epidermis is its more superficial layer.

537. The portion of a hair beneath the skin surface is called the
    a. Bulb
    b. Follicle
    c. Root
    d. Shaft

538. When a horse is standing on firm ground, the only portion of its hoof that normally contacts the ground is the
    a. Coronary band
    b. Sole
    c. Wall
    d. White line

539. The epidermis of the skin is composed of what kind of epithelium?
    a. Simple squamous, keratinized
    b. Simple squamous, nonkeratinized
    c. Stratified squamous, keratinized
    d. Stratified squamous, nonkeratinized

540. The number of teats on the mammary glands of different animals varies. List the correct number of teats for a mare.
    a. 2
    b. 4
    c. 12
    d. 14

541. List the correct number of teats for a cow.
    a. 2
    b. 4
    c. 12
    d. 14

542. List the correct number of teats for a sow.
    a. 2
    b. 4
    c. 12
    d. 14

543. List the correct number of teats for a rat.
    a. 2
    b. 4
    c. 12
    d. 14

544. The suspensory apparatus of the udder includes the
    a. Symphyseal tendon
    b. Urethralis muscle
    c. Deep digital flexor tendon
    d. Proximal digital annular ligament

545. In cows, the "milk vein" is the
    a. External pudendal
    b. Femoral
    c. Lateral thoracic
    d. Subcutaneous abdominal

546. Colostrum provides the neonate with
    a. Immunoglobulins
    b. Erythrocytes
    c. Granulocytes
    d. Glucocorticoids

547. Production of colostrum is initiated by
    a. Specialized endothelial cells
    b. The fetus
    c. A response to hormonal influences
    d. The portal hepatic system

548. Colostrum provides which type of immunity?
    a. Active
    b. Passive
    c. Cellular
    d. Acquired

549. In cows, production of colostrum begins
    a. During the last 2 to 3 weeks of gestation
    b. When the calf suckles
    c. During the first postparturient estrous cycle
    d. During the first trimester of pregnancy

550. The quality of a mare's colostrum can be evaluated by all of the following except
    a. Stickiness
    b. Specific gravity
    c. Smell
    d. Direct measurement of IgG in the fluid

551. Agalactia is a
    a. Commercially produced milk replacer
    b. Lack of milk production
    c. Rejection of a newborn by the dam
    d. Blood-tinged colostrum

552. A cow with mastitis should
    a. Be milked frequently
    b. Be milked from all quarters except the affected one
    c. Not be milked at all
    d. Be immediately sent to have her teat removed

553. The agent that aids in secretion and release of milk from the mammary gland after parturition is
    a. Oxytetracycline
    b. Progesterone
    c. Oxytocin
    d. Prednisolone

554. What is not a common cause of enlarged mammary glands in horses?
    a. Mastitis
    b. Abscess
    c. Periparturient udder edema (physiologic)
    d. Tuberculosis

555. The principal muscle of respiration is the diaphragm. Where is it located?
    a. Between the thorax and abdomen
    b. Between the ribs
    c. At the thoracic inlet
    d. Cranial to the heart

556. In general, muscles are divided into three major groups according to their cellular structure. They are
    a. Striated, skeletal, and visceral
    b. Smooth, unstriped, and visceral
    c. Striated, smooth, and cardiac
    d. Striped, skeletal, and smooth

557. What feature is unique to cardiac muscle?
    a. Tone
    b. Muscular fibers
    c. Purkinje fibers
    d. Striations

558. What word describes the action of a muscle that moves an extremity toward the midline?
    a. Flexion
    b. Adduction
    c. Extension
    d. Abduction

559. The function of Purkinje fibers is to
    a. Hold the heart in the proper shape
    b. Maintain proper valve shape during heart contractions
    c. Transmit the electrical signal for ventricular contractions
    d. Maintain ventricular size

560. What is the basic unit of function in a striated muscle?
    a. Dark bands
    b. Light bands
    c. Fiber
    d. Tendon

561. What muscle is the main extensor of the elbow?
    a. Biceps brachium
    b. Triceps brachium
    c. Trapezius
    d. Brachiocephalicus

562. What is the chief action of the biceps brachium?
    a. Extension of the elbow
    b. Flexion of the elbow
    c. Adduction of the shoulder
    d. Flexion of the neck

Correct answers are on pages 52-71.

563. A hip adductor is found on which side of the femur?
    a. Cranial
    b. Caudal
    c. Lateral
    d. Medial

564. What is the point of insertion for the four heads of the quadriceps femoris?
    a. Tibia
    b. Acetabulum
    c. Hock
    d. Elbow

565. Which abdominal muscle layer is the most superficial?
    a. External oblique
    b. Internal oblique
    c. Rectus
    d. Transversus

566. The maximum amount that a muscle fiber can contract is about what proportion of its resting length?
    a. One fourth
    b. One half
    c. Twice
    d. Four times

567. The least movable of the attachments of a muscle to bone is the
    a. Periosteum
    b. Origin
    c. Insertion
    d. Cortex

568. Muscles that tend to pull a limb away from the median plane are termed
    a. Flexors
    b. Extensors
    c. Adductors
    d. Abductors

569. The large muscle in the calf of the leg that flexes the stifle and extends the hock is the
    a. Gastrocnemius
    b. Biceps brachium
    c. Triceps brachium
    d. Sartorius

570. Muscles that attach to the skin and are responsible for skin movement are termed
    a. Flexors
    b. Extensors
    c. Epithelial
    d. Cutaneous

571. The spasmodic muscular contractions that produce heat to help maintain normal body temperature are called
    a. Convulsions
    b. Tonus
    c. Shivering
    d. Peristalsis

572. Skeletal muscles that are arranged circularly to constrict a body opening are termed
    a. Sphincters
    b. Circumflexors
    c. Abductors
    d. Adductors

573. Loss of nerve supply to a muscle results in
    a. Denervation hypertrophy
    b. Disuse hypertrophy
    c. Disuse hypoplasia
    d. Denervation atrophy

574. What triangular and flat muscle originates along the dorsal midline and inserts mainly on the spine of the scapula?
    a. Biceps brachii
    b. Trapezius
    c. Deltoideus
    d. Triceps brachii

575. What muscle is the main adductor of the shoulder?
    a. Omotransversarius
    b. Brachiocephalicus
    c. Biceps brachii
    d. Pectoralis

576. The biceps femoris, semitendinosus, and semimembranosus are known collectively as the
    a. Hamstring muscles
    b. Calf muscles
    c. Foreleg muscles
    d. Thigh muscles

577. With what type of tissue is muscle attached to bone?
    a. Ligaments
    b. Fat
    c. Cartilage
    d. Tendons

578. Tendons that are flat and usually attach to flat muscles are known as
    a. Diarthroses
    b. Aponeuroses
    c. Arthroses
    d. Platytenacea

579. The central nervous system encompasses what subdivisions?
    a. Brain and spinal cord
    b. Spinal cord and spinal nerves
    c. Sympathetic nerves
    d. Parasympathetic nerves

580. Nerve processes that conduct impulses toward the cell bodies are referred to as
    a. Axons
    b. Cytons
    c. Somas
    d. Dendrites

581. Intercalated disks are found between __ muscle cells
    a. Cardiac
    b. Skeletal
    c. Visceral smooth
    d. Multiunit smooth

582. From an evolutionary standpoint, which of the following is one of the oldest parts of the cerebrum? It is associated primarily with the sense of smell and is sometimes called the *olfactory brain.*
    a. Rhinencephalon
    b. Diencephalon
    c. Longitudinal fissure
    d. Telencephalon

583. Hydrocephalus (water on the brain) causes the cerebrum to become extremely thin and may impair or prevent parturition. The most frequent cause of this abnormality is
    a. Obstruction of the interventricular foramina
    b. Occlusion of the cerebral aqueduct
    c. A porous dura mater
    d. Fetal malpresentation

584. The ventral corticospinal tract connects the motor area of the cerebral cortex with motor cells in the ventral gray horns on the same and opposite sides of the spinal cord. The impulses are associated with
    a. Pain and temperature
    b. Pressure sensations
    c. Voluntary motor activity
    d. Tone of the extensor muscles

585. Each forelimb of animals is innervated by a brachial plexus that contains cervical and thoracic nerves. In what species is the brachial plexus not composed of the last three cervical nerves and the first thoracic nerve?
    a. Horses
    b. Cattle
    c. Pigs
    d. Dogs

586. Of the following nerves supplied by the brachial plexus, which one does not innervate muscles in the shoulder?
    a. Thoracodorsal
    b. Long thoracic
    c. Axillary
    d. Median

587. Which nerve is the largest peripheral nerve in the body and stimulates muscles of the thigh region?
    a. Tibial
    b. Femoral
    c. Sciatic
    d. Ulnar

588. Damage to what nerve, most commonly affected by dystocias, results in the inability to adduct the rear legs of a cow?
    a. Obturator
    b. Tibial
    c. Sciatic
    d. Radial

589. Of the 12 cranial nerves, which is a motor nerve to muscles in the shoulder and neck?
    a. Accessory
    b. Vestibulocochlear
    c. Trochlear
    d. Hypoglossal

590. What nerve (one of the longest in the body) supplies parasympathetic fibers to the heart and lungs and to nearly all of the abdominal viscera?
    a. Glossopharyngeal
    b. Facial
    c. Vagus
    d. Oculomotor

591. The most distal part of the digestive tract and most of the urogenital system are supplied with fibers from what portion of the parasympathetic nervous system?
    a. Sacral
    b. Cervical
    c. Thoracic
    d. Lumbar

592. The plasma membrane of the neuron in the resting state (electrically polarized) is very permeable to K+ but is almost impermeable to
    a. Na^+
    b. Cl^-
    c. Ca^{11}
    d. Mg^{++}

Correct answers are on pages 52-71.

593. When a sodium ion is rushing into a nerve cell, the cell is unable to produce another action potential regardless of how strong a stimulus is applied. This time is called the
    a. Absolute refractory period
    b. Relative refractory period
    c. Threshold stimulus period
    d. Action potential period

594. What term refers to the fact that a number of axonal endings synapse on a single cell and its dendrites?
    a. Convergence
    b. Propagation
    c. Orthodromic movement
    d. Divergence

595. Cranial nerves are unique in that some are responsible for performing multiple functions. Which cranial nerve has multiple functions?
    a. Trigeminal
    b. Oculomotor
    c. Vestibulocochlear
    d. Optic

596. If an animal loses its balance and develops nystagmus, the nerve most likely to be the cause is the
    a. Abducens
    b. Auditory
    c. Optic
    d. Vagus

597. If an animal is unable to control its fall and cannot right itself, which spinal tract is most likely affected?
    a. Dorsal white columns
    b. Ventral white columns
    c. Lateral white columns
    d. Adjacent white columns

598. The condition referred to as *sweeney* results from damage to the
    a. Axillary nerve
    b. Radial nerve
    c. Suprascapular nerve
    d. Supraspinatus muscle

599. Injury to what nerve is commonly seen with dystocias in cows that have a small or juvenile pelvis?
    a. Pudendal
    b. Obturator
    c. Perineal
    d. Femoral

600. The autonomic nervous system is directly responsible for innervation of
    a. Visceral organs
    b. Lumbar muscles
    c. Triceps muscles
    d. Somatic organs

601. Parasympathetic stimulation is distributed to visceral structures by what four cranial nerves?
    a. III, V, VII, X
    b. I, III, IV, X
    c. III, VII, IX, X
    d. IX, X, XI, XII

602. Which of the following is not a result of sympathetic nervous system stimulation?
    a. Decreased blood pressure
    b. Increased heart rate
    c. Increased activity of the respiratory–bronchiole dilator reflex
    d. Decreased gut motility

603. The terminal part of the spinal cord is called the
    a. Tail
    b. Cauda equina
    c. Terminus dendriticus
    d. Meningeal terminus

604. Soma is another term for
    a. Nerve cell cytoplasm
    b. Nerve cell body
    c. Nerve cell nucleus
    d. Nerve cell centrosome

605. What term is applied to inflammation of the covering layers of the spinal cord?
    a. Meningitis
    b. Encephalitis
    c. Myelitis
    d. Encephalomyelitis

606. Which of the following correctly lists the number of cervical nerves and corresponding number of cervical vertebrae?
    a. 7, 8
    b. 8, 7
    c. 7, 9
    d. 9, 7

607. What structure, whose Latin name means "little brain," is located at the caudal part of the brain and contains over half of the brain's nerves?
    a. Cerebral cortex
    b. Brainstem
    c. Medulla oblongata
    d. Cerebellum

608. Injury to what nerve results in knuckling of the forepaw onto its dorsal aspect?
   a. Median
   b. Musculocutaneous
   c. Axillary
   d. Radial

609. Complex reflexes are mediated through certain centers in the brain. The medulla oblongata contains reflex centers for all of the following except
   a. Heart contractions
   b. Swallowing
   c. Vomiting
   d. Knee jerk

610. Raising a horse's head prevents kicking by extending the neck, which increases the tone of the extensor muscles of the forelimbs and decreases the tone of the extensors in the hind limbs. This postural reaction is referred to as the
   a. Tonic eye reflex
   b. Extensor postural thrust
   c. Tonic neck reflex
   d. Auditory obtundation

611. What morphine-like substance found in the thalamus and hypothalamus acts as a natural analgesic?
   a. Endorphin
   b. Epinephrine
   c. Norepinephrine
   d. Acetylcholine

612. Any change in a nerve's environment that depolarizes the resting potential and leads to production of a nerve impulse is called
   a. Action potential
   b. Relative refractory period
   c. Repolarization
   d. Stimulus

613. What specialized structure of a neuron conducts impulses away from the cell body?
   a. Neurolemma
   b. Axon
   c. Dendrite
   d. Neuroglia

614. What is the normal average gestation period of horses?
   a. 63 days
   b. 148 days
   c. 285 days
   d. 336 days

615. What is an ectopic pregnancy?
   a. Fetus that is born dead
   b. Short-term pregnancy
   c. Pregnancy that takes place outside of the uterus
   d. Pregnancy that continues beyond the normal term

616. What two hormones influence the growth of lactating tissue?
   a. Estrogen and progesterone
   b. Estrogen and oxytocin
   c. Progesterone and oxytocin
   d. Testosterone and oxytocin

617. Where is the ovum fertilized?
   a. Uterus
   b. Oviducts
   c. Vagina
   d. Cervix

618. The correct order for the stages of the estrous cycle is
   a. Proestrus, anestrus, estrus, metestrus
   b. Anestrus, estrus, proestrus, metestrus
   c. Proestrus, estrus, metestrus, anestrus
   d. Anestrus, metestrus, estrus, proestrus

619. How often does estrus occur in normal, nonpregnant cows?
   a. Every 10 to 15 days
   b. Every 19 to 23 days
   c. Every 30 to 35 days
   d. Every 285 to 290 days

620. What is the normal average gestation period of guinea pigs?
   a. 75 days
   b. 63 days
   c. 21 days
   d. 10 days

621. How long do estrus and gestation normally last in mice?
   a. 4 to 5 days (estrus), 19 to 27 days (gestation)
   b. 16 days (estrus), 59 to 72 days (gestation)
   c. 21 days (estrus), 27 days (gestation)
   d. 32 days (estrus), 63 days (gestation)

622. Which is a response to estrogen?
   a. Inducing estrus via action on the brain
   b. Decreasing blood flow to the uterus
   c. Constricting the cervix
   d. Decreasing uterine contractions

Correct answers are on pages 52-71.

623. Which is a response to progestins?
    a. Dilating the cervix
    b. Decreasing motility of the uterine muscles
    c. Increasing blood flow to the uterus
    d. Inducing estrus via action on the brain

624. What is the main hormonal influence during proestrus?
    a. Follicle Stimulating Hormone (FSH)
    b. Luteinizing Hormone (LH)
    c. Progestins
    d. Prostaglandin

625. What term best describes the estrous cycle of cows?
    a. Biannually polyestrous
    b. Seasonally polyestrous
    c. Polyestrous
    d. Monestrous

626. The greatest amount of fetal growth occurs during the
    a. First trimester
    b. Second trimester
    c. Third trimester
    d. First week of gestation

627. The germinal layer in the early embryo that is responsible for most skin development is the
    a. Mesoderm
    b. Endoderm
    c. Keratoderm
    d. Ectoderm

628. Mammary glands are found in
    a. Males only
    b. Females only
    c. Males and females
    d. Sexually mature females only

629. How many mammary glands do cats have?
    a. 2
    b. 4
    c. 8
    d. 12

630. What hormone is not a prerequisite for lactation?
    a. Estrogen
    b. Prolactin
    c. Testosterone
    d. Progesterone

631. Where are the ovaries located?
    a. Caudal to the urinary bladder
    b. Near the diaphragm
    c. Near the kidneys
    d. Cranial to the liver

632. What is the literal definition of corpus luteum (CL)?
    a. Dead body
    b. Fluid-filled body
    c. Reproducing body
    d. Yellow body

633. The funnel-like structure of the oviduct adjacent to the ovary is the
    a. Infundibulum
    b. Corpus luteum
    c. Caruncle
    d. Fimbriae

634. When is puberty reached in a cow?
    a. When she is 6 months old
    b. When her reproductive organs become functional
    c. After her first act of copulation
    d. When she is 1 year old

635. During, or shortly after, what stage of the estrous cycle does ovulation occur?
    a. Metestrus
    b. Proestrus
    c. Anestrus
    d. Estrus

636. What is the relatively short period of quiescence (estrous inactivity) between estrous cycles in polyestrous animals?
    a. Diestrus
    b. Anestrus
    c. Triestrus
    d. Quadestrus

637. The luteal phase of the estrous cycle includes
    a. Estrus and diestrus
    b. Proestrus and metestrus
    c. Metestrus and diestrus
    d. Estrus and proestrus

638. Metritis is inflammation of the
    a. Uterus
    b. Mammary gland
    c. Fallopian tube
    d. Vagina

639. What is dystocia?
    a. Quiet birth
    b. Difficult birth
    c. Early birth
    d. Overdue birth

640. What is the major male sex hormone?
    a. Endorphin
    b. Estrogen
    c. Testosterone
    d. Progesterone

641. Where do spermatozoa mature?
   a. Testes
   b. Vas deferens
   c. Scrotum
   d. Epididymis

642. What is the term for reflex emptying of the epididymis, urethra, and accessory sex glands?
   a. Erection
   b. Ejaculation
   c. Copulation
   d. Spermatogenesis

643. Hormones with masculinizing effects are known as
   a. Gonadotropins
   b. Estrogens
   c. Progestins
   d. Androgens

644. What action is not associated with testosterone effects in males?
   a. Promotes development of accessory sex glands
   b. Promotes development of secondary sex characteristics
   c. Decreases protein anabolism
   d. Increases libido

645. Sperm can be fertile for up to how many hours in the reproductive tract of a ewe?
   a. 2
   b. 10
   c. 48
   d. 72

646. What gland secretes gonadotropin-releasing hormone?
   a. Anterior pituitary
   b. Hypothalamus
   c. Posterior pituitary
   d. Thyroid

647. The release of prostaglandin F2-alpha from the uterus, as a result of nonpregnancy, causes
   a. A rise in estrogen levels
   b. A rise in progesterone levels
   c. Lysis of the corpus callosum
   d. Lysis of the corpus luteum

648. What is the major hormonal influence during metestrus?
   a. Estrogen
   b. Progesterone
   c. Oxytocin
   d. Gonadotropin-releasing hormone

649. During what part of the estrous cycle is the female most receptive to the male?
   a. Proestrus
   b. Estrus
   c. Metestrus
   d. Anestrus or diestrus

650. When is the usual breeding season for ewes?
   a. Summer
   b. Fall
   c. Winter
   d. Spring

651. What hormone inhibits excessive uterine motility during gestation?
   a. Prostaglandin
   b. Oxytocin
   c. Estrogen
   d. Progesterone

652. What is the normal average length of gestation in a sow?
   a. 21 days
   b. 114 days
   c. 150 days
   d. 285 days

653. What is the term for the time from fertilization of the ovum until birth of the fetus?
   a. Implantation
   b. Parturition
   c. Gestation
   d. Dystocia

654. What does the term *multiparous* mean?
   a. Having given birth to viable offspring in more than one gestation
   b. Having more than one period of estrus during the year
   c. Having more than two viable offspring during one gestation
   d. Having viable offspring sired by more than one male during one gestation

655. In ruminants, the cotyledon of the placenta attaches to what structure on the uterus to form the placentome?
   a. Zonule
   b. Allantois
   c. Chorioallantois
   d. Caruncle

656. What structure produces the ovum?
   a. Ovary
   b. Uterus
   c. Fallopian tube
   d. Fimbria

Correct answers are on pages 52-71.

657. Rupture of a follicle releases
    a. Progesterone
    b. FSH
    c. An ovum
    d. Oxytocin

658. What is another name for fallopian tubes?
    a. Ureters
    b. Oviducts
    c. Uterine horns
    d. Broad ligaments

659. What structure produces LH?
    a. Hypothalamus
    b. Posterior pituitary
    c. Thyroid gland
    d. Anterior pituitary

660. LH promotes growth of the
    a. Fetus
    b. Mammary glands
    c. Uterus
    d. Corpus luteum

661. What hormone is released from the corpus luteum?
    a. Progesterone
    b. Estrogen
    c. LH
    d. FSH

662. Nymphomania is caused by
    a. Too much progesterone
    b. Not enough estrogen
    c. Cystic ovaries
    d. Hypertrophy of the uterus

663. What female is an induced or reflex ovulator?
    a. Cow
    b. Bitch
    c. Mare
    d. Queen

664. In the first stage of parturition, ACTH stimulates the fetal adrenal cortex to release
    a. Hydrocortisone
    b. Estrogen
    c. Progesterone
    d. FSH

665. What hormone results in strong uterine contractions?
    a. Progesterone
    b. Estrogen
    c. Prostaglandin
    d. Oxytocin

666. What is the normal average length of gestation in goats?
    a. 21 days
    b. 114 days
    c. 150 days
    d. 285 days

667. What is the cutaneous sac that contains the testes?
    a. Epididymis
    b. Labia
    c. Sheath
    d. Scrotum

668. In what two species is cryptorchidism most prevalent?
    a. Cats and dogs
    b. Cattle and goats
    c. Horses and pigs
    d. Sheep and dogs

669. The seminal plasma of all species contains
    a. Progesterone
    b. Fructose
    c. Urine
    d. Polysaccharides

670. Enlargement of what structure is responsible for prolonged retention of the penis within the vagina during coitus in canines?
    a. Prostate gland
    b. Bulbourethral glands
    c. Vasa deferentia
    d. Bulbus glandis

671. What is a photoperiod?
    a. Length of daylight and darkness
    b. Time needed for a photosynthetic reaction
    c. Time it takes for light to move a specific distance
    d. Estrus induced by light

672. What female has ovaries that resemble a cluster of grapes because of the large number of protruding follicles?
    a. Cow
    b. Ewe
    c. Sow
    d. Mare

673. The process by which ova are formed is termed
    a. Spermatogenesis
    b. Odontogenesis
    c. Oophorosis
    d. Oogenesis

674. Which of these is not a layer of the fetal placenta?
    a. Caruncle
    b. Amnion
    c. Chorion
    d. Allantois

675. Most conditioning of inspired air occurs in the
    a. Larynx
    b. Nares
    c. Nasal passages
    d. Pharynx

676. Which of the following is not a function of the respiratory system?
    a. Acid–base regulation
    b. Mastication
    c. Olfaction
    d. Phonation

677. The sites in the lung where gases are exchanged between the air and the blood are the
    a. Alveoli
    b. Bifurcations
    c. Bronchi
    d. Bronchioles

678. The short, irregular tubular structure in the neck region that acts as a valve to control airflow to the lungs is the
    a. Bronchus
    b. Larynx
    c. Pharynx
    d. Trachea

679. The transfer of oxygen and carbon dioxide between the air and blood in the lungs is accomplished by
    a. Blood pressure
    b. Diffusion
    c. Ion pumps
    d. Osmosis

680. The epithelium lining the alveoli is
    a. Pseudostratified columnar
    b. Simple cuboidal
    c. Simple squamous
    d. Stratified squamous

681. The main tubular structure in the neck region that carries air to and from the lungs is the
    a. Bronchus
    b. Larynx
    c. Pharynx
    d. Trachea

682. What structure is not part of the upper respiratory tract?
    a. Bronchiole
    b. Larynx
    c. Pharynx
    d. Trachea

683. When the diaphragm contracts, it
    a. Compresses the lungs
    b. Creates positive pressure in the thoracic cavity
    c. Increases the size of the abdominal cavity
    d. Increases the size of the thoracic cavity

684. Compared with blood entering the alveolar capillaries, air drawn into the alveoli of the lungs has
    a. Higher Pco2 and higher Po2
    b. Higher Pco2 and lower Po2
    c. Lower Pco2 and higher Po2
    d. Lower Pco2 and lower Po2

685. The epithelium lining the upper respiratory tract is
    a. Pseudostratified columnar
    b. Stratified squamous
    c. Simple squamous
    d. Transitional

686. External respiration takes place
    a. At the nares
    b. In the lungs
    c. In the upper respiratory tract
    d. Throughout the body tissues

687. Which of the following is a major function of the larynx?
    a. Filtering inspired air
    b. Olfaction
    c. Phonation
    d. Warming inspired air

688. Internal respiration takes place
    a. At the nares
    b. In the lungs
    c. In the upper respiratory tract
    d. Throughout the body tissues

689. The common passageway for the respiratory and digestive systems is the
    a. Larynx
    b. Nasal passage
    c. Pharynx
    d. Trachea

Correct answers are on pages 52-71.

690. Proceeding caudally, the trachea bifurcates into two
    a. Mainstem bronchi
    b. Primary bronchioles
    c. Alveoli
    d. Secondary bronchioles

691. The diaphragm is primarily made up of __.
    a. Elastic connective tissue
    b. Fibrous connective tissue
    c. Skeletal muscle
    d. Multiunit smooth muscle

692. Which of the following lists the respiratory structures in the order through which air passes during exhalation?
    a. Bronchi, trachea, larynx, pharynx, nasal passages
    b. Bronchi, trachea, pharynx, larynx, nasal passages
    c. Nasal passages, larynx, pharynx, trachea, bronchi
    d. Nasal passages, pharynx, larynx, trachea, bronchi

693. Exchange of oxygen and carbon dioxide between blood and the cells and tissues is termed
    a. External respiration
    b. Internal respiration
    c. Olfaction
    d. Phonation

694. Which cranial nerve mediates the sense of smell?
    a. Oculomotor
    b. Glossopharyngeal
    c. Olfactory
    d. Hypoglossal

695. What division of the nervous system contains the cranial nerves and paired spinal nerves?
    a. CNS (central)
    b. PNS (peripheral)
    c. ANS (autonomic)
    d. VNS (vagal)

696. Which cranial nerve innervates the throat area and the heart?
    a. Glossopharyngeal
    b. Spinal accessory
    c. Abducens
    d. Vagus

697. Which of the following is a response to increased sympathetic stimulation?
    a. Accelerated heart rate and amplitude
    b. Constricted bronchioles
    c. Dilated blood vessels in the intestinal tract
    d. Increased gastrointestinal secretions

698. What structure acts as a light receptor?
    a. Uvea
    b. Sclera
    c. Cone
    d. Cochlea

699. What portion of the ear is essential for hearing and equilibrium?
    a. Inner
    b. Middle
    c. External
    d. Eardrum

700. Which cranial nerve carries impulses from the ear to the brain?
    a. Acoustic (VIII)
    b. Olfactory (I)
    c. Optic (II)
    d. Vagus (X)

701. Which cranial nerve provides parasympathetic innervation to the heart, lungs, stomach, and small intestine?
    a. Trochlear (IV)
    b. Vagus (X)
    c. Abducens (VI)
    d. Trigeminal (V)

702. Birds recognize feed primarily by
    a. Sight
    b. Odor
    c. Taste
    d. Touch

703. What structure is not part of a nerve cell?
    a. Axon
    b. Dendrite
    c. Stoma
    d. Axolemma

704. Which cranial nerve conducts motor impulses to the tongue?
    a. Oculomotor (III)
    b. Trigeminal (V)
    c. Vestibulocochlear (VIII)
    d. Hypoglossal (XII)

705. Which cranial nerve provides parasympathetic innervation to the cranial three quarters of the body?
    a. Olfactory (I)
    b. Abducens (VI)
    c. Vagus (X)
    d. Spinal accessory (XI)

706. How many pairs of cranial nerves do dogs have?
    a. 6
    b. 8
    c. 10
    d. 12

707. Cerebrospinal fluid is found in the
    a. Kidney
    b. Central canal of the spinal cord
    c. Liver
    d. Anterior chamber of the eye

708. Outside of the brain and spinal cord, nerve cell bodies are usually found in clumps or aggregations called
    a. Receptors
    b. Ganglia
    c. Bundles
    d. Neuromas

709. The spinal cord is a communicating link between body tissues and the
    a. Brain
    b. Heart
    c. Liver
    d. Intestinal tract

710. Nerve fibers that carry information to the brain are termed
    a. Efferent
    b. Parasympathetic
    c. Motor
    d. Afferent

711. The presence of a myelin sheath on an axon tends to
    a. Accelerate all impulses
    b. Slow all impulses
    c. Accelerate only impulses to peripheral tissues
    d. Accelerate only impulses to the brain

712. The point at which the axon of one neuron meets the dendrite of another and over which nerve impulses can pass is called a
    a. Synapse
    b. Reflex arc
    c. Cyton
    d. Meninx

713. The eye converts light stimuli to nerve impulses via the
    a. Lens
    b. Pupil
    c. Retina
    d. Iris

714. The portion of the retina that is not sensitive to light stimuli is called the
    a. Optic nerve
    b. Choroid
    c. Ciliary body
    d. Cornea

715. In what order does light pass through ocular structures on its way to the retina?
    a. Lens, cornea, pupil
    b. Cornea, lens, pupil
    c. Cornea, pupil, lens
    d. Pupil, cornea, lens

716. What is the pigmented sphincter like structure of the eye that controls the amount of light entering the posterior eye?
    a. Sclera
    b. Iris
    c. Pupil
    d. Retina

717. An electrical charge moving along the membrane of a nerve fiber is called
    a. A stimulus
    b. An impulse
    c. A reflex
    d. A repolarization wave

718. Homeostasis or homeokinesis is the chief role of what part of the nervous system?
    a. Autonomic nervous system
    b. Central nervous system
    c. Cranial nerves
    d. Peripheral nervous system

719. What enzyme inactivates acetylcholine?
    a. Norepinephrine
    b. Cholinesterase
    c. Adrenolytic agent
    d. Acetylcholinesterase

720. What substance is a catecholamine?
    a. Acetylcholine
    b. Acetylcholinesterase
    c. Norepinephrine
    d. Nicotine

Correct answers are on pages 52-71.

721. The scientific term for the white of the eye is
    a. Iris
    b. Retina
    c. Cornea
    d. Sclera

722. The central nervous system consists of the brain and the
    a. Sympathetic nerves
    b. Parasympathetic nerves
    c. Spinal cord
    d. Cranial nerves

723. Nerve fibers encased in a white sheath of fatty material are termed
    a. Parasympathetic
    b. Myelinated
    c. Sympathetic
    d. Ganglia

724. Which of these is not one of the three major subdivisions of the brain?
    a. Cerebrum
    b. Brainstem
    c. Cerebellum
    d. Occipital lobe

725. Which of these is not a layer of the meninges?
    a. Pons
    b. Dura mater
    c. Pia mater
    d. Arachnoid

726. How many pairs of thoracic nerves does a dog have?
    a. 2
    b. 10
    c. 13
    d. 21

727. Spinal nerves are what type of nerve?
    a. Sensory (afferent)
    b. Motor (efferent)
    c. Autonomic
    d. Mixed

728. Branch like structures that conduct impulses toward the nerve cell body are called
    a. Dendrites
    b. Axons
    c. Synapses
    d. Neurons

729. Articular cartilage consists of a thin layer of
    a. Periosteum
    b. Endosteum
    c. Epiphyseal cartilage
    d. Hyaline cartilage

730. One of the primary functions of long bones is
    a. Mineral manufacture
    b. Formation of a protective cavity for the brain
    c. Formation of a protective cavity for the thorax
    d. Hematopoiesis

731. The study of skeletal systems with bones as the chief structures is called
    a. Angiology
    b. Osteology
    c. Esthesiology
    d. Arthrology

732. The axial skeleton includes all of the following except the
    a. Skull
    b. Sternum
    c. Appendages
    d. Vertebral column

733. Which of these joint types is found mainly in the skull?
    a. Suture
    b. Syndesmosis
    c. Gomphosis
    d. Synchondrosis

734. Most synovial joints are similar in structure and include all of the following except
    a. Articular cartilage
    b. Ligaments
    c. Joint capsule
    d. Tendons

735. Arthritis may lead to an increased production of
    a. Peritoneal fluid
    b. Synovial fluid
    c. Plasma
    d. Serum

736. A major function of osteoblasts is to
    a. Aid in bone growth and fracture repair
    b. Decrease bone resorption
    c. Increase bone calcification
    d. Aid in vitamin D synthesis

737. What structure is a passage or a tube like opening through bone?
    a. Fissure
    b. Fovea
    c. Fossa
    d. Meatus

738. Which of the following is a separate cranial bone of horses and cats but in other species is present only in the fetus and fuses with surrounding bones before birth?
  a. Temporal bone
  b. Interparietal bone
  c. Frontal bone
  d. Occipital bone

739. What term describes movement of a part away from the median plane or a digit away from the axis of the limb?
  a. Flexion
  b. Extension
  c. Abduction
  d. Circumduction

740. Which joint type can, through a simple sliding motion, move in one (uniaxial) direction only?
  a. Plane
  b. Hinge
  c. Pivot
  d. Condyloid

741. The os penis of the dog and cat and the ossa cordis found in the heart of ruminants are examples of
  a. Pneumatic bones
  b. Sesamoid bones
  c. Splanchnic bones
  d. Flat bones

742. Which of the following is an example of a saddle joint?
  a. Distal interphalangeal in a dog
  b. Scapulohumeral in a horse
  c. Atlantoaxial in a cow
  d. Metacarpophalangeal in an elephant

743. What term describes implantation of a tooth into the alveolus of the mandible?
  a. Syndesmosis
  b. Gomphosis
  c. Diarthrosis
  d. Synchondrosis

744. What enzyme is necessary for deposition of calcium salts in osteoid tissue to form true bone?
  a. Rennin
  b. Enterokinase
  c. Phosphatase
  d. Ribonuclease

745. What areas of bone fuse early in life but cause bones to continue to increase in size as a result of the hereditary condition known as achondroplasia?
  a. Proximal epiphyses
  b. Distal epiphyses
  c. Diaphyses
  d. Metaphyses

746. Oversecretion by what gland causes demineralization of the skeleton called *osteitis fibrosa* or *von Recklinghausen disease*?
  a. Parathyroid gland
  b. Endocrine gland
  c. Thymus gland
  d. Adrenal gland

747. Functions of long bones include all of the following except
  a. Providing support
  b. Absorbing concussion
  c. Aiding in locomotion
  d. Acting as levers

748. Functions of flat bones include all of the following except
  a. Protecting the brain
  b. Providing large areas for muscle attachment
  c. Shielding the heart and lungs
  d. Reducing friction

749. Nonarticular depressions or holes in bones include all of the following except
  a. Fossa
  b. Facet
  c. Fovea
  d. Foramen

750. Osteocytes are located in small cavities in bone called
  a. Centers of ossification
  b. Canaliculi
  c. Lacunae
  d. Haversian canals

751. Extracapsular (periarticular) ligaments are those outside the joint capsule and include all of the following except
  a. Collateral ligament
  b. Dorsal ligament
  c. Palmar ligament
  d. Proximal ligament

Correct answers are on pages 52-71.

752. What type of joint in the front limb has no connection with the bony thorax?
   a. Syndesmoid
   b. Sphenoid
   c. Ginglymoid
   d. Arthrodial

753. Red marrow persists in what bone throughout life and is thus a convenient place for aspiration and examination?
   a. Scapula
   b. Maxilla
   c. Sternum
   d. Atlas

754. A vertebra consists of all of the following except
   a. Body
   b. Arch
   c. Processes
   d. Girdle

755. Which of the following gives bones rigidity and makes them more opaque on radiographs?
   a. Enamel
   b. Bone marrow
   c. Inorganic salts
   d. Electrolytes

756. Within bone, blood vessels from the periosteum and endosteum communicate with those of the Haversian system via what canals?
   a. Volkmann
   b. Alar
   c. Condyloid
   d. Syndesmoid

757. Articular, spinous, and transverse processes are all found on the
   a. Clavicle
   b. Vertebrae
   c. Ribs
   d. Pelvic girdle

758. Which of the following is pivot joint?
   a. Carpometacarpal
   b. Atlantoaxial
   c. Antebrachiocarpal
   d. Interphalangeal

759. The mandible forms synovial joints with the
   a. Frontal bone
   b. Parietal bone
   c. Occipital bone
   d. Temporal bone

760. The frontal and lacrimal sinuses have small openings into which meatus?
   a. Acoustic
   b. Ethmoidal
   c. Temporal
   d. Osseous

761. The ilium, ischium, and pubis have bodies that meet to form the
   a. Pelvic symphysis
   b. Tuber coxae
   c. Acetabulum
   d. Obturator foramen

762. What is the primary function of the urinary system?
   a. Removal of all liquid from the body
   b. Extraction of excess glucose from the blood
   c. Extraction of waste products from the blood
   d. Addition of glucose to the blood

763. The major force that affects filtration pressure through the kidneys is
   a. Hormone levels
   b. Blood pressure
   c. Osmotic pressure
   d. Oxygen levels

764. The urinary bladder is lined with what type of epithelium?
   a. Stratified squamous
   b. Cuboidal
   c. Transitional
   d. Stratified columnar

765. What is the basic functional unit of the kidney?
   a. Nephron
   b. Efferent tubule
   c. Afferent tubule
   d. Glomerulus

766. The hormone that regulates sodium resorption in the nephron is
   a. ADH
   b. Estrogen
   c. Progesterone
   d. Aldosterone

767. Which of these species has a lobulated kidney?
   a. Horses
   b. Sheep
   c. Goats
   d. Cattle

768. Most absorption in the kidney is
   a. Active
   b. Passive
   c. By electrolyte pump
   d. By diapedesis

769. Where is the main filtration mechanism in the kidney?
    a. Collection ducts
    b. Glomerulus
    c. Loop of Henle
    d. Efferent convoluted tubules

770. The vessel that carries blood to the nephron is the
    a. Glomerular artery
    b. Efferent arteriole
    c. Afferent arteriole
    d. Renal vein

771. Most domestic animals have kidneys that are shaped like a
    a. Tulip
    b. Pea
    c. Bean
    d. Heart

772. Which of these tubular structures conveys urine from the kidney to the bladder?
    a. Urethra
    b. Ureter
    c. Loop of Henle
    d. Nephron

773. Increased excretion of urine is termed
    a. Diuresis
    b. Polyphagia
    c. Polydipsia
    d. Hypertrophy

774. What two hormones normally have the greatest influence on the kidneys?
    a. Progesterone and aldosterone
    b. Progesterone and ADH
    c. Oxytocin and ADH
    d. Aldosterone and ADH

775. What is the general term for inflammation of the kidney?
    a. Cystitis
    b. Nephritis
    c. Rhinitis
    d. Glomerulitis

776. What structure lies between the proximal and distal convoluted tubules of the kidney?
    a. Bowman capsule
    b. Malpighian corpuscle
    c. Loop of Henle
    d. Glomerulus

777. What hormone is secreted by the kidneys?
    a. ADH
    b. Aldosterone
    c. Angiotensin
    d. Renin

778. What structure conveys urine from the bladder to the exterior?
    a. Ureter
    b. Urethra
    c. Loop of Henle
    d. Nephron

779. Urine cannot be expelled from the urinary bladder without relaxation of the
    a. External sphincter
    b. Prostate
    c. Urethra
    d. Ureter

780. Angiotensin II promotes resorption of
    a. Calcium
    b. Phosphorus
    c. Sodium
    d. Nitrogen

781. What hormone increases the permeability of renal tubular cells to water?
    a. LH
    b. ADH
    c. ACTH
    d. GnRH

782. What is the scientific term for emptying of the bladder?
    a. Defecation
    b. Polydipsia
    c. Polyphagia
    d. Micturition

783. The odor of urine is probably most influenced by an animal's
    a. Body temperature
    b. Body weight
    c. Diet
    d. Age

784. What is the scientific term for lack of urine production?
    a. Polyuria
    b. Oliguria
    c. Anuria
    d. Dysuria

785. What is normally the most plentiful chemical buffer in the body?
    a. Hemoglobin
    b. Nitrogen
    c. Amylase
    d. ADH

Correct answers are on pages 52-71.

ANSWERS

1. **d** The stomach wall, uterus, urinary bladder, intestine, and ciliary body all have smooth muscles.

2. **c** Diastolic blood pressure is present when the ventricles are relaxed and therefore is a lower pressure than systolic blood pressure.

3. **a** A stronger palpated pulse is due to a greater pulse pressure.

4. **a** Exercise increases blood pressure because of vasoconstriction.

5. **b**

6. **b**

7. **d** PR interval is the length of time for the impulse to travel through the AV node. T wave is ventricular repolarization, and the QRS complex is ventricular depolarization.

8. **c** The SA node is the heart's dominant pacemaker.

9. **a** The cardia is the sphincter between the esophagus and stomach. Chyme is the digested stomach content that moves through the pylorus. Rugae are long folds found in the stomach.

10. **c** Neuroglia protect and support the nervous system. Schwann cells are specialized glial cells in the peripheral nerves. Oligodendrocytes are specialized glial cells in the brain and spinal cord.

11. **a**

12. **d**

13. **b**

14. **d** Afferent nerves conduct impulses from sensory receptors to the central nervous system. Motor nerves are efferent nerves that send impulses to the skeletal muscles, organs, glands, and so forth from the central nervous system.

15. **b**

16. **a**

17. **d** Molecules of the local anesthetic block the sodium channels so depolarization cannot occur, and the sensation of pain will not reach the brain.

18. **b** Smooth muscles are found in the walls of many soft internal organs. They can also be found in various structures of the eyes, blood vessels, and small passageways in the lungs.

19. **c** Skeletal muscle cells have multiple nuclei.

20. **a** Cattle and swine continuously cycle throughout the year.

21. **c** Dogs cycle twice a year: in the spring and in the fall.

22. **d** Cats will remain in prolonged estrus if not bred.

23. **c** The corpus luteum develops after ovulation.

24. **a** The corpus luteum produces progesterone. Prolactin is produced by the anterior pituitary gland, and oxytocin by the posterior pituitary gland.

25. **d**

26. **a** Endometrium is the lining of the uterus.

27. **a**

28. **c** Estrogens prepare the animal for breeding and pregnancy. Progesterone prepares the uterus for implantation and maintains pregnancy. Oxytocin causes contractions for parturition.

29. **d** Most ruminants have cotyledonary placental attachments.

30. **a** The cotyledon is the fetal side of the placenta, and the placentoma is the structure that results when the caruncle and cotyledon are joined.

31. **c**

32. **a**

33. **d**

34. **a**

35. **b**

36. **a** The number varies but typically there are four thoracic mammae, four abdominal mammae, and two inguinal mammae.

37. **d** Sympathetic stimulation elicits the "fight or flight" response that is seen with the other three reactions.

38. **b** The other three reactions are the result of parasympathetic nervous system stimulation.

39. **c** Postganglionic sympathic neurons release epinephrine or norepinephrine.

40. **a**

41. **a**

42. **d**

43. **a**

44. **b** In ventricular fibrillation, there is effectively no blood being pumped by the heart.

45. **a** Lidocaine, a local anesthetic, is a Na^+ channel blocker, that is, it does the opposite of increasing permeability to Na^+.

46. **d**

47. **b** Albumin is the primary constituent of blood responsible for the oncotic pressure of blood. Oncotic pressure is a form of osmotic pressure exerted by proteins in blood plasma. It pulls water into the circulatory system.

48. **d**

49. **a**

50. **a**

51. **d**

52. **c** Caused by a buildup of CO_2

53. **d**

54. **b**

55. **c**

56. **c**

57. **d**

58. **d**

59. **a** Increased concentration of fatty acids in the blood will elicit insulin resistance.

60. **c** Long-term use of glucocorticoids will suppress immune function.

61. **d**

62. **d**

63. **a**

64. **c**

65. **c**

66. **a**

67. **d**

68. **d** The other conditions are common to hyperthyroidism.

69. **d** The other three drugs would inhibit oxytocin release.

70. **a**

71. **c**

72. **c**

73. **a**

74. **a**

75. **b**

76. **a**

77. **c**

78. **b** Approximately 8% of an animal's body weight is blood, and 1 ml of blood weighs approximately 1 g.

79. **a** There are only muscular connections between the scapula and the torso.

80. **a**

81. **d** *Lipogenesis* is a term used to describe the storing of fatty acids that are already formed.

82. **b** Glucose is the primary nutrient used in anaerobic metabolism.

83. **a** If adipose were composed entirely of fat, the correct answer would be higher (~9000 kcal/kg); however, adipose is also constructed of connective tissue (protein) and blood vessels (water), all of which decrease the caloric density of adipose tissue.

84. **c**

85. **b**

86. **d** The primary function of high-density lipoprotein (HDL) is to carry cholesterol from peripheral tissues to the liver.

87. **c** (LDLs)

88. **a** Hormone-sensitive lipase (HSL) is the rate-limiting enzyme responsible for mobilizing fatty acids from adipose tissue.

89. **a**

90. **d** Glucagon is the primary hormone that stimulates gluconeogenesis.

91. **a** Elicited by atrial depolarization

92. **b** The islets contain cells that produce insulin (beta cells) and glucagon (alpha cells) along with three other types of cells.

93. **a**

94. **d** Increasing the rate of contractions does not increase the strength of contractions.

95. **c**

96. **b**

97. **b**

98. **b**

99. **a** To compensate for the moderate anemia, blood pressure would be normal to increased.

100. **a**

101. **b** The carpus in the horse is called a *knee joint*, which is equivalent to the wrist joint in a person.

102. **a**

103. **b**

104. **b**

105. **c** Two seconds or less is a normal value for capillary refill time.

106. **b** The greater trochanter is a large, flat projection found lateral to the head of the femur. It is the attachment site for the large gluteal muscles.

107. **b**

108. **c** Proximal refers to the beginning of a structure or the part nearest the midline.

109. **c** Palmar refers to the bottom of the front foot or hoof (distal to the carpus).

110. **a** The physis (epiphyseal plate) is the segment of bone that involves growth of bone.

111. **a** Periosteum is a tough, fibrous tissue that forms the outer covering of bone.

112. **d**

113. **c** The mitral valve is located between the left atrium and left ventricle. The tricuspid valve is located between the right atrium and right ventricle.

114. **b** The pulmonic valve is the right ventricular outflow valve, and the aortic valve is the left ventricular outflow valve.

115. **a** The adult cat has 30 teeth; the upper jaw contains 16 teeth and the lower jaw contains 14 teeth.

116. **b** At the thoracic inlet of a bird, the ventral wall of the esophagus expands greatly to form the crop that bulges to the right and lies against the breast muscle.

117. **c** Chickens have eight air sacs; single cervical and clavicular sacs and paired cranial thoracic, caudal thoracic, and abdominal sacs.

118. **d**

119. **b** The gizzard or ventriculus is the muscular stomach of birds.

120. **b** The boundaries of the femoral triangle are the sartorius muscle cranial, the pectineus muscle caudal, and the vastus medialis and iliopsoas deep laterally.

121. **d** The choroid is the middle layer of the eyeball that contains blood vessels and supplies blood for the entire eye.

122. **b**

123. **c**

124. **a**

125. **d** Although all are important arteries, the aorta is the only one associated directly with the left ventricle.

126. **d** The femoral vein is in the caudal part of the body and would be associated with the caudal vena cava not the cranial vena cava.

127. **b**

128. **b** The right atrium receives all venous blood with the exception of blood in the pulmonary vein.

129. **b**

130. **a** The systemic circulation is under high pressure; the pulmonary and coronary circulations are under low pressure.

131. **c**

132. **b** The ilium (with a second "i") is part of the pelvis.

133. **b** The horse and rat are two species that lack gall bladders.

134. **a** Ruminants lack upper incisors and canines. They have a dental pad that helps them break up grassy materials as they chew.

135. **a**

136. **d**

137. **c**

138. **d**

139. **c** The G cells are found in the antrum of the stomach.

140. **d** Luteinizing hormone, oxytocin, and growth hormones are all pituitary hormones.

141. **b** The endocrine system is ductless.

142. **d**

143. **b** The corpus luteum is responsible for the initial secretion of the hormones necessary to maintain pregnancy.

144. **a**

145. **c**

146. **a**

147. **b**

148. **d**

149. **c** Carbohydrate transport is not a function of the lymph system.

150. **d**

151. **b** Lacteals are intestinal lymph tissue that transports fats that are too large to be transported by the circulatory system.

152. **d**

153. **c**

154. **b**

155. **b**

156. **a**

157. **c**

158. **a**

159. **c**

160. **b**

161. **a** Estrous is the time period from the start of one heat cycle to the start of the next. Estrus is the actual heat period.

162. **b**

163. **d**

164. **a**

165. **c**

166. **b**

167. **c**

168. **d** The thorax is under negative pressure. This pulls the lungs against the thoracic wall, allowing the lungs to move with the thorax as it expands or contracts.

169. **a** Skeletal muscles are under voluntary control. The other three answers apply to smooth muscle.

170. **c** Calcium and phosphate crystals are deposited to form bone.

171. **d**

172. **b** Parathyroid hormone prevents hypocalcemia by stimulating bone degradation.

173. **c** Calcitonin prevents hypercalcemia by depositing excess calcium in the bones.

174. **a**

175. **d**

176. **c** The four types of bones are flat, short, long, and irregular.

177. **d**

178. **b**

179. **c**

180. **a** The sphenoid bone forms the bottom of the cranium and contains the pituitary fossa. The other three are the bones of the ear.

181. **b**

182. **b**

183. **d**

184. **a**

185. **a**

186. **d** The hoof grows on the average 1/4 inch per month.

187. **c** Cattle lack upper incisors.

188. **d**

189. **c**

190. **a**

191. **d**

192. **d**

193. **a**

194. **b**

195. **d** The trunk is the part of the body that the head and limbs are attached to.

196. **a** Correct veterinary medical terminology should always be used, and animals do not have arms.

197. **d** Phalanges are named proximal, middle, and distal from the point closest to the trunk of the body.

198. **d** The humerus, radius, and ulna are jointed at the animal's elbow. The carpus is distal to the elbow.

199. **d** In a normally positioned animal with a normal liver, the liver sits cranial in the abdomen, and the kidneys are in the midlumbar region.

200. **a** All of the leg bones support substantial weight except the fibula, which is primarily used for tendon and ligament attachments and in some species is vestigial.

201. **d** In humans this is the "calf" muscle. In dogs it is the largest bellied muscle on the back of the lower hind leg.

202. **c** The latissimus dorsi is part of the musculature that aids in thoracic limb movement.

203. **b** Triceps : *tri* means *three*.

204. **b** Fascia can be found in several parts of the body but is always a sheet or band of fibrous connective tissue.

205. **a** The deltoid muscles are a group of muscles at the lateral edge of the scapula; they are triangular in shape and help flex the shoulder and abduct the foreleg.

206. **c** Under = sub or infra; the eye = orbit.

207. **b** The cardiac sphincter lies in the proximal end of the stomach closest to the heart (hence the name), and the pyloric sphincter lies at the distal end of the part of the stomach called the *pylorus,* where the stomach joins the duodenum.

208. **a** The dorsal plane divides the body into dorsal and ventral portions.

209. **a** Spelling counts. This is the only one of the small intestinal divisions that ends in *-unum*. The *e* at the beginning of the word is for "eat."

210. **d** Remember that *visceral* always refers to an organ.

211. **d** The glottis is the opening between the vocal folds through which an endotracheal tube passes.

212. **b** *Serratus* means "saw like."

213. **a** This is most common in species with penile sheaths and may be used when discussing abnormalities with clients, because it is a term they would recognize.

214. **d** The cardiovascular system includes the heart, blood, blood circulation, and blood vessels.

215. **c** The other bones are part of the visceral skeleton.

216. **d** No ungulates (hoofed animals) have an os penis.

217. **b** Short bones are somewhat cuboidal or approximately equal in all dimensions. They have no large marrow cavity, but the interior is filled with spongy bone and marrow spaces. The exterior is a thin layer of compact bone. Their function is to absorb concussion forces, and they are found in complex joints such as the carpus and tarsus.

218. **c** Flat bones are thin, expand in two dimensions, and consist of two plates of compact bone separated by spongy material. They protect vital organs such as the brain (skull), heart and lungs (scapula), pelvic viscera (pelvis), and thoracic organs (ribs).

219. **a** Irregular bones are on the median plane—vertebrae or in the skull. They do not fit into any other classification and function as protection, support, and for muscle attachment.

220. **b** The axial skeleton includes the skull, vertebral column, ribs, and sternum.

221. **c** Most cloven-hoofed animals have no first digit, and their second and fifth digits are either vestigial or missing.

222. **c**

223. **a** Navicular disease is a chronic degeneration of the equine navicular bone and includes damage to the flexor surface and overlying flexor tendon in the front feet.

224. **b** The skull suture is an example of a fibrous or synarthrotic joint in which fibrous tissue unites bones and permits no movement.

225. **d** The pivot joint is a rotary joint, and the only example in the body is the joint at C1–C2.

226. **a** Trochanters are found on the femur only.

227. **d** A facet is a smooth, nearly flat articular surface. The rest are holes or channels.

228. **c** *Costo* = rib; *chondral* = cartilage.

229. **d** A normal dog has 7 cervical, 13 thoracic, and 7 lumbar vertebrae.

230. **b** The dentition of a cow is I 0/3, C 0/1, PM 3/3–4, M 3/3.

231. **d** All of the other valves are within the heart. The semilunar valves are inside the arteries.

232. **b** The fibers that lie along the bottom and sides of the inner ventricles are named after J. E. Purkinje, a Bohemian anatomist (1787–1869).

233. **a** Diastole is the relaxation period between contractions; conversely, systole describes the contraction phases, first of the atria, then of the ventricles.

234. **a**

235. **c**

236. **b** Systole is the contraction that provides the blood pressure in the arteries and is more easily measured.

237. **a** Systemic refers to blood circulation outside the thorax.

238. **d** The closed-up foramen ovale is called the *fossa ovalis* in an adult.

239. **b** Lymph is made up of 95% water, plasma proteins, and chemical substances from the blood plasma. Its sparse cellular content contains mostly lymphocytes.

240. **c** The tricuspid valve is also known as the right atrioventricular valve or right A-V valve.

241. **b** The thymus is lymph tissue located in the mediastinum, cranial to the heart, and produces cells that destroy foreign substances and the formation of lymphocytes. It is most easily seen in young animals, because it begins to atrophy as the animal ages.

242. **b** The medical term for the eardrum is *tympanic membrane.*

243. **a** The spleen's major functions are hemopoiesis, phagocytosis, and storage of blood in the splenic pulp.

244. **b** Association neurons, also called *interneurons,* link sensory neurons with motor neurons or other association neurons.

245. **a** *Efferent* neurons are neurons that respond to afferent stimulus and create an *effect.* A simple example is touching something hot: the afferent neurons relay a message to the brain to pull away, and the efferent neurons stimulate the action to pull away, which is a motor function.

246. **c** *Afferent* neurons are the sensing neurons that *affect* the brain to respond. A simple example is touching something hot: the afferent neurons relay a message to the brain to pull away, and the efferent neurons stimulate the action to pull away, which is a motor function.

247. **c**

248. **b** The pulmonary artery carries deoxygenated blood from the heart to the lungs, where it is oxygenated.

249. **d**

250. **a**

251. **b**

252. **d**

253. **c**

254. **c**

255. **a**

256. **b**

257. **a**

258. **d**

259. **c** Cardiac output = Stroke volume $\times$ Heart rate

260. **a**

261. **c** The QRS complex represents depolarization of the ventricles.

262. **b** Platelets help plug defects in blood vessels and start the clotting process.

263. **b** Decreased osmotic pressure in the blood would result in fluid moving out into the tissues.

264. **c** Albumin is one of the plasma proteins.

265. **c** Erythropoietin is produced by the kidneys.

266. **b**

267. **c**

268. **c**

269. **a**

270. **b**

271. **c**

272. **b**

273. **a**

274. **b** Amylase breaks down carbohydrates and is contained in the saliva.

275. **c**

276. **b**

277. **d** Villi, which also contain the microvilli, are adaptations of the mucosa to increase surface area for absorption of nutrients.

278. **c**

279. **b**

280. **b**

281. **d**

282. **b**

283. **a**

284. **d**

285. **c**

286. **b** Mitochondria are the "power plants" of the cell.

287. **c** The nuclei appear at different levels within the cells, and the cells look to be multilayered but actually are not.

288. **b**

289. **d**

290. **b**

291. **d**

292. **d** Synovial fluid is produced by the synovial membrane that lines the joint capsules.

293. **d**

294. **c** Mammals have seven cervical vertebrae.

295. **a**

296. **c** Carpal bones 1 and 5 are present in a minority of horses.

297. **b**

298. **b** The main function of the muscles of the quadriceps is to extend the stifle.

299. **c** It is the only muscle fiber type that does not have striations. Both cardiac and smooth are involuntary muscle types, and Purkinje fibers are found in cardiac muscle.

300. **a** Acetylcholinesterase is an enzyme that breaks down acetylcholine.

301. **c** The acetylcholine within the synaptic cleft would continue to stimulate the muscle.

302. **b**

303. **a**

304. **d**

305. **b**

306. **b** Antidiuretic hormone causes the kidney to conserve water when the body gets dehydrated.

307. **d**

308. **a** Estrogen is responsible for inducing estrus.

309. **c** Oxytocin stimulates uterine contractions and milk let-down.

310. **c** Aldosterone is a mineralocorticoid hormone produced in the adrenal cortex.

311. **b**

312. **d**

313. **a**

314. **c**

315. **b** Bovine somatotropin is the naturally occurring growth hormone of cattle.

316. **a**

317. **b**

318. **c**

319. **b**

320. **b**

321. **c** FSH = follicle-stimulating hormone

322. **a**

323. **b** The proximal phalanx is not included as part of the foot of the horse.

324. **c** The subcutis is also called the *hypodermis.*

325. **a** The dermis layer contains sebaceous and sweat glands.

326. **d** The sebaceous glands are responsible for lubricating the skin and hair.

327. **d** The ceruminous glands are found in the ear canal.

328. **b** The circumoral glands are found on the lips of cats.

329. **a**

330. **c** The arrector pili muscles are responsible for raising the hackles of a dog.

331. **c** The epidermis is the most superficial layer. The hypodermis is the deepest layer.

332. **a** The ergot is the listed structure located most distal on the horse's limb.

333. **d** The secondary hairs are also called *wool hairs,* and they make up the undercoat in mammals.

334. **c** The white line should not be penetrated with the nail during shoeing, because the nail will enter the sensitive laminae layer.

335. **b** Sex of the animal does not influence body temperature.

336. **c** Panting and sweating represent the most common type of water evaporation from the body.

337. **c** *Mastitis* is defined as inflammation of the mammary glands.

338. **a** *Vibrissa* is another name for cat whiskers.

339. **b** *Albinism* is a term used to describe an absence of normal skin pigment.

340. **b** *Laminitis* is a term used to describe founder in horses.

341. **b** *Thrush* is defined as a degenerative condition of the frog associated with standing in wet, filthy, and contaminated grounds.

342. **c** *Gravel* is a term used to describe a drainage tract up the sensitive laminae caused by a crack in the hoof wall.

343. **b** The diaphysis is the shaft or body of a long bone.

344. **a** The epiphyses are the enlarged ends of a long bone.

345. **c** The periosteum is the fibrous layer that surrounds bone used for attachment of ligaments and tendons.

346. **b** The medullary cavity is the innermost part of a bone that contains the bone marrow.

347. **d** Flexion decreases the angle between bones.

348. **c** The hip joint is a synovial joint classified as a ball-and-socket joint capable of universal movement.

349. **a** The elbow joint is a compound hinge joint that moves at right angles, causing flexion and extension; it is also a synovial joint.

350. **d** The stifle joint articulates the femur, patella, and tibia.

351. **b**

352. **d** The xiphoid process is found at the caudal end of the sternum.

353. **d** The obturator foramen helps reduce the weight of the pelvis.

354. **b** The coffin bone (distal phalanx) may rotate during chronic episodes of laminitis. This is also called a *dropped sole.*

355. **d** The hip joint is also described as the coxofemoral joint.

356. **c** Fascia is a sheet of fibrous membrane that separates layers of muscles.

357. **c** The action of an extensor increases the angle between bones.

358. **b** The large lateral cheek muscle that elevates the mandible to aid in chewing is the masseter muscle.

359. **c** The lumbodorsal fascia is the extensive aponeurosis that covers the lower back.

360. **a** The clavobrachialis is located on the shoulder and works to flex the forearm or brachium.

361. **c** The pylorus is the distal opening of the stomach, which empties into the duodenum.

362. **d** The caudofemoralis is included in the gluteal muscle group.

363. **a** This sequence describes the abdominal muscle layers, from superficial to deep.

364. **c** The rectus abdominis is found in this region and extends from the pubis to the upper ribs.

365. **b**

366. **b** Atrophy is described as a decrease in muscle size resulting from lack of use.

367. **a** The gracilis is a broad superficial muscle extending down the medial surface of the thigh to insert on the tibia.

368. **b** The quadriceps muscles include the rectus femoris, vastus lateralis, vastus medialis, and vastus intermedius that act to extend the stifle and flex the hip.

369. **a** The triceps brachii muscles, which include the long, lateral, and medial heads, work to extend the elbow or forearm.

370. **a** The muscular system does not act to protect the body. This is the function of the integumentary system.

371. **b** The antagonist works in opposition to the prime mover.

372. **a** The cecum is described as a huge comma-shaped structure on the right side of the horse's abdomen.

373. **d** The sections of the small intestines, from cranial to caudal, include the duodenum, jejunum, and the ileum.

374. **c** The rumen is called the *fermentation vat* and is responsible for the majority of the fermentation.

375. **b** The trocar is a sharp instrument used to relieve bloat in ruminants by puncturing the abdominal wall into the rumen to release gas.

376. **d** Rumination is a four-stage process consisting of eructation, reinsalivation, remastication, and redeglutition.

377. **b** The cecum and colon act as areas of fermentation in the horse.

378. **a** The liver is located immediately behind the diaphragm in the carnivore.

379. **a** The reticulum is the most proximal portion of the ruminant stomach and collects the hardware swallowed during grazing.

380. **b** The cow and small ruminants, such as the goat, have a dental pad in place of the upper incisors and canines.

381. **a** The *visceral peritoneum* is the name of the serosa that covers the abdominal organs.

382. **a** The mesentery is the connecting peritoneum, which contains blood vessels, nerves, and lymphatics that supply these areas.

383. **d** The soft palate divides the rostral part of the pharynx into oropharynx and nasopharynx regions.

384. **d** A red blood cell loses its nucleus as it matures.

385. **b** Three layers make up a cell membrane; a lipid layer is sandwiched between the two protein layers.

386. **d**

387. **b**

388. **a**

389. **c**

390. **d** Keratin is an insoluble protein, which makes stratified squamous epithelium very protective of underlying tissues.

391. **c**

392. **a** The wave like motion of cilia helps move mucus and debris out of the respiratory system.

393. **c** Transitional epithelium is cuboidal when tissue is not in a contracted state, but it may become flattened when an organ is distended.

394. **c** Calcium is involved in the breakage and recoupling of cross linkages between myofilaments in a striated muscle fiber.

395. **d** (a.) skeletal muscle, (b.) smooth muscle, (c.) no such thing

396. **b** (a.) attachment between columnar epithelial cells, (c.) terminal area of the axon of a motor nerve fiber at the neuromuscular junction, (d.) site of impulse transmission between neurons

397. **c** (a.) skeletal muscle fibers may regenerate in this manner, (b.) mitotic division of smooth muscle fibers possible, (d.) possible means of smooth muscle regeneration

398. **d** The peritoneum, pleura, and pericardium all consist of flat expanded arrangements of loose connective tissue covered by mesothelium.

399. **a**

400. **c** The right atrium receives carbon dioxide–rich blood from the systemic circulation.

401. **b** The mitral valve is the left atrioventricular valve.

402. **d** The right ventricle pumps blood to the pulmonary circulation.

403. **a** The aortic valve is the left ventricular outflow valve.

404. **a** The first heart sound is produced by closure of the two atrioventricular valves. The second heart sound is produced by closure of the two ventricular outflow valves.

405. **d** All of the others carry oxygen-rich blood.

406. **d** Removal of the spleen is not life threatening. Removal of any of the other organs listed is fatal.

407. **d**

408. **c**

409. **c** The monocyte is a macrophage and is important in the process of inflammation.

410. **c** Chordae tendineae are present on the atrioventricular valves.

411. **a**

412. **c** The pulmonary valve is the right ventricular outflow valve.

413. **a** All of the other blood vessels carry carbon dioxide–rich blood.

414. **c**

415. **a**

416. **c**

417. **b** Simple squamous epithelium forms the very smooth endothelium that lines the entire circulatory system.

418. **d**

419. **d** The right ventricle pumps blood to the pulmonary circulation.

420. **a** Fresh, oxygenated blood from the lungs flows back to the left atrium.

421. **b** The left ventricle pumps blood out to the systemic circulation.

422. **d** The tricuspid valve is the right atrioventricular valve.

423. **c** The pulmonary valve is the right ventricular outflow valve.

424. **b**

425. **a**

426. **a**

427. **a** The bundle of His conducts impulses from the atrioventricular node to the Purkinje fibers at the apex of the heart.

428. **a**

429. **d**

430. **d** The pulmonary valve is the right ventricular outflow valve.

431. **a** The mitral valve is the left atrioventricular valve.

432. **c** The aortic valve is the left ventricular outflow valve.

433. **b** The tricuspid valve is the right atrioventricular valve.

434. **d** The sinoatrial node is the pacemaker of the heart.

435. **a** The ductus arteriosus shunts blood from the pulmonary artery to the aorta of a fetus.

436. **a** The aortic valve is the left ventricular outflow valve.

437. **b** The Purkinje fibers conduct impulses from the bundle of His to the walls of the ventricles.

438. **d** Blood returning to the heart through the vena cava enters the right atrium and then passes through the right atrioventricular (tricuspid) valve.

439. **d** The vena cava returns blood to the heart from the systemic circulation.

440. b

441. c The pulmonary vein returns blood from the lungs to the left atrium.

442. b All of the other choices are bony foramina.

443. d

444. c

445. d The mitral valve is the left atrioventricular valve.

446. a Blood from the pulmonary vein enters the left atrium.

447. a The general effect of the parasympathetic portion of the autonomic nervous system is to depress cardiac function.

448. b Pressure in the right atrium is higher than in the left atrium, resulting in right-to-left blood flow.

449. b Serum does not contain fibrinogen, which is essential for blood clotting.

450. b

451. b

452. b Blood flows from the heart through arteries, then through capillaries, then veins, and back to the heart.

453. d

454. a Platelets and red blood cells do not normally have intact nuclei, and lymphocytes have single, roundish nuclei.

455. d

456. a Herbivores rely on microbial fermentation to digest plant material.

457. a

458. c

459. b

460. c

461. a

462. b From proximal to distal, sections of the small intestine are the duodenum, jejunum, and ileum. The *ilium* is a bone of the pelvis.

463. b

464. b

465. c

466. d

467. b

468. d The rumen is where most of the microbial fermentation occurs in a ruminant.

469. c

470. d

471. b

472. b The duodenum is the first (most proximal) segment of the small intestine.

473. d

474. a

475. a

476. b The exocrine secretion of the pancreas consists primarily of various digestive enzymes.

477. a

478. b

479. c

480. b The anus and the esophagus are lined by stratified squamous epithelium. The pancreas is an accessory digestive organ.

481. b Chyme is the semifluid homogeneous material produced by the action of digestive enzymes and acid on the food in the stomach.

482. b Newborn ruminants are functionally simple-stomached animals. Until their forestomachs become active at weaning, the esophageal groove prevents milk from fermenting in the forestomach compartments.

483. **c** The ileum is the last segment of the small intestine.

484. **c** The villi of the small intestine increase the surface area of its lining, improving the efficiency of nutrient absorption.

485. **b** Blood cells are not normally formed in the liver of adult animals.

486. **b**

487. **c** Microbial fermentation is most important in digestion by herbivorous animals, (e.g., horses).

488. **a**

489. **a**

490. **c** The pharynx is the common passageway for both the respiratory and the digestive systems.

491. **c** Although saliva does contain some digestive enzymes, it contributes little to the digestive process.

492. **a** The esophagus merely conducts swallowed food from the pharynx to the stomach.

493. **a** The gas that results from microbial fermentation in a ruminant must be periodically eliminated by eructation (burping) to prevent ruminal tympany (bloat).

494. **a**

495. **c** The pituitary hormones function chiefly to regulate the activity of other endocrine glands.

496. **d** FSH is secreted by the anterior pituitary gland.

497. **b** Glucocorticoids are produced by the adrenal glands.

498. **c** Insulin is produced by the beta cells of the islets of Langerhans in the pancreas.

499. **d**

500. **d** Thyroxine (T4) and calcitonin (Ca-regulating hormone) are produced by the thyroid gland, insulin is produced by the pancreas, and parathormone is produced by the parathyroid gland.

501. **c** The release of oxytocin stimulates milk flow and milk let-down.

502. **b** (a.) pituitary gland location, (c.) adrenal gland location, (d.) pancreas location

503. **a** The secretory products of exocrine glands are transported via ducts. Salivary and sweat glands are exocrine glands.

504. **b** Addisons disease results from insufficient adrenocortical hormones.

505. **d** Epinephrine and norepinephrine are secreted by the adrenal medulla, hence their name, *adrenergics*.

506. **c** Iodine is necessary for production of T3 and T4.

507. **a** Loss of weight is associated with hyperthyroidism; the others are related to hypothyroidism.

508. **b** Enlargement of the thyroid gland is termed *goiter.*

509. **a** *Potentiation* (or synergism) is the term used to describe an increased effect.

510. **c**

511. **d** ADH helps control water loss by facilitating resorption of water from the distal portion of the nephron.

512. **a**

513. **c** The adrenal glands are located adjacent to the kidneys.

514. **d** A decrease in parathyroid hormone results in decreased blood calcium levels, and an increase in parathyroid hormone levels increases blood calcium levels.

515. **d** There are usually two, but the exact number and location vary among species.

516. **a** Diabetes mellitus is caused by lack of insulin or inability to use insulin.

517. **b** Glucagon is produced by the alpha cells. It has the opposite effect of insulin.

518. **c** Paracrine transmission uses interstitial fluid to diffuse hormones in the body; endocrine uses blood; neurocrine uses the synaptic clefts between neurons; and exocrine uses ducts to secrete to the exterior of the body.

519. **a** Pancreatic juices are not endocrine hormones.

520. **c** Keratinized epithelium makes up the dry skin surface.

521. **d** Although long and coiled, the sweat glands are simple tubes.

522. **a** The cells that produce the hoof wall are located in the coronary band.

523. **d** The hoof wall has the lowest water content and thus the firmest consistency.

524. **c** Sebaceous glands are simple sac like (alveolar) structures.

525. **b** Salivary glands are part of the digestive system.

526. **a** The other three answers are true of the epidermis.

527. **c** The hair follicle is a "gland" of sorts, whose product is the keratinized cylinder that we call a *hair.*

528. **a** The chestnut is a small vestigial mass of horn located in the vicinity of the carpus and tarsus.

529. **c** Vitamin E is not synthesized in the skin.

530. **c**

531. **d**

532. **a** Granules of melanin are deposited in the cortex of pigmented hairs by melanocytes in the hair follicles.

533. **a** Guard hairs are pulled into a more erect position by contraction of the arrector pili muscles. This creates more air spaces among the adjacent wool hairs, which are stretched up by the erect guard hairs.

534. **d**

535. **c**

536. **c** The dermis consists of connective tissue only.

537. **c**

538. **c**

539. **c**

540. **a**

541. **b**

542. **d**

543. **c**

544. **a** In addition to providing a common origin for the gracilis and adductor muscles of each limb, the symphyseal tendon also gives rise to part of the suspensory apparatus.

545. **d**

546. **a**

547. **c** Secretion of colostrum takes place around the time of parturition, coinciding with an inordinately rapid drop in plasma levels of progesterone, and plasma estrogen increases to the highest levels observed during gestation.

548. **b**

549. **a** The levels of IgG-1 decrease in maternal plasma 2 to 3 weeks before calving; from this time until parturition, maximum concentrations of IgG-1 are present in lacteal secretions.

550. **c**

551. **b**

552. **a** Frequent milkings throughout episodes of acute mastitis can help remove inflammatory mediators that might be harmful if allowed to persist for extended periods.

553. **c**

554. **d** Tuberculosis is an even less common cause of enlarged mammary glands in horses.

555. **a** The intercostal muscles between the ribs enlarge the diameter of the chest when they contract, but the principal respiratory muscle is the diaphragm. This thin membranous sheet separates the thorax from the abdomen.

556. **c** Striated is striped or skeletal; smooth is unstriped or visceral; cardiac is found in the heart and is also striated.

557. **c** Purkinje fibers are specialized cardiac muscle cells.

558. **b**

559. **c** Purkinje fibers carry the message from the sinoatrial node to the ventricles to contract.

560. **c** Fiber is the basic unit of structure and function in striated muscle and is made of normal sarcomeres.

561. **b** The triceps brachium is the main extensor of the elbow.

562. **b** The main action of the biceps brachium is to flex the elbow.

563. **d** Hip adductors are found on the medial side of the femur.

564. **a** The tibial tuberosity is the point of insertion for the quadriceps femoris on the tibia.

565. **a** The external oblique is the most superficial abdominal muscle.

566. **b** The maximum amount a muscle fiber can contract is one half its resting length.

567. **b** The least movable attachment is called the *origin* and the most movable is called the *insertion*.

568. **d** Abductors are generally muscles that pull a limb away from the body axis.

569. **a** The gastrocnemius is the large muscle that flexes the stifle and extends the hock.

570. **d** Cutaneous muscles attach to the skin and are responsible for movement of the skin.

571. **c** Spasmodic muscle contractions used to maintain body temperature are called *shivering*.

572. **a** Sphincter muscles constrict a body opening as a result of their circular arrangement.

573. **d** Denervation atrophy results from loss of nerve supply to a muscle.

574. **b** The trapezius is the flat, triangular muscle found in the neck.

575. **d** The pectoral muscle (superficial and deep) is the main adductor of the shoulder.

576. **a** These muscles are known as *hamstring* muscles.

577. **d** Tendons are the connective tissue that attaches muscles to bone.

578. **b** Flat sheets of tendons are known as aponeuroses.

579. **a**

580. **d**

581. **a**

582. **a**

583. **a**

584. **c**

585. **a**

586. **d**

587. **c**

588. **a**

589. **a**

590. **c**

591. **a**

592. **a**

593. **a**

594. **a**

595. **a**

596. **b**

597. **c**

598. **c**

599. **b**

600. **a**

601. **c**

602. **a**

603. **b**

604. **b**

605. **a**

606. **b**

607. **d**

608. **d**

609. **d**

610. **c**

611. **a**

612. **d**

613. **b**

614. **d** a. bitch, b. ewe, c. cow

615. **c** An ectopic pregnancy takes place outside of the uterus, such as in a fallopian tube.

616. **a** Oxytocin stimulates milk let-down; testosterone is the major male hormone.

617. **b** Sperm fertilizes the ovum in an oviduct.

618. **c**

619. **b** A cow's average estrous cycle is 19 to 23 days.

620. **b** The guinea pig's pregnancy lasts approximately 63 days.

621. **a**

622. **a** Estrogen works via the brain to cause estrual behavior (heat); estrogen would result in the opposite effects of *b, c,* and *d.*

623. **b** Progestin maintains pregnancy by keeping the uterus quiescent; the other answers are responses to estrogen.

624. **a** FSH targets the ovary to bring about the growth and maturity of the follicles, which in turn secrete estrogen to stimulate the onset of estrus.

625. **c** Cows cycle throughout the year with approximately 21-day estrous cycles.

626. **c** The fetus grows the most during the third trimester.

627. **d** Ectoderm gives rise to many tissues and organs, including the skin.

628. **c** Males and females are both born with mammary glands, although these glands fully develop in sexually mature females only.

629. **c** Cats have two thoracic and two abdominal pairs of mammary glands.

630. **c** Testosterone plays no major role in lactation.

631. **c** The ovaries are located adjacent to the kidneys.

632. **d** The literal definition is "yellow body."

633. **a** The infundibulum is the structure of the oviduct adjacent to the ovary.

634. **b** Puberty is reached when reproductive organs first become functional. This is true for all species.

635. **d** During or shortly after estrus, ovulation occurs.

636. **a** Diestrus is the relatively short period of quiescence (rest) between estrous cycles in polyestrous animals; anestrus is a longer period of quiescence, as in seasonally polyestrous animals.

637. **c** Metestrus and diestrus make up the luteal phase of the estrous cycle.

638. **a** Because *metr-* refers to "uterine tissue" and *-itis* means "inflammation," metritis is inflammation of the uterus.

639. **b** Because *dys-* means "painful, bad, or difficult" and *-tocia* relates to birth, *dystocia* is defined as a difficult birth.

640. **c** Testosterone is the major male sex hormone.

641. **d** The epididymes serve as a place for spermatozoa to mature before they are expelled by ejaculation.

642. **b** Ejaculation, the rhythmic contraction of the sex glands, results in expelling semen, which consists of sperm and secondary sex gland secretions.

643. **d** Androgens, such as testosterone, are hormones that have masculinizing effects.

644. **c** Testosterone promotes protein anabolism, resulting in increased male body size as compared with the female's body.

645. **c** Sperm may remain fertile in a ewe's reproductive tract for 30 to 48 hours.

646. **b** The hypothalamus releases GnRH in response to low levels of progesterone.

647. **d** This results in rapid regression, or lysis, of the corpus luteum.

648. **b** Progesterone is released from the corpus luteum, which is present during metestrus.

649. **b** Estrus is known as the "heat" period.

650. **b** Most are polyestrous only in the fall, so they will give birth in the spring.

651. **d** Progesterone maintains a quiescent (quiet) uterus during gestation.

652. **b** Gestation in a sow lasts 114 days, or 3 months, 3 weeks, and 3 days.

653. **c** *Gestation* is the term used for the time an animal is pregnant.

654. **a** A multiparous female has given birth after each of multiple pregnancies.

655. **d** The cotyledon attaches to the caruncle to form the placentome.

656. **a** The ovaries produce and expel ova.

657. **c** Rupture of a follicle releases an ovum.

658. **b** Fallopian tubes are also known as *oviducts* or *uterine tubes*.

659. **d** The anterior pituitary gland releases LH.

660. **d** LH promotes the growth of the corpus luteum after the follicles rupture.

661. **a** The corpus luteum is the main source of pro-gesterone during metestrus.

662. **c** Cystic ovaries may cause persistent estrual behavior as a result of continued estrogen release.

663. **d** Ovulation is stimulated by coitus in the cat.

664. **a** Fetal hydrocortisone crosses the placental barrier to stimulate uterine contractions that signal the onset of labor.

665. **d** Oxytocin brings about strong uterine contractions, which expel the fetus.

666. **c** The average length of gestation for goats is 150 days, the same as for sheep.

667. **d** The scrotum is the cutaneous sac that contains the testes.

668. **c** Horses and pigs seem to have more cases of cryptorchidism, or undescended testes, than the other species listed.

669. **b** Fructose is a component of seminal plasma in all species.

670. **d** Enlargement of the bulbus glandis results in prolonged retention of the penis during coitus, or "the tie."

671. **a** A photoperiod is the length of daylight, which regulates the heat cycles in some species.

672. **c** A sow has an ovary that resembles a cluster of grapes, because the animal is litter bearing.

673. **d** Oogenesis is the process by which ova are formed.

674. **a** The caruncle is not a layer of the fetal placenta; it is a maternal structure.

675. **c** The inhaled air is warmed, humidified, and filtered by the lining of the nasal passages.

676. **b** Mastication, the chewing of food, is a digestive system function.

677. **a** The alveoli are tiny grape like clusters of air sacs, which are surrounded by capillary networks.

678. **b**

679. **b** The gases diffuse from areas of high concentration (pressure) to areas of low concentration (pressure).

680. **c**

681. **d** The trachea is commonly called the *windpipe*.

682. **a** Bronchioles are part of the lower respiratory system.

683. **d** Flattening of the diaphragm when it contracts increases the size (volume) of the thoracic cavity.

684. **c** Inhaled air contains more oxygen and less carbon dioxide than does blood entering the alveolar capillaries.

685. **a**

686. **b** External respiration is the exchange of oxygen and carbon dioxide between the blood and inspired air.

687. **c** None of the other choices is a significant function of the larynx.

688. **d** Internal respiration is the exchange of oxygen and carbon dioxide between the blood and the body's cells and tissues.

689. **c** The pharynx is a common passageway for both the respiratory and digestive systems.

690. **a**

691. **c** The diaphragm is made up of skeletal muscle.

692. **a** Exhaled air passes from the alveoli to the bronchi to the trachea to the larynx to the nasal passages.

693. **b**

694. **c** The olfactory nerve mediates the sense of smell.

695. **b** The peripheral nervous system consists of 12 paired cranial nerves and paired spinal nerves that pass through the intervertebral foramina to supply the body and limbs.

696. **d** The vagus nerve (X) controls the pharynx, larynx, and heart.

697. **a** The sympathetic nervous system is used in emergency situations for rapid energy release to meet critical demands.

698. **c** Cones are the receptors for color and bright light.

699. **a** The inner ear contains the semicircular canals, which include the organs for balance, and the cochlea, which holds the hearing organs).

700. **a** The acoustic nerve is also known as *cranial nerve VIII,* or the *vestibulocochlear nerve,* and it carries impulses from the ear to the brain.

701. **b** The vagus nerve provides parasympathetic fibers for most of the cranial half to two thirds of the body.

702. **a** Sight is the primary way birds recognize food.

703. **c** *Stoma* refers to a mouth, as opposed to a *soma,* which is the nerve cell body.

704. **d** The hypoglossal nerve conducts motor impulses to the tongue; the trigeminal nerve sends some sensory impulses.

705. **c** The vagus nerve provides parasympathetic innervation to the heart, lungs, and most of the abdominal viscera.

706. **d**

707. **b** Cerebrospinal fluid is produced in the lateral ventricles and choroid plexus of the third ventricle and in the subarachnoid space and all tissues of the central nervous system.

708. **b** Groups of nerve cell bodies outside of the brain and spinal cord are usually called *ganglia.*

709. **a** The spinal cord links the peripheral body to the brain.

710. **d** Afferent fibers carry information to the brain.

711. **a**

712. **a** A synapse is a gap between one nerve cell's axon and another's dendrites, across which the nerve impulse must be conducted.

713. **c** The retina has specialized receptors (rods and cones with rhodopsin) that, when stimulated by photons from light, create an electrical impulse to pass along the optic nerve.

714. **a** The location at which the optic nerve enters the eye and spreads to make up the retina is also called the *blind spot.* There are no light receptors at this point.

715. **c** Passing posteriorly from the corneal surface, light passes through these structures.

716. **b** The iris is the pigmented structure that surrounds the pupil.

717. **b** An impulse is an electrical charge moving along a nerve fiber.

718. **a** The chief role of the autonomic nervous system is to maintain a stable internal body environment.

719. **d** Acetylcholinesterase aids in dissipation of acetylcholine.

720. **c** Norepinephrine is a catecholamine, as is epinephrine.

721. **d** The sclera, or white of the eye, is the fibrous tunic of the eyeball.

722. **c** The central nervous system consists of the brain and spinal cord.

723. **b** Nerve fibers surrounded by a white sheath of fatty material are termed *myelinated.*

724. **d** The occipital lobe is a division of the cerebrum.

725. **a** The layers (from outer to inner) are the dura mater, arachnoid, and pia mater. The pons is located in the brainstem and transmits sensory information between the cerebellum and cerebrum.

726. **c** There are the same number of thoracic nerve pairs as there are thoracic vertebrae.

727. **d** Spinal nerves are known as *mixed* (i.e., both sensory and motor fibers).

728. **a** Dendrites are nerve processes that conduct impulses toward the cell body.

729. **d** Articular cartilage is a thin layer of hyaline cartilage that covers the articular surface of a bone.

730. **d** Blood cell formation takes place in the red marrow of long bones.

731. **b**

732. **c**

733. **a** *Suture* refers to the junction between bones of the skull that are united by fibrous tissue early in life but may ossify after maturity.

734. **d**

735. **b**

736. **a**

737. **d**

738. **b**

739. **c**

740. **a**

741. **c** Splanchnic bones develop in soft organs, remote from the rest of the skeleton.

742. **a** The distal interphalangeal joint in dogs is a saddle joint.

743. **d**

744. **c**

745. **d**

746. **a**

747. **b** Absorbing concussion is a function of short bones.

748. **d**

749. **b** A facet is a relatively flat articular surface, as found between adjacent carpal bones.

750. **c**

751. **d**

752. **a**

753. **c**

754. **d**

755. **c**

756. **a**

757. **b**

758. **b**

759. **d**

760. **b**

761. **c**

762. **c**

763. **b** Blood pressure directly affects the glomerular filtration rate (GFR). A decrease in blood pressure reduces the GFR.

764. **c**

765. **a**

766. **d** Aldosterone secreted by the adrenal gland is considered a mineralocorticoid. Its primary function is to increase Na+ resorption from the distal nephron.

767. **d**

768. **b**

769. **b** The glomerulus filters substances from blood plasma. Secretory and resorptive processes of the nephron then alter the filtrate to form urine.

770. **c** Separated by the glomeruli, the afferent arterioles bring arterial blood to the glomeruli.

771. **c**

772. **b** The ureters convey urine from the renal pelves to the bladder.

773. **a**

774. **d** Aldosterone and ADH normally have the most influence on the kidneys.

775. **b**

776. **c** The loop of Henle lies between the proximal and distal convoluted tubules.

777. **d**

778. **b**

779. **a** The external sphincter must relax for urine to be released from the bladder.

780. **c** Sodium resorption is promoted by angiotensin II, along with water resorption to increase blood pressure.

781. **b** ADH increases the tubular cells' permeability to water, thus increasing water resorption.

782. **d**

783. **c**

784. **c**

785. **a** Hemoglobin (protein of red blood cells) is normally the most plentiful chemical buffer in the body, although sodium bicarbonate is the chief chemical buffer in the body.

Hospital Management

Joann Colville

QUESTIONS

1. Contaminated gloves and gauze are disposed of
   a. In the sharps container
   b. In the biohazard waste disposal
   c. In the restroom trash receptacle
   d. In any trash receptacle that is dated

2. When referring to the use of hazardous products in the workplace, it is imperative to always do what first?
   a. Check the proper psi of the fire extinguisher
   b. Confirm the status of insurance
   c. Read the label for cautions, handling procedures, and directions
   d. Confirm that duties are in your job description

3. SOAP is the acronym for
   a. Symptoms, observations, assessment, plan
   b. Subjective, objective, assessment, plan
   c. Streamlined operation action plan
   d. Synergistic outline alternative for prognosis

4. MSDS is the acronym for
   a. Modified systemic dental systems
   b. Main surgery and dental supplies
   c. Material safety data sheet
   d. Mandatory safety detail score

5. OSHA is the acronym for
   a. Occupational Safety and Health Administration
   b. Occupational Solicitation Hazards Administration
   c. Occupational Storage of Hazardous Agents
   d. Occupational Signs for Health Associations

6. Which of the following tasks is not legal for veterinary technicians?
   a. Venipuncture
   b. Patient restraint
   c. Parking clients' cars
   d. Prescribing medications

7. The optimal temperature for housing most mammals and birds is
   a. 55° F
   b. 65° F to 84° F
   c. 98.6° F
   d. 100° F

8. Which of the following diseases/conditions warrants isolation of the affected animal?
   a. *Bordetella bronchiseptica*
   b. Diabetes
   c. Renal disease
   d. Lyme disease

9. How many sides/surfaces are there to an animal cage?
   a. 7
   b. 6
   c. 5
   d. 4

10. Washing your hands immediately after completing a procedure is most important in which of the following situations?
    a. Exposure to radiation from the x-ray machine
    b. Holding an animal that may have *Microsporum canis* infection
    c. Invoicing a file for a cat with feline leukemia
    d. Bathing a dog with demodectic mange

11. How should you dispose of used needles and syringes?
    a. Syringes must be disposed of in a sharps container; needles should be cut off and thrown in the garbage.
    b. Needles and syringes should be autoclaved and placed in the garbage.
    c. A needle should be cut off a syringe and placed in the sharps container; the syringe may be cleaned, sterilized, and reused or discarded.
    d. Needle and attached syringe should be disposed of in the sharps container.

73

Correct answers are on pages 82-85.

12. *Universal precautions* refers to
    a. Sterile surgical packs
    b. Blood-borne pathogens
    c. Disinfectants with a red label
    d. The safe handling of MSDS

13. Offensive language in the workplace may be an example of
    a. Infringement of privacy
    b. Freedom of speech
    c. Sexual harassment
    d. Medical interpretation

14. Why should the lid of a sample never be used as the primary label?
    a. There is not enough room to write
    b. Lids can get misplaced
    c. It is too difficult to read instructions
    d. Ink may become smudged

15. When clients are instructed to bring in a fecal sample, how much are they told to collect?
    a. 1 pint
    b. 1 to 2 teaspoons
    c. 1 cup
    d. 60 ml

16. Examples of PPEs are
    a. Needles and syringes
    b. Masks, gowns, gloves, and goggles
    c. Drapes and towels
    d. Surgical scrub and alcohol

17. If you found a 2-liter ventilation bag in the reception area, you would return it to
    a. The x-ray department
    b. The lab
    c. The surgery suite
    d. The kennel

18. A shipment of Sodasorb arrives. You should deliver it to
    a. The surgery suite to be placed in surgical packs
    b. The surgery suite for use in the autoclave
    c. The surgery suite for cleaning the instruments
    d. The surgery suite for use in the anesthesia machine

19. What is the most appropriate "cloth" to use on the microscope lens?
    a. Kim wipes
    b. Lens paper
    c. Tissue paper
    d. Gauze

20. Surgical drapes, towels, and gowns should be washed
    a. With the kennel laundry
    b. With the dishes
    c. With the instruments
    d. Alone

21. According to the American Animal Hospital Association, *SOP* refers to
    a. Synopsis of procedure
    b. Standard operating procedure
    c. Station of preference
    d. Situation of patients

22. The employees' "right to know" is part of
    a. The Animal Welfare Act of 1973
    b. The Institutional Animal Care and Use Committee by laws
    c. OSHA guidelines
    d. Life insurance plans

23. *OTC* refers to
    a. Owner's top complaint
    b. Over the counter
    c. Obstructed trachea condition
    d. Obese tomcat

24. The term *informed consent* usually is in reference to
    a. The purchase of pharmaceuticals
    b. Hospital discharges
    c. Anesthesia and/or procedures, surgical or otherwise, that have been explained to the owner
    d. Permission to initiate a diet change

25. For a veterinarian to prescribe treatment or medication, there must be a
    a. Prescription pad and pen available in the exam room
    b. Documented patient
    c. Confirmed diagnosis
    d. Patient, veterinarian, and client relationship

26. All documentation in the patient's medical record should be signed
    a. Using red ink
    b. With the initials of the person doing the documentation
    c. At the end of the hospitalization
    d. By the owner

27. Legible and thorough documentation validates patient care and is the responsibility of
    a. The patient
    b. The owner
    c. Each member of the veterinary team
    d. The doctor only

28. What color ink is most appropriate to use when marking in medical records?
    a. Red because it is more noticeable
    b. Black because it photocopies well
    c. Green because it is easy to read
    d. Any color that is available

29. Changing a medical record in any way is illegal and constitutes
    a. Harassment
    b. Tampering
    c. Poor care
    d. An approach to neatness

30. To correct a mistake in a medical record
    a. Use liquid paper and start over
    b. Erase it as best you can and write over the erased area
    c. Draw a line through it, label it as an error, and initial it
    d. Strike it out with red ink

31. Discussion of a patient's records with outside parties
    a. Is okay as long as you do not benefit financially
    b. Is a normal and common practice
    c. Is a breach of confidentiality
    d. May benefit the patient's well-being

32. Cage cards should contain all of the following information, with the exception of
    a. Species/breed, gender, date of birth
    b. Reason for visit
    c. Name
    d. Date of last visit

33. Medical records must be maintained for a certain amount of time. Although this varies from state to state, the generally accepted minimum storage time is
    a. 3 years
    b. 2 years
    c. 7 years
    d. 1 year

34. Health records issued for small-animal interstate travel are valid for how many days?
    a. 10 days
    b. 30 days
    c. 15 days
    d. 21 days

35. If consent forms are signed by a minor, they
    a. Are not legally binding
    b. Are frequently not legible
    c. Are valid only if the minor is the client
    d. Are valid only after a 10-day waiting period

36. Which of the following aspects of a written job description would you deem most important?
    a. Performance of essential skills
    b. Educational requirements
    c. Amount of experience
    d. Physical requirements and personality traits

37. Which of the following statements is the least appropriate use of a job description?
    a. To recruit and select new employees
    b. To review performance of employees
    c. To determine salary
    d. To determine disciplinary action by personnel when needed

38. Which of the following would be the least profitable place to advertise a professional position for a licensed veterinary technician?
    a. Local newspaper
    b. Employment agency
    c. Professional school
    d. Professional journal or magazine

39. Which term is defined as a vocation or occupation that requires advanced education and training and involves intellectual skills?
    a. Professionalism
    b. Professional expectations
    c. Professional ethics
    d. Profession

40. The most important skill that a successful hospital manager can have is the ability to
    a. Hire new employees
    b. Communicate well with others
    c. Terminate employees
    d. Schedule work hours so that all busy times and areas are well staffed

41. Written job descriptions
    a. Do not change for a specific job
    b. Should be general guidelines rather than detailed descriptions
    c. Cannot legally state that a disability would make a job candidate unacceptable
    d. Should detail only the responsibilities of the position and not the special skills required

42. Which of the following questions should not be asked on a job application or during a job interview?
    a. Do you have any children?
    b. Why did you leave your last place of employment?
    c. How does this position fit into your long-term goals?
    d. Do you prefer working alone or working with others? Why?

Correct answers are on pages 82-85.

43. Good client communication skills require that you
    a. Ask probing, leading questions to attain information on medical history
    b. Be a good listener but do not make eye contact with the client
    c. Use the patient's name only, not the client's name, in conversation
    d. Be skillful in the use of words and observe appropriate body language

44. When obtaining the medical history on a new patient, which information is of least importance?
    a. Dates of previous immunizations and heartworm prevention
    b. Previous veterinarian/clinic used
    c. History of previous illnesses or surgical procedures
    d. History of allergies

45. Most new clients with companion animals select a veterinarian based on
    a. A recommendation from a friend
    b. Discounted fees
    c. Convenience of practice location
    d. Personality of staff

46. Which of the following is the least appropriate reason to terminate an employee?
    a. Unsatisfactory performance of duties
    b. Elimination of a position
    c. Excessive tardiness or absenteeism
    d. Dishonest or unethical behavior in the performance of duties

47. Concerning personnel files, which statement is least accurate?
    a. Employee files should be kept in a locked, secure cabinet that is accessible to management only
    b. Each employee should have a separate file in which all materials related to employment are stored
    c. An employee should have access to his or her personnel file at any time without supervision
    d. Any grievance against an employee should be kept in his or her file

48. A personnel record should contain all of the following except
    a. The original application, reference letters, and résumé
    b. An employee record form with date of hire, salary, and employment history
    c. A record of benefits, vacation times, and places visited
    d. Performance evaluations and pay raises

49. Staff meetings
    a. Should be held regularly during a lunch or dinner break
    b. Should include full-time employees only
    c. Should be very informal and unstructured
    d. Should be part of every employee's compensation package

50. Some interview questions are unlawful or discriminatory and must not be asked. All of the following topics would be considered unlawful questioning except
    a. Age
    b. National origin
    c. Gender
    d. Religion

51. Concerning management of a veterinary practice, which of the following is least likely to influence client compliance and satisfaction?
    a. Quality communication to inform and educate the client on treatment options
    b. Delivery of quality medical care for the patient
    c. The caring attitude of the veterinary team
    d. Cost-cutting practices for medical services

52. Good management of hospital areas aids the efficiency of a veterinary practice. Lack of attention to facility maintenance can lead to any of the following except
    a. Staff frustrations
    b. Increase in profitability
    c. Loss of income
    d. Decrease in client service and patient care

53. Which of the following professional agencies accredits veterinary hospitals based on standards of excellence concerning facility design, equipment, patient care, medical records, inventory control, client communication, and marketing?
    a. AVMA
    b. DHEC
    c. AAHA
    d. CVTEA

54. In accepting checks as payment for veterinary services, you should record or verify certain items. Which of the following is not considered essential?
    a. Client's name and current address
    b. His or her driver's license number
    c. The initials of the employee who accepted the check
    d. Home or work telephone number or place of employment

55. Which of the following is not considered a legal reason for maintaining medical records?
    a. Hospital-employed accountants and attorneys require them
    b. They are essential in the defense of legal actions for malpractice or incompetence
    c. They are used to establish that a legal contract existed for the care of a patient and collection of a fee
    d. Many states and some professional associations require them

56. This schedule of controlled substances has the least potential for abuse and is primarily antitussive and antidiarrheal drugs.
    a. Schedule I
    b. Schedule III
    c. Schedule IV
    d. Schedule V

57. Upon the loss of a controlled substance, the veterinarian or veterinary technician must
    a. Notify the local veterinary clinics and hospitals
    b. Alert the local police department and the FBI in your area
    c. Notify the local police department and DEA field office
    d. Notify other veterinary clinics/hospitals within a 50-mile radius

58. The duties of the veterinary technician, as related to controlled substances, typically include all of the following except
    a. Ordering
    b. Dispensing
    c. Record keeping
    d. Storage procedures

59. Extremely popular during the past few years, what may be the greatest cost-saving feature ever developed for the filing and retrieval of records?
    a. Digital phasing
    b. Color coding
    c. Chronologic filing
    d. Geographic filing

60. What filing system operates generally by state or country and then alphabetically or numerically by account name or number?
    a. Geographic filing
    b. Subject filing
    c. Numeric filing
    d. Open filing

61. Which system's greatest benefit is speed of filing and finding? Although this system requires a cross index, it can increase efficiency by 40% to 50%.
    a. Alphabetic system
    b. Numeric filing
    c. Subject filing
    d. Chronologic filing

62. Which item is usually not included in a patient's medical record?
    a. History and physical examination forms
    b. Laboratory and radiology reports
    c. Special procedure reports
    d. Photographs of the client

63. The most immediate and tangible increase in income from hospital computer use may result from the reminder and recall system. Evidence has shown a return rate increase of what percentage range with follow-up contact with clients via reminder cards or calls?
    a. 10% to 20%
    b. 80% to 90%
    c. 1% to 5%
    d. 40% to 50%

64. Basic considerations in planning the physical arrangement of veterinary hospital include all of the following, except
    a. Efficient flow of traffic
    b. Economy of time
    c. Economy of energy
    d. Avant-garde design

65. If an incorrect entry is made in a medical record, the accepted procedure is to
    a. Erase the entire entry and start again
    b. Draw an ink line through the incorrect entry, initial it, and insert the date of the change in the margin; the correct entry is then made on the following line
    c. Begin a new medical record, copying all previous entries
    d. Erase the incorrect entry only; initial and follow with the correct entry on the following line

66. The original medical record, along with x-ray films and laboratory reports or electrodiagnostics tests, is the property of the
    a. Patient
    b. Veterinary hospital and its owner
    c. Owner of the practice and his or her legal representative
    d. Client

Correct answers are on pages 82-85.

67. A comprehensive medical record should contain all of the following except
    a. Clinical signs
    b. Patient's pedigree history
    c. Vaccination status
    d. Discharge summary

68. Which of the following medical record formats takes more time to compile? Because it makes available more historical data and other information, this format supports case planning and provides protection in the event of litigation.
    a. Problem-oriented medical records
    b. Conventional method
    c. Situation method
    d. Master problem list

69. Each practice or clinic sets its own rules for purging active records. How long are records generally kept in a practice?
    a. 3 years
    b. 5 years
    c. 1 year
    d. 10 years

70. In which form of color coding is one color assigned to each digit from 0 to 9, and the colors vary on the record according to the number? This system prevents chart misfiles.
    a. Alphabetic
    b. Sequential
    c. Numeric
    d. Microlegal

71. A signed authorization form from the patient's owner is not needed before any information in the medical record can be released to
    a. The owner
    b. Another veterinarian
    c. The insurance company
    d. A coworker veterinary technician

72. Which separate financial record consists of a chronologic listing of every daily transaction? This includes client and patient identification, service rendered, fee charged, and amount paid.
    a. Daybook
    b. Ledger card
    c. Business record form
    d. Charge or fee slip

73. Which of the following is not an ingredient of the inventory control system?
    a. Supply ledger or card file
    b. Want sheet
    c. Actual count of items in the hospital
    d. Ledger sheet

74. This document arrives with supplies and usually includes a list of items in the package. It is checked against the contents to ensure that everything is enclosed.
    a. Bill
    b. Packing slip
    c. Invoice
    d. Inventory record

75. In routine processing of veterinary product shipments, what is the usual sequence of document handling?
    a. Packing slip, bill, invoice, and inventory record
    b. Invoice, bill, packing slip, and inventory record
    c. Packing slip, invoice, inventory record, and bill
    d. Inventory record, packing slip, invoice, and bill

76. The bill usually lists all of the following except
    a. Invoice numbers
    b. Total amount of each invoice
    c. Total amount of purchases made during the month
    d. Packing slip numbers and dates shipped

77. A veterinarian who dispenses or regularly administers controlled substances must take an inventory of all substances on hand on the same date every
    a. year
    b. 5 years
    c. 2 years
    d. 3 years

78. Records for what schedule of drugs must be kept separate from all other controlled substance records?
    a. Schedule II
    b. Schedule I
    c. Schedule III
    d. Schedule IV

79. When might a veterinary technician's error result in the veterinarian being found guilty of malpractice?
    a. When the error endangers a patient or a client
    b. When the veterinarian is aware of the error
    c. When the veterinarian is not present when the error is made
    d. A veterinary technician's error would never result in the veterinarian's liability

80. If a client insists on restraining his or her animal and is then injured, are there grounds for a malpractice suit against the veterinary clinic?
   a. Yes; the veterinary clinic has an obligation to always protect clients from injury
   b. Yes, but only if the animal was previously known to be vicious
   c. Yes, but only if the injury occurs as a direct result of the animal's being frightened by examination or treatment
   d. No; there is no potential liability in such a case

81. In which of the following situations would the veterinarian definitely not be held liable for damages?
   a. During rectal palpation, a mare becomes excited and fractious and her rectum is torn, resulting in peritonitis and death
   b. A dog escapes from a clinic's outdoor run and is never seen again
   c. A 2-year-old child opens a Ziploc bag that contains medication for a dog, eats several tablets, and is poisoned
   d. An animal dies as a result of the client's not following written directions relating to treatment

82. Prescriptions
   a. Need not be signed
   b. Are not considered legal documents
   c. Should be recorded, and records should be maintained
   d. Are not necessary for extra label drug dispensing

83. Which of the following is appropriate when a disgruntled client alleges malpractice that may precipitate a law suit?
   a. Apologize and state that the mistake can be corrected
   b. Respond angrily and indignantly to the client; these types of people understand forceful language only
   c. Offer to waive the charges for the procedure and care in question
   d. Show concern for the client

84. Medical records
   a. Are the undisputed property of the client and must be sent to any client who is moving from the area
   b. Do not include radiographic films and laboratory reports
   c. Should be retained even if the client moves away
   d. Can be shared with anyone requesting copies

85. The recommended procedure for an unvaccinated dog with a known exposure to a rabid animal is
   a. Quarantine for 10 days
   b. Quarantine for 30 days
   c. Immediate vaccination, then quarantine for 10 days
   d. Euthanasia

86. Which of the following label statements indicates a prescription product?
   a. Sold to graduate veterinarians only
   b. Caution: Federal law restricts this drug for use by or on the order of a licensed veterinarian
   c. For veterinary use only
   d. Caution: Use only as directed

87. According to a recent clarification from the federal government, who may sign health certificates and other official veterinary documents?
   a. The veterinarian only
   b. The veterinarian or a veterinary technician on the advice of the veterinarian
   c. Any employee of the clinic, as long as the employee has power of attorney and the signature is initialed by the employee
   d. Any employee of the clinic may apply the veterinarian's signature stamp

88. To issue an interstate health certificate, a veterinarian must be accredited and
   a. Have seen the animal within the last 7 days
   b. Have seen the animal within the last 30 days
   c. Have seen the animal on the day the certificate is signed
   d. Familiar with the herd of origin, even though the specific animal in question has not been seen

89. To be moved across most state lines or into Canada, dogs must be vaccinated against
   a. Parvovirus infection
   b. Rabies
   c. Canine distemper
   d. Lyme disease

90. Which of the following does not require a valid veterinarian–client–patient relationship for dispensing?
   a. Dimethylsulfoxide (DMSO)
   b. Prostaglandins
   c. Canine parvovirus vaccine
   d. Oxytocin

Correct answers are on pages 82-85.

91. Brucellosis vaccination tags are what color and are applied to which ear of cattle?
    a. Silver, right
    b. Green, left
    c. Blue, left
    d. Orange, right

92. If an entire cattle herd is tested negative for brucellosis on two occasions, __ months apart, it may qualify as a certified *brucellosis-free* herd
    a. 2
    b. 12
    c. 10 to 14
    d. 6 to 8

93. Which federal government agency is responsible for monitoring and enforcing regulations on the interstate shipment of livestock?
    a. Department of the Interior
    b. Animal and Plant Health Inspection Service
    c. Drug Enforcement Administration
    d. Food and Drug Administration

94. Cattle are tested for tuberculosis by injection with tuberculin in what site and are reexamined how long after the injection?
    a. Neck, 24 hours
    b. Caudal fold, 24 hours
    c. Neck, 48 hours
    d. Caudal fold, 72 hours

95. What is the longest period some rabies vaccines provide protection for dogs and cats?
    a. 6 months
    b. 3 years
    c. 5 years
    d. The life of the animal

96. Rabies vaccines licensed to be administered only intramuscularly are to be injected
    a. In the thigh
    b. In the gluteals
    c. In the pectorals
    d. Over the crest of the shoulders

97. When may a rabies tag be issued without completing a rabies certificate?
    a. If the tag replaces a lost tag
    b. If the owner does not want or need a certificate
    c. If the owner is simply using the tag for identification
    d. It should never be issued without completing a rabies certificate, even in the case of a lost tag

98. The recommended procedure for a dog that has just bitten a person is
    a. Quarantine and observe for 10 days
    b. Quarantine and observe for 30 days
    c. Advise the owner to closely observe the dog for 15 days
    d. Immediate euthanasia

99. Chloramphenicol is
    a. Legal for use in calves and baby pigs less than 2 weeks old
    b. Legal for use in food animals when the requirements of extra label drug use are met
    c. Illegal for use in any food animals
    d. Illegal for use in all animals

100. The FDA checks and licenses drugs and biologics before they can be sold. Which aspects are evaluated by the FDA?
    a. Cost-effectiveness and probable demand
    b. Safety and efficacy
    c. Profit margin (markup) and packaging
    d. Market niche

101. Who can purchase an over-the-counter (OTC) drug?
    a. Anyone
    b. Veterinarians only
    c. Veterinarians and pharmacists only
    d. Veterinarians and veterinary technicians only

102. If a drug has been identified as a carcinogen, what would you expect the residue tolerance to be?
    a. One part per million
    b. One part per billion
    c. One part per trillion
    d. Residues detected at any level would not be tolerated

103. After being cited for a first-time residue violation, a feedlot must
    a. Pay a fine not to exceed $10,000
    b. Send five head of cattle to be slaughtered and tested for residues before sending the next load of cattle to slaughter
    c. Eliminate use of all drugs at the feedlot
    d. Do nothing; there is no required action after a first-time violation

104. Extra label use of feed medications is
    a. Permitted by veterinary prescription
    b. Strictly illegal
    c. Permitted if a Form 1900 is secured
    d. Permitted under the guidelines of Form FD 2656

105. Controlled substances with no accepted medical use are classified as
    a. Schedule I
    b. Schedule II
    c. Schedule IV
    d. Schedule V

106. How long must controlled substance records be maintained?
    a. 90 days
    b. 1 year
    c. 2 years
    d. 5 years

107. Which species may be legally vaccinated against rabies using an injectable rabies vaccine?
    a. Ferret
    b. Skunk
    c. Wolf
    d. Raccoon

108. Which bovine brucellosis ear tattoo is incorrect?
    a. 3V8
    b. 5V2
    c. 4V1
    d. 1V0

109. A written consent form
    a. Is not considered part of a patient's medical record
    b. Is not necessary for surgery when verbal consent has been given
    c. Should be used when a client requests that a child proof container not be used for dispensed medication
    d. Is not necessary for euthanasia when the owner is a recognized client

110. Which of the following would be considered ethical and appropriate on the part of a veterinary technician?
    a. Telling a client that Mrs. J, another client, owns an animal that has a contagious disease
    b. Confiding to a client that Dr. A has had recent mishaps in surgery and suggesting that Dr. B perform the requested surgical procedure
    c. Explaining that the reason service fees are higher than those of the clinic down the street is because they do not do things as well at that clinic
    d. Refusing to reduce the charges for professional services without the approval of the veterinarian

111. Which of the following may be legally performed by a veterinary technician?
    a. Canine castration
    b. Diagnosing feline epilepsy
    c. Administering isoflurane
    d. Prescribing ampicillin

112. The accrediting body for veterinary technology education programs in the United States is the
    a. North American Veterinary Technician Association (NAVTA)
    b. AVMA Committee on Veterinary Technician Education and Activities (CVTEA)
    c. United States Department of Agriculture (USDA)
    d. Association of Veterinary Technician Educators (AVTE)

113. A client takes a Rottweiler to a two-veterinarian clinic for castration. The client indicates to the receptionist that the dog has a bad disposition, and the receptionist records this information on the patient's medical record. Dr. X castrates the dog without incident. When the client returns the next day to pick up the dog, Dr. Y asks the veterinary technician to take the dog to the reception area, which is crowded with other clients. As the dog's leash is handed to the client, the dog jerks away and attacks another client's dog. Who is least liable for damages claimed by the second client?
    a. The owner of the Rottweiler
    b. The veterinary technician
    c. Dr. X
    d. Dr. Y

114. If a veterinarian who is your employer commits acts that you as a veterinary technician consider to be unethical, you should
    a. Do or say nothing
    b. Warn clients
    c. Discuss your concerns with the veterinarian
    d. Immediately report the veterinarian to the State Board of Examiners

115. A client brings in a dog for a parvovirus vaccination. The only canine parvovirus vaccine in the clinic has an expiration date that indicates it expired 2 months earlier. What should be done?
    a. The vaccine should be used at the recommended dose
    b. The vaccine should be used at twice the recommended dose
    c. Feline panleukopenia vaccine should instead be used
    d. A new appointment should be made for a date after a shipment of new vaccine has arrived

Correct answers are on pages 82-85.

116. Ethically speaking, veterinary technicians involved in animal research should
    a. Avoid unnecessary suffering and pain in their subjects
    b. Avoid any use of live animals
    c. Become active in militant animal rights organizations and sabotage any research techniques with which he or she disagrees
    d. Use only invertebrates and amphibians in research

117. Which statement concerning ethics is most accurate?
    a. Because declawing cats is excessively painful and considered unethical, euthanasia should be performed when cats cannot be discouraged from causing damage with their front claws.
    b. Clients should not be allowed to be present when their pet is euthanized.
    c. A client's request for euthanasia of a terminally ill pet should always be denied; euthanasia is never ethical.
    d. It is appropriate to send a sympathy card to the client following the death of a pet.

ANSWERS

1. **b** Universal precautions; the box must also be dated.

2. **c** Emphasized in ACT and AAHA training videos

3. **b** S = information from the owner; O = data gathered; A = conclusions from S & O; P = strategy

4. **c** These give information about the properties of chemicals, drugs, and so forth.

5. **a** OSHA is the federal agency charged with ensuring safety in the workplace. Veterinary practices fall under OSHA jurisdiction.

6. **d** Individual state laws vary, but in general, veterinary technicians may not diagnose diseases, prescribe medications, or perform surgery.

7. **b**

8. **a** It can be transmitted by airborne particles sneezed or coughed out by the affected animal.

9. **a** One top, three sides, one bottom, two front bars (inside and outside)

10. **b** Fungal contaminant

11. **c** Cutting off the needle increases the chance of injury and possible aerosol contamination.

12. **b** Treat all blood as though it were contaminated.

13. **c**

14. **b** Write on the container only.

15. **b** This volume is more than enough for most in-house diagnostic procedures.

16. **b** Personal protection equipment

17. **c** The ventilation bag is part of an anesthesia machine that is most likely located in the surgical suite.

18. **d** Sodasorb is used in inhalant anesthesia machines to absorb carbon dioxide exhaled by the patient.

19. **b** These are less likely to scratch the lens surface.

20. **d** To prevent hair and other debris from clinging to it

21. **b** Used in office procedures

22. **c**

23. **b** Commonly used term for products that can be purchased without a prescription

24. **c** Pertains to signed permits and waivers used in a clinic or hospital

25. **d** This is mandated by state and/or national governing bodies.

26. **b** Accountability is important.

27. **c** All those involved in the care of patient

28. **b** Black ink photocopies most clearly and therefore is more acceptable in a court of law.

29. **b** It is considered misrepresentation, hiding what might be evidence.

30. **c** It must not appear as though one is trying to hide something.

31. **c** You must first have the client's written permission.

32. **d** Least likely to be pertinent information

33. **c**

34. **c** A veterinarian from the originating state must examine the animal within 15 days of travel.

35. **a** Only an adult can sign consent forms.

36. **a** The inability to perform the essential skills would make a prospective employee unqualified for the position. This is usually the most detailed portion of a job description and is used as an initial screening device to hire an employee well trained in the required skills who will need only minimal additional training by the hospital staff.

37. **d** Disciplinary action for an employee by personnel should be stated in a hospital policies and procedures manual that discusses reasons for termination of employment.

38. **a** Newspaper advertising is the most commonly used source when seeking nonprofessional employees. If the position to be filled is for a professional employee, you will want to advertise the position in the appropriate professional journal or with an agency.

39. **d** Definition of *profession* provided by NAVTA

40. **b** Effective communication skills include verbal and listening skills, which encourage adequate flow of information and create a trusting environment among staff. Developing good communications between staff and management is your most important challenge as a hospital manager.

41. **c** Job descriptions should state the intellect and skill functions of the job as well as the physical, time, and stress demands. If an individual, except for limitations caused by a disability, is qualified to perform the essential functions of a job, the employer must consider whether or not the individual could perform these functions with the assistance of a reasonable accommodation. Refer to the Americans with Disabilities Act for further details.

42. **a** This is an unlawful application or interview question. It is not pertinent to the individual's potential employability.

43. **d** The employee should not ask leading questions pertaining to medical history, because it might minimize the descriptions and answers given by the client concerning the medical condition.

44. **b** Information concerning the client's previously used veterinary hospital is of little importance when obtaining medical history on a patient, unless records must be obtained from that clinic.

45. **c** When new clients are searching for a veterinarian, a convenient location is considered to be important in the initial selection by most clients.

46. **b** When the need arises to terminate an employee, it should be based on poor job performance and unethical behavior.

47. **c** An employee should have access to only his or her personnel files when requested and may only review them in the presence of management.

48. **c** A personnel record should contain all information pertinent to the employee's hiring, job performance, benefits, and record of firing.

49. **d** It is recommended to include all staff for staff meetings, and part-time personnel should be paid for their time to attend such meetings.

50. **a** It is not unlawful to ask questions concerning the age of the candidate during an interview.

51. **d** Clients receive greater satisfaction in the treatment of their pets through genuine concern, communication, and quality service rather than the cheapest prices.

52. **b** Poor facility maintenance can lead to downtime of equipment and loss of services offered. This would not increase profitability but instead would cause loss of income, staff frustration, and client dissatisfaction.

53. **c** The American Animal Hospital Association (AAHA) is the agency responsible for accrediting veterinary hospitals based on standards of excellence.

54. c

55. a

56. d

57. d

58. b

59. b

60. a

61. b

62. d

63. a

64. d

65. b

66. d

67. b

68. a

69. a

70. c

71. d

72. a

73. d

74. b

75. c

76. d

77. c

78. a

79. a The veterinary technician is an agent of the veterinarian.

80. a

81. d By issuing written directions, the clinic fulfills its obligation. The client has an obligation to follow those written directions. The veterinarian could reasonably be found liable for damages in the other three situations: injury to a patient, disappearance of a patient in his or her custody, and failure to dispense medication in child proof packaging.

82. c Prescriptions are legal documents and must be signed, and records of prescriptions should be maintained. Drugs dispensed for "extra label use" must be handled on a prescription basis.

83. d The AVMA Professional Liability Insurance Trust recommends that potential fault not be acknowledged. It is appropriate to empathize with the client in an unfortunate situation.

84. c Medical records are the property of the clinic and are strictly confidential.

85. d

86. b

87. a

88. a

89. b

90. c DMSO, prostaglandins, and oxytocin are prescription products and, as such, require a valid veterinary–client–patient relationship to dispense.

91. d

92. c

93. b

94. d

95. b Rabies vaccine may not be dispensed. It may be used by a veterinarian only or, in some states, under the direct supervision of a veterinarian.

96. a

97. d If a client has lost a rabies tag, a new one may be issued; however, a new certificate should be issued (including the original vaccination information) with the new tag number.

98. a

99. c Chloramphenicol is specifically forbidden for use in food animals by the FDA because of the potential of fatal aplastic anemia in some people consuming tissues of treated animals.

100. b

101. a

102. d

103. b

104. b Label dosage regimens and indications of feed additives must be strictly observed in all cases by all individuals, including veterinarians.

105. a

106. c

107. a

108. b The first digit indicates the quarter of the year of brucellosis vaccination. The digit following the V shield indicates the year of vaccination. For example, a heifer vaccinated in November of 1995 would have a tattoo of 4V5.

109. c A written consent form should be used for surgery, euthanasia, and other risky or expensive procedures. A completed and signed written consent form is considered part of the medical record from a legal standpoint.

110. d Confidentiality should be maintained at all times. It is not ethical to criticize professional colleagues, and it is not appropriate for a veterinary technician to reduce fees without the veterinarian's approval.

111. c According to the AVMA Model Practice Act, veterinary technicians may not perform surgery, make diagnoses, or prescribe treatments.

112. b

113. a The veterinary hospital is usually considered responsible for the safety of clients and patients on the premises and should take appropriate steps to minimize any possible risk. The owner of the dog has met his obligation under the law by informing the hospital of the dog's disposition.

114. c Ethical concerns should first be discussed with the person involved. It would be inappropriate to voice the concerns to clients.

115. d Outdated products should never be used. Panleukopenia vaccine is not a satisfactory substitute for canine parvovirus vaccine.

116. a

117. d Euthanasia is a viable, ethical option in a number of situations. Declawing cats is considered by many veterinarians to be an ethical alternative to needless euthanasia. It is appropriate for the client to be present when a pet is euthanized if requested.

Section 3

Medical Calculations

Eloyes Hill • Thomas Colville

QUESTIONS

1. How many milligrams of a drug should be given to a patient who weighs 22 lb if the dose is 0.2 mg/kg?
   a. 2
   b. 4.4
   c. 20
   d. 44

2. A 75-lb dog must be dewormed. If the daily dose of the dewormer is 1 tsp/25 lb of body weight for 3 days, approximately how much should be given each day?
   a. 3 tbs
   b. 1 tbs
   c. 5 tsp
   d. 1 tsp

3. A cat on intravenous fluids must receive 30 ml/hr normal saline. If this cat has a drip set that provides 60 drops/ml, what should the drip rate be?
   a. 1 drop/2 sec
   b. 1 drop/6 sec
   c. 3 drops/sec
   d. 16 drops/sec

4. The concentration of furosemide (Lasix) is 5%. How many milligrams are in 0.5 ml?
   a. 150
   b. 2.5
   c. 25
   d. 50

5. How many milliliters of a drug with a concentration of 100 mg/ml should be given to a 75-lb dog at a dose of 1 mg/lb?
   a. 75
   b. 100
   c. 0.75
   d. 0.34

6. A prescription in which 3 ml of lactulose are given orally twice daily will require how many ounces to last at least 30 days?
   a. 3
   b. 6
   c. 90
   d. 180

7. A commercial dog food is 420 kcal/cup. A dog weighing 60 lb fed at a rate of 70 kcal/lb/day should be fed how many cups at each meal if you feed him twice a day?
   a. 5
   b. 10
   c. 2
   d. 1

8. A cockatiel needs 100 mg/kg piperacillin via intramuscular injection. If the bird weighs 80 g, and the concentration of piperacillin is 100 mg/ml, how many milliliters should be given?
   a. 0.08
   b. 0.8
   c. 80
   d. 1.6

9. A rabbit needs 300 µg/kg of a 1% ivermectin solution. If the rabbit weighs 8 lb, how many milliliters of ivermectin should be given?
   a. 8
   b. 10
   c. 0.1
   d. 0.8

10. How many milliliters of a 50% dextrose solution are needed to make 1000 ml of a 5% dextrose solution?
    a. 1
    b. 10
    c. 50
    d. 100

Correct answers are on pages 100-104.

11. Six 12-oz puppies need deworming medication. If the dose is 1 ml/lb, how many milliliters do you dispense?
    a. 12
    b. 4.5
    c. 6
    d. 3

12. To make a solution with a concentration of 15 mg/ml, how many milliliters of sterile water should be added to 30 g of powdered drug?
    a. 5
    b. 200
    c. 150
    d. 2000

13. How many tablets would you dispense for a 30-day supply of a drug with a dose of one and one-half tablets three times daily?
    a. 500
    b. 45
    c. 135
    d. 90

14. One gram of powdered drug diluted with how many milliliters of sterile water will make a concentration of 20 mg/ml?
    a. 0.05
    b. 0.2
    c. 100
    d. 50

15. You regularly order six 10-ml vials per month of a drug that has a concentration of 50 mg/ml. Now that same drug is available in only 20-ml vials of 10 mg/ml. How many vials should you order this month to get the same total amount of drug?
    a. 150
    b. 60
    c. 10
    d. 15

16. If a dog that receives fluids at a rate of 120 ml/hr has a rate reduction of 20%, what would be the new rate in milliliters per hour?
    a. 1.6
    b. 0.4
    c. 24
    d. 96

17. A cat that weighs 5 kg is given 0.1 ml of a drug with a concentration of 10 mg/ml. What dose did this cat receive?
    a. 0.05 mg/kg
    b. 0.2 mg/kg
    c. 2 mg/kg
    d. 25 mg/kg

18. You give 5 mg of a drug to a 10-kg animal. What is the dose of the drug in mg/kg?
    a. 2
    b. 10
    c. 0.5
    d. 50

19. A bird that weighs 50 g requires a particular drug at 4 mg/kg divided twice a day. What is the morning dose?
    a. 1 mg
    b. 4 mg
    c. 0.1 mg
    d. 100 mg

20. How long will it take to give a whole blood transfusion of 60 ml at a rate of 2 ml/min?
    a. 30 hours
    b. 3 hours
    c. 1/2 hour
    d. 1.8 hours

21. If a prescription calls for one tablet to be given for 3 days bid, then one tablet for 5 days sid, then one-half tablet given every other day for 2 weeks, how many tablets should be dispensed?
    a. 15
    b. 18
    c. 20
    d. 11

22. Fifty milliliters of a solution of 50% dextrose is added to a liter of 0.45% NaCl with 2.5% dextrose to yield a solution with a final dextrose concentration of what percent?
    a. 3%
    b. 4.8%
    c. 5%
    d. 10%

23. A dog consumes five bowls of water in a 24-hour period. Each bowl contained exactly 100 ml. If you collect 475 ml of urine over the same 24-hour period, approximately how many milliliters constitute insensible loss?
    a. 475
    b. 500
    c. 25
    d. 5

24. If you measure an animal and set the x-ray machine at 70 kVp and 1/60 second and the resulting radiograph is 20% too light, what should the new kVp be increased to?
    a. 84
    b. 87
    c. 90
    d. 114

25. Tidal volume for a dog is 15 ml/kg. If a 10-kg male dog is taking 10 breaths per minute, what is his minute volume?
    a. 150 ml/min
    b. 1500 ml/min
    c. 15 ml/min
    d. 10 ml/min

26. The 10-kg dog in the previous question has a diaphragmatic hernia, and his tidal volume is now only 10 ml/kg. If this dog were on a ventilator, what should his breathing rate be changed to?
    a. 15 breaths/min
    b. 5 breaths/min
    c. 8 breaths/min
    d. 100 breaths/min

27. An anesthesia machine is set to deliver 1 L/min oxygen and 3% isoflurane. Approximately how many milliliters of isoflurane will be used for a 1-hour procedure?
    a. 30
    b. 180
    c. 2400
    d. 1800

28. A 300-g bird must be tube fed 2 ml liquid formula per 100 g body weight three times daily. One gram of powdered formula will yield 15 ml of liquid formula after reconstitution, which is good for 24 hours only. How many grams of powdered formula should you measure out for a 24-hour period, assuming no waste?
    a. 0.8
    b. 0.4
    c. 2.5
    d. 1.2

29. A cat with a gastrotomy tube must receive 300 kcal daily. A 15-oz can of the prescribed diet has 1500 kcal. The prescribed diet must be diluted 50:50 with water to flow through the tube, and a maximum of 45 ml can be given at one feeding. Approximately how many feedings does this cat need daily?
    a. 10
    b. 8
    c. 4
    d. 2

30. If the cat in the previous question requires an additional 160 ml water daily, how many additional 45-ml boluses of water must be given?
    a. 3.5
    b. 2.5
    c. 1.5
    d. 5.5

31. Five tonometer readings in millimeters of mercury are 14, 15, 19, 14, and 18. What is the average (mean) reading?
    a. 17
    b. 18
    c. 16
    d. 15

32. A patient requires 3 units of insulin every 12 hours. If the concentration of insulin is 100 units/ml, how many milliliters should be given at each administration?
    a. 0.3
    b. 30
    c. 0.03
    d. 0.15

33. If the concentration of the insulin in the previous question were 30 units/ml, what would the volume of insulin given at each administration be?
    a. 0.1
    b. 10
    c. 0.05
    d. 0.01

34. A diagnostic laboratory requires 1 ml of serum to run a chemistry panel. A bird with a PCV of 50% would need how many full HCT tubes collected to have enough serum for the est? (Each HCT tube holds 0.1 ml of whole blood.)
    a. 100
    b. 20
    c. 10
    d. 5

35. A 20-kg dog with a PCV of 40% has 300 ml of blood collected. The red blood cells are separated from the serum. What volume of saline would you add to the red cells to make a PCV of 50%?
    a. 360 ml
    b. 240 ml
    c. 180 ml
    d. 120 ml

36. You are taking the heart rate of a cat. If you count 10 beats in 5 seconds, what is the rate in beats per minute?
    a. 50
    b. 120
    c. 300
    d. 220

Correct answers are on pages 100-104.

37. Six blood pressure readings are 115, 120, 123, 121, 121, and 112 mm Hg. What is the average (mean) value?
    a. 123
    b. 120
    c. 121
    d. 119

38. A growth in the skin is 2 inches in diameter. What is the diameter of the growth in centimeters?
    a. 2.5
    b. 30
    c. 20
    d. 5

39. The veterinary dermatologist is having you prepare a dog for a patch test. Forty antigens need to be tested, and each antigen must be 1 cm from the next. What size patch should you shave on the dog?
    a. 4 cm × 4 cm
    b. 20 cm × 20 cm
    c. 8 cm × 5 cm
    d. 16 cm × 10 cm

40. A 16-oz bottle contains how many milliliters?
    a. 480
    b. 240
    c. 40
    d. 1.6

41. Four hundred pounds is how many kilograms?
    a. 880
    b. 182
    c. 600
    d. 18

42. A commercial poultry diet contains 18 g of calcium per pound of feed on an as-fed basis. If calcium carbonate, the sole calcium source, is 60% elemental calcium, how much calcium carbonate is in 1 ton of feed?
    a. 21.6 kg
    b. 30 g
    c. 6000 g
    d. 18 kg

43. In a feed that has 20 lb of corn, 5 lb of beet pulp, 1 lb bone meal, and 2 lb of whey, approximately what percent is corn?
    a. 98%
    b. 28%
    c. 40%
    d. 71%

44. Approximately how many ounces of bleach diluted with water make 1 gallon of a 30% bleach solution (1 qt = 32 oz)?
    a. 19
    b. 38
    c. 3
    d. 76

45. A dose of 30 mEq KCl has been added to 1 L of normal saline. What drip rate would provide a patient with 2 mEq KCl/hr?
    a. 15 ml/hr
    b. 67 ml/hr
    c. 6.7 ml/hr
    d. 60 ml/hr

46. You have an injectable calcium solution that is 30 mg/ml. How much do you add to 1 L of lactated Ringer solution to deliver 4 mg/hr of calcium at a fluid rate of 30 ml/hr?
    a. 133
    b. 13.3
    c. 4.4
    d. 0.67

47. A 5% dextrose solution is diluted with sterile water. The volume of the sterile water added is 40% of the volume of the 5% dextrose solution. What approximately is the new dextrose concentration?
    a. 1.4%
    b. 2.3%
    c. 3.6%
    d. 6.5%

48. The volume of an injection for a small iguana is 0.005 ml. This amount is too small to measure accurately. What dilution would allow you to give a volume of 0.05 ml?
    a. 1:10
    b. 1:100
    c. 1:1000
    d. 1:50

49. Ten cockatiels consume a total of approximately 60 ml of water per day. How many milligrams of tetracycline powder should you add to the daily measured drinking water so each 100-g bird gets 10 mg/kg/day?
    a. 100
    b. 10
    c. 60
    d. 36

50. You need to deworm 100 head of cattle with a pour-on product that is applied at a rate of 1 ml/100 lb and is sold in 250-ml bottles. The cattle weigh 825 to 1050 lb each. Approximately how many bottles of dewormer should you purchase?
    a. 4
    b. 8
    c. 10
    d. 16

51. The level of fluid in the 1-L IV bag reads halfway between the 4 and 5 marks. How much fluid remains in the bag?
    a. 1000 ml
    b. 550 ml
    c. 450 ml
    d. 0.5 L

52. The level of fluid in the 1-L IV bag reads at the 700 mark. How much fluid has been given?
    a. 700 ml
    b. 300 ml
    c. 0.3 L
    d. 300 cc

53. How many milligrams of dextrose does 1 ml of 50% dextrose solution contain?
    a. 5 mg/ml
    b. 50 mg/ml
    c. 500 mg/ml
    d. 5000 mg/ml

54. The "French" unit is commonly used to express the diameter of a urinary catheter. Each French unit is equivalent to 1/3 mm. What is the diameter of a 12 French catheter in millimeters?
    a. 3 mm
    b. 4 mm
    c. 18 mm
    d. 36 mm

55. What is the correct volume of epinephrine, in milliliters, to administer to a 28-lb dog, if the dose is 0.1 mg/kg and the concentration in the bottle is 1:1000 (1 mg/ml)?
    a. 2.8
    b. 1.4
    c. 1.3
    d. 0.28

56. How many milligrams of epinephrine are administered in the previous calculation?
    a. 0.13
    b. 2.8
    c. 0.41
    d. 1.3

57. How many milligrams of doxapram (Dopram) should be administered to a 7-lb cat, if the dose range is 1 to 5 mg/kg IV and the concentration in the bottle is 20 mg/ml?
    a. 9.5
    b. 0.59
    c. 21
    d. 0.21

58. How many milliliters will be administered in the previous calculation?
    a. 1.3
    b. 2.1
    c. 0.95
    d. 0.48

59. How many milliliters of a 50:50 mixture of diazepam and ketamine at a dose of 1 ml/20 lb should be given to an 8-lb cat?
    a. 0.4 ml diazepam; 0.4 ml ketamine
    b. 0.2 ml diazepam; 0.2 ml ketamine
    c. 2 ml diazepam; 2 ml ketamine
    d. 1 ml diazepam; 1 ml ketamine

60. The suggested oxygen flow rate for a circle rebreathing system is 25 to 50 ml/kg/min and 130 to 300 ml/kg/min for a nonrebreathing system. What is the most appropriate flow setting for a 10-lb cat?
    a. 0.3 L
    b. 900 ml
    c. 3 L
    d. 0.9 ml

61. Using the same suggested oxygen flow rates as in the previous question, what is the most appropriate oxygen flow rate for a 32-lb spaniel?
    a. 8 L
    b. 1.6 L
    c. 435 ml
    d. 0.435 ml

62. You have just administered an injection of 0.02 ml of acepromazine (10 mg/ml). How many milligrams did you give?
    a. 2
    b. 0.2
    c. 20
    d. 200

63. You have just administered one tablet of 64.8 mg of phenobarbital. How many grains of drug did you deliver?
    a. 0.25
    b. 0.5
    c. 0.6
    d. 1

Correct answers are on pages 100-104.

64. A 0.25 gr (grain) of phenobarbital is how many milligrams?
    a. 15.2
    b. 14
    c. 16.2
    d. 32.4

65. Lidocaine of 2% is prescribed for a 13-lb beagle at a dose of 2 mg/kg IV. How many milliliters will you deliver?
    a. 1.6
    b. 0.16
    c. 0.6
    d. 6

66. You just administered 1.2 ml of penicillin (300,000 U/ml). How many units did you administer?
    a. 260,000
    b. 360,000
    c. 360
    d. 0.26

67. What unit of measure is most commonly used for serum potassium?
    a. French
    b. mEq
    c. International units
    d. German

68. Your patient is a 42-lb Shepherd mix with a history of vomiting. The order reads: metoclopramide HCl (5 mg/ml); give 0.3 mg/kg IM q6h prn. How many milliliters will you deliver?
    a. 8
    b. 1
    c. 5
    d. 2

69. In the situation in the previous question, how many milligrams will you deliver?
    a. 8
    b. 1
    c. 5.7
    d. 2

70. NPH insulin is labeled 100 units/ml. The order is for a 12-lb poodle and reads: NPH insulin 1 unit/kg qd. How many units do you deliver?
    a. 4
    b. 3
    c. 5.5
    d. 6

71. How many milliliters will you draw up to deliver the number of units in the previous question?
    a. 4
    b. 3
    c. 6
    d. 0.05

72. You are preparing an insulin drip. If you add 1 unit of insulin per 100 ml of IV fluid, how many units will you add to the 1-L bag of fluids?
    a. 100
    b. 1
    c. 10
    d. 1000

73. The insulin drip prepared in the previous question is to be administered at 1 unit/hr. How many milliliters will this be per hour?
    a. 1
    b. 10
    c. 0.01
    d. 100

74. What would be the drip rate per second for 6 units of insulin using the drip prepared in Question 72 (1 unit/100 ml) administered over a 2-hour period using a 60 gtt (drops)/ml administration set?
    a. 1 gtt/sec
    b. 0.5 gtt/sec
    c. 1.5 gtt/sec
    d. 5 gtt/sec

75. A cat in end-stage renal disease is receiving epoetin (2000 units/ml). The dose is 100 units/kg. Your patient weighs 5.5 lb. How many units will you deliver?
    a. 250
    b. 25
    c. 0.25
    d. 100

76. How many milliliters will you draw up to administer 25 units of epoetin (2000 units/ml)?
    a. 2.5
    b. 0.25
    c. 0.01
    d. 0.1

77. Potassium gluconate is administered 1/4 tsp per 4.5 kg po bid. How many milliliters will you deliver in 1 day to a 10-lb cat?
    a. 4.5
    b. 2
    c. 0.15
    d. 2.5

78. If the potassium is labeled 5 mEq/5 ml, how many milliequivalents of potassium are delivered in 2 ml?
    a. 2.0
    b. 0.2
    c. 20
    d. 5.5

79. Chemotherapy medications are dosed by
    a. ml/kg
    b. cc/lb
    c. Body surface area
    d. mg/ml

80. What is the fluid deficit in milliliters for a 33-lb dog with 9% dehydration?
    a. 297
    b. 1350
    c. 135
    d. 330

81. To prepare 128 oz of a 1:7 dilution of iodine and alcohol, you would use
    a. 480 oz iodine, 3360 oz alcohol
    b. 12.8 oz of iodine, 115.2 oz of alcohol
    c. 128 ml of iodine, 896 ml alcohol
    d. 480 ml iodine, 3360 ml alcohol

82. What is the fluid deficit for a 10-lb cat with 12% dehydration?
    a. 120 ml
    b. 60 ml
    c. 545 ml
    d. 1200 ml

83. To prepare 1 cup of instrument milk using the suggested 1:6 dilution ratio, yo would use
    a. 1 oz milk, 6 oz water
    b. 34.3 ml milk, 205.7 ml water
    c. 30 ml milk, 210 ml water
    d. 1 ml milk, 6 ml water

84. You need to deliver 450 ml of 5% glucose. You have on hand a liter of sterile water and a 500-ml bottle of 50% glucose. Which of the following is the correct preparation?
    a. 45 ml of 50% glucose in 405 ml sterile water
    b. 0.45 ml of 50% glucose in 40.5 ml sterile water
    c. 90 ml of 50% glucose in 360 ml of sterile water
    d. 4.5 ml of 50% glucose in 445.5 ml sterile water

85. A 25% solution of sulfamethazine contains how many milligrams of sulfamethazine per milliliter?
    a. 2500 mg/ml
    b. 250 mg/ml
    c. 25 mg/ml
    d. 2.5 mg/ml

86. How much sodium chloride is required to produce 5 L of 0.85% saline solution?
    a. 42.5 mg
    b. 4.25 kg
    c. 425 mg
    d. 42.5 g

87. What volume of a 1.2% sodium hydroxide (NaOH) solution can be made from 600 mg of NaOH?
    a. 50 ml
    b. 5 ml
    c. 250 ml
    d. 500 ml

88. What volume of distilled water must be added to a 5-g vial of thiopental sodium to create a 2.5% solution?
    a. 40 ml
    b. 200 ml
    c. 250 ml
    d. 500 ml

89. A stock solution was diluted 1:5, then 1:3, then 1:2, and finally 1:6 to produce a final concentration of 0.4 mg/ml. The original concentration of the stock solution was
    a. 0.025%
    b. 6.4 mg/ml
    c. 7.2%
    d. 7.2 mg/ml

90. What volume of water must be added to 12.5 ml of a 6% stock solution to produce a 0.5% solution?
    a. 150 ml
    b. 137.5 ml
    c. 37.5 ml
    d. 6.25 ml

91. A 30% stock solution of potassium permanganate ($KMnO_4$) was diluted four times as follows: 0.1 ml of stock was added to 0.4 ml of distilled water; 4.5 ml of distilled water was added; the resulting solution was diluted 1:3; the resulting solution was again diluted to 0.06 L. The final concentration of the solution was
    a. 1.36%
    b. 50 mg/ml
    c. 5 mg/ml
    d. 0.05%

92. What volume of 4.5% potassium chloride (KCl) solution is needed to prepare 0.75 L of a 9-mg/ml KCl solution?
    a. 15 ml
    b. 375 ml
    c. 1.5 ml
    d. 150 ml

Correct answers are on pages 100-104.

93. The concentration of a culture medium produced by dissolving 2.5 g in 0.4 L of distilled water is
    a. 0.15%
    b. 0.625%
    c. 0.16%
    d. 6.25%

94. The amount of glucose to be weighed out to produce 500 ml of a 4.5% solution is
    a. 22.5 g
    b. 2.25 g
    c. 0.225 kg
    d. 22.5 mg

95. A stock solution was diluted four times as follows: 18 ml of distilled water was added to 2 ml of stock; the resulting solution was diluted 1:3; 240 ml of distilled water was added; the resulting solution was diluted to 0.9 L. If the final concentration of the diluted solution was determined to be 100 μg/ml, the original concentration of the stock solution was
    a. 4.5 mg/ml
    b. 4.5%
    c. 60 mg/ml
    d. 0.21%

96. What volume of sulfuric acid (H_2SO_4) is in 275 ml of a 12% v/v solution?
    a. 33 ml
    b. 22.9 ml
    c. 3.3 ml
    d. 4.36 ml

97. The concentration of a glucose solution produced when 4500 mg of glucose is dissolved in 3.6 L of water is
    a. 0.8%
    b. 0.008%
    c. 0.125%
    d. 1.25%

98. The basic unit of mass in the metric system is the
    a. Kilogram
    b. Gram
    c. Milligram
    d. Microgram

99. 50 g is equal to
    a. 0.005 kg
    b. 0.05 kg
    c. 500,000 mg
    d. 5,000,000 μg

100. The mean cellular hemoglobin (MCH) for a particular blood sample is calculated to be 24.3 pg. This is equal to
    a. 24,300 mg
    b. 2430 μg
    c. 24.3×10^{12} g
    d. 24.3×10^{-12} g

101. The mean corpuscular volume (MCV) for a particular blood sample is calculated to be 66.5 femtoliter (fl). This is equal to
    a. 66.5×10^{-15} L
    b. 66.5×10^{15} ml
    c. 66.5×10^{-3} μl
    d. 66.5×10^{-9} L

102. The basic unit of length in the metric system is the
    a. Millimeter
    b. Centimeter
    c. Meter
    d. Kilometer

103. 485 km is equal to
    a. 4.85×10^3 m
    b. 485×10^4 mm
    c. 4.85×10^8 mm
    d. 48,500 cm

104. 250 cc is equal to
    a. 25 ml
    b. 0.25 L
    c. 25,000 μl
    d. 2.5 L

105. One metric ton of livestock feed is equal to
    a. 1000 lb
    b. 10,000 g
    c. 2204 lb
    d. 1,000,000 mg

106. One centimeter is
    a. Greater than 1 mm but shorter than 1μ (1 micron)
    b. Shorter than both 1 m and 1 mm
    c. Greater than both 1 mm and 1μ
    d. Shorter than 1 km but greater than 1 m

107. A dog weighs 55 lb. Its weight can also be stated as
    a. 121 kg
    b. 25 g
    c. 121 mg
    d. 25 kg

108. 8 oz is equal to approximately
     a. 227,200 mg
     b. 454 g
     c. 227 mg
     d. 2.27 kg

109. 10 inches is equal to approximately
     a. 25 mm
     b. 4 cm
     c. 25 cm
     d. 0.04 m

110. The volume of a stock solution required to prepare 3.5 L of a 1:40 dilution is
     a. 0.14 L
     b. 87.5 ml
     c. 630 ml
     d. 0.875 L

111. A stock solution of atropine sulfate has a concentration of 2.2 mg/ml. It may also be used clinically as a 0.05% solution. The volume of the more concentrated atropine solution required to prepare 40 ml of the dilute solution is
     a. 17.6 ml
     b. 9.1 ml
     c. 4.4 ml
     d. 0.91 ml

112. The volume of a 1:25 dilution that can be prepared from 150 ml of stock solution is
     a. 3750 ml
     b. 6 L
     c. 6000 ml
     d. 75 ml

113. If a 0.75% solution results from the addition of 380 ml of water to 20 ml of stock solution, the concentration of the stock solution is
     a. 15%
     b. 0.375 mg/ml
     c. 14.25%
     d. 300 mg/ml

114. If you are asked to administer 0.1 mg of epinephrine to an animal with threatened cardiac collapse, how much of a 1:10,000 solution should you inject?
     a. 10 ml
     b. 0.01 ml
     c. 0.1 ml
     d. 1 ml

115. When the doctor orders an intravenous infusion, you need three pieces of information to calculate the flow rate in drops per minute. Which of the following is not relevant to this calculation?
     a. Total volume to be infused
     b. Type of fluid to be delivered
     c. Calibration of the administration set being used (in drops per milliliter)
     d. Duration of the infusion

116. The doctor orders an intravenous infusion to run at 20 ml/hr. Calculate the flow rate using an administration set that delivers 60 drops/ml.
     a. 30 drops/min
     b. 33 drops/min
     c. 20 drops/min
     d. More information is needed

117. Calculate the flow rate for an intravenous infusion of 1 L of fluid to run over 8 hours with a set calibrated at 20 drops/ml.
     a. 20 drops/min
     b. 42 drops/min
     c. 50 drops/min
     d. 125 drops/min

118. Calculating drug dosages involves routine conversion between units of measure within the metric system. Which of the following conversions is not correct?
     a. 3 cc = 3 ml
     b. 1 µg = 1000 mg
     c. 1 kg = 1000 g
     d. 1 L = 1000 ml

119. Which metric conversion is not correct?
     a. 3500 ml = 3.5 L
     b. 520 mg = 0.52 g
     c. 950 µg = 9.5 mg
     d. 750 cc = 0.75 L

120. Which common equivalent is not correct?
     a. 1 tbs = 3 tsp = 15 ml
     b. 1 oz = 30 ml = 2 tbs
     c. 1/2 gr = 64 mg
     d. 1 L of H_2O = 1000 g of H_2O

121. Which equivalent is not correct?
     a. 1 tbs = "1 tablespoonful" = 15 ml
     b. 1 tsp = "1 teaspoonful" = 5 ml
     c. 1 gtt = 1 drop
     d. 1 gr = "1 gram" = 30 ml

Correct answers are on pages 100-104.

122. A doctor's order calls for prednisone at a dosage of 2 mg/kg to be delivered orally to a 7.5-kg cat. How many 5-mg tablets of prednisone would you give the cat?
    a. 1/4
    b. 1
    c. 2
    d. 3

123. You are asked to give a patient phenobarbital po at 2.2 mg/kg. The medication is available in 1/2-gr tablets. How many tablets should you give a 35-lb dog?
    a. 1/4
    b. 1/2
    c. 1
    d. 2

124. A prescription reads "amoxicillin, 750 mg, po bid, × 10 days." The drug is available in 500-mg tablets. How many tablets must you count out to fill this prescription?
    a. 30
    b. 60
    c. 90
    d. 120

125. Diphenhydramine elixir, 25 mg po, is ordered for a 12-year-old, 12.5-kg beagle. The solution contains 12.5 mg/5 ml. What volume should you give to this patient?
    a. 0.5 ml
    b. 2 ml
    c. 10 ml
    d. 20 ml

126. You are asked to give a dog with head trauma 20% mannitol at 0.5 g/kg by slow intravenous injection. You check the record and see that the dog weighs 44 lb. What volume should you give?
    a. 10 ml
    b. 25 ml
    c. 50 ml
    d. 250 ml

127. How much drug does 100 ml of a 10% solution contain?
    a. 0.1 g
    b. 1 g
    c. 10 g
    d. More information is needed

128. You are asked to draw up 2 ml of 50% dextrose in water to give to a hypoglycemic kitten. What volume should you draw into the syringe?
    a. 1 ml
    b. 2 ml
    c. 10 ml
    d. More information is needed

129. To mix a 4% solution in a bottle that contains 5 g of drug powder, how much water should you add?
    a. 12.5 ml
    b. 50 ml
    c. 125 ml
    d. 500 ml

130. To prepare a dose of 0.2 mg of atropine using a solution that contains 400 µg/ml, how much do you draw into the syringe?
    a. 0.05 ml
    b. 0.2 ml
    c. 0.5 ml
    d. 2 ml

131. You are asked to give intravenously 20 mg of furosemide. The solution contains 25 mg/ml. What volume should you draw into the syringe?
    a. 0.8 ml
    b. 1.25 ml
    c. 2.5 ml
    d. The weight of the patient must be known

132. You are asked to prepare 20 mEq of KCl for addition to a 1-L bag of lactated Ringer solution. The solution contains 30 mEq/15 ml. How much should you draw into a syringe to add to the fluid bag?
    a. 10 ml
    b. 20 ml
    c. 30 ml
    d. 40 ml

133. You are asked to infuse fluids intravenously at 50 ml/h. The administration set is calibrated at 60 drops/ml. How fast should you set the drip rate?
    a. 1 drop/min
    b. 10 drops/min
    c. 50 drops/min
    d. 60 drops/min

134. You are asked to infuse intravenously 3 L of 0.9% saline during 24 hours. The administration set is calibrated at 15 drops/ml. How fast should you set the drip rate?
    a. 200 drops/min
    b. 125 drops/min
    c. 31 drops/min
    d. 15 drops/min

135. You are asked to infuse fluids intravenously at 60 drops/min. The drip rate is currently at 7 drops/15 sec. What adjustment in the drip rate is necessary?
    a. No adjustment is necessary
    b. Double the flow rate
    c. Reduce the flow rate by 50%
    d. Increase the flow rate by 25%

136. You are asked to infuse intravenously 1 L of fluids at 25 drops/min over 10 hours. After 5 hours you observe that 650 ml have been given. What adjustment in the drip rate is necessary?
    a. No action is necessary; the IV infusion will be completed on schedule
    b. Rate must be slowed from 25 drops/min to 18 drops/min to complete the infusion as ordered
    c. Rate must be increased from 25 drops/min to 32 drops/min to complete the infusion as ordered
    d. Rate must be slowed from 100 ml/hr to 60 ml/hr to complete the infusion as ordered

137. You are asked to infuse intravenously 750 ml of fluids over 6 hours. The administration set is calibrated at 20 drops/ml. After 2 hours you observe that 300 ml have been infused. What should the adjusted drip rate be?
    a. 8 drops/min
    b. 19 drops/min
    c. 27 drops/min
    d. 38 drops/min

138. You are asked to infuse intravenously 500 ml of fluids over 6 hours. The administration set is calibrated at 20 drops/ml. After 4 hours you observe that only 150 ml have been given. What should the adjusted drip rate be?
    a. 19 drops/min
    b. 25 drops/min
    c. 39 drops/min
    d. 58 drops/min

139. How much 50% dextrose must be added to 1 L of lactated Ringer solution to make a solution that contains 5% dextrose?
    a. 5 ml
    b. 50 ml
    c. 55 ml
    d. 110 ml

140. Diphenhydramine elixir is prescribed at 12.5 mg po q8h. The drug is available in 30-ml bottles that contain 25 mg/5 ml. How long will one bottle last?
    a. 2 days
    b. 4 days
    c. 6 days
    d. 1 week

141. You are asked to prepare a bottle of heparinized saline with a concentration of 4 IU heparin/ml to flush indwelling catheters. The stock sodium heparin solution contains 1000 IU/ml. How much of heparin must be added to each 250-ml bottle of sterile physiologic saline (0.9% NaCl) to make the flushing solution?
    a. 1 ml
    b. 2 ml
    c. 3 ml
    d. 4 ml

142. You are asked to prepare a solution that contains potassium chloride at 20 mEq/L. How much of a 2 mEq/ml solution of KCl should be added to a 500-ml bag of fluids to comply with this order?
    a. 5 ml
    b. 10 ml
    c. 20 ml
    d. 30 ml

143. What is the fluid deficit for a 50-lb dog estimated to be approximately 8% dehydrated?
    a. 500 ml
    b. 1 L
    c. 2 L
    d. 4 L

144. A 1-L sample contains
    a. 1 ml
    b. 10 ml
    c. 100 ml
    d. 1000 ml

Correct answers are on pages 100-104.

145. A 10-cc syringe can hold
  a. 1 ml
  b. 10 ml
  c. 100 ml
  d. 1000 ml

146. A 5-kg dog weighs approximately
  a. 2.5 lb
  b. 5 lb
  c. 7.5 lb
  d. 11 lb

147. A 354-g rat weighs
  a. 0.0354 kg
  b. 0.354 kg
  c. 3.54 kg
  d. 35.4 kg

148. A 450-µg sample contains
  a. 4.5 g
  b. 0.45 g
  c. 0.045 g
  d. 0.00045 g

149. A 3700-cc sample contains
  a. 370 ml
  b. 37 L
  c. 0.37 L
  d. 3.7 L

150. An 11-lb cat weighs approximately
  a. 22 kg
  b. 5 kg
  c. 500 g
  d. 5000 g

151. A 6.2-g sample contains
  a. 3 kg
  b. 3100 mg
  c. 6,200,000 µg
  d. 6200 µg

152. A 0.5 g/ml sample contains
  a. 5 mg/ml
  b. 50 g/100 ml
  c. 5 g/100 ml
  d. 500 mg/100 ml

153. A 500-kg horse weighs approximately
  a. 250 lb
  b. 750 lb
  c. 1100 lb
  d. 1000 lb

154. A 20-dr vial of digitalis contains approximately
  a. 1.5 oz
  b. 2 oz
  c. 2.5 oz
  d. 4 oz

155. A 120-gr aspirin contains approximately
  a. 7.8 mg
  b. 78 mg
  c. 780 mg
  d. 7800 mg

156. A solution of 45 gr/30 ml contains approximately
  a. 100 mg/ml
  b. 450 mg/ml
  c. 10 g/ml
  d. 1 g/100 ml

157. A 12-fl dr bottle contains approximately
  a. 36 ml
  b. 45 ml
  c. 68 ml
  d. 120 ml

158. A 1/120-gr tablet contains approximately
  a. 0.005 mg
  b. 0.05 mg
  c. 0.5 mg
  d. 5 mg

159. A 2-qt container holds
  a. 12 oz
  b. 18 oz
  c. 32 oz
  d. 64 oz

160. A 14-oz bottle contains approximately
  a. 420 ml
  b. 210 ml
  c. 105 ml
  d. 56 ml

161. A 6-tbs dose given bid requires
  a. 2 oz/day
  b. 240 ml/day
  c. 1.8 L for a 10-day supply
  d. 2.6 L for a 2-week supply

162. A dosage of 1 tbs daily requires
  a. 2 oz for a 14-day supply
  b. 5 oz for a 14-day supply
  c. 7 oz for a 14-day supply
  d. 10 oz for a 14-day supply

163. A dosage of 2 tbs bid requires approximately
  a. 16 oz for a 16-day supply
  b. 1 qt for a 16-day supply
  c. 36 oz for a 16-day supply
  d. 2.5 pt for a 16-day supply

164. A dosage of 1.5 tsp bid requires
  a. 8 tbs for a 2-week supply
  b. 1 oz for a 2-week supply
  c. 10 tbs for a 2-week supply
  d. 14 tbs for a 2-week supply

165. A dosage of 5 ml tid equals approximately
  a. 1 tsp/day
  b. 2 tsp/day
  c. 3 tsp/day
  d. 5 tsp/day

166. A dosage of 1 tbs every other day requires approximately
  a. 45 ml for a 2-week supply
  b. 90 ml for a 2-week supply
  c. 105 ml for a 2-week supply
  d. 210 ml for a 2-week supply

167. A 554-kg mare needs sulfadimethoxine at 10 mg/lb daily. It is available as a 40% solution. How much sulfadimethoxine should be administered daily?
  a. 13.85 ml
  b. 138.5 ml
  c. 45.32 ml
  d. 30.5 ml

168. Fenbendazole liquid is available as a 22.2% concentration, and a 45-lb German shorthaired pointer needs 50 mg/lb. How many teaspoons does it require?
  a. 1 tsp
  b. 1.5 tsp
  c. 2 tsp
  d. 3 tsp

169. Procaine penicillin is available in a concentration of 300,000 IU/ml and is administered at 20,000 IU/kg. How much do you give a 900-lb Arabian gelding?
  a. 2.7 ml
  b. 27 ml
  c. 60 ml
  d. 132 ml

170. Altrenogest for horses is available as a 0.22% solution. The daily dosage is 0.044 mg/kg. If you treated a 990-lb Morgan mare for 15 days, how much would you dispense for the client?
  a. 9 ml
  b. 135 ml
  c. 165 ml
  d. 254 ml

171. A 9-month-old female Great Dane is admitted for a routine ovariohysterectomy. The animal weighs 65 lb, and the veterinarian wants to use the following preanesthetic regimen: butorphanol (10 mg/ml) IM at 0.2 mg/kg; acepromazine (10 mg/ml) IM at 0.05 mg/kg; and atropine (0.02% solution) SC at 0.02 mg/kg. How much butorphanol should be administered?
  a. 0.6 ml
  b. 1.3 ml
  c. 2.9 ml
  d. 6 ml

172. A 9-month-old female Great Dane is admitted for a routine ovariohysterectomy. The animal weighs 65 lb, and the veterinarian wants to use the following preanesthetic regimen: butorphanol (10 mg/ml) IM at 0.2 mg/kg; acepromazine (10 mg/ml) IM at 0.05 mg/kg; and atropine (0.02% solution) SC at 0.02 mg/kg. How much acepromazine should be administered?
  a. 0.16 ml
  b. 0.3 ml
  c. 0.7 ml
  d. 1.5 ml

173. A 9-month-old female Great Dane is admitted for a routine ovariohysterectomy. The animal weighs 65 lb, and the veterinarian wants to use the following preanesthetic regimen: butorphanol (10 mg/ml) IM at 0.2 mg/kg; acepromazine (10 mg/ml) IM at 0.05 mg/kg; and atropine (0.02% solution) SC at 0.02 mg/kg. How much atropine should be administered?
  a. 1.43 ml
  b. 3.0 ml
  c. 6.5 ml
  d. 14.3 ml

174. A yearling paint colt is admitted for castration. The animal weighs 700 lb, and the veterinarian wants to use the following regimen: butorphanol (10 mg/ml) IV at 0.02 mg/kg; xylazine (10 mg/ml) IV at 0.2 mg/kg; and ketamine (100 mg/ml) IV at 2.2 mg/kg. How much butorphanol should be administered?
  a. 0.6 ml
  b. 1.4 ml
  c. 3.1 ml
  d. 6 ml

Correct answers are on pages 100-104.

175. A yearling paint colt is admitted for castration. The animal weighs 700 lb, and the veterinarian wants to use the following regimen: butorphanol (10 mg/ml) IV at 0.02 mg/kg; xylazine (10 mg/ml) IV at 0.2 mg/kg; and ketamine (100 mg/ml) IV at 2.2 mg/kg. How much xylazine should be administered?
    a. 3.2 ml
    b. 6.4 ml
    c. 14 ml
    d. 31 ml

176. A yearling paint colt is admitted for castration. The animal weighs 700 lb, and the veterinarian wants to use the following regimen: butorphanol (10 mg/ml) IV at 0.02 mg/kg; xylazine (10 mg/ml) IV at 0.2 mg/kg; and ketamine (100 mg/ml) IV at 2.2 mg/kg. How much ketamine should be administered?
    a. 2.8 ml
    b. 7.0 ml
    c. 15.4 ml
    d. 34 ml

ANSWERS

1. **a** 22 lb ÷ 2.2 lb/kg × 0.2 mg/kg = 2 mg

2. **b** 1 tbs = 3 tsp

3. **a** (30 ml/h) × (60 dr/sec) ÷ (3600 sec/h) = 0.5 drop/sec or 1 drop/2 sec

4. **c** 5% = 50 mg/1 ml or 25 mg/0.5 ml

5. **c** 75 lb × 1 mg/lb ÷ 100 mg/ml = 0.75 ml

6. **b** (3 ml × 2 per day) × 30 days = 180 ml ÷ 30 ml/oz = 6 oz

7. **a** (60 lb) × (70 kcal/lb/day) ÷ (420 kcal/cup) ÷ 2 feedings/day = 5 cups

8. **a** 80 g ÷ 1000 g/kg × 100 mg/kg ÷ 100 mg/ml = 0.08 ml

9. **c** 8 lb ÷ 2.2 lb/kg × 300 μg/kg ÷ 1000 μg/mg ÷ 10 mg/ml = 0.1 ml

10. **d** 5% = 50 mg/ml × 1000 ml/L = 50,000 mg/L; 50,000 mg/L ÷ 500 mg (50% = 500 mg/ml) = 100 ml; (100 ml 50% dextrose + 900 ml water = 1000 ml of 5% dextrose)

11. **b** 12 oz ÷ 16 oz/lb × 1 ml/lb × 6 puppies = 4.5 ml

12. **d** 30 g × 1000 mg/g ÷ 15 mg/ml = 2000 ml

13. **c** 1.5 tablets/dose × 3 doses/day × 30 days = 135 tablets

14. **d** 1 g × 1000 mg/g ÷ 20 mg/ml = 50 ml

15. **d** 6 vials × 10 ml × 50 mg/ml = 3000 mg; 20 ml × 10 mg/ml = 200 mg; 3000 ÷ 200 = 15 vials

16. **d** 20% of 120 ml/hr = 0.2 × 120 ml/hr = 24 ml/hr; 120 ml/hr − 24 ml/hr = 96 ml/hr

17. **b** 0.1 ml ÷ 5 kg × 10 mg/ml = 0.2 mg/kg

18. **c** 5 mg ÷ 10 kg = 0.5 mg/kg

19. **c** 50 g ÷ 1000 g/kg × 4 mg/kg = 0.2 mg ÷ 2 = 0.1 mg

20. **c** 60 ml ÷ 2 ml/min ÷ 60 min/hr = 0.5 hr

21. **a** 6 + 5 + (7 × 0.5) = 14.5

22. **b** (500 mg/ml × 50 ml) + (25 mg/ml × 1000 ml) = (50,000 mg)/1050 L = 47.6 mg/ml = 4.76%

23. **c** 500 − 475 = 25

24. **a** (70 kVp × 20/100) = 14; 70 + 14 = 84

25. **b** (15 ml/breath) × 10 kg = (150 ml/breath) × 10 breaths/min = 1500 ml/min

26. **a** (10 kg) × (10 ml/kg) = 100 ml/breath; 1500 ml/min ÷ 100 ml/breath = 15 breaths/min

27. **d** 3% = (30 ml/1000 ml) × 1000 ml/min × 60 min/hr = 1800 ml/hr

28. **d** 2 ml/100 g × 300 g × 3 = (18 ml) ÷ (15 ml/g) = 1.2 g

29. **c** 1500 kcal/15 oz ÷ 15 = 100 kcal/oz; 300 kcal needed ÷ 100 kcal/oz = 3 oz needed; 3 oz × 30 ml/oz = 90 ml × 2 (dilution) = 180 ml; 180 ml ÷ 45 ml/feeding = 4 feedings

30. **a** 160 ml ÷ 45 ml/feeding = 3.5

31. c (15 + 14 + 14 + 19 + 18) ÷ 5 = 16 mm Hg

32. c 3 units ÷ 100 units/ml = 0.03 ml

33. a 3 units ÷ 30 units/ml = 0.1 ml

34. b 0.1 ml × 50/100 (50%) = 0.05 ml; 1 ml/0.05 ml = 20 tubes

35. d 300 ml × 40/100 (40%) = 120 ml ÷ 0.5 (50%) = 240 ml − 120 ml cells = 120 ml saline

36. b 10 beats/5 sec × 60 sec/min = 120 beats per minute

37. d (115 + 120 + 123 + 121 + 121 + 112) ÷ 6 = 118.66 mm Hg

38. d 2.5 cm/in. × 2 in. = 5 cm

39. c 8 × 5 = 40 cm

40. a 16 oz × 30 ml/1 oz = 480 ml

41. b 400 lb ÷ 2.2 lb/kg = 181.8 kg round up to 182 kg

42. a 18 g × 60/100 (60%) = 10.8 g/lb × 2000 lb/ton = 21,600 g/ton ÷ 1,000 g/kg = 21.6 kg/ton

43. d (20 + 5 + 1 + 2) = 28 total lb; 20 lb of corn ÷ 28 lb total = 71.4%

44. b 32 oz/qt × 4 qt/gal = (128 oz/gal) × 30/100 = 38.4 oz

45. b 30 mEq/L = 0.03 mEq/ml; 2 mEq/hr ÷ 0.03 mEq/ml = 66.667 round up to 67 ml/hr

46. c 4 mg/hr at 30 ml/hr = 4 mg/30 ml = 133.3 mg/1000 ml; 133.3 mg ÷ 30 mg/ml = 4.4 ml

47. c 5% = 50 mg/ml × 100 ml = 5000 mg ÷ (100 ml + 40 ml) = 35.7 mg/ml = 3.57% round up to 3.6%

48. a 0.005 ml × 10 = 0.05 ml

49. b 10 mg/kg/day ÷ 1000 g/kg × 100 g/bird = 1 mg/day × 10 birds = 10 mg

50. a 1050 lb + 825 lb ÷ 2 = 938 lb × 100 head of cattle = 93,800 lb ÷ 100 lb/ml = 938 ml ÷ 250 ml/bottle = 3.75 bottles

51. b

52. a

53. c 50% = 50 g/100 ml or 50,000 mg/100 ml; 50,000 mg/100 ml ÷ 100 ml = 500 mg/ml

54. b French size ÷ 3 = diameter in millimeters, so 12 French ÷ 3 = 4 mm

55. c 28 lb ÷ 2.2 lb/kg × 0.1 mg = 1.27 mg ÷ 1 mg/ml = 1.27 ml

56. d 1.27 ml × 1 mg/ml = 1.27 mg

57. a 7 lb ÷ 2.2 lb/kg × 1 to 5 mg/kg = 3.18 mg to 16 mg

58. d 3.18 to 16 mg ÷ 20 mg/ml = 0.16 ml to 0.8 ml

59. b 8 lb ÷ 20 = 0.4 ml total ÷ 2 = 0.2 ml each

60. b 10 lb ÷ 2.2 lb/kg × (130 − 300 ml/kg/min) = (590 − 1364 ml); the nonrebreathing system should be used because of the animal's size.

61. c 32 lb ÷ 2.2 lb/kg × (25 to 50 ml/kg/min) = 364 ml to 727 ml; the circle system may be used for an animal of this size.

62. b 0.02 ml × 10 mg = 0.2 mg

63. d 1 gr = 64.8 mg

64. c 64.8 mg ÷ 4 = 16.2 mg

65. c 13 lb ÷ 2.2 lb/kg × 2 mg/kg = 11.8 mg ÷ 20 mg/ml = 0.59 ml

66. b 1.2 ml × 300,000 U/ml

67. b

68. b 42 lb ÷ 2.2 lb/kg × 0.3 mg = 5.7 mg ÷ 5 mg/ml = 1.1 ml

69. c 42 lb ÷ 2.2 lb/kg × 0.3 mg/kg = 5.7 mg

70. c 12 lb ÷ 2.2 lb/kg × 1 unit/kg

71. d 5.5 units ÷ 100 units/ml = 0.05 ml

72. c 1000 ml ÷ 100 ml = 10

73. d 1 unit/100 ml

74. d 6 units × 100 ml/unit = 600 ml × 60 gtt/ml = 36,000 gtt ÷ 7200 seconds = 5 gtt/sec

75. a 5.5 lb ÷ 2.2 lb/kg × 100 units/kg = 250 units

76. **c** 25 units ÷ 2000 units/ml = 0.0125 ml

77. **d** 10 ÷ 2.2 = 4.5 kg; 1/4 tsp = 1.25 ml (1 tsp = 5 ml) per dose × 2 = 2.5 ml/day

78. **a** 5 mEq ÷ 5 ml = 1 mEq/ml; 2 ml × concentration (1 mEq/ml) = 2 mEq

79. **c** square meters = conversion from body weight to body surface area

80. **b** 33 lb ÷ 2.2 lb/kg = 15 kg × 0.09 (deficit) = 1.35 kg fluid loss × 1000 ml/kg of fluid

81. **d** 128 × 30 ml/oz = 3840 ml ÷ 8 = 480 ml iodine; 3840 ml total volume − 480 ml of iodine = 3360 ml of alcohol

82. **c** 10 lb ÷ 2.2 lb/kg × 0.12 (deficit) × 1000 ml/kg

83. **b** 1 cup = 8 oz × 30 ml/oz = 240 ml divided by 7 total parts = 34.3 ml milk; 240 ml total − 34.3 ml = 205.7 ml water

84. **a** 450 ml × 50 mg/ml (5%) ÷ 500 mg/ml (50%) = 45 ml 50% glucose

85. **b** 25% solution = 25 g/100 ml = 250 mg/ml

86. **d** 0.85% solution = 8.5 mg/ml × 5000 ml = 42,500 mg ÷ 1000 mg/g = 42.5 g

87. **a** 1.2% solution = 1.2 g/100 ml = 1200 mg/100 ml = 600 mg/50 ml

88. **b** 2.5% solution = 2.5 g/100 ml = 5 g/200 ml

89. **c** Total dilution = (1:5) × (1:3) × (1:2) × (1:6) = 1:180. Total dilution factor (DF) = 180. Original concentration = Final concentration × DF; 0.4 mg/ml (final concentration × 180 [DF]) = 72 mg/ml = 7.2%

90. **b** $C_1V_1 = C_2V_2$; 6% × 12.5 ml = 0.5% × V_2; V_2 (final volume) = 150 ml; 150 ml − 12.5 ml stock = 137.5 ml water

91. **d** Total dilution = (1:5) × (1:10) × (1:3) × (1:4) = 1:600; [F] = [O] × 1/D = 30% × 1/600 = 0.05%

92. **d** $C_1V_1 = C_2V_2$; 45 mg/ml × V_1 = 9 mg/ml × 750 ml; V_1 (volume of stock) = 150 ml

93. **b** 2.50 g/400 ml = 0.625 g/100 ml = 0.625%

94. **a** 4.5% solution = 4.5 g/100 ml; 4.5 × 5 = 22.5 g/500 ml

95. **b** Total dilution = (1:10) × (1:3) × (1:5) × (1:3) = 1:450; Total dilution factor = 450; [O] = [F] × DF = 100 μg/ml × 450 = 45,000 μg/ml = 45 mg/ml = 4.5%

96. **a** 12% v/v solution = 12 ml/100 ml = Xml/275 ml; 100X = 12 × 275; 12 × 275 = 3,300/100 = 33 ml

97. **c** 4500 mg/3.6 L = 4.5 g/3600 ml = 0.125 g/100 ml = 0.125%

98. **b** The gram is the basic unit of mass in the metric system; 1 kilogram = 10^3 grams; 1 milligram = 10^{-3} grams; 1 microgram = 10^{-6} grams

99. **b** 1 kg = 1000 g

100. **d** pg = picogram; 1 pg = 10^{-12} g; 24.3 pg = 24.3 × 10^{-12} g

101. **a** fl = femtoliter; 1 fl = 10^{-15} L; 66.5 fl = 66.5 × 10^{-15} L

102. **c** The meter is the basic unit of length in the metric system; 1 millimeter = 10^{-3} meters; 1 centimeter = 10^{-2} meters; 1 kilometer = 10^3 meters

103. **c** 1 km = 10^3 m or 10^6 mm; so 485 km = 4.85 × 10^8 mm

104. **b** 250 cc = 250 ml = 0.25 L

105. **c** 1 ton = 1000 kg; 1 kg = 2.204 lb

106. **c** 1 cm = 10 mm = 10,000 μ (microns)

107. **d** 2.204 lb = 1 kg

108. **a** 1 oz = 28.4 g; 1 g = 1000 mg

109. **c** 1 in = 2.5 cm

110. **b** 3.5 L = 3500 ml; 3500 ml/40 = 87.5 ml

111. **b** $C_1V_1 = C_2V_2$; 2.2 mg/ml × V_1 = 0.5 mg/ml × 40 ml; V_1 = 9.1 ml

112. **a** 150 ml × 25 = 3750 ml

113. **a** 20 ml + 380 ml = 400 ml; dilution = 20:400 = 1:20. [O] = [F] × DF = 0.75% × 20 = 15%

114. **d** 1:10,000 = 0.01% = 0.1 mg/ml; volume = 1.0 ml

115. **b** The calculation is performed the same regardless of the type of fluid.

116. **c** 20 ml/h × 1 h/60 min × 60 drops/ml = 20 drops/min

117. **b** 125 ml/h × 1 h/60 min × 20 drops/ml = 42 drops/min

118. **b** Know your metric conversions and watch your decimal places: 1 mg = 1000 μg

119. **c** 1 mg = 10^3 μg

120. **c** Study apothecary and household measurements, as well as the metric system. 1 gr = 64 mg, so 1/2 gr = 32 mg

121. **d** Do not confuse abbreviations: g = gram; gr = grain; 1 gr = 64 mg

122. **d** 7.5 kg × 2 mg/kg × 1 tablet/5 mg = 3 tablets

123. **c** 35 lb × 1 kg/2.2 lb × 2.2 mg/kg = 35 mg; each 1/2 gr tablet = 32 mg

124. **a** 750 mg × 1 tablet/500 mg; 1-1/2 tablets twice daily = 3 tablets/day × 10 days = 30 tablets

125. **c** 25 mg × 5 ml/12.5 mg = 10 ml

126. **c** 44 lb × 1 kg/2.2 lb × 500 mg/kg (0.5 g/kg)/200 mg/ml (20% = 200 mg/ml) = 50 ml

127. **c** "%" means "grams per hundred milliliters"

128. **b** The order tells you what volume to draw up.

129. **c** 4% = 4 g/100 ml = 5 X = 125 ml

130. **c** 0.2 mg = 200 μg; 200 μg/400 μg/ml = 0.5 ml

131. **a** 20 mg × 1 ml/25 mg = 0.8 ml

132. **a** 20 mEq/L × 15 ml/30 mEq = 10 ml

133. **c** 50 ml/h × 1 h/60 min × 60 drops/ml = 50 drops/min

134. **c** 3000 ml/24 h = 125 ml/h × 1 h/60 min = 2 ml/min × 15 drops/ml = 31 drops/min

135. **b** 7 drops/15 sec = X drops/60 sec = 28 drops/60 sec

136. **b** 1000 − 650 = 350 ml remain; 10 − 5 = 5 hr remain; 350 ml/5 hr × 1 hr/60 min × 15 drops/ml = 17.5 drops/min

137. **d** 750 − 300 = 450 ml remain; 6 − 2 = 4 hr remain; 450 ml/4 hr × 1 hr/60 min × 20 drops/ml = 37.5 drops/min

138. **d** 500 − 150 = 350 ml remain; 6 − 4 = 2 hr remain; 350 ml/2 hr × 1 hr/60 min × 20 drops/ml = 58 drops/min

139. **d** $C_1V_1 = C_2V_2$; 50 × X = 5 × (1000 + X); solve for X

140. **b** 12.5 mg × 5 ml/25 mg = 2.5 ml per dose = 7.5 ml per day; 30 ml/7.5 = 4 days

141. **a** 4 IU/ml × 250 ml × 1 ml/1000 IU = 1 ml heparin per 250-ml bottle

142. **a** 20 mEq/L × 1 ml/2 mEq = 10 mEq/L; thus, add 5 ml per 500-ml bag

143. **c** 55 lb × 1 kg/2.2 lb × 1 L/1 kg × 0.08 (1 kg = 1 L; 8% = 0.08) = 2 L

144. **d** 1 L = 1000 ml

145. **b** Cubic centimeters and milliliters are equivalent.

146. **d** 1 kg = 2.2 lb

147. **b** 1 kg = 1000 g

148. **d** 1,000,000 μg = 1 g

149. **d** 1 L = 1000 ml = 1000 cc

150. **b** 1 kg = 2.2 lb

151. **c** 1 g = 1,000,000 μg

152. **b** 0.5 g/ml = 50 g/100 cc = 50 g/100 ml

153. **c** 1 kg = 2.2 lb

154. **c** 1 dr (dram) = 1/8 oz

155. **d** 1 gr = 65 mg

156. **a** 1 gr = 65 mg

157. **b** 1 fl dr = 1/8 oz or 3.7 ml

158. **c** 1 gr = 65 mg

159. **c** 1 qt = 32 oz

160. **a** 1 oz = 30 ml

161. **c** 1 tbs = 1/2 oz = 15 ml

162. **c** 1 tbs = 1/2 oz

163. **b** 1 tbs = 1/2 oz; 16 oz = 1 pt; 32 oz = 1 qt

164. **d** 3 tsp/day = 1 tbs/day

165. **c** 1 tsp = 5 ml

166. **c** 1 tbs = 15 ml

167. **d** Example of percent calculations: In performing percent calculations, the important aspect to remember is that % is equal to grams per 100 ml. Therefore, in this case, sulfadimethoxine is 40% or 40 g/100 ml or 400 mg/ml. The mare weighs 554 kg, which is equal to 1218.8 lb (554 kg × 2.2 lb/kg), and the dosage is 10 mg/lb. Thus, the mare requires 12,188 mg of sulfadimethoxine/day (1218.8 lb/mare × 10 mg/lb). We know that 40% sulfadimethoxine is equal to 400 mg/ml, so the mare needs a daily dose of 30.5 ml (12,188 mg ÷ 400 mg/ml).

168. **c** 45 lb × 50 mg/lb × 1 ml/222 mg (22.2% = 222 mg/ml) = 10 ml = 2 tsp

169. **b** 900 lb × 1 kg/2.2 lb × 20,000 IU × 1/300,000 IU/ml = 27 ml

170. **b** 990 lb × 1 kg/2.2 lb × 0.044 mg/kg × 1 ml/2.2 mg (0.22% = 2.2 mg/ml) × 15 days = 135 ml

171. **a** Sample calculation: The problem should be divided into three parts.
    1. Calculate the correct weight. The dog weighs 65 lb or 29.5 kg (2.2 lb/kg).
    2. Calculate the total amount of medication needed. The dosage for butorphanol is 0.2 mg/kg. Thus, a 29.5-kg animal needs 5.9 mg of butorphanol (29.5 kg × 0.2 mg/kg) for the total dose.
    3. Calculate the actual volume to be administered, which requires knowing the concentration of the medication. In this case, butorphanol is available in a concentration of 10 mg/ml. Thus, the animal needs approximately 0.6 ml (5.9 mg ÷ 10 mg/ml).

172. **a** 65 lb × 1 kg/2.2 lb × 0.05 mg/kg × 1 ml/10 mg = 0.16 ml

173. **b** 65 lb × 1 kg/2.2 lb × 0.02 mg/kg × 1 ml/0.2 mg/ml = 2.95 ml

174. **a** 700 lb × 1 kg/2.2 lb × 0.02 mg/kg × 1 ml/10 mg = 0.6 ml

175. **b** 700 lb × 1 kg/2.2 lb × 0.2 mg/kg × 1 ml/10 mg = 6.4 ml

176. **b** 700 lb × 1 kg/2.2 lb × 2.2 mg/kg × 1 ml/100 mg = 7 ml

Medical Terminology

Sarah Wagner • *Joann Colville*

QUESTIONS

1. What is the correct term for blood in the urine?
   a. Hemolysis
   b. Uremia
   c. Hematuria
   d. Hemocentesis

2. What is the correct term for an increased leukocyte count not due to cancer?
   a. Leukemia
   b. Leukopenia
   c. Leukophilia
   d. Leukocytosis

3. What organ or area is affected by mastitis?
   a. Uterus
   b. Testicle
   c. Hands
   d. Mammary gland

4. What is the correct term for sticking a needle into a lymph node and aspirating cells for examination?
   a. Punch biopsy
   b. Lymphostomy
   c. Lymphocentesis
   d. Histopathology

5. What is the correct term for an inflammation of the urinary bladder?
   a. Nephritis
   b. Cystitis
   c. Cystocentesis
   d. Cystouritis

6. What is the correct term for the surgical removal of a mammary gland?
   a. Mastotomy
   b. Mastostomy
   c. Mastectomy
   d. Mammotomy

7. What does the term *anorexia* mean?
   a. Low erythrocyte count
   b. Not eating
   c. Depressed
   d. Abnormal heart rhythm

8. What is the correct term for an instrument used to examine ears?
   a. Ophthalmoscope
   b. Laryngoscope
   c. Laparoscope
   d. Otoscope

9. What term means "fever"?
   a. Hypothermia
   b. Pyrexia
   c. Hyperthermitis
   d. Caliente

10. What is the term for an inflammation of the brain and spinal cord?
    a. Hydrocephalus
    b. Encephalitis
    c. Encephalomyelitis
    d. Epilepsy

11. What is the term that refers to a benign black tumor?
    a. Melanoma
    b. Melanocarcinoma
    c. Melanosis
    d. Xanthoma

12. What is the name of the device used to count blood cells?
    a. Hematoscope
    b. Hemocytometer
    c. Hematometer
    d. Leukocytometer

Correct answers are on pages 116-120.

13. A dog's spleen is enlarged. What is the correct term for this condition?
    a. Splenomegaly
    b. Hypoplasia
    c. Analgesia
    d. Splenoplasia

14. What is the correct term for a radiograph taken with air in the urinary bladder?
    a. Cystogram
    b. Aerocystogram
    c. Electrocystogram
    d. Pneumocystogram

15. What is the correct term for surgically creating a new opening into the urethra?
    a. Urethrotomy
    b. Ureterostomy
    c. Urethrostomy
    d. Urethrectomy

16. What is the correct term for heart muscle disease?
    a. Pericarditis
    b. Electrocardiopathy
    c. Endocarditis
    d. Cardiomyopathy

17. What is the term that means "a condition of death"?
    a. Autolysis
    b. Pathosis
    c. Necritis
    d. Necrosis

18. Sometimes lymph nodes enlarge because of an increase in the number of cells. What is the term for overdevelopment because of an increase in the number of cells?
    a. Hypertrophy
    b. Adenopathy
    c. Hyperplasia
    d. Metastasis

19. What term refers to an inflammation of the kidney?
    a. Nephritis
    b. Nephrosis
    c. Renalitis
    d. Uremia

20. What structure is inflamed in a keratitis?
    a. Prostate
    b. Retina
    c. Conjunctiva
    d. Cornea

21. A dog is born with a soft, swollen area over the anterior cranium. The veterinarian suspects "water on the brain." What is the correct medical term for this condition?
    a. Hydroencephalitis
    b. Cephalohydrosis
    c. Hydronephrosis
    d. Hydrocephalus

22. Orthopedics is the medical specialty concerned with
    a. Muscle and bone
    b. Neoplasia
    c. The reproductive system
    d. Aged animals

23. Which of the following cells is normally found in the red bone marrow?
    a. Oocyte
    b. Squamous cell
    c. Myocyte
    d. Myelocyte

24. What is the term for a blood clot that travels through the circulation?
    a. Thrombus
    b. Thromboembolus
    c. Embolus
    d. Stroke

25. Which of the following literally means the "study of no feeling"?
    a. Analgesiology
    b. Analgia
    c. Hypoesthesiology
    d. Anesthesiology

26. What is the name of the area where the upper and lower eyelids meet?
    a. Conjunctiva
    b. Cornea
    c. Uvea
    d. Canthus

27. A collie is born with eyes smaller than normal. What is this called?
    a. Hyperophthalmia
    b. Anophthalmia
    c. Microphthalmia
    d. Ophthalmitis

28. A cataract is found in what structure?
    a. Kidney
    b. Lens of the eye
    c. Brain
    d. Reproductive tract

29. Which of the following terms means "difficult breathing"?
    a. Dystrophy
    b. Tachypnea
    c. Pneumothorax
    d. Dyspnea

30. What is the term for a malignant bone tumor?
    a. Osteodystrophy
    b. Osteosarcoma
    c. Osteomyelitis
    d. Osteomalacia

31. What is the term for the procedure in which a sterile needle is inserted into the chest and fluid is withdrawn into a syringe?
    a. Cystocentesis
    b. Thoracorrhagia
    c. Pneumogenesis
    d. Thoracocentesis

32. What term refers to the medical specialty that deals primarily with tumors?
    a. Oncology
    b. Neoplasology
    c. Neonatology
    d. Cancerology

33. The veterinarian has noted in a dog's record that alopecia is present. This means which of the following conditions is present?
    a. Itching
    b. Diarrhea
    c. Not eating
    d. Hair loss

34. What term refers to an animal drinking more water than normal?
    a. Hydrophilia
    b. Polydipsia
    c. Polyphagia
    d. Multihydrosis

35. A dog has had a cast on its leg for 5 weeks. When the cast is removed, the muscles on the affected leg are smaller than on the other leg. What is the term used to describe this condition?
    a. Muscular dystrophy
    b. Muscular atrophy
    c. Muscular dysplasia
    d. Muscular hyperplasia

36. Which of the following terms refers to a white blood cell count below normal?
    a. Leukopenia
    b. Leukocytosis
    c. Leukemia
    d. Anemia

37. A dog has swallowed a ball, and it is stuck in its stomach. What is the name of the surgical procedure performed to remove it?
    a. Gastrectomy
    b. Gastrostomy
    c. Gastrotomy
    d. Gastropexy

38. What is the correct term for a drug administered to relieve pain?
    a. Analgesic
    b. Anesthetic
    c. Antipyretic
    d. Antitussive

39. A cat that has already delivered two kittens has another kitten stuck in the birth canal and is having difficulty giving birth to it. What term is used to describe this condition?
    a. Pyometra
    b. Hysterectomy
    c. Dystocia
    d. Paronychia

40. What does the term *pathogenic* refer to?
    a. Neoplasia
    b. Disease causing
    c. Unknown cause
    d. Road to nowhere

41. The veterinarian indicates in the record that a cat has otitis. What structure is affected?
    a. Eye
    b. Bone
    c. Nose
    d. Ear

42. An anesthetized cat's heart rate has slowed to an abnormally low 30 beats per minute. Which of the following terms best describes this condition?
    a. Arrhythmia
    b. Murmur
    c. Bradycardia
    d. Tachycardia

43. The veterinarian aspirates pus from the chest of a cat. What is the term for this condition?
    a. Pyothorax
    b. Pneumonia
    c. Peritonitis
    d. Pyoderma

Correct answers are on pages 116-120.

44. An anesthetized dog has a blue color to its mucous membranes. What is the term used to describe this condition?
    a. Icterus
    b. Lipemia
    c. Cyanosis
    d. Xanthosis

45. What term refers to a benign fatty tumor?
    a. Lipocarcinoma
    b. Lipoma
    c. Obesioma
    d. Liposarcoma

46. What is an electrocardiogram?
    a. A surgical procedure on the heart
    b. Looking at sound waves from the heart
    c. An electrical recording of the heart
    d. A radiograph of the heart

47. A cat is exhibiting anisocoria. What is occurring?
    a. The cat is not eating
    b. The cat is lame
    c. The cat is scratching
    d. The cat's pupils are different sizes

48. The granules in the cytoplasm of an eosinophil are
    a. Purple
    b. Blue
    c. Red
    d. Black

49. To *torse* means
    a. To have decreased circulation
    b. To fill with gas
    c. To twist
    d. To displace

50. The word part that means "long" is
    a. Dolicho
    b. Meso
    c. Brachy
    d. Trophy

51. The word part that means "growth" is
    a. Dolicho
    b. Meso
    c. Brachy
    d. Trophy

52. The word part that means "middle" is
    a. Dolicho
    b. Meso
    c. Brachy
    d. Trophy

53. The word part that means "short" is
    a. Dolicho
    b. Meso
    c. Brachy
    d. Trophy

54. Inflammation of the gums is
    a. Stomatitis
    b. Glossitis
    c. Gingivitis
    d. Pharyngitis

55. Inflammation of all or any of the mucous membranes of the mouth is
    a. Stomatitis
    b. Glossitis
    c. Gingivitis
    d. Pharyngitis

56. Inflammation of the tongue is
    a. Stomatitis
    b. Glossitis
    c. Gingivitis
    d. Pharyngitis

57. Inflammation of the throat is
    a. Stomatitis
    b. Glossitis
    c. Gingivitis
    d. Pharyngitis

58. Inflammation of the salivary glands is
    a. Sialoschesis
    b. Sialogen
    c. Sialoadenitis
    d. Sialocele

59. A salivary cyst is a
    a. Sialoschesis
    b. Sialogen
    c. Sialoadenitis
    d. Sialocele

60. Suppression of the flow of saliva is
    a. Sialoschesis
    b. Sialogen
    c. Sialoadenitis
    d. Sialocele

61. An agent that induces salivation is a
    a. Sialoschesis
    b. Sialogen
    c. Sialoadenitis
    d. Sialocele

62. Difficulty standing is
    a. Dyschezia
    b. Dyspnea
    c. Dysphagia
    d. Ataxia

63. Difficulty swallowing is
    a. Dyschezia
    b. Dyspnea
    c. Dysphagia
    d. Ataxia

64. Difficulty defecating is
    a. Dyschezia
    b. Dyspnea
    c. Dysphagia
    d. Ataxia

65. Difficulty breathing is
    a. Dyschezia
    b. Dyspnea
    c. Dysphagia
    d. Ataxia

66. A displaced or malpositioned organ is referred to as
    a. Epistaxis
    b. Ecchymosis
    c. Ectopic
    d. Ectropion

67. An eyelid that is turning outward is described as an
    a. Epistaxis
    b. Ecchymosis
    c. Ectopic
    d. Ectropion

68. Blood under the skin produced by ruptured blood vessels in the area is known as
    a. Epistaxis
    b. Ecchymosis
    c. Ectopic
    d. Ectropion

69. A nose-bleed is also known as an
    a. Epistaxis
    b. Ecchymosis
    c. Ectopic
    d. Ectropion

70. Accumulation of water in the thorax is known as
    a. Chylothorax
    b. Pyothorax
    c. Hydrothorax
    d. Pneumothorax

71. Accumulation of fatty fluid in the thorax is known as
    a. Chylothorax
    b. Pyothorax
    c. Hydrothorax
    d. Pneumothorax

72. Accumulation of purulent fluid in the thorax is known as
    a. Chylothorax
    b. Pyothorax
    c. Hydrothorax
    d. Pneumothorax

73. Accumulation of air in the thorax is known as
    a. Chylothorax
    b. Pyothorax
    c. Hydrothorax
    d. Pneumothorax

74. Inflammation of the lacrimal gland is
    a. Dacryoadenalgia
    b. Dacryoadenitis
    c. Dacryocystoptosis
    d. Dacryoma

75. A tumor of the lacrimal gland would be identified as a
    a. Dacryoadenalgia
    b. Dacryoadenitis
    c. Dacryocystoptosis
    d. Dacryoma

76. A painful lacrimal gland is described as
    a. Dacryoadenalgia
    b. Dacryoadenitis
    c. Dacryocystoptosis
    d. Dacryoma

77. Prolapse of the lacrimal gland is described as
    a. Dacryoadenalgia
    b. Dacryoadenitis
    c. Dacryocystoptosis
    d. Dacryoma

78. A pug, with its very short nose, is an example of a __ breed.
    a. Dolichocephalic
    b. Mesaticephalic
    c. Brachiocephalic
    d. Prognathous

79. A greyhound, with its very long nose, is an example of a __ breed.
    a. Dolichocephalic
    b. Mesaticephalic
    c. Brachiocephalic
    d. Brachygnathous

Correct answers are on pages 116-120.

80. The term *marsupialization* refers to
    a. Creation of a communication between two vessels
    b. Creation of opening into an organ
    c. Creation of opening from a cyst to the body surface
    d. Creation of incision into an organ

81. Retinomalacia refers to
    a. Inflammation of the retina
    b. Softening of the retina
    c. Tumor of the retina
    d. Splitting of the retina

82. Tenesmus refers to
    a. Paralysis of the anal sphincter
    b. Straining to defecate
    c. Uncontrollable defecation
    d. Copious amounts of diarrhea

83. Steatorrhea refers to
    a. Fat in the stool
    b. Blood in the stool
    c. Mucus in the stool
    d. Plant material in the stool

84. Coprophagia refers to
    a. Increased appetite
    b. Ingesting feces
    c. Excessive amount of stool
    d. Difficulty eating

85. Osteomalacia refers to
    a. Inflammation of the bone
    b. Cancer of the bone
    c. Infection of the bone
    d. Softening of the bone

86. Epiphora refers to
    a. Excessive urination
    b. Excessive salivation
    c. Excessive tear flow
    d. Excessive defecation

87. Hyperesthesic animals are
    a. Abnormally sensitive to stimuli
    b. Abnormally unresponsive to stimuli
    c. Abnormally sensitive to anesthesia
    d. Abnormally unresponsive to anesthesia

88. Hypernatremia refers to a/an
    a. Deficiency of sodium in the blood
    b. Deficiency of sodium in the urine
    c. Excessive amount of sodium in the urine
    d. Excessive amount of sodium in the blood

89. A condition in which voluntary muscular movements overreach the intended goal is
    a. Hypermetria
    b. Hyperorexia
    c. Hypermastia
    d. Hypermetropia

90. Mastication refers to the process of
    a. Defecating
    b. Swallowing
    c. Chewing
    d. Urinating

91. A meatus is
    a. The body of a muscle
    b. The area distal to the tarsus
    c. The joining of two vessels
    d. An opening or passage

92. Prehension refers to
    a. Retaining
    b. Grasping
    c. Comprehending
    d. Releasing

93. The term that pertains to a jaundice color is
    a. Ichthyoid
    b. Icteric
    c. Idiopathic
    d. Ichor

94. Atelectasis results in a/an
    a. Agglutination
    b. Nose-bleed
    c. Collapsed lung
    d. Failure of muscle coordination

95. Oliguria refers to
    a. Difficult urination
    b. No urination
    c. Excessive amount of urination
    d. Small amount of urination

96. Otoplasty refers to
    a. Reconstruction of the ear
    b. Removal of the ear
    c. Reconstruction of the eye
    d. Removal of the eye

97. The term that means "itching" is
    a. Puritis
    b. Pruritus
    c. Putrid
    d. Psoriasis

98. The term *myositis* refers to
    a. Inflammation of the uterus
    b. Inflammation of the heart
    c. Inflammation of the kidney
    d. Inflammation of the muscle

99. The endosteum is found on
    a. The interior surfaces of bones
    b. The outer surfaces of bones
    c. The interior of the heart
    d. The interior of the thorax

100. The term for an undersized brain is
    a. Dystrophy
    b. Hydrocephaly
    c. Microcephaly
    d. Hypertrophy

101. What is the term used to describe treatment using ultracold liquids?
    a. Lithotripsy
    b. Hydrotherapy
    c. Microsurgery
    d. Cryotherapy

102. The prefix that relates to water is
    a. Hidro-
    b. Hydro-
    c. Xantho-
    d. Pyo-

103. The term that means "impaired or difficult breathing" is
    a. Dyspnea
    b. Tachypnea
    c. Stridor
    d. Rales

104. The suffix that means "inflammation" is
    a. -osis
    b. -itis
    c. -opathy
    d. -emia

105. The term that refers to an excision or surgical removal of the kidney is
    a. Hepatopexy
    b. Hepatectomy
    c. Nephrectomy
    d. Nephropexy

106. An animal that suffers from this condition is having difficulty ingesting or swallowing food.
    a. Dysphagia
    b. Dyspnea
    c. Dystrophy
    d. Indigestion

107. A condition characterized by a decrease in red blood cells is
    a. Anencephaly
    b. Anorexia
    c. Angina
    d. Anemia

108. The surgical removal of a retained testicle is called
    a. Cryptectomy
    b. Cryptorchidectomy
    c. Orchidectomy
    d. Monorchidectomy

109. The term that refers to surgically creating a new opening in the intestines and connecting it to the outside of the body or to another hollow organ is
    a. Enterotomy
    b. Enterostomy
    c. Enterorrhaphy
    d. Enteropexy

110. The term that refers to making an incision through the abdominal wall is
    a. Laparostomy
    b. Enterotomy
    c. Enterostomy
    d. Laparotomy

111. The procedure used to achieve surgical fixation of the true stomach compartment of a cow is
    a. Abomasotomy
    b. Rumenotomy
    c. Abomasopexy
    d. Rumenopexy

112. The term that means "joint pain" is
    a. Arthralgia
    b. Arthropathy
    c. Arthritis
    d. Arthrogryposis

113. The term that refers to an animal infected with yeast of the family *Candida* is
    a. Candidalgia
    b. Candidopathy
    c. Candiditis
    d. Candidiasis

114. Dilatation, expansion, or distention of the lungs results in
    a. Emphysema
    b. Empyema
    c. Pleurisy
    d. Pleuritis

Correct answers are on pages 116-120.

115. A disorder or disease of a bone is a/an
    a. Ostealgia
    b. Osteopathy
    c. Chondralgia
    d. Chondropathy

116. A slow heart rate is described as
    a. Anacardia
    b. Bradycardia
    c. Microcardia
    d. Tachycardia

117. Lack of any urine flow is described as
    a. Anuria
    b. Dysuria
    c. Oliguria
    d. Polyuria

118. The term that refers to low blood pressure is
    a. Hypertension
    b. Hypocardia
    c. Hypotension
    d. Hypercardia

119. What condition involves pus?
    a. Chylothorax
    b. Nephritis
    c. Cystitis
    d. Pyoderma

120. The surgical removal of the uterus is
    a. Salpingectomy
    b. Orchiectomy
    c. Hysterectomy
    d. Episiectomy

121. The combining form related to the testes is
    a. Salpingo-
    b. Orchi-
    c. Hystero-
    d. Episio-

122. The combining form related to the oviducts is
    a. Salpingo-
    b. Orchi-
    c. Hystero-
    d. Episio-

123. The term that refers to the removal of the testes is
    a. Vasectomy
    b. Orchidectomy
    c. Hysterectomy
    d. Spaying

124. The two word parts that have the same meaning are
    a. Costo- and chondro-
    b. Adipo- and lipo-
    c. Cephalo- and cranio-
    d. Mandibulo- and maxillo-

125. The medical description used to classify flat-faced breeds such as bulldogs and Persian cats is
    a. Hyperocular
    b. Dyspneic
    c. Pediatric
    d. Brachygnathia

126. The junction where the ribs join the cartilage from the sternum is
    a. Costochondral
    b. Thoracosternal
    c. Thoracoabdominal
    d. Thoracochondral

127. The surgical procedure that involves cutting the eardrum to drain exudate is a
    a. Costotomy
    b. Ototomy
    c. Myringotomy
    d. Pinnotomy

128. The medical term for declawing is
    a. Phalangectomy
    b. Digitectomy
    c. Plicectomy
    d. Onychectomy

129. Two words or word parts that mean the same thing are
    a. Micro- and megalo-
    b. Spondylo- and chondro-
    c. Pilo- and tricho-
    d. Ankylo- and tarso-

130. Any localized, abnormal change in tissue structure is called a
    a. Lesion
    b. Nidus
    c. Nevus
    d. Ulcer

131. A disease of the vertebrae or the spinal column is called a/an
    a. Neurosis
    b. Spondylosis
    c. Encephalosis
    d. Osteosis

132. The condition of being bent, looped, or fused is
   a. Sclerosis
   b. Megalosis
   c. Ankylosis
   d. Atelectasis

133. The procedure used to destroy a stone or calculus is
   a. Sclerotripsy
   b. Nephrotomy
   c. Cystotomy
   d. Lithotripsy

134. The term used to describe pathologic hardening of the arteries is
   a. Arteriosclerosis
   b. Atherosclerosis
   c. Vasoectasia
   d. Vasodura

135. The term used to describe enlargement of the liver is
   a. Microhepatitis
   b. Hepatitis
   c. Hepatomegaly
   d. Cholelithiasis

136. The suffix that means "paralysis" is
   a. -liasis
   b. -lysis
   c. -phagia
   d. -plegia

137. The term that means "abnormal growth" is
   a. Paresis
   b. Hyperplasia
   c. Dysplasia
   d. Dysplegia

138. The condition that is described as a weakness or paralysis of one side of the body is
   a. Hemiparesis
   b. Paralysis
   c. Quadriplegia
   d. Diplegia

139. The enlargement of tissue due to increased cell numbers is a
   a. Hypertrophy
   b. Hyperlysis
   c. Hyperplasia
   d. Hyperplegia

140. A plane parallel to the median plane is
   a. Transverse
   b. Axial
   c. Sagittal
   d. Oblique

141. The surface of a tooth closest to the tongue is
   a. Lingual
   b. Mesial
   c. Buccal
   d. Occlusal

142. The foot is __ relative to the knee.
   a. Proximal
   b. Distal
   c. Medial
   d. Oblique

143. The skeleton of a limb is part of the __ skeleton.
   a. Appendicular
   b. Axial
   c. Sagittal
   d. Proximal

144. Where on an animal is an ectoparasite found?
   a. Stomach
   b. Intestines
   c. Lungs
   d. Skin

145. Where is the submandibular lymph node found?
   a. Next to the ear
   b. Under the arm
   c. Under the jaw
   d. Behind the knee

146. The inside of a horse's leg is the __ surface of the leg.
   a. Dorsal
   b. Ventral
   c. Medial
   d. Lateral

147. Where are the parathyroid glands located?
   a. Above the thyroid glands
   b. Below the thyroid glands
   c. Next to the thyroid glands
   d. On the thyroid glands

148. A purulent condition always involves
   a. Bacteria
   b. Viruses
   c. Injury
   d. Pus

149. What does *hypodermic* mean?
   a. For injection
   b. Under the skin
   c. Single use
   d. Sterile

Correct answers are on pages 116-120.

150. When describing bone fractures, the two terms that mean the same thing are
    a. *Closed* and *compound*
    b. *Compound* and *comminuted*
    c. *Comminuted* and *open*
    d. *Open* and *compound*

151. Spherical bacterium found grouped in pairs is
    a. Staphylococcus
    b. Bacillus
    c. Streptococcus
    d. Diplococcus

152. The condition in which the tissues turn blue is
    a. Leukosis
    b. Cyanosis
    c. Melanosis
    d. Xanthosis

153. The condition in which the skin hardens and is replaced with connective tissue is
    a. Dermatitis
    b. Dermatophytosis
    c. Scleroderma
    d. Xanthoderma

154. The cancerous condition of an overproduction of white blood cells is
    a. Leukemia
    b. Leukocytosis
    c. Leukocyte
    d. Leukopenia

155. The cancerous condition that involves black skin lesions is
    a. Leukosis
    b. Lymphoma
    c. Melanoma
    d. Dermatosis

156. An intra articular injection is given
    a. In the joint
    b. Between two joints
    c. In the cartilage
    d. Between two vertebrae

157. The prefix that means "within" or "inside" is
    a. Intra-
    b. Syn-
    c. Toco-
    d. Aniso-

158. Another term with the same meaning as "clot cell" is
    a. Acanthocyte
    b. Erythrocyte
    c. Leukocyte
    d. Thrombocyte

159. A permanent, surgically created opening into the stomach through the body wall is a/an
    a. Enterotomy
    b. Enterostomy
    c. Gastrostomy
    d. Gastrotomy

Answer questions 160-163 based on the following case history:

A 6-year-old spayed female mixed-breed dog with a history of chronic emesis and occasional ataxia is brought to a veterinarian. The veterinarian prescribes metoclopramide at 0.3 mg/kg po tid.

160. What clinical sign is present in this dog?
    a. Soft and bloody stool
    b. Vomiting
    c. Irregular heartbeat
    d. Increased salivation

161. This dog's gait is occasionally
    a. Uncoordinated
    b. Sluggish
    c. Lame
    d. Frenzied

162. The prescribed medication should be given by what route?
    a. Rectally
    b. Intramuscularly
    c. Orally
    d. Subcutaneously

163. The client gives the medication at 7 A.M. one morning; the next dose should be given at
    a. 7 A.M. the next day
    b. 7 P.M. the same day
    c. 1 P.M. the same day
    d. 3 P.M. the same day

164. A medication that is prescribed *prn* should be given on which of the following schedules?
    a. Indefinitely, until the veterinarian orders it stopped
    b. As needed
    c. Twice daily
    d. Only in conjunction with another medication

165. An adenocarcinoma is best described as a
    a. Malignant tumor derived from glandular tissue
    b. Benign growth found on the intestine
    c. Malignant tumor of the reproductive organs
    d. Benign tumor found in the oral cavity

166. Which dermatologic clinical sign would
you expect to be associated with an allergic
reaction to an ointment placed on the
skin?
    a. Pruritus
    b. Hematochezia
    c. Ptyalism
    d. Nystagmus

167. *Proptosis* refers to a/an
    a. Cherry eye syndrome
    b. Protrusion of the rectal mucosa
    c. Displacement or bulging of the eye
    d. Inversion of the right atrioventricular valve

168. The medical term for protrusion of an organ
through the body wall is
    a. Torsion
    b. Volvulus
    c. Hernia
    d. Hemorrhoid

169. An acute disease is one that
    a. Involves the gastrointestinal tract
    b. Involves the skin
    c. Comes on slowly
    d. Comes on quickly

170. What is a laparotomy?
    a. A surgical procedure to discover the cause of
    abdominal pain
    b. Incision through the abdominal wall
    c. Removal of part of the gastrointestinal tract
    d. Search for a foreign body in the small
    intestine

171. An intussusception can be described
as a/an
    a. Prolapse of one part of the intestine into the
    lumen of an adjacent part of the intestine
    b. Torsion of the mesentery, resulting in
    strangulation of the intestine
    c. Obstruction of the intestine by a foreign body
    d. Cancerous growth on the intestine

172. A surgical anastomosis can be best
described as
    a. An incision into the lumen of an organ
    b. Removing unnecessary or diseased tissue
    c. Suturing together two separate structures
    d. Changing the shape of an organ

173. Necrotic tissue is tissue in which
    a. Inflammation is present
    b. Cancer cells are present
    c. A color change has occurred
    d. The cells have died

174. What is pulmonary edema?
    a. Presence of free fluid between the chest wall
    and the lungs
    b. Effusion of fluid into the alveoli
    c. Stagnant blood circulation in the lungs
    d. Parasitic infection of the lungs

175. Proud flesh is the
    a. Persistence of the spermatic cord following
    castration of a horse
    b. Exuberant granulation tissue developing in a
    wound
    c. Cutaneous neoplasm found in a horse
    d. Crest of a stallion's neck

176. Ischemia occurs when a tissue lacks
    a. Heat
    b. Cells
    c. Firmness
    d. Blood flow

177. An arthrotomy is a surgical procedure in which
    a. An incision is made into a joint
    b. The interior of a joint is examined with an
    arthroscope
    c. Cartilage is removed from the joint surface
    d. Fluid is aspirated from a joint

178. Blepharospasm is a spasm or twitching of the
    a. Prepuce
    b. Thigh
    c. Facial nerve
    d. Eyelids

179. Glossitis is inflammation of the
    a. Oviduct
    b. Bile duct
    c. Tongue
    d. Superficial layers of skin

180. Rhinoplasty is
    a. Looking into the throat
    b. Surgical repair of the throat
    c. Looking into the nose
    d. Surgical repair of the nose

181. What is an infarct?
    a. Traveling blood clot
    b. Blood-filled area of tissue
    c. Area of dead tissue
    d. Heart attack

182. A nephrotoxic drug is one that can
damage the
    a. Kidneys
    b. Liver
    c. Nervous tissue
    d. Gall bladder

Correct answers are on pages 116-120.

183. Cryptorchidism is
   a. Removal of the testicles
   b. Repair of a scrotal hernia
   c. Having one testicle only
   d. Having one or more ectopic testicles

Use the following scenario to answer questions 184-186:

A horse is suffering from nystagmus, photophobia, and fasciculations. The veterinarian believes the animal may have ingested a toxic plant and prescribes an oral vitamin and mineral solution to be given qid.

184. The term *nystagmus* is best defined as
   a. A condition in which the horse appears to be unusually sleepy
   b. A behavioral state in which the female appears to be in heat
   c. An involuntary deviation of the eye
   d. Rhythmic movement of both eyeballs in unison

185. *Fasciculation* refers to
   a. Seizure like movements
   b. Small, local, involuntary muscular contractions
   c. Generalized, increased muscle tone
   d. Inability to move

186. If the client gives the prescribed medication at 8 A.M., the next treatment should be given at
   a. 8 P.M. the same day
   b. 8 A.M. the next morning
   c. 2 P.M. the same day
   d. 4 P.M. the same day

187. When used in reference to food, *tdn* refers to
   a. Total determined nutrition
   b. Tested digestible nutrition
   c. Total digestible nutrients
   d. Tested determined nutrients

188. A specific-pathogen–free (SPF) pig is one that is known to be free of
   a. Inherited defects
   b. Gastrointestinal parasites
   c. Nutritional deficiencies
   d. Certain infectious microorganisms

189. An endoscope is an instrument used to
   a. Administer pills or boluses
   b. Open a body cavity to allow inspection or medication
   c. Allow direct observation of internal organs, such as the stomach
   d. Prevent an animal from kicking

190. What is the difference between an emasculatome and an emasculator?
   a. The emasculatome removes the testicle, whereas the emasculator does not.
   b. A skin incision is not made before using the emasculator but is required when using the emasculatome.
   c. The emasculatome crushes the spermatic cord, whereas the emasculator crushes and cuts the spermatic cord.
   d. The emasculator is used for cattle only; the emasculatome is used for horses only.

ANSWERS

1. **c** Hemolysis is the breakdown of blood cells. Uremia refers to urea in the blood.

2. **d** Leukemia is a neoplasia of blood cells. Leukopenia is a decrease in white blood cells.

3. **d**

4. **c**

5. **b**

6. **c**

7. **b**

8. **d** The ophthalmoscope is used to examine the eyes. The laryngoscope is used to examine the larynx and aid in the placement of an endotracheal tube. A laparoscope is used to examine the abdomen.

9. **b**

10. **c** Encephalitis is an inflammation of the brain only.

11. **a**

12. **b**

13. **a**

14. **d**

15. **c** Urethrotomy is when an incision is made in the urethra but is then sutured.

16. **d** Pericarditis is an inflammation of the area around the heart. Endocarditis is an inflammation of the inner lining of the heart.

17. **d**

18. **c** Hypertrophy is the enlargement of a tissue because of an increase in the size of the cells such as seen in muscle. Metastasis is the spread of malignant cells from a neoplasm somewhere else in the body. Metastasis often occurs to lymph nodes that filter lymph from the area of the neoplasm and results in enlargement of the affected node(s).

19. **a**

20. **d**

21. **d**

22. **a**

23. **d** The myelocyte is an immature granulocyte white blood cell normally found in the bone marrow.

24. **b** A thrombus is a blood clot; an embolus is any undissolved substance that travels through the blood vessels. Thromboembolus is an undissolved blood clot that travels through the blood vessels.

25. **d**

26. **d**

27. **c**

28. **b**

29. **d** *Dystrophy* refers to a poorly formed tissue or organ. *Tachypnea* means "fast breathing." Pneumothorax is when there is air in the chest outside of the lungs and often results in dyspnea.

30. **b**

31. **d**

32. **a**

33. **d**

34. **b**

35. **b**

36. **a** Leukocytosis is a white blood cell count above normal. Leukemia is a neoplasia of blood cells. Anemia is an erythrocyte count below normal.

37. **c** A gastrotomy is when an incision is made in the stomach, which allows foreign bodies to be removed. A gastrectomy is when a portion of the stomach is surgically removed. A gastrostomy is when a new opening is made in the stomach (and not sutured). A gastropexy is when the stomach is sutured to the body wall (to prevent twisting).

38. **a**

39. **c**

40. **b**

41. **d**

42. **c** A murmur is an abnormal heart sound. Tachycardia is a heart rate above normal.

43. **a** Pneumonia is an inflammation of the lungs. Peritonitis is an inflammation of the peritoneum or lining of the abdomen. Pyoderma is areas of pus in the skin.

44. **c** Icterus is a yellowing of the mucous membranes resulting from increased bilirubin in the blood. Lipemia is a fat in the blood that gives a white color to the serum or plasma.

45. **b**

46. **c**

47. **d** A nisocoria is a condition that is often seen after severe head trauma.

48. **a** *Eosin-* refers to the color red.

49. **c**

50. **a**

51. **d**

52. **b**

53. **c**

54. **c**

55. **a** The prefix *stoma-* refers to a mouth like opening or the mouth.

56. **b** *Gloss(o)* is a word element that refers to the tongue.

57. **d** *Pharyng(o)* refers to the pharynx or throat.

58. **c** *Aden(o)* is a word element that refers to the gland; *-itis* refers to inflammation.

59. **d** *-cele* is a word element that can mean "tumor" or "cavity."

60. **a**

61. **b** *-gen* is a word element that means "agent that produces."

62. **d**

63. **c** *-phagia* is a word element that means "eating or swallowing."

64. **a**

65. **b** *-pnea* is a word element that means "breathing or respiration."

66. **c**

67. **d**

68. **b**

69. **a**

70. **c** *Hydr(o)* is a word element that means "water or hydrogen."

71. **a** *Chyl(o)* is a word element that pertains to chyle, a milky fluid consisting of lymph and fat.

72. **b** *Py(o)* is a word element that means "pus."

73. **d**

74. **b** *-aden* is a word element that means "gland"; *-itis* refers to inflammation.

75. **d** *-oma* is a word element that means "tumor or neoplasm."

76. **a** *-adenalgia* means "pain in a gland."

77. **c**

78. **c** *Brachy(o)* is a word element that means "short."

79. **a** *Dolich(o)* is a word element that means "long."

80. **c**

81. **b** The suffix *-malacia* means a softening or softness of a part or tissue.

82. **b**

83. **a** *Steat(o)* is a word element that means "fat or oil." The suffix *-orrhea* pertains to flow or discharge.

84. **b**

85. **d**

86. **c**

87. **a** *Hyper-* is a word element that means "abnormally increased or excessive"; *-esthesic* pertains to sensation.

88. **d**

89. **a**

90. **c**

91. **d**

92. **b**

93. **b**

94. **c**

95. **d** *Olig(o)* is a word element that means "few, little, or scant."

96. **a**

97. **b**

98. **d**

99. **a**

100. **c**

101. **d**

102. b

103. a

104. b

105. c

106. a

107. d

108. c

109. b

110. d

111. c

112. a

113. d

114. a

115. b

116. b

117. a

118. c

119. d

120. c

121. b

122. a

123. b

124. b

125. d

126. a

127. c

128. d

129. c

130. a

131. b

132. c

133. d

134. a

135. c

136. d

137. c

138. a

139. c

140. c

141. a

142. b

143. a

144. d

145. c

146. c

147. c

148. d

149. b

150. d *Open and compound* are used to describe fractures in which bone penetrates the skin.

151. d

152. b

153. c

154. a

155. c

156. a

157. a

158. d

159. c

160. b

161. a

162. c

163. **d** The medication is to be given three times a day or every 8 hours.

164. b

165. a

166. a

167. c

168. c

169. d

170. b

171. a

172. c

173. d

174. b

175. b

176. d

177. a

178. d

179. c

180. d

181. c

182. a

183. d

184. d

185. b

186. **c** The medication is to be given four times a day or every 6 hours.

187. c

188. d

189. c

190. c

Part Two

VTNE REVIEW

Pharmacology

Sarah Wagner • *Joann Colville*

Questions

1. Neonatal animals are less tolerant of some drugs than older animals, because in neonates the drugs are
   a. Biotransformed (metabolized) more rapidly
   b. Absorbed more slowly from the gastrointestinal tract
   c. Not biotransformed
   d. Biotransformed (metabolized) more slowly

2. Decreased function of what organ would have the greatest effect on biotransformation of most drugs?
   a. Kidney
   b. Liver
   c. Pancreas
   d. Spleen

3. The generic name for a drug is also called the
   a. Trade name
   b. Chemical name
   c. Proprietary name
   d. Nonproprietary name

4. You are asked to administer a drug that is supplied as an enteric-coated tablet at 100 mg, 50 mg, and 25 mg; you require 25 mg but have available 50-mg tablets only. You should
   a. Use a pill splitter to divide the 100-mg tablet into quarters to have the smallest piece.
   b. Use a pill splitter to divide the 50-mg tablet into halves to have the most accurate dose.
   c. Administer the 50-mg tablet but then skip the next scheduled dosing.
   d. Order or purchase 25-mg tablets for the dosing schedule.

5. A prescription reads "2 tab q4h po prn until gone." The translation of these instructions is
   a. Two tablets are to be taken four times per day for pain until all tablets are gone.
   b. Two tablets are to be taken four times per day under supervision by the veterinarian until all tablets are gone.
   c. Two tablets are to be taken every 4 hours with food and water until all tablets are gone.
   d. Two tablets are to be taken every 4 hours by mouth as needed until all tablets are gone.

6. Ten milliliters of a 2.5% solution of thiopentone contains
   a. 250 mg of thiopentone
   b. 25 mg of thiopentone
   c. 100 mg of thiopentone
   d. 2.5 mg of thiopentone

7. The percentage of the total dose that ultimately reaches the bloodstream is called
   a. Absorption
   b. Distribution
   c. Bioavailability
   d. Clearance

8. Cholinergic agents do all of the following except
   a. Slow heart rate
   b. Increase blood flow to intestinal tract
   c. Decrease diameter of bronchioles
   d. Cause peripheral vasodilation

9. The nonsteroidal antiinflammatory drug (NSAID) that is extremely toxic to cats is
   a. Aspirin
   b. Acetaminophen
   c. Carprofen
   d. Flunixin

123

Correct answers are on pages 147-160.

10. The most common adverse side effects of aminoglycoside antimicrobials are
    a. Nephrotoxicity
    b. Nephrotoxicity and ototoxicity
    c. Ototoxicity and neurotoxicity
    d. Nephrotoxicity, ototoxicity, and neurotoxicity

11. Which statement regarding tetracyclines is true?
    a. They are bactericidal.
    b. They alter the permeability of the cell wall and cause lysis.
    c. Currently many bacteria are resistant to them.
    d. They are unable to penetrate the bacterial cell wall.

12. To what other drug class is a cephalosporin-class drug closely related?
    a. Tetracyclines
    b. Sulfas
    c. Penicillins
    d. Fluoroquinolones

13. Because of the manner in which they are excreted, sulfonamides are often effective against infections of
    a. Nervous tissue
    b. Urinary tract
    c. Skin
    d. Joint capsules

14. The use of fluoroquinolones as antiinfective agents should be done with great caution or not at all in
    a. Dogs
    b. Cats
    c. Horses
    d. Birds

15. The antiinfective drug that should be avoided in all food-producing animals is
    a. Lincosamides
    b. Cephalexin
    c. Enrofloxacin
    d. Chloramphenicol

16. Penicillins are primarily excreted by the
    a. Small intestine
    b. Liver
    c. Kidney
    d. Stomach

17. Acepromazine must be used with caution or not at all in
    a. Bitches
    b. Tomcats
    c. Cows
    d. Stallions

18. The benzodiazepine derivative diazepam is often administered in combination with
    a. Droperidol
    b. Morphine
    c. Ketamine
    d. Xylazine

19. If using a regular disposable-type syringe, which of the following drugs should not be preloaded and left for a time?
    a. Acepromazine
    b. Atropine
    c. Diazepam
    d. Ketamine

20. A 10-kg dog has inadvertently been administered a dose of xylazine hydrochloride intended for a 30-kg dog. The correct reversal agent for this overdose is
    a. Yohimbine
    b. Atipamezole
    c. Noradrenalin
    d. Atropine

21. Griseofulvin acts on
    a. Gram-positive bacteria
    b. Gram-negative bacteria
    c. Gram-negative and gram-positive bacteria
    d. Dermatophytes

22. What is not true of sulfonamides?
    a. They can cause renal failure.
    b. They can cause skin eruptions.
    c. They can cause keratoconjunctivitis sicca.
    d. They can cause hepatitis.

23. What antiinfective compounds, when given to juvenile animals, can impair cartilage development?
    a. Cephalosporins
    b. Fluoroquinolones
    c. Penicillins
    d. Macrolides

24. Potentiated penicillins
    a. Have a narrow spectrum of action relative to regular penicillins
    b. Include cephalosporins
    c. Are active against b-lactamase–producing bacteria
    d. Are not used in treating mastitis

25. If you are instructed to give a medication IP, you inject the medication
    a. Into the jugular vein
    b. Into the popliteal artery
    c. Into the abdominal cavity
    d. Into a major muscle mass

26. Xylazine
    a. Is safe in all dogs
    b. Can be reversed with naloxone
    c. Provides some analgesia
    d. Can cause priapism in stallions

27. Propofol
    a. Is a potent analgesic
    b. Can be given via the IM and IV routes
    c. Is best administered as a single bolus
    d. Can be given in incremental doses

28. Butorphanol
    a. Is an antibiotic
    b. Is an antitussive
    c. Can be reversed using yohimbine
    d. Is contraindicated in the cat

29. An iodophor
    a. Has a longer action than basic iodine compounds
    b. Is not inactivated by organic materials
    c. Is not an irritant at concentrations generally used
    d. Provides adequate disinfection with a single application

30. Heartgard contains ivermectin, which
    a. Prevents dogs from developing congestive heart failure
    b. Is also effective in treating tapeworms
    c. Is used to prevent heartworm infection
    d. Can be administered orally only

31. The active drug in ProHeart is moxidectin, a member of the drug class
    a. Arsenical
    b. Organophosphate
    c. Avermectin
    d. Pyrantel

32. A risk to veterinary technicians who administer prostaglandins is
    a. Acne
    b. Liver failure
    c. Kidney damage
    d. Inducing an asthma attack

33. Loop diuretics such as furosemide
    a. Cause dehydration in normal animals
    b. Cannot be used simultaneously with ACE inhibitors
    c. Are unsafe for use in animals with pulmonary edema
    d. May cause hypokalemia with chronic use

34. Pain receptors are called
    a. Nociceptors
    b. C fibers
    c. Proprioceptors
    d. Prostaglandins

35. If it is accidentally administered as an IV bolus, lidocaine may cause
    a. Full body numbness
    b. Seizures
    c. Bradyarrhythmia
    d. Polyuria

36. Which of these opioids is an agonist/antagonist?
    a. Oxymorphone
    b. Meperidine
    c. Butorphanol
    d. Fentanyl

37. Acepromazine maleate causes
    a. Respiratory depression
    b. Tachycardia
    c. Hypotension
    d. Reduced salivation

38. What is the ratio between the toxic dose and therapeutic dose of a drug used as a measure of the relative safety of the drug for a particular treatment?
    a. Toxic index
    b. LD50
    c. ED50
    d. Therapeutic index

39. Aspirin may be safely used in cats as an NSAID, but it should be noted that its half-life in this species approximates
    a. 2 hours
    b. 8 hours
    c. 15 hours
    d. 30 hours

40. Which statement is most accurate pertaining to insect growth regulators?
    a. They prevent the female from laying eggs.
    b. They effectively kill all adult stages.
    c. They are insecticidal with very low risk of toxic effects in mammals.
    d. They are neurotoxic to mammals.

41. What drug is approved for the treatment of old dog dementia?
    a. Clomicalm
    b. Metacam
    c. Diazepam
    d. Anipryl

Correct answers are on pages 147-160.

42. What is not a short-term effect of corticosteroid therapy?
    a. Polyuria
    b. Polyphagia
    c. Delayed healing
    d. Osteoporosis

43. A common side effect of antihistamine drugs such as diphenhydramine is
    a. Polyuria
    b. Sedation
    c. Pruritus
    d. Panting

44. The H_2 receptors are found in the
    a. Gastric mucosa
    b. Saliva
    c. Carotid arteries
    d. Aortic arch

45. Thiobarbiturates should be administered with great care or not at all to
    a. Collies
    b. Greyhounds
    c. Rottweilers
    d. Spaniels

46. What drug is contraindicated in the treatment of glaucoma?
    a. Atropine sulfate
    b. Carbachol
    c. Miotics
    d. Pilocarpine

47. A chronotropic agent affects the
    a. Force of a contraction
    b. Rate of a contraction
    c. Rhythm of a contraction
    d. Rate of relaxation

48. Puppies born via cesarean section that are not breathing well may benefit from __ drops administered sublingually.
    a. Dobutamine
    b. Digitalis
    c. Doxapram
    d. Diazepam

49. Parenteral administration of phenylbutazone should be via __ only.
    a. Subcutaneous injection
    b. Intramuscular injection
    c. Subcutaneous or intramuscular injection
    d. Intravenous injection

50. Intradermal injections are used primarily for
    a. Insulin injections
    b. Antibiotic injections
    c. Vaccinations
    d. Allergy testing

51. Most biotransformation of drugs occurs in the
    a. Liver
    b. Kidney
    c. Lungs
    d. Spleen

52. The main reason that generic forms of drugs are less expensive than trademark name drugs is because generic brands
    a. Use less expensive ingredients
    b. Are not advertised heavily
    c. Do not incur the expense of developing a new drug
    d. Do not work as well as trademark name drugs

53. Repository forms of parenteral drugs
    a. Contain a special coating that protects the drug from the harsh, acidic environment of the stomach
    b. Are formulated to prolong absorption of the drug from the site of administration
    c. Are composed of specially prepared plant or animal parts rather than being manufactured from chemicals
    d. Are extremely irritating to the tissues

54. All of the following organs may facilitate the elimination of drugs except the
    a. Kidneys
    b. Liver
    c. Lungs
    d. Spleen

55. What liquid form of drug is most commonly administered intravenously?
    a. Emulsion
    b. Solution
    c. Suspension
    d. Elixir

56. When a drug is said to have a narrow therapeutic range, it means that
    a. Its effective and toxic doses are close to each other.
    b. It may be used for treatment of a few disorders only.
    c. It must be dosed frequently.
    d. It must be given in greater concentrations to be effective.

57. The regulatory agency that oversees the development and approval of animal topical pesticides is the
    a. FDA
    b. EPA
    c. USDA
    d. DEA

58. A drug that has extreme potential for abuse and no approved medicinal purpose in the United States is classified as
    a. C-I
    b. C-II
    c. C-IV
    d. C-V

59. A drug given by which of the following routes reaches its peak plasma concentration the fastest?
    a. Orally
    b. Intramuscularly
    c. Subcutaneously
    d. Intravenously

60. Which of these drugs is not an antifungal drug?
    a. Griseofulvin (Fulvicin)
    b. Clotrimazole (Otomax)
    c. Ketoconazole (Nizoral)
    d. Sulfadimethoxine (Albon)

61. An example of an antibiotic that is considered to be a β-lactamase inhibitor is
    a. Amoxicillin
    b. Clavamox
    c. Tetracycline
    d. Penicillin

62. In what class of antibiotic drugs are nephrotoxicity and ototoxicity potential side effects?
    a. Barbiturates
    b. Aminoglycosides
    c. Phenothiazine tranquilizers
    d. Dissociative anesthetics

63. The best means of assuring that a particular antibiotic treatment will be successful is to
    a. Treat for no less than a full 2-week course.
    b. Collect a sample from the infected area for culture and sensitivity.
    c. Use the highest dose that is considered nontoxic.
    d. Use a broad-spectrum antibiotic.

64. Dr. Blackman prescribed a particular antibiotic for a rabbit with a *Pasteurella* infection and asked you to educate the client regarding special instructions for administration of the drug. You told the client that she should wear gloves when handling this medication, because it has been associated with a rare adverse reaction in humans: aplastic anemia. Based on this information, the drug that you dispensed was most likely
    a. Gentamicin
    b. Tetracycline
    c. Erythromycin
    d. Chloramphenicol

65. The term *anaphylaxis* refers to
    a. A severe, life-threatening hypersensitivity reaction
    b. The development of resistance to a particular antimicrobial drug
    c. The disruption of bacteria's normal metabolic activity, causing cell death
    d. Bacterial cell death as a result of impaired production of nucleic acids

66. A very useful group of broad-spectrum drugs, whose popularity has more recently declined because of numerous potential side effects, including keratoconjunctivitis sicca, polyarthritis (especially in Doberman pinschers), hematuria, photosensitivity, and hypothyroidism, is the
    a. Sulfonamides
    b. Macrolides
    c. Tetracyclines
    d. Fluoroquinolones

67. Which of the following statements about tetracyclines is true?
    a. Tetracyclines are bacteriocidal.
    b. Oral absorption of tetracyclines is increased in the presence of food.
    c. Tetracyclines are potentially nephrotoxic and ototoxic.
    d. Tetracyclines may lead to bone or teeth problems if given to young animals.

68. A 50-lb dog is to be given 1 mg/kg dose of diazepam. How many milligrams will he be given?
    a. 50 mg
    b. 22.7 mg
    c. 500 mg
    d. 2.27 mg

Correct answers are on pages 147-160.

69. Amoxicillin (Amoxi-Drop) was prescribed for Tallulah, a 4-year-old female Chihuahua, who was being discharged after a hospitalization. Dr. Segal asks you to give her owner discharge instructions. You advise the client of all of the following except
    a. She should call if she notices any adverse side effects as a result of the medication.
    b. She should complete all the medication dispensed, even if Tallulah is feeling well and her symptoms have resolved.
    c. She should administer the medication on an empty stomach.
    d. The medication should be refrigerated.

70. Antimicrobial drugs like enrofloxacin (Baytril), marbofloxacin (Zeniquin), and orbifloxacin (Orbax) all belong to which group of antibiotics?
    a. Penicillins
    b. Cephalosporins
    c. Fluoroquinolones
    d. Aminoglycosides

71. Which of the following drugs is least likely to kill the normal flora in the gut of a rabbit, causing severe diarrhea?
    a. Sulfonamide (Tribrissen)
    b. Amoxicillin with clavulanic acid (Clavamox)
    c. Cephalothin (Keflin)
    d. Enrofloxacin

72. Guaifenesin is an example of a(n)
    a. Expectorant
    b. Antitussive
    c. Bronchodilator
    d. Mucolytic agent

73. Which of these drugs is available over the counter as an antitussive?
    a. Codeine
    b. Dextromethorphan
    c. Hydrocodone
    d. Butorphanol

74. Dr. Charles is performing a C-section on Sadie, a 3-year-old Dalmatian. The smallest pup was not breathing spontaneously, so the doctor asked you give the following respiratory stimulant.
    a. Theophylline (Theo-Dur)
    b. Albuterol
    c. Doxapram HCl (Dopram)
    d. Terbutaline

75. Butorphanol tartrate is an example of a drug that functions on more than one body system. It is both an
    a. Antitussive and narcotic analgesic
    b. Expectorant and narcotic analgesic
    c. Analgesic and expectorant
    d. Analgesic and barbiturate

76. The type of drug that would be most helpful for a patient with a productive cough is
    a. Antitussive
    b. Antihistamine
    c. Expectorant
    d. Analgesic

77. The anticoagulant diluted in saline or sterile water for injection to form a flush solution for preventing blood clots in intravenous catheters is
    a. Heparin
    b. EDTA
    c. Coumarin
    d. Acid citrate dextrose (ACD)

78. Sox, a 10-year-old M/C Siamese X, was brought to the emergency hospital, crying in pain and unable to walk. He was diagnosed with an arterial thromboembolism secondary to cardiomyopathy. The treatment for this condition is a(n)
    a. Hematinic drug
    b. Anticoagulant drug
    c. Hemostatic drug
    d. Fibrinolytic drug

79. The diuretic drug used most commonly in patients with congestive heart failure is
    a. Mannitol
    b. Spironolactone
    c. Chlorothiazide
    d. Furosemide

80. Epinephrine
    a. Increases the heart rate
    b. Decreases the heart rate
    c. Decreases the blood pressure
    d. Should be used to reverse the effects of acepromazine

81. The most common side effect of drugs that cause vasodilation is
    a. Cardiac arrhythmias
    b. Anorexia, vomiting, and diarrhea
    c. Hypotension
    d. Bradycardia

82. Cosmo, an 11-year-old M/C pug, has recently been diagnosed with mitral insufficiency and was referred to a veterinary cardiologist. The specialist decided to initiate treatment with digoxin, a positive inotrope and negative chronotrope. This means that it
    a. Increases the blood pressure and decreases the cardiac output
    b. Increases the peripheral vascular resistance and decreases the cardiac output
    c. Increases the force of contraction and decreases the heart rate
    d. Increases the heart rate and decreases the blood pressure

83. Scooter, a 13-year-old miniature schnauzer, has arrested under anesthesia for routine dentistry. You run to the crash cart and grab what you know to be the drug of choice for cardiac arrest, which is
    a. Epinephrine
    b. Lidocaine
    c. Digoxin
    d. Dobutamine

84. A 3-month-old chow chow is presented to the pet emergency clinic because it has eaten a box of warfarin-based rat poison. Which of the following would be most useful to treat this toxicity?
    a. Protamine sulfate
    b. Coumarin
    c. Streptokinase
    d. Vitamin K

85. Which of the following statements about drugs used for cancer chemotherapy is true?
    a. They are usually given by mouth.
    b. They usually have relatively low margins of safety.
    c. They are available over the counter.
    d. They are all nephrotoxic.

86. Which of the following side effects is commonly seen with many cancer chemotherapeutic drugs?
    a. Hyperglycemia
    b. Immunosuppression
    c. Constipation
    d. Hyperphagia

87. Which of the following would be the least common side effect expected with common cancer chemotherapeutic drugs?
    a. Myelosuppression
    b. Vomiting and diarrhea
    c. Pruritus
    d. Alopecia

88. Common drugs of plant origin, such as digoxin and atropine, are ineffective in a cow when administered orally because of
    a. Eructation
    b. The large size of the rumen
    c. Methane gas
    d. Digestive microorganisms

89. Which of these tissues is not a normal site for drugs to accumulate to be released later, thereby prolonging the effect of the drug?
    a. Pancreas
    b. Fat
    c. Muscle
    d. Liver

90. Chronic use of moderate-to-high doses of glucocorticoids may result in the development of
    a. Addisons disease
    b. Cushings disease
    c. Diabetes mellitus
    d. Insulinoma

91. Glucocorticoids are often used in veterinary medicine for treatment of all of the following conditions except
    a. Allergies
    b. Musculoskeletal problems
    c. Infections
    d. Immune-mediated disease

92. Glucocorticoids have different durations of activity, a fact that plays an important role in their risk of side effects with long-term use. Which of the following glucocorticoids has the shortest duration of activity?
    a. Hydrocortisone
    b. Prednisone
    c. Dexamethasone
    d. Triamcinolone

93. Which of the following statements about glucocorticoids is true?
    a. If adverse effects are seen after long-term administration, treatment should be discontinued immediately.
    b. They are generally considered safer to use than NSAIDs.
    c. They are a type of NSAID.
    d. They may cause immune system suppression.

94. What drug is not an NSAID?
    a. Prednisone
    b. Flunixin
    c. Phenylbutazone
    d. Aspirin

Correct answers are on pages 147-160.

95. Two relatively new NSAIDs used frequently in dogs for the relief of pain and inflammation, especially those associated with osteoarthritis, are
    a. Meclofenamic acid (Arquel) and dimethyl sulfoxide (DMSO)
    b. Orgotein (superoxide dismutase) and phenylbutazone
    c. Carprofen (Rimadyl) and etodolac (EtoGesic)
    d. Dipyrone and acetaminophen (Tylenol)

96. Flunixin meglumine (Banamine) is an NSAID most commonly used
    a. In dogs for the treatment of chronic osteoarthritis
    b. In horses for treatment of colic
    c. In horses for reducing fever
    d. In dogs for its anticoagulant activity

97. The species that generally clears NSAIDs most slowly is
    a. Dog
    b. Cat
    c. Horse
    d. Ruminant

98. What NSAID is administered to cats with a dosing interval of 2 days or more?
    a. Aspirin
    b. Ibuprofen (Advil)
    c. Carprofen (Rimadyl)
    d. Naproxen (Naprosyn)

99. The most common side effect of NSAIDs is
    a. Polyuria
    b. Gastrointestinal ulceration
    c. Diarrhea
    d. Constipation

100. What precautions should you take when applying DMSO to an animal's skin?
    a. Wear a facial mask to avoid inhaling the fumes.
    b. Apply a bandage to cover the area of application.
    c. DMSO is irritating and should not be applied to skin.
    d. Wear latex gloves to avoid contact with the drug.

101. The surgeon has completed Buffy's surgical procedure and asks you to discontinue the inhalant anesthesia. What is absolutely necessary to do when terminating anesthesia in a patient that has been receiving nitrous oxide?
    a. Give an injection of the reversal agent.
    b. Observe carefully for signs of seizures.
    c. Allow the patient to recuperate in a quiet, dark area.
    d. Oxygenate for 5 to 10 minutes.

102. All of the following drugs are controlled substances, and their use must be logged except
    a. Propofol (PropoFlo)
    b. Diazepam (Valium)
    c. Ketamine (Ketaset)
    d. Oxymorphone (Numorphan)

103. Malignant hyperthermia is a phenomenon associated primarily with the use of what inhalant anesthetic?
    a. Nitrous oxide
    b. Sevoflurane (SevoFlo)
    c. Halothane (Fluothane)
    d. Isoflurane (AErrane)

104. What drug is in the same class as thiopental?
    a. Ketamine
    b. Diazepam
    c. Phenobarbital
    d. Atropine

105. An opioid analgesic often used in transdermal patches to control postsurgical pain is
    a. Fentanyl
    b. Pentazocine (Talwin)
    c. Meperidine (Demerol)
    d. Butorphanol (Torbugesic)

106. Mrs. Stillman's poodle Roxy has been diagnosed with idiopathic epilepsy. The doctor has decided to dispense what drug, which Mrs. Stillman can administer per rectum, in the event of a seizure at home?
    a. Pentobarbital
    b. Phenobarbital
    c. Diazepam (Valium)
    d. Acepromazine (PromAce)

107. A recent graduate veterinary technician is concerned that a sedated patient has a heart rate of 50 beats/min when the heart rate in a dog is normally 60 to 120 beats/min. You ask her which sedative the veterinarian used and were not at all surprised when she told you that the drug used was
    a. Medetomidine (Domitor)
    b. Diazepam (Valium)
    c. Ketamine (Ketaset)
    d. Acepromazine (PromAce)

108. All of the following drugs are antagonists, used to reverse the effects of another drug except
    a. Yohimbine (Yobine)
    b. Detomidine (Dormosedan)
    c. Atipamezole (Antisedan)
    d. Naloxone (Narcan)

109. You are asked to work in the surgical recovery area. Oreo, a cat, is recovering from an exploratory laparotomy. Oreo was given morphine, in addition to other drugs. You anticipate all of the following except that
    a. Oreo will be hypersensitive to sounds.
    b. Oreo may vomit and defecate from being given opioids.
    c. Oreo most likely will have an elevated respiratory rate.
    d. Oreo would be most comfortable recovering in a dark, quiet room.

110. What gas anesthesia demands the greatest degree of patient monitoring, because anesthetic depth changes occur most rapidly?
    a. Nitrous oxide
    b. Sevoflurane (SevoFlo)
    c. Halothane (Fluothane)
    d. Isoflurane (AErrane)

111. Norepinephrine, epinephrine, and dopamine are the primary neurotransmitters for the
    a. Parasympathetic nervous system
    b. Sympathetic nervous system
    c. Central nervous system
    d. Peripheral nervous system

112. Beuthanasia solution is back ordered at the distributor, so your employer asks you to order a different euthanasia solution. In researching the available drugs, you are reminded that the active ingredient in most euthanasia solutions is
    a. Phenobarbital
    b. Pentobarbital
    c. Methohexital (Brevane)
    d. Thiopental (Pentothal)

113. You are working with an equine veterinarian on a breeding farm. You will be sedating a young stallion for an oral examination. You are well aware that the veterinarian will probably *not* be using what tranquilizer for the procedure?
    a. Xylazine (Rompun)
    b. Diazepam (Valium)
    c. Detomidine (Dormosedan)
    d. Acepromazine (PromAce)

114. The newly hired veterinary assistant is cleaning up after a procedure and returns an opened bottle of propofol (PropoFlo) to the refrigerator, stating that it can be used tomorrow on another patient. You explain to her that
    a. Propofol should be stored at room temperature rather than in the refrigerator.
    b. The bottles are designed to contain only enough drug for one patient, and there likely will not be enough drug left to anesthetize another patient tomorrow.
    c. Bacteria will readily grow in propofol and will produce endotoxins, so it is unwise to use the remains of an opened bottle.
    d. The bottle has been contaminated from the first patient, and there is a possibility that contagious diseases can be transmitted in this way.

115. You are out on an ambulatory call with Dr. Burrows to Milkman's Dairy. You are asked to bring the xylazine from the truck to sedate the patient. You are well aware that when using this drug in the bovine, you must
    a. Use adequate doses, because cattle tend to be resistant to its effects
    b. Always use it concurrently with a barbiturate to achieve adequate analgesia
    c. Not use xylazine because it is contraindicated in this species
    d. Use it at about 1/10 of the equine dose

116. You were assigned to work the front office at the hospital today. When you walk back to the treatment area, you notice a cat under anesthesia. The cat has eyes wide open and unblinking and limbs stiffly distended and is salivating profusely. Your highly educated guess is that this cat was anesthetized using which of the following drugs?
    a. Xylazine (Rompun)
    b. Medetomidine (Domitor)
    c. Ketamine (Ketaset)
    d. Propofol (PropoFlo)

117. A cow is accidentally dosed with an equine dose of xylazine. What drug should be immediately administered?
    a. None; the equine and bovine doses of xylazine are the same
    b. Epinephrine
    c. Naloxone
    d. Yohimbine

Correct answers are on pages 147-160.

118. Acepromazine should be avoided in
    a. Patients with a history of seizures
    b. Aggressive patients
    c. Geriatric patients
    d. Doberman pinschers

119. The behavioral drug group that may be used to stimulate appetite in cats is
    a. Benzodiazepines
    b. Tricyclic antidepressants
    c. Selective serotonin reuptake inhibitors
    d. Progestins

120. A progestin, often used in the past for the treatment of inappropriate elimination in cats, that has now fallen out of favor because of serious potential side effects, including mammary hyperplasia and adenocarcinoma, is
    a. Megestrol acetate (Ovaban)
    b. Oxazepam (Serax)
    c. Amitriptyline (Elavil)
    d. Fluoxetine (Prozac)

121. Which tricyclic antidepressant is now approved for used in dogs and cats to control separation anxiety?
    a. Buspirone (BuSpar)
    b. Selegiline (Anipryl)
    c. Paroxetine (Paxil)
    d. Clomipramine (Clomicalm)

122. A 12-year-old spayed female golden retriever is brought into your clinic with a history of waking up in her bed in a puddle of urine. A complete blood count (CBC), profile, and urinalysis reveal no sign of urinary tract disease. The doctor tells you to fill a prescription for phenylpropanolamine. The doctor is choosing this drug because
    a. It treats bladder atony by increasing bladder tone.
    b. It treats urinary incontinence by decreasing urethral sphincter tone.
    c. It treats urinary incontinence by increasing urethral sphincter tone.
    d. It treats bladder atony by decreasing bladder tone.

123. Erythropoietin (Epogen) is primarily used in the following feline patients:
    a. Cats with anemia due to chronic renal failure
    b. Cats with anemia due to rodenticide toxicity
    c. Cats with aortic thromboembolism secondary to cardiomyopathy
    d. Cats suffering from Tylenol toxicity

124. Which of the following drugs is used to decrease gastric acid production by blocking histamine receptors in the stomach?
    a. Famotidine (Pepcid)
    b. Sucralfate (Carafate)
    c. Omeprazole (Prilosec)
    d. Erythropoietin (Epogen)

125. Amphojel and Basaljel are drugs in the general category of
    a. Potassium supplements
    b. Antihypertensives
    c. Urinary acidifiers
    d. Phosphate binders

126. Mr. Williams just adopted a mixed-breed puppy from the local animal shelter, and it was suggested that he bring it to a veterinarian to treat the worms noticed in its feces. Mr. Williams wanted to save some money and went to the local pet shop to buy a dewormer. The product that he purchased was most likely
    a. Pyrantel pamoate (Nemex)
    b. Piperazine (Pipa-tabs)
    c. Fenbendazole (Panacur)
    d. Ivermectin (Ivomec)

127. A heartworm preventive that is also approved for the treatment of ear mites and sarcoptic mange is
    a. Diethylcarbamazine (Filaribits)
    b. Milbemycin (Interceptor)
    c. Ivermectin (Heartgard)
    d. Selamectin (Revolution)

128. If a drug package insert states that the drug is a coccidiostat, against what group of parasites will this drug be effective?
    a. Ascarids *(Toxocara, Toxascaris)*
    b. Tapeworms *(Taenia)*
    c. Protozoa *(Eimeria, Isospora)*
    d. Flukes (liver fluke, lung fluke)

129. Which of the following drugs can cause severe tissue necrosis if given perivascularly?
    a. Phenylbutazone (Butazolidin)
    b. Oxymorphone (Numorphan)
    c. Propofol (PropoFlo)
    d. Ketamine (Ketaset)

130. Which statement about organophosphates is incorrect?
    a. They are neurotoxic.
    b. They are used for control of endoparasites and ectoparasites.
    c. They have a narrow margin of safety.
    d. They have relatively few side effects.

131. By what route is insulin usually administered in cases of uncomplicated diabetes?
   a. Intramuscular
   b. Subcutaneous
   c. Intravenous
   d. Oral

132. Insulin concentration is measured in
   a. Milligrams per milliliter
   b. Milliequivalents per milliliter
   c. Units per milliliter
   d. Grams per milliliter

133. Oral hypoglycemic drugs, such as glipizide (Glucotrol), are used to treat
   a. Diabetic ketoacidosis
   b. Non–insulin-dependent diabetes
   c. Hypoglycemia
   d. Pancreatitis

134. The primary function of insulin is to
   a. Regulate the metabolic processes of the body
   b. Regulate digestion through secretion of gastrointestinal hormones
   c. Facilitate the entry of glucose into cells
   d. Control reproductive function

135. Resuspension of NPH insulin is done by
   a. Gently rolling the bottle
   b. Vigorous shaking of the bottle
   c. Gentle heating of the bottle in warm water
   d. Refrigeration of the bottle

136. Altrenogest, which is used for estrus synchronization in female animals, is a synthetic
   a. Estrogen
   b. Androgen
   c. Progestin
   d. Follicle-stimulating hormone (FSH)

137. Serious potential side effects of estrogen administration include
   a. Hemorrhage and thromboembolism
   b. Bone marrow suppression and pyometra
   c. Cardiac arrhythmias and pulmonary edema
   d. Renal failure and gastric ulcers

138. When diethylstilbestrol (DES), a synthetic estrogen, is used at higher doses, it can have the potentially dangerous side effect of
   a. Gastric ulceration
   b. Cardiac arrhythmias
   c. Bone marrow suppression
   d. Hepatopathy

139. Kaolin and pectin (Kaopectate) and bismuth subsalicylate (Pepto-Bismol) are examples of
   a. Narcotic analgesics
   b. Antispasmodics
   c. Anticholinergics
   d. Protectants

140. Psyllium and Metamucil are examples of
   a. Saline cathartics
   b. Bulk laxatives
   c. Lubricants
   d. Irritant cathartics

141. What is *not* a potential side effect of the phenothiazine antiemetics?
   a. CNS depression
   b. Diarrhea
   c. Lowering of the seizure threshold
   d. Hypotension

142. A stool softener often helpful in patients recovering from anal surgery is
   a. Docusate sodium succinate (DSS, Colace)
   b. Magnesium hydroxide
   c. Mineral oil
   d. Bran

143. The most widely used type of antiemetic drugs used to prevent motion sickness in dogs and cats are the
   a. Phenothiazines
   b. Antihistamines
   c. Anticholinergics
   d. Antispasmodics

144. The emetic of choice in cats is
   a. Xylazine
   b. Syrup of ipecac
   c. Apomorphine
   d. Hydrogen peroxide

145. The emetic of choice in dogs is
   a. Xylazine
   b. Syrup of ipecac
   c. Apomorphine
   d. Hydrogen peroxide

146. Spike the dog ingested his owner's cardiac medication about half an hour ago. The veterinarian instructs you to give him an emetic that may be administered into the conjunctival sac, then flush as necessary. The name of the drug is
   a. Xylazine
   b. Syrup of ipecac
   c. Apomorphine
   d. Hydrogen peroxide

Correct answers are on pages 147-160.

147. A coating agent that forms an ulcer-adherent complex at the ulcer site is
    a. Kaopectate
    b. Sucralfate
    c. Cimetidine
    d. Misoprostol

148. Fleet (sodium phosphate) enemas are contraindicated in what species?
    a. Horses
    b. Ruminants
    c. Cats
    d. Pigs

149. The principal site of drug biotransformation is the
    a. Liver
    b. Kidney
    c. Stomach
    d. Small intestine

150. What drug is most likely to be prescribed to prevent motion sickness in dogs and cats?
    a. Apomorphine
    b. Syrup of ipecac
    c. Atropine
    d. Acepromazine

151. A veterinarian prescribes erythropoietin (Epogen) for use in a dog in terminal renal failure. Why was this drug prescribed?
    a. For its fibrinolytic activity
    b. For its immunosuppressive activity
    c. For its ability to stimulate red blood cell production and release
    d. For its ability to reduce hypertension

152. Which of the following drugs is considered a biologic response modifier?
    a. Interferon
    b. Streptokinase
    c. Cephalosporin
    d. EDTA

153. Atropine is often given as a preanesthetic agent. It is classified as an anticholinergic drug. That means that it will likely have the following effects on an animal receiving the drug:
    a. Decreased heart rate, decreased salivation, and decreased GI motility
    b. Increased heart rate, increased salivation, and increased GI motility
    c. Increased heart rate, decreased salivation, and decreased GI motility
    d. Decreased heart rate, increased salivation, and increased GI motility

154. A drug classified as an *antagonist* may exert its influence by
    a. Mimicking the activity of the neurotransmitter used in the impulse
    b. Preventing the breakdown of the neurotransmitter used in the impulse
    c. Blocking the neurotransmitter receptor on the effector organ
    d. Enhancing the release of the neurotransmitter used in the impulse

155. A client is advised to discontinue aspirin therapy in his dysplastic dog before the dog undergoes surgery to remove a mammary tumor. The client asks you why this request was made. You tell him
    a. Aspirin decreases platelet aggregation and may increase the likelihood of hemorrhage.
    b. Aspirin may result in gastrointestinal ulceration.
    c. Aspirin may adversely affect hepatic biotransformation.
    d. Aspirin has an antiinflammatory effect.

156. Duragesic (Fentanyl) transdermal patches are used most commonly in veterinary medicine to control
    a. Diarrhea
    b. Vomiting
    c. Seizures
    d. Pain

157. Acetylcysteine (Mucomyst) is an antidote for what type of drug toxicity?
    a. Opioid
    b. Acetaminophen
    c. Lidocaine
    d. Digoxin

158. An *expectorant* is a drug that acts to
    a. Suppress a productive cough
    b. Liquefy and dilute viscous secretions in the respiratory tract
    c. Suppress inflammatory cells in the respiratory tract
    d. Reduce the allergic component of respiratory disease

159. The *therapeutic range* of a drug refers to which of the following?
    a. The plasma concentration at which therapeutic benefits should be observed
    b. The relationship of a drug's ability to achieve a desired effect versus causing a toxic effect
    c. The range of curative properties that a drug may exhibit
    d. The frequency of idiosyncratic reactions

160. Which of the following drugs are contraindicated in a patient that has a history of seizures?
    a. Diazepam
    b. Thiopental
    c. Acepromazine
    d. Fentanyl

161. *Nutraceuticals* is a category of drugs with which of the following characteristics?
    a. Genetically derived materials that enhance immune function
    b. Drugs that are derived from humans for use in animal
    c. Drugs that are undergoing clinical trials before FDA approval
    d. Nontoxic food components that have proven health benefits

162. What is the reversal agent for xylazine (Rompun)?
    a. Fentanyl
    b. Naloxone (Narcan)
    c. Acepromazine
    d. Yohimbine (Yobine)

163. The reversal agent used for opioid toxicity is
    a. Naloxone (Narcan)
    b. Yohimbine
    c. Acetylcysteine
    d. Diazepam

164. One of the adverse side effects of opioid administration is
    a. Increased seizure activity in epileptic animals
    b. Induction of cardiac arrhythmias
    c. Significant respiratory depression
    d. Systemic hypertension

165. In which of the following circumstances should a thiobarbiturate drug be avoided?
    a. In a patient with respiratory alkalosis
    b. In obese patients
    c. In sight hounds and very thin patients
    d. In hyperproteinemic animals

166. What is a potential electrolyte imbalance that can occur as a result of administering a loop diuretic to a small animal?
    a. Hypokalemia
    b. Hyperkalemia
    c. Hypercalcemia
    d. Hypocalcemia

167. Which of the following drugs is used to treat feline hypertension?
    a. Amlodipine (Norvasc)
    b. Erythromycin
    c. Amitriptyline (Elavil)
    d. Atropine

168. A cat is given ketamine as an anesthetic induction agent. The veterinary technician monitoring this animal may observe which of the following side effects?
    a. Bradycardia
    b. Hypotension
    c. Apneustic breathing
    d. Flaccid muscle tone

169. The category of drugs classified as ACE inhibitors has which of the following effects on the body?
    a. Increases preload and afterload on the heart
    b. Decreases preload and afterload on the heart
    c. Enhances fluid retention in the body
    d. Enhances the production of angiotensin II

170. Nitroglycerin is given primarily to achieve which of the following effects?
    a. Vasodilation
    b. Vasoconstriction
    c. Antiarrhythmic
    d. ACE inhibitor

171. For cats diagnosed with hypertrophic cardiomyopathy, a calcium channel blocker is often prescribed to relax the heart in an attempt to improve cardiac output. Which of the following drugs falls in this category?
    a. Procainamide
    b. Diltiazem
    c. Lidocaine
    d. Digoxin

172. Lidocaine is primarily used to control which of the following abnormalities?
    a. Atrial bradyarrhythmias
    b. Ventricular tachyarrhythmias
    c. Hypertension
    d. Excessive urine output

173. In dogs that have been receiving long-term glucocorticoid therapy (months to years), a sudden discontinuation of the drug may result in which of the following medical problems?
    a. Immunosuppression
    b. Iatrogenic addisonian crisis
    c. Polyuria and polydipsia
    d. Iatrogenic thyroid disease

174. In dogs that have been receiving long-term glucocorticoid therapy (months to years), which of the following endocrinopathies can occur?
    a. Hypothyroidism
    b. Hyperthyroidism
    c. Iatrogenic Cushings disease/ hyperadrenocorticism
    d. Estrogen-responsive incontinence

Correct answers are on pages 147-160.

175. Which of the following is/are *not* a side effect of oral glucocorticoid administration in dogs?
    a. Polyuria and polydipsia
    b. Polyphagia
    c. Hyperglycemia
    d. Vomiting

176. Glucocorticoids are often used to treat all but which of the following conditions?
    a. Autoimmune skin disease
    b. Asthma
    c. Lymphocytic neoplasias
    d. Hyperadrenocorticism

177. An example of an anticholinergic drug is
    a. Acetylcholine
    b. Pilocarpine
    c. Atropine
    d. Nicotine

178. The term *drug compounding* refers to which of the following activities?
    a. Diluting or combining drugs for ease of administration
    b. Delivering a drug via a different route than is directed on the label
    c. Delivering a drug at a different dose than is directed on the label
    d. Delivering the drug to a different species than is directed on the label

179. Which of the following drugs is most commonly used to treat urinary incontinence in dogs?
    a. Phenylpropanolamine
    b. Diethylcarbamazine
    c. Acepromazine
    d. Bethanechol

180. Which of the following drugs is classified as an osmotic diuretic and is often used to reduce intracranial pressure or treat oliguric renal failure?
    a. Furosemide
    b. Propranolol
    c. Mannitol
    d. Bethanechol

181. Which of the following drugs does not have an antiemetic action?
    a. Phenothiazines (Chlorpromazine)
    b. Metoclopramide (Reglan)
    c. Antihistamines (Meclizine)
    d. Apomorphine

182. An animal that demonstrates an allergic response to penicillin administration should not be given which of the following antibiotics?
    a. Clindamycin
    b. Cephalosporins
    c. Sulfonamides
    d. Fluoroquinolones

183. Griseofulvin (Fulvicin) is used in cats, dogs, and horses to treat which of the following disorders?
    a. Dermatophytosis
    b. Staphylococcus pyoderma
    c. Rickettsial disease
    d. Nematode infection

184. Which of the following drugs provides analgesic relief to a patient who undergoes a painful procedure?
    a. Acepromazine
    b. Diazepam
    c. Thiopental
    d. Fentanyl

185. Which of the following drugs is used as an adulticide to treat a heartworm-positive dog?
    a. Melarsomine (Immiticide)
    b. Ivermectin (Heartgard)
    c. Milbemycin (Interceptor)
    d. Moxidectin (ProHeart)

186. The antidote for warfarin (Dicumarol) poisoning is
    a. Vitamin C
    b. Naloxone
    c. Vitamin K
    d. Primidone

187. An example of an α_2-agonist is
    a. Xylazine
    b. Propranolol
    c. Hydralazine
    d. Epinephrine

188. The number of species of bacteria that are affected by an antibiotic is known as the antibiotic's
    a. Effectiveness
    b. Efficacy
    c. Spectrum
    d. Sphere

189. Which of the following statements correctly describes multidrug chemotherapeutic protocols?
    a. Drugs are usually selected that work in the same part of the cell cycle.
    b. Drugs are usually selected that work in different parts of the cell cycle.
    c. Drugs are selected that produce similar adverse side effects.
    d. Most chemotherapy drugs are dosed on a milligram/kilogram basis.

190. Which of the following drugs does not have an immunosuppressive effect?
    a. Cyclosporine
    b. Azathioprine (Imuran)
    c. Prednisone
    d. Ivermectin

191. An example of an aminoglycoside antibiotic is
    a. Erythromycin
    b. Ampicillin
    c. Neomycin
    d. Doxycycline

192. A recently reported side effect of fluoroquinolone administration (Baytril) in cats given SID dosing at a higher dosing schedule is
    a. Retinal damage
    b. Hypertension
    c. Renal failure
    d. Hepatic failure

193. Which of the following clinical signs may indicate that an animal is experiencing lidocaine toxicity?
    a. CNS signs: drowsiness, ataxia, muscle tremors
    b. Renal signs: oliguria
    c. Hepatic signs: jaundice, clotting problems
    d. Respiratory signs: labored respirations, bronchoconstriction

194. An asthmatic cat may receive which of the following drugs for its bronchodilatory effect?
    a. Histamine
    b. Digoxin
    c. Prednisone
    d. Theophylline

195. The class of antibiotics most commonly prescribed to treat rickettsial infections, such as Rocky Mountain spotted fever, is
    a. Tetracyclines
    b. Penicillins
    c. Aminoglycosides
    d. Sulfonamides

196. What drug will not cause nephrotoxicity?
    a. Aminoglycosides
    b. Banamine (Flunixin Meglumine)
    c. Cisplatin (Platinol)
    d. Oxymorphone

197. Why is it an accepted practice for cats receiving aspirin therapy to be dosed on a 2-day interval schedule only (i.e., a minimal dose every 2 days)?
    a. Liver metabolism of salicylates occurs at a very slow rate in comparison to other species, thereby making cats extremely susceptible to overdose in comparison to dogs.
    b. Salicylates cause severe respiratory depression in cats.
    c. Salicylates often result in severe hypertension.
    d. Salicylates may result in hypercoagulable states in cats.

198. A cat diagnosed with hyperthyroidism may be offered a number of treatment options, including all but which of the following?
    a. Radioactive iodine-131 treatment
    b. Methimazole (Tapazole) medical management
    c. Thyroidectomy surgery
    d. Fenbendazole medical management

199. Butorphanol is an opioid that is often used for its analgesic properties but is also used in other clinical scenarios as
    a. An antidiarrheal agent
    b. An antitussive agent
    c. An antiemetic
    d. A bronchodilator

200. Triple sulfas were developed to the avert __ that was/were seen with single sulfonamide toxicity.
    a. Diarrhea
    b. Crystalluria
    c. Bronchospasms
    d. Seizures

201. A dog diagnosed with a mast cell tumor is scheduled for surgery. The veterinarian chooses to pretreat the dog with an H_1 blocker to prevent the negative effects of histamine release when the tumor is manipulated. Which of the following drugs may be chosen?
    a. Diphenhydramine
    b. Methimazole
    c. Vincristine
    d. Sulfasalazine

Correct answers are on pages 147-160.

202. Which of the following drugs is used for its sedative, antiseizure, and appetite stimulant effects?
    a. Diazepam (Valium)
    b. Cyproheptadine
    c. Ketamine
    d. Potassium bromide

203. A cat is given a drug (methionine) to alter the pH of his urine in an effort to dissolve his struvite stones. The drug has which of the following intended effects?
    a. Acidification of the urine
    b. Alkalinization of the urine
    c. Dilution of urine
    d. Concentration of the urine

204. Which of the following types of insulin provides the longest duration of action?
    a. NPH insulin
    b. Regular insulin
    c. Ultralente insulin
    d. Semilente insulin

205. It is essential for veterinary technicians to educate clients expected to treat their pets with insulin. Which of the following statements is true?
    a. Insulin can be stored at room temperature in between uses.
    b. The bottle of insulin should be shaken before use.
    c. The injection is given in the same site each time.
    d. Insulin should be given with a meal.

206. Antimicrobial (antibiotic) drugs are classified according to the type of organisms they affect. Which type of antimicrobial drug would be effective against organisms like *Giardia* or *Eimeria*?
    a. Bactericidal
    b. Virucidal
    c. Antiprotozoal
    d. Fungistatic

207. Many antibiotic drug inserts (information included in packages of drugs) make reference to the MIC at which the antibiotic is effective. What is the MIC?
    a. Minimum inflammatory concentration
    b. Maximum infusion concentration
    c. Minimum inhibitory concentration
    d. Maximum inhalation concentration

208. Antimicrobial drugs like neomycin, gentamicin, and amikacin each belong to what group of antibiotics?
    a. Penicillins
    b. Cephalosporins
    c. Quinolines
    d. Aminoglycosides

209. Aminoglycosides, if given at high dosages or by continuous IV infusion, cause damage to the
    a. Lungs and liver
    b. Liver and inner ear
    c. Kidney and liver
    d. Inner ear and kidney

210. Bacterial resistance to antibiotics is a significant problem in veterinary medicine. What factor is not considered to be a significant contributor to development of bacterial resistance?
    a. Prolonged levels of higher-than-recommended dosages of antibiotics
    b. Normal dosages of antibiotics for half the recommended duration
    c. Low dosages of antibiotics in the feed for prolonged periods
    d. Antibiotics that do not reach the infection site in concentrations that exceed MIC

211. Which of the following drug groups is most likely to provoke an allergic reaction in treated animals?
    a. Aminoglycosides
    b. Quinolines
    c. Penicillins
    d. Tetracyclines

212. Antimicrobial drugs that work against bacterial deoxyribonucleic acid (DNA) have the potential for causing birth defects or other problems in the host animal if they also alter mammalian DNA. One group of antimicrobial agents known for this tendency is
    a. Antifungals
    b. Antibacterials
    c. Antivirals
    d. Antiprotozoals

213. Unlike many other penicillins, penicillin G is not recommended for use by mouth (po). Why?
    a. It upsets the stomach.
    b. It is destroyed by gastric acid.
    c. It causes severe diarrhea and intestinal cramping.
    d. It is ineffectively absorbed from the gastrointestinal tract.

214. Which type of adverse reaction is most commonly observed when penicillins are administered to rabbits?
    a. Kidney damage and subsequent change in urine production
    b. Hives and swelling of the face from allergic reaction
    c. High fever and severe depression
    d. Severe diarrhea

215. Certain bacteria, especially Staphylococcus, produce an enzyme (β-lactamase) that destroys many penicillin drugs. Which is one of the penicillins not destroyed by β-lactamase?
    a. Penicillin G
    b. Cloxacillin
    c. Amoxicillin
    d. Hetacillin

216. What is added to amoxicillin to make it resistant to the penicillin-destroying β-lactamase enzymes produced by some bacteria?
    a. Trimethoprim
    b. Clavulanic acid
    c. Piperonyl butoxide
    d. Ormetoprim

217. Some penicillin G injectable products contain procaine or benzathine, and some penicillin G products contain neither. What effect do procaine and benzathine have on penicillin G?
    a. They act as a local anesthetic to decrease the pain of injection.
    b. They prolong absorption of penicillin G from the injection site.
    c. They increase the rate at which penicillin G enters the bloodstream.
    d. They enhance the bacterial killing activity of the penicillin.

218. Ceftiofur is classified on the package insert as a third-generation cephalosporin antibiotic; cefadroxil is classified as a first-generation cephalosporin. How do third-generation cephalosporins differ from first-generation cephalosporins?
    a. Third-generation drugs are better absorbed when given orally.
    b. Third-generation drugs have better gram-negative activity.
    c. Third-generation drugs last longer in the body; they are given once daily only.
    d. Third-generation drugs have fewer side effects and adverse reactions.

219. Aminoglycoside antibiotics (e.g., amikacin and gentamicin) are powerful agents against bacteria. Unfortunately, they do not seem to work well in deep puncture wounds or in the lumen of the colon. Why?
    a. These are anaerobic sites, and bacteria require oxygen to take up aminoglycosides.
    b. These sites often have enzymes that inactivate aminoglycosides.
    c. Gram-positive bacteria commonly infect these sites, and aminoglycosides are ineffective against gram-positive bacteria.
    d. The DNA of bacteria at these sites is resistant to aminoglycosides.

220. How can a drug like neomycin, which has severe risk of nephrotoxicity when administered by injection, have little risk when administered topically or orally?
    a. Some species are resistant to kidney damage that may result from the drug.
    b. Little of the drug is absorbed through the skin.
    c. Absorbed drug is excreted so quickly that it does not have time to damage the kidneys.
    d. Subcutaneous enzymes inactivate the drug.

221. What antibiotic is most likely to cause damage to the ear?
    a. Amoxicillin
    b. Gentamicin
    c. Tetracycline
    d. Enrofloxacin

222. What route of administration of amikacin or gentamicin causes the highest risk for nephrotoxicity (kidney toxicity)?
    a. Per os
    b. Intramuscular
    c. Continuous intravenous infusion
    d. Intravenous bolus

223. What can a technician do to recognize early signs of nephrotoxicity in an animal that receives aminoglycosides?
    a. Monitor blood urea nitrogen (BUN) and creatinine levels
    b. Monitor the CBC and total protein level
    c. Monitor feces for change in consistency
    d. Monitor urine for casts and protein

Correct answers are on pages 147-160.

224. Why is it important that pus-filled wounds or ear canals with purulent debris be thoroughly cleaned before applying a topical aminoglycoside (e.g., gentamicin)?
    a. Purulent material shields bacteria from the antibiotic.
    b. The alkaline nature of the purulent material reduces bacterial uptake of the drug.
    c. Nucleic acids in the cellular debris (pus) bind the aminoglycoside.
    d. Irritation from the purulent material causes the tissue to produce enzymes against the aminoglycoside.

225. What drugs are considered fluoroquinolones?
    a. Oxytetracycline, doxycycline
    b. Danofloxacin, enrofloxacin
    c. Sulfadimethoxine, sulfamethazine
    d. Chloramphenicol, lincomycin

226. What organ blocks entrance of many drugs because of a barrier similar to the blood-brain barrier?
    a. Prostate gland
    b. Thyroid gland
    c. Pancreas
    d. Spleen

227. In what animal is use of enrofloxacin safest?
    a. 1-year-old Dutch rabbit
    b. 3-month-old Doberman puppy
    c. 6-month-old quarter horse colt
    d. 2-year-old Siamese cat

228. What is the drug group of choice for treating Lyme disease (borreliosis)?
    a. Antifungal
    b. Antiviral
    c. Antibiotic
    d. Antiprotozoal

229. With what type of diet should oral tetracyclines not be administered?
    a. High fat
    b. Low sodium
    c. High calcium
    d. Low potassium

230. Why should tetracycline use be avoided in pregnant bitches?
    a. It may cause changes in the joint cartilage that may result in arthritis at an older age in the pup.
    b. It may be deposited in dental enamel and give the pup's teeth a mottled yellow appearance.
    c. It may impair normal central nervous system development in the pups that may show up as behavioral changes later in life.
    d. It may damage the developing pups and may result in liver impairment later in life.

231. What is the effect of prostaglandin F2 alpha on the reproductive system?
    a. Ovulation
    b. Luteolysis
    c. Follicle stimulation
    d. Corpus luteum formation

232. What drug readily penetrates the blood-brain barrier and achieves therapeutic concentrations of antibiotic in the central nervous system?
    a. Amoxicillin
    b. Enrofloxacin
    c. Oxytetracycline
    d. Chloramphenicol

233. Chloramphenicol is metabolized by specific enzymes in the liver. Consequently, it interferes with or influences how rapidly other drugs metabolized by the same liver enzymes are eliminated from the body. This is important to remember to prevent accidental overdose of a simultaneously administered drug. Metabolism of what drug is affected by simultaneous use of chloramphenicol?
    a. Phenobarbital
    b. Aspirin
    c. Sulfadimethoxine
    d. Enrofloxacin

234. Why is chloramphenicol used with extreme caution in cats and neonates?
    a. It can bind with dietary calcium (milk) and become deactivated.
    b. The liver is unable to metabolize chloramphenicol effectively in these animals.
    c. It can alter developing bone, enamel, and cartilage.
    d. It may drastically alter gut bacterial flora, resulting in fatal diarrhea.

235. What fatal reaction to chloramphenicol has been reported in cats and people?
    a. Kidney failure
    b. Aplastic anemia
    c. Pulmonary edema
    d. Liver failure

236. What antimicrobial is banned from use in any food animal because of the risk to human health?
    a. Oxytetracycline
    b. Dicloxacillin
    c. Chloramphenicol
    d. Sulfadimethoxine

237. When are drugs like sulfadimethoxine, sulfadiazine, and other sulfa drugs most likely to cause kidney problems?
    a. When an animal is receiving intravenous fluids and they have a diuretic effect on the kidneys
    b. When an animal is dehydrated
    c. When an animal has only one functional kidney
    d. When an animal has a bladder infection

238. What are trimethoprim and ormetoprim?
    a. Agents that are growth regulators
    b. Agents that enhance bactericidal activity of sulfa drugs
    c. Agents that enhance the spectrum of activity of penicillins
    d. Agents that reduce the risk of liver damage from hepatotoxic drugs

239. Within the past few years there have been reports of dogs having adverse reactions to sulfadiazine, a very commonly used sulfonamide. What reaction should clients and veterinary professionals watch for?
    a. Cardiac arrest
    b. Sudden liver failure
    c. Decreased tear production
    d. Increased urination

240. What antibacterial drug is also effective against protozoa such as *Giardia*?
    a. Clindamycin
    b. Griseofulvin
    c. Metronidazole
    d. Sulfasalazine

241. Ketoconazole, miconazole, and griseofulvin are effective against
    a. Viruses
    b. Flukes
    c. Intestinal nematodes
    d. Fungi

242. What drug is used intravenously to treat status epilepticus?
    a. Primidone
    b. Phenytoin
    c. Diazepam
    d. Phenobarbital

243. What anticonvulsant drug is converted by the liver primarily to phenobarbital, which accounts for most of its anticonvulsant activity?
    a. Diazepam
    b. Primidone
    c. Phenytoin
    d. Clonazepam

244. What traditional anticonvulsant is now being used simultaneously with phenobarbital in dogs that are nonresponsive to phenobarbital alone?
    a. Diazepam
    b. Potassium bromide
    c. Phenytoin
    d. Strychnine

245. What drug is a respiratory stimulant?
    a. Oxytocin
    b. Dobutamine
    c. Propranolol
    d. Doxapram

246. Drugs that effectively block the cough reflex are called
    a. Mucolytics
    b. Expectorants
    c. Antitussives
    d. Antihistamines

247. Drugs that reduce the viscosity of secretions in the respiratory tract are called
    a. Antiinflammatories
    b. Expectorants
    c. Antitussives
    d. Antihistamines

248. Drugs used to increase airflow through respiratory passageways narrowed by the contraction of smooth muscle around them are called
    a. Bronchodilators
    b. Expectorants
    c. Antitussives
    d. Antihistamines

249. Butorphanol and hydrocodone are examples of
    a. Mucolytics
    b. Expectorants
    c. Antitussives
    d. Antihistamines

250. Drugs that are described as β_2-adrenergic receptor stimulators have what effect on the respiratory tree?
    a. Increase the volume of watery secretions
    b. Increase the volume of sticky mucoid secretions
    c. Cause bronchoconstriction
    d. Cause bronchodilatation

Correct answers are on pages 147-160.

251. Terbutaline, albuterol, and metaproterenol are described as selective β_2-adrenergic agonists. They are used in veterinary medicine to
    a. Treat feline asthma or other bronchoconstrictive diseases
    b. Treat low blood pressure caused by shock
    c. Suppress a productive cough, such as in bronchopneumonia
    d. Stimulate secretions within the respiratory tree to aid the mucociliary apparatus

252. Methylxanthines are often used to improve breathing in cardiac patients and patients with respiratory disease. What drugs are methylxanthines used for this purpose?
    a. Theophylline and aminophylline
    b. Codeine and dextromethorphan
    c. Hydrocodone and butorphanol
    d. Guaifenesin and propranolol

253. Most drugs that control arrhythmias of the heart are said to be "negative inotropes." What does this mean?
    a. They increase the heart rate.
    b. They decrease the heart rate.
    c. They increase the force of contractions.
    d. They decrease the force of contractions.

254. What drug reduces tachyarrhythmias by decreasing conduction of the impulse that causes cardiac contraction through the heart?
    a. Propranolol
    b. Lidocaine
    c. Procainamide
    d. Digoxin

255. Hyperthyroid cats have heart rates of over 200 beats per minute because of large numbers of β_1-sympathetic receptors in their heart that make the heart more sensitive to epinephrine and norepinephrine. This high heart rate is an anesthetic risk. What drug is used to slow the heart rate and decrease arrhythmias associated with β_1-receptor stimulation?
    a. Lidocaine
    b. Propranolol
    c. Quinidine
    d. Digoxin

256. Digoxin has a narrow therapeutic index. What does this mean?
    a. Plasma drug concentrations that produce toxicity are very low.
    b. Plasma drug concentrations required to achieve a beneficial effect are very high.
    c. Plasma drug concentrations that produce toxicity are very close to the minimum concentration at which a beneficial effect occurs.
    d. Plasma drug concentrations are extremely variable from animal to animal.

257. Because digoxin has a narrow therapeutic index, veterinary technicians and owners of animals that receive digoxin must be able to detect early signs of digoxin toxicity, such as
    a. Increased urination and increased water consumption
    b. Increased coughing and difficulty breathing
    c. Decreased appetite, anorexia, diarrhea, and vomiting
    d. Wobbly gait, fainting (syncope), and disorientation

258. Some drugs commonly used to treat veterinary patients with cardiovascular disease alter the electrolyte levels (Na^+, K^+, Cl^-) within the body. Which electrolyte change greatly enhances the risk of digoxin toxicity?
    a. Increased sodium (hypernatremia)
    b. Increased potassium (hyperkalemia)
    c. Decreased chloride (hypochloremia)
    d. Decreased potassium (hypokalemia)

259. What drug would be most effective against dermatophytes?
    a. Tylosin
    b. Enrofloxacin
    c. Sulfadimethoxine
    d. Itraconazole

260. Drugs classified as ACE inhibitors have what effect on the body?
    a. Increase the strength of heart contractions
    b. Cause vasodilatation
    c. Cause bronchodilatation
    d. Increase the heart rate

261. Captopril is an example of a(n)
    a. Positive inotrope
    b. Antiarrhythmic
    c. Bronchodilator
    d. Vasodilator

262. Nitroglycerin is sometimes used as a paste applied to the pinna or to the abdominal skin in dogs with cardiovascular disease. Nitroglycerin has what therapeutic effect?
    a. Increases strength of heart contractions
    b. Causes vasodilation
    c. Causes bronchodilation
    d. Decreases the heart rate

263. Spironolactone, chlorothiazide, and furosemide are classified as
    a. Diuretics
    b. Positive inotropes
    c. Antiarrhythmics
    d. Vasodilators

264. Dogs with heartworm disease are treated with aspirin because it
    a. Increases the diuretic effect of drugs like furosemide
    b. Decreases the risk of clot formation and proliferation of the pulmonary arterial lining
    c. Increases the ability of vasodilators to keep the coronary arterioles fully dilated
    d. Decreases oxygen consumption by the weakened cardiac muscle

265. What controlled substance rating indicates the drug with the greatest potential for abuse?
    a. C-III
    b. C-II
    c. C-V
    d. C-IV

266. For what reason is apomorphine used in canine patients in emergency veterinary medicine?
    a. To keep blood pressure elevated in animals in shock
    b. To alleviate pain
    c. To produce emesis after ingestion of a toxin
    d. To maintain kidney function during periods of reduced blood flow to the kidneys

267. What drug is most likely to be prescribed to prevent motion sickness?
    a. Apomorphine
    b. Syrup of ipecac
    c. Atropine
    d. Diphenhydramine

268. For what is syrup of ipecac used?
    a. To stimulate defecation to flush out poisons from the distal bowel
    b. To induce vomiting
    c. To stimulate duodenal movement to overcome constipation
    d. To increase blood supply to the gastrointestinal tract

269. Why should syrup of ipecac and activated charcoal (the universal antidote) not be given simultaneously?
    a. The resultant vomiting is too severe and too prolonged.
    b. They cancel out the beneficial effects of each other.
    c. Neither is absorbed in sufficient quantity to be of any benefit.
    d. Severe diarrhea and intestinal cramping result.

270. Anticholinergic drugs like atropine, aminopentamide (Centrine), or isopropamide (Darbazine) are expected to have what effect on the gastrointestinal tract?
    a. Increase secretions by the bowel
    b. Increase movement of feces through the bowel
    c. Decrease ability of compounds to irritate the bowel wall
    d. Decrease bowel motility

271. Opioid drugs such as paregoric and loperamide are often used as antidiarrheals. What is their main effect on the gastrointestinal tract?
    a. Decrease diarrhea by decreasing peristaltic waves
    b. Decrease diarrhea by relaxing segmental mixing contractions
    c. Decrease diarrhea by increasing segmental mixing contractions
    d. Decrease constipation by increasing intestinal secretions

272. Bismuth subsalicylate is the active ingredient in a common over-the-counter (OTC) preparation used for some types of gastrointestinal disease for what effect?
    a. Mild laxative
    b. Antiemetic
    c. Antidiarrheic
    d. Emetic

273. Drugs like flunixin meglumine, ibuprofen, and other NSAIDs often produce side effects in the gastrointestinal tract with long-term use or high-dosage use, especially in dogs. What are the side effects?
    a. Increased bowel motility, resulting in fluid diarrhea
    b. Decreased ability to digest fat, resulting in fatty stool (steatorrhea)
    c. Ulcers or gastritis from decreased mucus production
    d. Decreased bowel motility, resulting in constipation

Correct answers are on pages 147-160.

274. Cimetidine and ranitidine are often called H 2 blockers, traditionally referred to as *histamine receptors*. For what effect are they used?
    a. Antidiarrheal
    b. Laxative
    c. Rumen stimulant
    d. Antacid

275. What type of medication is sucralfate (Carafate)?
    a. Antiulcer
    b. Antidiarrheal
    c. Antibloat
    d. Anticonstipation

276. The drug most commonly used in treating animals with hypothyroidism is
    a. Thyroid-stimulating hormone (TSH)
    b. Thyroid extract
    c. Synthetic levothyroxine (T$_4$)
    d. Synthetic liothyronine (T$_3$)

277. For what disease are methimazole and propylthiouracil used?
    a. Hypothyroidism in dogs
    b. Cushings disease (hyperadrenocorticism) in dogs
    c. Hyperthyroidism in cats
    d. Addisons disease (hypoadrenocorticism) in dogs

278. What drug is used to return a mare to proestrus from diestrus through lysis of the corpus luteum?
    a. Progesterone
    b. Estrogen
    c. Prostaglandin
    d. Gonadotropin

279. What hormone is given to mares or cows for several days to mimic diestrus and then withdrawn to mimic natural lysis of the corpus luteum and a return to proestrus?
    a. Estradiol cypionate (ECP)
    b. Prostaglandin-F2-alpha (dinoprost tromethamine)
    c. Human chorionic gonadotropin (HCG)
    d. Progestin (Altrenogest)

280. What reproductive hormone can produce pyometra in dogs? It is also used in the pregnant mare in an attempt to keep it from prematurely aborting its fetus.
    a. Estrogen
    b. Progesterone
    c. Gonadotropin
    d. Prostaglandin

281. What reproductive hormone can cause severe (and sometimes fatal) aplastic anemia or open-cervix pyometra several weeks after it has been given?
    a. Estradiol cypionate
    b. Prostaglandin-F2-alpha (dinoprost tromethamine)
    c. Human chorionic gonadotropin
    d. Progestin (Altrenogest)

282. What drug is used as a contraceptive in dogs and sometimes for correction of behavioral problems in cats (e.g., inappropriate urination)?
    a. Altrenogest
    b. Megestrol acetate
    c. Estradiol cypionate
    d. Dinoprost tromethamine

283. What drug does not cause the adverse gastro-intestinal effects associated with most NSAIDs?
    a. Aspirin (salicylate)
    b. Flunixin meglumine
    c. Acetaminophen
    d. Phenylbutazone

284. The glucocorticoid drug commonly used orally to treat inflammatory conditions in dogs and cats is
    a. Hydrocortisone
    b. Prednisone
    c. Triamcinolone
    d. Dexamethasone

285. Predictable, short-term side effects of glucocorticoid therapy of which every client should be aware are
    a. Polyuria and polydipsia
    b. Cough and nasal discharge
    c. Anorexia and diarrhea
    d. Dry skin and skin irritations

286. Commonly used glucocorticoids affect the CBC. What are the effects of glucocorticoid use on the CBC?
    a. Neutrophils decreased, eosinophils increased, lymphocytes decreased
    b. Neutrophils increased, eosinophils increased, lymphocytes increased
    c. Neutrophils increased, eosinophils decreased, lymphocytes decreased
    d. Neutrophils decreased, eosinophils decreased, lymphocytes increased

287. Chronic administration of high doses of glucocorticoids can cause iatrogenic
    a. Renal failure
    b. Addisons disease
    c. Cushings disease
    d. Johnes disease

288. In what species might glucocorticoid administration lead to abortion during the last few weeks of gestation?
    a. Horses and cattle
    b. Pigs and dogs
    c. Dogs and cats
    d. Horses and cats

289. NSAIDs are most likely to cause side effects in what two organ systems?
    a. Renal and pulmonary
    b. Renal and gastrointestinal
    c. Pulmonary and cardiac
    d. Cardiac and hepatic

290. Which NSAID, when given perivascularly in horses, can cause skin necrosis and sloughing?
    a. Phenylbutazone
    b. Etodolac
    c. Ketoprofen
    d. Meclofenamic acid

291. One of the following antiinflammatory drugs is sometimes applied topically. Care must be taken to clean the area where it is applied because it readily penetrates the skin and can carry bacterial toxins or other chemicals with it into the body. What drug is this?
    a. Dexamethasone
    b. Dimethyl sulfoxide
    c. Flunixin meglumine
    d. Hydrocortisone

292. Which of these opioid drugs is not a controlled substance?
    a. Butorphanol
    b. Loperamide
    c. Buprenorphine
    d. Fentanyl

293. A drug's package insert states that the drug is an anticestodal. Against what type of parasite will this drug be effective?
    a. Ascarids *(Toxocara, Toxascaris)*
    b. Tapeworms *(Taenia)*
    c. Protozoa *(Eimeria, Giardia)*
    d. Flukes (liver fluke, lung fluke)

294. What breed of dog has a blood-brain barrier that allows ivermectin to reach toxic concentrations within the brain more readily than in other breeds?
    a. German shepherd
    b. Collie
    c. Schnauzer
    d. Cocker spaniel

295. What drug is used most commonly as a microfilaricide in treatment of heartworm disease?
    a. Thiacetarsemide
    b. Diethylcarbamazine
    c. Ivermectin
    d. Piperazine

296. If an animal receives an overdose of organophosphate insecticide (from dips, powders, sprays), what is the treatment of choice?
    a. Diphenhydramine (Benadryl)
    b. Corticosteroids (glucocorticoids)
    c. Intravenous fluids to aid elimination of the compound through the urine
    d. Atropine

297. What insecticide is effective in treating demodectic mange?
    a. Fenoxycarb
    b. Amitraz
    c. Pyrethrin
    d. Allethrin

298. Methoprene and fenoxycarb are ingredients found increasingly in flea and other insect products. What are they?
    a. Insecticides
    b. Repellents
    c. Insect growth regulators
    d. Synergists

299. The following information was provided for a prescription written by a veterinarian: Dr. Pete Bill, Veterinary Associates, Inc., 325 Sentry Highway West Lafayette, IN 47907. Indiana License Number #4xxx. (317) 555-8636. For: Mr. R. K. Jones, 111, Melrose Place, Loomisville, IN 47905. Canine patient, Amoxicillin 100 mg tablets, Sig: 1 tab q8h po prn 2 refills. Date: 1/5/96. Signature: Pete Bill. What vital information is missing from this prescription?
    a. Veterinarian's Drug Enforcement Administration (DEA) license number
    b. Pet's name
    c. Owner's telephone number
    d. Number of tablets

300. The following information was provided for a prescription written by a veterinarian: Canine patient, Amoxicillin 100 mg tablets, Sig: 1 tab q8h po prn 2 refills. Date: 1/5/96. In the prescription what does *po* mean?
    a. Administer every other day
    b. Administer by mouth
    c. Administer as needed
    d. Administer on an empty stomach

Correct answers are on pages 147-160.

301. The following information was provided for a prescription written by a veterinarian: Canine patient, Amoxicillin 100 mg tablets, Sig: 1 tab q8h po prn 2 refills. Date: 1/5/96. How many times a day is this medication to be given?
    a. Once
    b. Twice
    c. Three times
    d. Four times

302. The following information was provided for a prescription written by a veterinarian: Canine patient, Amoxicillin 100 mg tablets, Sig: 1 tab q8h po prn 2 refills. Date: 1/5/96. What does *prn* mean?
    a. Administer every other day
    b. Administer by mouth
    c. Administer as needed
    d. Administer on an empty stomach

303. The abbreviations *od* and *os* on a prescription refer to
    a. Administer by mouth and by rectum
    b. Administer every other day and every 3 days
    c. Right eye and left eye
    d. Administer with food and without food

304. What do *15 gr* and *10 g* mean on a prescription?
    a. 15 grains and 10 grams
    b. 15 grains and 10 grains
    c. 15 grams and 10 grams
    d. 15 grams and 10 grains

305. Most pharmaceutical agents that are measured in grains have how many milligrams per grain?
    a. 30
    b. 60
    c. 100
    d. 120

306. Which of the following is a concentration of a drug solution?
    a. 15 mg/kg
    b. 1000 U/ml
    c. 20 gr/mg
    d. 250 g/lb

307. How many milliliters are in a teaspoon?
    a. 1
    b. 3
    c. 5
    d. 10

308. How many cubic centimeters are in a tablespoon?
    a. 5
    b. 15
    c. 25
    d. 30

309. Which equivalent is correct?
    a. q12h = QD
    b. q6h = QID
    c. q4h = TID
    d. q8h = BID

310. A 10-kg animal weighs how many pounds?
    a. 2
    b. 15
    c. 18
    d. 22

311. What dosage form must be shaken before administration to an animal?
    a. Solution
    b. Ointment
    c. Gel
    d. Suspension

312. When a drug is used by a route, in a species, or for another indication other than that specified by the manufacturer, this use is
    a. A felony offense
    b. An extra label use
    c. Prohibited by the AVMA
    d. An implied consent from the manufacturer

313. Each drug approved for use in food-producing animals has a time period given on the label between the last dose and when the animal can be slaughtered for food or when the milk can be sold. What is this period called?
    a. Elimination half-life
    b. Secretion period
    c. Refractory period
    d. Withdrawal time

314. Sometimes drugs are first administered in a large dose and then given as a series of smaller doses. What is the first dose called?
    a. Initial dose
    b. Loading dose
    c. Distribution dose
    d. Bolus dose

315. Many drugs do not have X mg/ml listed on their labels but instead have their concentrations listed as a percent (e.g., X% solution). Which of the following most accurately reflects the conversion of a percentage of a solution to a weight per volume format?
    a. X% = X g/ml
    b. X% = X g/10 ml
    c. X% = X g/100 ml
    d. X% = X mg/10 ml

316. How many milligrams are in each milliliter of a 24% solution?
   a. 24
   b. 2.4
   c. 240
   d. 0.24

317. What class of drugs generally poses the greatest potential health threat to those handling the medication?
   a. Antibiotics
   b. Antineoplastics
   c. Antinematodals
   d. Antiprotozoals

318. What effect does renal failure or compromised liver function have on the pharmacokinetics of many drugs?
   a. Decreased absorption of drugs given orally
   b. Increased elimination rate of drugs from the body
   c. Decreased volume of distribution of drugs
   d. Increased half-life of drugs

319. Controlled substances are drugs that
   a. Cannot be used in any animal intended for use as human food
   b. Have a high potential for abuse
   c. Are very hazardous to anyone handling them
   d. Are environmentally hazardous

320. Drugs that are administered intra articularly are injected into
   a. The abdominal cavity
   b. The globe of the eye
   c. The ear canal
   d. A joint

321. If a drug that is very irritating to tissues is accidentally given outside of the cephalic vein (perivascularly), you should immediately
   a. Apply a tourniquet to prevent movement of the drug up the leg
   b. Infiltrate the area with sterile saline or other sterile isotonic fluid
   c. Aspirate the area with a needle and syringe to remove as much drug as possible
   d. Inject epinephrine into the area to constrict the capillaries and decrease drug absorption

322. Generally 1 fluid ounce is equal to approximately how many milliliters of liquid?
   a. 1
   b. 15
   c. 30
   d. 60

Answers

1. **d** The neonatal liver is not equipped to deal efficiently with the biotransformation of most drugs until approximately 1 month of age.

2. **b** The majority of the biotransformation of most drugs occurs in the liver.

3. **d** Generic and nonproprietary names are interchangeable; no single company owns the rights to these types of names.

4. **d** Sustained-release and enteric-coated medicines should not be divided, because they are meant to dissolve at a specified rate and in a uniform manner; this dissolution is dependent on the outer surface of the tablet being intact.

5. **d** Sig, instructions; q4h, every 4 hours; po, by mouth; and prn, as needed.

6. **a** 2.5% = 25 mg/ml; therefore in 10 ml there is 250 mg of thiopentone.

7. **c** Bioavailability is the percentage of administered drug that gains access to the systemic circulation.

8. **d** Cholinergic agents mimic the effects of the parasympathetic nervous system; sometimes it is referred to as the "rest and restore" system; it has minimal effect on peripheral vessels.

9. **b** Administration of even small doses of acetaminophen (Tylenol) to cats may be fatal.

10. **b** Aminoglycoside drugs tend to concentrate in the kidneys and inner ears.

11. **c** Tetracyclines have been in use for many years, and, as a result, the resistance to them is proportionately greater than with many other antiinfectives.

12. **c** Cephalosporins and penicillins are both β-lactam drugs; animals with an allergy to one class are usually also allergic to the other class.

13. **b** Sulfonamide antibiotics are excreted in the urine and can be useful for urinary tract infections with susceptible organisms.

14. **b** At some doses, the fluoroquinolone drug Enrofloxacin has been associated with blindness in cats.

15. **d** Chloramphenicol use is banned in food animals in the United States, because it may cause irreversible aplastic anemia in humans.

16. **c** Some metabolism of penicillins occurs in the liver, but penicillins are mainly excreted intact by the kidneys.

17. **d** Acepromazine may cause paraphimosis in stallions.

18. **c** "KetVal," ketamine and Valium (diazepam), is a commonly used drug combination.

19. **c** Diazepam has a potential to react with plastic. Prolonged exposure should be avoided.

20. **a** Xylazine hydrochloride is an α_2-adrenergic receptor agonist that is antagonized by Yohimbine.

21. **d** Griseofulvin is a superficial antifungal agent.

22. **d** Potential for renal disease but no adverse effects on liver

23. **b** Fluoroquinolones have been associated with cartilage damage in young horses and puppies.

24. **c** Potentiated penicillins are resistant to inactivation by β-lactamase.

25. **c** IP is the abbreviation for "intraperitoneal."

26. **c** Xylazine is an α_2-adrenergic receptor agonist.

27. **d** Propofol has a wide margin of safety and may be used as continuous infusion or as repeated boluses.

28. **b** Butorphanol's original use was as a cough suppressant.

29. **a** Iodophors are iodine combined with a carrier molecule; the effect is that the iodine is released over time, so there is a prolonged effect.

30. **c** Ivermectin is a proven preventive for *Dirofilaria immitis*.

31. **c** Moxidectin is a member of the avermectin drug class.

32. **d** Prostaglandins cause smooth-muscle contraction and may be absorbed across the skin. Asthmatics should wear gloves when administering prostaglandins or avoid them entirely.

33. **d** Long-term loop diuretics may often lead to hypokalemia; potassium supplements are often administered. They increase the excretion of water by increasing the excretion of the electrolytes (salts), especially potassium.

34. **a**

35. **c** Lidocaine diminishes nerve conduction; when given as an IV bolus, it may slow nerve conduction through the heart and cause bradyarrhythmia.

36. **c** Butorphanol is used alone and can be used to reverse the depressant effects of other opioid drugs.

37. **c** Acepromazine is a phenothiazine derivative that has the effect of vasodilation; therefore the blood pressure falls, resulting in hypotension.

38. **d**

39. **d** Aspirin has a long half-life in cats, 30 hours, because it is excreted by the liver (albeit slowly).

40. **c** Insect growth regulators (IGRs) affect immature stages and are generally considered safe.

41. **d** Anipryl administration allows dopamine levels to increase; reduced dopamine levels are associated with canine cognitive dysfunction.

42. **d** Osteoporosis is a *long-term* effect.

43. **b** Mild sedation or drowsiness is a common side effect of most antihistamine drugs.

44. **a**

45. **b** Sight hounds such as greyhounds, have minimal fat, so the thiobarbiturates will remain in the circulation at high concentrations.

46. **a** Atropine is a mydriatic and cycloplegic and is used to facilitate examination of the eye.

47. **b** *Chronotropic* relates to rate; *inotropic* relates to force.

48. c Doxapram is a respiratory stimulant.

49. d Subcutaneous and intramuscular injections may lead to sloughing of tissue.

50. d

51. a Biotransformation, or drug metabolism, is the altering of a drug before its elimination from the body. The liver is the primary organ involved in biotransformation.

52. c The federal government requires rigorous testing of any new animal health product before its marketing. This is a very time-consuming and expensive process, taking anywhere from 7 to 10 years at a cost ranging from $15 to $20 million. Generic drugs are often chemically identical to trademark name drugs.

53. b Repository forms of injectable drugs are not necessarily irritating to tissues and are formulated specifically to prolong absorption from the site of administration. Enteric coatings protect drugs from the acidic environment of the stomach.

54. d The two major routes of drug elimination are via the kidney into the urine and via the liver into the bile and subsequently into the feces. Certain drugs, for example, inhalant anesthetics, are mostly eliminated via the lungs.

55. b Drugs administered intravenously are generally clear, rather than cloudy or thick, and they contain suspended particles. Elixirs are intended for oral administration.

56. a Therapeutic range is the plasma concentration of drug considered to provide the most beneficial results. If this range is narrow, the difference between a therapeutic dose and a potentially toxic dose is very small.

57. b The Environmental Protection Agency (EPA) is the regulatory agency that oversees the development and approval of animal topical pesticides, and the Food and Drug Administration (FDA) oversees the development and approval of new animal drugs and feed additives. The United States Department of Agriculture (USDA) regulates the development and approval of vaccines and sera. The Drug Enforcement Administration (DEA) strictly enforces the regulations for the prescribing, handling, and storing of controlled substances.

58. a

59. d Drugs administered intravenously, directly into the bloodstream, reach their peak plasma concentration virtually instantaneously as compared to those administered and absorbed through other routes.

60. d Albon is a coccidiostat and antibacterial drug. All other drugs listed have antifungal activity.

61. b Clavulanic acid is added to penicillin drugs such as amoxicillin, producing a potentiated compound. This combination drug is active against a wider spectrum of bacteria, including those that produce enzymes called *β-lactamase*, which attack and break down penicillin's β-lactam ring, rendering it inactive.

62. b The aminoglycoside group of antibiotics is successfully used in the treatment of severe bacterial infections, although a great deal of care must be taken because of their potential to cause serious side effects.

63. b By collecting a sample for bacterial culture and sensitivity and sending it to the laboratory, a veterinarian will be able to determine the causative agent for the infection, as well as the specific antibiotics that will be most successful in eradicating that infection.

64. d Chloramphenicol is a broad-spectrum antibiotic often used for the treatment of infections in rabbits and pocket pets, because penicillins and cephalosporins are potentially toxic in these species. Chloramphenicol has been found to cause myelosuppression in mammals, including humans, resulting in nonregenerative anemia and leukopenia. Care must be taken in handling this drug to minimize repeated contact with or inhalation of the powder.

65. a Anaphylactic reactions may occur in response to a variety of substances, including drugs, vaccines, diagnostic agents such as radiographic contrast media, protein foods, and insect venom.

66. a Sulfonamides—including Tribrissen, Primor, and Albon—are still often used for treatment of infections, although it is important that veterinary professionals be able to recognize the potentially serious side effects of these drugs.

67. d

68. b

69. **c** Although the bioavailability of most penicillins is decreased in the presence of food, amoxicillin is an exception to this rule and need not be administered on an empty stomach.

70. **c**

71. **d** Enrofloxacin is commonly used in pocket pets, because it is not active against the anaerobic flora of the gut.

72. **a** Guaifenesin is also administered intravenously for muscle relaxation in equine anesthesia.

73. **b** Dextromethorphan is generally not as effective as prescription antitussives.

74. **c** Acute respiratory failure is generally best managed by intubation and mechanical support of respiration. In certain instances, however, it may be desirable to stimulate respiration with drugs. One indication for use of a respiratory stimulant drug is when the respiratory efforts of neonates are adversely affected by general anesthesia of the bitch during cesarean section.

75. **a** Butorphanol is a narcotic analgesic drug used in preanesthetic protocols and to control pain, as well as an antitussive.

76. **c** An expectorant helps loosen phlegm and thin bronchial secretions associated with a cough that is producing mucus. It is best not to suppress a productive cough with an antitussive, because coughing helps the body clear its airways.

77. **a**

78. **d** Fibrinolysis is the dissolution of a fibrin clot or thromboembolus. The fibrinolytic drug used most often in the treatment of thromboembolism is streptokinase.

79. **d** By definition, congestive heart failure involves fluid congestion or accumulation in the body. This usually occurs in the abdominal cavity in the form of ascites or in the thoracic cavity or lungs in the form of pulmonary edema. Diuretics are indicated to rid the body of this excess fluid. Furosemide (Lasix) is the treatment of choice in both the acute and chronic forms of cardiac failure.

80. **a** Epinephrine or adrenalin is an adrenergic (sympathomimetic) agent that stimulates all receptors to cause an increase in heart rate and cardiac output.

81. **c** Vasodilators relax blood vessels, allowing blood to flow more freely out of the congested heart. Because these vascular walls dilate, the pressure of the blood within may drop, resulting in hypotension.

82. **c** Inotropy is the force of cardiac contraction, and chronotropy is the frequency of cardiac contraction.

83. **a** Epinephrine is the initial drug of choice for treating bronchoconstriction and hypotension resulting from anaphylaxis, as well as all forms of cardiac arrest.

84. **d** Warfarin is an oral anticoagulant that binds vitamin K and is used in many rodenticides. Vitamin K is essential in the synthesis of several clotting factors, and so the management of this toxicity involves the administration of vitamin K.

85. **b** Chemotherapeutic agents usually have low margins of safety; consequently, doses must be calculated with care, and treatment must be closely monitored.

86. **b** Most cancer chemotherapeutic drugs suppress components of the immune system.

87. **c** Antineoplastic compounds produce characteristic toxicity to various body tissues that are related to tissue growth rate. Lymphocytes and bone marrow cells are most profoundly affected, followed by the mucosal cells of the gastrointestinal tract and cells of the hair follicles. Pruritus is a less frequently anticipated side effect of chemotherapy.

88. **d** Drugs of plant origin may be inactivated by the digestive microorganisms in the rumen.

89. **a**

90. **b** High levels of glucocorticoids cause Cushings disease. When the glucocorticoids are exogenous, the disease is called *iatrogenic*.

91. **c** Glucocorticoids are contraindicated in patients with infections, because they are potentially immune-suppressive.

92. **a**

93. **d** Glucocorticoids may cause immune suppression.

94. **a** Prednisone is a steroid drug of the glucocorticoid type.

95. **c** Carprofen and etodolac selectively target inhibition of the enzyme cyclooxygenase-2 (COX-2), thereby reducing inflammation without blocking the prostaglandins associated with protection of the gastrointestinal tract and renal vascularity and blood flow.

96. **b** Flunixin meglumine is primarily used in equine patients with colic for its antiinflammatory, analgesic, and antiendotoxin effects.

97. **b** Most NSAIDs have a long half-life in cats compared to other species.

98. **a** Cats are deficient in the liver enzyme glucuronyl transferase and thus metabolize aspirin very slowly.

99. **b** Most NSAIDs inhibit the enzyme cyclooxygenase, which leads to a reduction in the synthesis of both inflammatory prostaglandins and those prostaglandins that act to protect the mucosa of the gastrointestinal tract.

100. **d** DMSO has the ability to penetrate intact skin; this is prevented if the person applying it wears gloves.

101. **d** This is necessary to minimize the effects of diffusion hypoxia, which occurs when nitrous oxide diffuses from the bloodstream into the lungs, thus diluting the oxygen concentration within the alveoli.

102. **a**

103. **c** Malignant hyperthermia, a potential side effect of halothane anesthesia, is a greatly increased body temperature that can result in brain damage or death.

104. **c** Thiopental and phenobarbital are both barbiturate drugs.

105. **a**

106. **c** Diazepam, usually administered intravenously, is the anticonvulsant drug of choice in the emergency treatment of seizures. It is also absorbed well through the mucosal lining of the rectum, thereby providing the ability to treat a pet before arrival at the emergency facility.

107. **a** Although most anesthetic agents cause cardiovascular depression, medetomidine characteristically produces a profound bradycardia.

108. **b** Yohimbine is an antagonist to xylazine, atipamezole antagonizes the action of medetomidine (Domitor), and naloxone is a narcotic antagonist.

109. **c** Side effects of narcotic drugs include hypersensitivity to noise, vomiting, and defecation. Morphine will likely depress Oreo's respiratory system, thus producing a decreased rather than an elevated respiratory rate.

110. **b**

111. **b**

112. **b**

113. **d** A potential side effect of acepromazine and other phenothiazine tranquilizers is penile prolapse (paraphimosis). It is therefore contraindicated for use in breeding stallions.

114. **c** Propofol contains no preservatives, and the emulsion promotes bacterial growth. Strict aseptic technique should be applied when withdrawing propofol, and it should be used within 6 hours of opening the container.

115. **d** Ruminants are extremely sensitive to xylazine when compared with horses, dogs, or cats, generally requiring approximately one-tenth the equine dose to exhibit the same effect.

116. **c** Ketamine is a dissociative anesthetic. It does not induce the muscle relaxation found in most other anesthetics. The eyes of feline patients remain open, necessitating the use of lubricating ophthalmic ointment; to reduce the effects of hypersalivation, atropine is often used.

117. **d** Yohimbine is a specific antagonist for xylazine and reverses its depressant effects.

118. **a** In veterinary medicine it is generally felt that phenothiazines should not be used in epileptic animals or in those susceptible to seizures because they lower the convulsive threshold and may precipitate seizures.

119. **a** Benzodiazepines may cause appetite stimulation in cats.

120. a

121. d Clomicalm is a relatively new tricyclic antidepressant drug used in dogs and cats for obsessive compulsive disorders, including separation anxiety.

122. c Phenylpropanolamine is used chiefly for the treatment of hypotonus of the urethral sphincter and resulting incontinence in dogs and cats.

123. a Erythropoietin is a hormone that regulates erythropoiesis (the production of red blood cells). It is used for treatment of the anemia associated with chronic renal failure.

124. a Famotidine is an H_2 receptor blocker that decreases gastric acid production.

125. d Patients with chronic renal failure often have hyperphosphatemia. Amphojel and Basaljel bind phosphates in the diet when given with food. This reduces the phosphorus intake from the GI tract and helps normalize the blood phosphorus level.

126. b Piperazine is the vermifuge most commonly found in over-the-counter worming preparations. All other medications listed require a veterinarian's prescription.

127. d All listed medications are used for the prevention of heartworm infection. Only selamectin is additionally approved for the treatment of both ear mites and scabies.

128. c Coccidia are protozoan parasites. A coccidiostat is a drug that controls this type of infection.

129. a All of these drugs may be administered intravenously. Of the listed drugs, only Phenylbutazone (Butazolidin) requires extreme care when injecting to avoid perivascular leakage.

130. d Organophosphate parasiticides have a very narrow margin of safety. Numerous side effects include vomiting, tremors, hyperexcitability, salivation, and diarrhea.

131. b

132. c

133. b Glipizide is a human oral antidiabetic agent that may be used in certain non–insulin-dependent diabetic cats. More often, the use of insulin is necessary.

134. c

135. a Clients must be instructed in proper techniques for withdrawing insulin into the syringe, including rolling the vial rather than shaking it before drawing it into the syringe.

136. c Progestins or progesterones usually have *-gest* in their drug name.

137. b

138. c

139. d Kaolin and pectin (Kaopectate) and bismuth subsalicylate (Pepto-Bismol) coat the intestinal mucosa, thereby protecting it from bacterial enterotoxins and other irritating substances.

140. b

141. b Phenothiazine drugs characteristically cause central nervous system depression, hypotension, and a lowering of the seizure threshold.

142. a Docusate is used in small animals when feces are hard or dry or in anorectal conditions when passing firm feces would be painful or detrimental to the animal's recovery.

143. a Phenothiazine antiemetics include acepromazine, chlorpromazine, and prochlorperazine.

144. a An adverse effect of xylazine when used as a sedative in cats is emesis. It is a safer and more effective emetic in cats than the other three drugs/compounds listed.

145. c Apomorphine is a rapidly acting, centrally mediated emetic used often in dogs that have ingested a potentially toxic substance.

146. c Apomorphine is administered as a tablet in the conjunctival sac.

147. b After oral administration, sucralfate reacts with hydrochloric acid in the stomach to form a paste like complex that binds to ulcer sites, forming a barrier that protects the ulcer from further damage.

148. c Cats may be particularly sensitive to the electrolyte imbalance effects of sodium phosphate enema solutions, and these products are not recommended for use in this species.

149. **a** Drug biotransformation is the inactivation or metabolism of a drug.

150. **d** Acepromazine is a sedative drug often used to help prevent motion sickness in dogs and cats.

151. **c** Animals in terminal renal failure are often anemic because of a deficit of endogenous erythropoietin. The administration of Epogen (a human-derived product) can stimulate the bone marrow to produce and release red blood cells.

152. **a** Interferon is administered to animals in an effort to enhance the function of the immune system. They are believed to have antiviral and antitumor activity. Interferon is derived from white blood cells and other cells of the body. It is recognized for its immunoregulatory effect.

153. **c** Atropine is given as a preanesthetic agent to maintain heart rate and decrease oral secretions. Some less desirable effects include decreased GI motility and decreased lacrimal secretions.

154. **c** An antagonist acts to reduce the likelihood of an activity (or impulse) from occurring. By blocking the receptor on an effector organ, an impulse is blocked. The other answers all describe the activity of an agonist.

155. **a** Aspirin therapy is discontinued before surgery because of concerns related to hemorrhage intraoperatively and postoperatively.

156. **d** Fentanyl patches are being increasingly used in veterinary medicine to control post-surgical pain. This is an example of a topical application producing systemic effects.

157. **b** Acetylcysteine is a mucolytic agent that is administered as an antidote for acetaminophen toxicity.

158. **b** By liquefying and diluting mucous secretions in the respiratory tract, an animal is better able to mobilize secretions and may actually demonstrate an increase in a productive cough.

159. **a** Drugs that achieve plasma, urine, and CSF concentrations in the therapeutic range are expected to have their desired therapeutic effect in an animal. Choice **b** is the definition for therapeutic index.

160. **c** Acepromazine can act to lower the seizure threshold, thereby increasing the likelihood of seizure activity in epileptic animals. Diazepam is used to treat seizure activity.

161. **d** Nutraceuticals are nutrients or naturally occurring substances in food (which are often purified or extracted) that have demonstrated health benefits. These agents may not make health claims in their advertising. There is controversy over whether these represent drugs or foods. Their use is gaining in popularity in veterinary medicine.

162. **d**

163. **a** Naloxone is a pure opioid antagonist and can be used to reverse the effects of opioids.

164. **c** Opioids often cause respiratory depression in animals; thus, careful monitoring of respiratory parameters is required.

165. **c** Thiobarbiturates redistribute to fat stores. In animals that are very thin (sight hounds, young animals, debilitated animals), this redistribution cannot occur; therefore blood levels remain high, increasing the likelihood of toxicity. Acidotic and hypoproteinemic animals also demonstrate increased sensitivity to thiobarbiturates.

166. **a** Hypokalemia may result from long-term use of loop diuretics such as Salix because of increased excretion of potassium.

167. **a** Norvasc is a calcium channel blocker that acts as an arteriolar vasodilator, thereby reducing cardiac afterload.

168. **c** Cats that receive ketamine as part of an anesthetic protocol demonstrate apneustic breathing (breath holding). They may also experience tachycardia and rigid muscle tone.

169. **b** ACE inhibitors prevent angiotensin converting enzyme (ACE) from converting angiotensin I to angiotensin II. This indirectly prevents sodium and water retention and also prevents vasoconstriction. This, in turn, results in a decreased preload and afterload on the heart in congestive heart failure cases.

170. **a** Nitroglycerin is a potent venodilator, it and at higher doses, it may also act as an arteriodilator. It is given to improve cardiac output by decreasing cardiac preload.

171. b Diltiazem is a calcium channel blocker used in hypertrophic cardiomyopathy (HCM) cases to relax a heart with thickened walls and poor contractility.

172. b Lidocaine is used to control premature ventricular contractions and ventricular tachycardia.

173. b The sudden withdrawal of long-term glucocorticoids can precipitate an iatrogenic (caused by the treatment) addisonian (hypoadrenocorticism) crisis, because the animal has received exogenous steroids for such a long time that the hypothalamic-pituitary-adrenal axis is suppressed and cannot resume endogenous steroid production immediately when exogenous steroids are suddenly withdrawn.

174. c Dogs that have received long-term exogenous steroids may develop the array of clinical signs associated with Cushings disease/hyperadrenocorticism.

175. d Emesis is not a commonly reported side effect of steroid administration in dogs.

176. d Glucocorticoids are the primary treatment in autoimmune, allergic/inflammatory, and some neoplastic diseases. Iatrogenic hyperadrenocorticism can actually be caused by glucocorticoid administration.

177. c All of the other drugs listed are cholinergic drugs.

178. a A veterinarian may alter a drug or medication for ease of administration by diluting, mixing drugs, and mixing drugs in a more palatable solution; this is referred to as *compounding*. Choices **b** to **d** define extra label drug use.

179. a

180. c Mannitol is osmotically active and is therefore effective at pulling fluid into the intravascular space.

181. d Choices **a** to **c** all have antiemetic action; apomorphine is used as an emetic agent in dogs.

182. b Animals that have an allergic reaction to penicillin often cross-react with cephalosporins as well.

183. a With nonlocalized or refractory infections, oral griseofulvin is used to treat dermatophytosis in addition to topical therapy with an antifungal agent.

184. d The only drug in this list that provides analgesia is the opioid fentanyl. The other drugs (acepromazine, diazepam, and thiopental) may be used as preinduction or induction agents but do not provide analgesia.

185. a Choices **b** to **d** are all microfilaricides that are used 6 weeks after the administration of an adulticide such as Immiticide.

186. c Vitamin K is administered in rodenticide toxicity cases in an effort to restore the hemostatic cascade.

187. a Propranolol is a β-adrenergic blocking agent, hydralazine is an α-adrenergic blocking agent, and epinephrine is a sympathomimetic drug.

188. c An antibiotic with a broad spectrum will be useful against a large number of microorganisms.

189. b Ideally a multidrug chemotherapy protocol aims to provide an array of drugs that attack the neoplasm in different parts of the cell cycle. There is also an attempt to select drugs that do not all result in the same adverse effects (e.g., bone marrow suppression). Most chemotherapy drugs are based on body surface area (meters squared) to achieve more accurate dosing because of the narrow margin of safety.

190. d Cyclosporine, azathioprine (Imuran), and prednisone are all used for their immunosuppressive effects.

191. c Erythromycin is a macrolide antibiotic, ampicillin is a penicillin, and doxycycline is a tetracycline.

192. a Retinal damage was reported in cats receiving SID dosing using the high end of the labeled dose range. Divided (BID) or using the lower end of the dosing range has been recommended.

193. a Cats are especially sensitive to lidocaine and may develop central nervous system (CNS) signs indicating toxicity. All animals, especially those receiving a constant rate infusion, should be carefully monitored for these signs.

194. d Theophylline and aminophylline are methylxanthines that demonstrate a bronchodilatory effect in addition to cardiac stimulation. Prednisone is used to treat asthmatics, but it is used primarily for its antiinflammatory properties and alone does not directly stimulate bronchodilation.

195. **a** Tetracyclines (oxytetracycline, doxycycline) are most commonly used as a first-line approach to treating rickettsial infections.

196. **d** Choices **a** to **c** are drugs that can potentially result in renal damage if used inappropriately.

197. **a** Cats can metabolize aspirin but do so at a very slow rate and thus must be dosed accordingly. It is best to avoid salicylates in cats when alternative drug choices exist.

198. **d** Hyperthyroid cats may receive radioactive iodine therapy (especially cats with ectopic thyroid tissue) or thyroidectomy surgery, or they may be managed medically with Tapazole. Fenbendazole is an antiparasitic drug.

199. **b** Butorphanol can be used to inhibit a nonproductive cough.

200. **b** The solubility of one sulfa in a triple sulfa is not dependent on the solubility of the other sulfas, so a smaller amount of each sulfa is used, thereby reducing the possibility of toxicity.

201. **a** An antihistamine such as diphenhydramine (Benadryl) or hydroxyzine (Atarax) is given to prevent histamine from binding to receptors and causing a detrimental histamine response (bronchoconstriction, tachycardia, etc.).

202. **a** Diazepam is used for the properties listed in the question. Cyproheptadine is an appetite stimulant often used in cats. Potassium bromide is an antiseizure medication used in refractory cases in conjunction with oral phenobarbital therapy. Ketamine is a dissociative anesthetic agent.

203. **a** Methionine (Methigel) is prescribed to promote the production of low pH (acidified) urine; this should assist with prevention and dissolution of struvite uroliths.

204. **c** Ultralente is the longest acting insulin product. NPH and Lente insulin demonstrate intermediate duration of action with regular and Semilente insulins providing the shortest duration of activity in patients.

205. **d** Insulin should be given around the time of a meal to prevent hypoglycemia.

206. **c** *Giardia and Eimeria* are protozoa.

207. **c** The minimum inhibitory concentration (MIC) for each pathologic organism can give an idea as to how high an antibiotic concentration will be necessary for it to be effective.

208. **d** Aminoglycosides are a diverse and commonly used group of antimicrobial drugs.

209. **d** Aminoglycosides are nephrotoxic (toxic to the kidney) and ototoxic (toxic to the ear).

210. **a** High dosages may increase the risk of toxicity, but they usually are sufficient to kill bacteria and prevent the selection for resistant strains of bacteria that occurs when low dosages or ineffective antibiotics are used.

211. **c** The most common adverse reaction to penicillin administration in most species is allergy (usually urticaria).

212. **a** Antifungal agents (e.g., griseofulvin) can cause birth defects if given to pregnant animals.

213. **b** Penicillin G is readily destroyed by the acidic environment in the stomach.

214. **d** Penicillins destroy the normal flora in the gut of rabbits, which may result in fatal diarrhea.

215. **b** Cloxacillin, dicloxacillin, and oxacillin are types of penicillin used in veterinary medicine that are effective against β-lactamase-producing bacteria.

216. **b** Penicillins with an added compound that destroys β-lactamase are called *potentiated penicillins*.

217. **b** Procaine penicillin G may be dosed less frequently than penicillin G. Whereas procaine is indeed a weak local anesthetic, its addition to penicillin G is for the repository effect and not for its anesthetic quality.

218. **b** The latter generations tended to shift their spectrum of activity to a greater extent against gram-negative bacteria and slightly away from gram-positive bacteria. In severe infections with gram-negative bacteria, the concept of generation when selecting a cephalosporin becomes very important.

219. **a** It is important to remember that aminoglycosides are largely ineffective against anaerobic bacteria.

220. **b** Aminoglycoside molecules are very hydrophilic, which means they do not effectively penetrate intact cellular membranes, such as those lining the gastrointestinal tract. Thus, neomycin, for the most part, remains in the bowel lumen and does not reach the kidneys.

221. **b** Aminoglycosides tend to accumulate in the fluid of the inner ear. If these concentrations rise high enough, they can damage the cells involved with hearing and balance.

222. **c** The risk of nephrotoxicity is diminished by ensuring that during the time between doses, the concentration of aminoglycoside in the body decreases below a certain critical level. A continuous intravenous infusion (drip) would not allow the concentrations to drop below this critical level.

223. **d** Casts and protein appear in the urine during the early stages of kidney insult. BUN and creatinine levels do not increase until 66% to 75% of the kidney have already been severely damaged.

224. **c** Aminoglycosides work by binding to ribosomes (made from ribonucleic acid or RNA). If there are lysed white blood cells (WBCs) present, the nucleic acid from the cellular debris binds to the aminoglycosides and prevents them from acting against the bacteria.

225. **b** Fluoroquinolone drug names typically end with *-floxacin*.

226. **a** The prostate has a blood-tissue barrier that blocks entrance of many antibiotics in a way similar to the way in which the blood-brain barrier prevents many substances from entering the brain.

227. **a** Enrofloxacin may adversely affect developing joint cartilage in dogs and horses. It has been associated with retinal blindness in cats. It is a good choice for rabbits because it does not destroy normal gut flora.

228. **c** Antibiotics, particularly tetracyclines, are effective against the spirochete bacterium *Borrelia,* which causes Lyme disease. Penicillins are also effective against this organism.

229. **c** Calcium and other minerals in the gastrointestinal tract chelates (combines with) tetracycline in such a way that the drug cannot be absorbed and is rendered ineffective. This is the reason oral tetracycline should not be given with milk products.

230. **b** The same attraction that chelates calcium to tetracycline binds tetracycline to bone and enamel in the developing fetus. The yellow mottling of otherwise white dental enamel can be unsightly.

231. **b** Luteolysis in polyestrus animals, such as cattle, can be used to synchronize breeding.

232. **d** Chloramphenicol exists largely in a non-ionized (lipophilic) form that can readily cross membranes. Most other antibiotics exist in an ionized (hydrophilic) form at normal body pH. Thus, they are prevented from readily crossing lipid membranes.

233. **a** Barbiturates rely heavily on the liver for their removal from the body. Any alteration in liver enzyme function is likely to affect barbiturate elimination and duration of action (e.g., prolongation of barbiturate anesthesia).

234. **b** The neonatal liver is not fully capable of functioning for several weeks. Thus, the neonate is unable to metabolize chloramphenicol very readily. The same is true for cats of any age.

235. **b** Chloramphenicol attaches to mitochondrial ribosomes in the bone marrow and can result in suppression of marrow blood cell formation. The result is severe anemia.

236. **c** The Food and Drug Administration (FDA) has banned use of chloramphenicol in any animal to be used for food production due to the risk of bone marrow toxicity with consumption of drug residues in foods of animal origin.

237. **b** When an animal is dehydrated, there is less water passing through the kidneys, resulting in possible precipitation of sulfate crystals that, in turn, can damage the kidneys.

238. **b** Ormetoprim and trimethoprim enhance the bactericidal effects of killing by sulfa drugs.

239. **c** Keratoconjunctivitis sicca, or dry eye, has been reported.

240. **c** Metronidazole is commonly prescribed as a therapeutic trial for suspected giardiasis, even if the organism cannot be demonstrated on fecal examinations.

241. **d** These drugs are used to treat dermatophyte infections such as ringworm.

242. **c** Diazepam (Valium) is not very effective when given PO, but it is commonly used via IV to stop ongoing seizure activity.

243. **b** Approximately 85% of primidone is converted to phenobarbital, which, in turn, constitutes the major drug-controlling seizure activity.

244. **b** This was the first anticonvulsant used in the late 1800s in people. Much of its mechanism of action is still unknown.

245. **d** Doxapram stimulates the brainstem respiratory centers.

246. **c**

247. **b**

248. **a** Bronchodilators are often used in the treatment of asthma.

249. **c** Butorphanol and hydrocodone are opioid drugs with antitussive properties.

250. **d** β_2-adrenergic receptors relax the smooth muscles that encircle the bronchioles.

251. **a** These drugs quickly reverse the bronchoconstriction caused by allergic insult, such as occurs in asthma.

252. **a** Aminophylline is actually made of 80% theophylline and 20% salt to decrease the gastrointestinal irritation when given PO.

253. **d** Many antiarrhythmic drugs may decrease the heart rate.

254. **b** Lidocaine blocks nervous conduction; this is also the reason for its local anesthetic effects.

255. **b** Propranolol is a rather nonspecific beta blocker (it blocks both β_1- and β_2-receptors). Blocking the receptors prevents the sympathetic nervous system from stimulating the heart and allows the parasympathetic system to naturally slow the heart rate.

256. **c** The therapeutic index measures how close toxic concentrations are to minimal therapeutic concentrations. If there is not much difference between the toxic dose and the beneficial dose, the therapeutic index is narrow or small.

257. **c** The gastrointestinal tract usually shows the first signs of digoxin toxicity.

258. **d** Hypokalemia, which may be caused by some diuretics used in patients with cardiovascular disease, increases the risk of digoxin toxicity. Low magnesium concentrations also do this. Sometimes patients that receive diuretics plus digoxin are given potassium supplementation to reduce the risk of digoxin toxicity.

259. **d** Dermatophytes are fungi. Choices a, b, and c are antibacterial drugs.

260. **b** ACE inhibitors block the angiotensin-converting enzyme, which is an enzyme that normally produces angiotensin II, a very potent vasoconstrictor. By blocking formation of the vasoconstrictor, the ACE inhibitor allows vasodilation.

261. **d** Captopril dilates arterioles and venules.

262. **b** Nitroglycerin is a venodilator, and, perhaps more importantly, it also dilates cardiac arterioles, providing improved blood supply to the cardiac muscle.

263. **a** These three diuretics work on different parts of the renal nephron to promote diuresis (increased urine production).

264. **b** Aspirin is used in heartworm disease to decrease clot formation and proliferation of the pulmonary arterial lining, both of which can significantly narrow the pulmonary arteries in dogs with heartworm disease.

265. **b** C-II are drugs with the highest potential for abuse that can be prescribed without special permission. C-I drugs have no proven or accepted medical application (heroin, marijuana, cocaine). C-V drugs have the lowest potential for abuse.

266. **c** Apomorphine is a potent emetic (stimulator of vomiting). It is usually administered via drops (crushed tablet in saline or water) or by placing the tablet directly into the conjunctival sac of the eye.

267. **d** Dimenhydrinate (Dramamine) and diphenhydramine (Benadryl) are antihistamines. Because histamine release is involved with vestibular stimulation of vomiting (vestibular function controls balance, sense of motion), blocking histamine receptors decreases vomiting caused by motion sickness. Acepromazine and other phenothiazine tranquilizers are also prescribed.

268. **b** Syrup of ipecac is an emetic. It is important to remember that syrup of ipecac takes up to 20 minutes to work, because it has to move into the duodenum to stimulate the gastrointestinal tract and be absorbed. Once absorbed it stimulates the chemoreceptor-trigger zone.

269. **b** Syrup of ipecac tends to coat the charcoal, preventing the toxicant from being absorbed by the charcoal. The charcoal tends to keep the syrup of ipecac away from the gastrointestinal wall, thus preventing it from irritating the gastrointestinal tract and inducing the desired emetic effect.

270. **d** These drugs are anticholinergic; that is, they work against acetylcholine. Acetylcholine is the neurotransmitter heavily involved with the parasympathetic nervous system. Blocking acetylcholine impairs the parasympathetic nervous system, which stimulates gastrointestinal movement, secretion, and blood flow.

271. **c** Opioid drugs (narcotics) are used to treat diarrhea by increasing segmental contractions of the bowel, thus increasing the resistance to feces flow.

272. **c** Pepto-Bismol contains this ingredient. The salicylate blocks prostaglandin formation in the gastrointestinal tract. Prostaglandins normally stimulate fluid secretions; therefore, blocking prostaglandin formation decreases the fluid consistency of the feces.

273. **c** Naturally occurring prostaglandins have a protective effect on the gastrointestinal tract. They increase intestinal secretions (including gastric mucus) and maintain normal perfusion of tissues. NSAIDs block prostaglandin formation, including the good prostaglandins that normally protect the stomach and intestinal tract.

274. **d** H_2 receptors are located on the cells that secrete hydrochloric acid into the stomach. When these receptors are blocked, the amount of acid dumped into the stomach is reduced.

275. **a** This drug forms a sticky paste when exposed to the acidic pH of the stomach. The paste adheres to ulcer sites and covers them like a Band-Aid, protecting the ulcer from the acidic environment of the stomach.

276. **c** TSH is available in injectable form only. Thyroid extract is made from pulverized thyroid glands, and its potency is somewhat inconsistent from dose to dose. T_3 is the active hormone, but using it as a supplement bypasses the normal regulatory mechanism that tissues have for converting just enough T_4 to T_3 to meet their metabolic needs. Therefore, T_4 is the best drug to use.

277. **c** These drugs prevent formation of new thyroid hormone, thus allowing concentrations of T_3 and T_4 to drop to normal levels.

278. **c** Prostaglandins are used to promote luteolysis in cows and mares.

279. **d**

280. **b** Progesterone increases uterine secretions and causes the endometrium to become a better incubation site for bacteria, which can lead to pyometra.

281. **a** Pyometra occurs because high levels of estrogens, such as estradiol cypionate, cause the uterine cells to produce more receptors to progesterone, essentially making the uterus more susceptible to pyometra.

282. **b** This is known by the trade name Ovaban.

283. **c** Acetaminophen is not an NSAID drug, so its mechanism of action and adverse-effect risks differ from the NSAID drugs.

284. **b** Prednisone is commonly administered orally to cats and dogs.

285. **a** Increased water consumption necessitates that the owner make accommodations for greater urinary frequency if the pet is an indoor animal.

286. **c** Glucocorticoids cause eosinophils and lymphocytes to be sequestered (taken up or hidden) from the general circulation; as a result, their numbers in the CBC decrease. Neutrophils, by contrast, come off the walls of the blood vessels and reenter the general circulation, causing neutrophilia. This pattern is commonly called a *stress leukogram*.

287. **c** Iatrogenic means "caused by the treatment itself." Cushings disease is hyperadrenocorticism, or the condition caused by excessive glucocorticoids.

288. **a** Dexamethasone is used to induce parturition in late-term or overdue cows.

289. **b** NSAIDs block prostaglandins; blocked prostaglandin formation predisposes an animal to gastritis, potential ulcer formation, and renal damage from inadequate blood and oxygen supplies.

290. **a** Phenylbutazone injection outside the vein can cause severe skin sloughing in horses.

291. **b** Dimethyl sulfoxide (DMSO) is also known for its potent garlic or raw oyster odor.

292. **b** Loperamide is the active ingredient in the over-the-counter antidiarrheal drug Imodium.

293. **b** Anticestodals are also sometimes referred to as *cestocides*.

294. **b** Collies, collie mixes, and collie-type dogs such as Australian shepherds are more susceptible to CNS toxicity after administration of avermectin drugs such as ivermectin.

295. **c** Although not officially approved for this use, ivermectin is the drug of choice for clearing *Dirofilaria* microfilariae from the blood of dogs.

296. **d** Organophosphates stimulate the parasympathetic nervous system, producing gastrointestinal hyperactivity (vomiting and diarrhea), bronchoconstriction, increased urination, and constricted pupils. Atropine blocks the parasympathetic nervous system receptor sites and therefore counteracts the parasympathetic effects.

297. **b** Amitraz (Mitaban) was developed to treat demodectic mange, a traditionally difficult condition to manage. Fenoxycarb is an insect growth regulator. Pyrethrin and allethrin are pyrethroid insecticides.

298. **c** Insect growth regulators prevent growth of the insect, which results in the death of the insect. Synergists (piperonyl butoxide) are compounds added to insecticides (like pyrethrins) to improve their insecticidal activity. Repellents used in veterinary products include butoxypolypropylene glycol (Butox PPG) and diethyltoluamide (DEET).

299. **d** The pharmacist is not likely to know how many tablets must be dispensed. The DEA number is not required except for prescriptions for controlled substances (barbiturates, tranquilizers), in which case some states require that a different prescription form be submitted.

300. **b** PO stands for the Latin *per os*, which means "by mouth."

301. **c** q8h = every 8 hours or three times daily (tid).

302. **c** PRN stands for the Latin *pro re nata*, which means "as needed."

303. **c** OD = oculus dexter (dexter means "right") and OS = oculus sinister (sinister means "left").

304. **a** The abbreviation *gr* is grain, and *g* is gram.

305. **b** Although traditionally 65 mg = 1 grain, many products (phenobarbital, aspirin) that are measured in grains use the conversion 60 mg = 1 grain.

306. **b** The concentration of a solution is a weight (mg, kg, g, gr, IU, u) per volume (ml, L, cc); units per ml (sometimes expressed as IU/ml) is commonly used for penicillin and insulin.

307. **c**

308. **b** 1 cc = 1 ml, so there are 15 milliliters in a tablespoon.

309. **b** Every 6 hours = 4 times daily (or per 24 hr); the abbreviation for four times daily (QID) should not be confused with the abbreviation for every day (QD).

310. **d** There are 2.2 lb in each kg (10 × 2.2 = 22).

311. **d** A suspension must be stirred up or shaken before dispensing to ensure uniform distribution of the drug throughout the liquid vehicle.

312. **b** Any manner of use other than that specified on the drug label is termed *extra label*.

313. **d** Any time a medication is administered to food animals, the withdrawal time must be clearly indicated on the label and to the livestock owner.

314. **b** The loading dose establishes adequate initial concentrations of the drug in the body. The smaller maintenance doses are then designed to keep the concentrations within the therapeutic range.

315. **c** A 5% solution contains 5 g/100 ml.

316. **c** There are 24 grams per 100 milliliters, which is 0.24 g per ml; 0.24 g = 240 mg.

317. **b** Antineoplastic drugs are cancer-fighting agents. They are potent and lethal to rapidly dividing cells, regardless of what animal (including the technician) they contact.

318. **d** Because many drugs leave the body through the kidneys and/or liver, a decrease in the function of these organs decreases the rate at which the drugs leave the body. Elimination rate is decreased, and half-life (the time it takes for half of the drug to leave the body) is prolonged or increased.

319. **b** Drugs are rated from C-I (most potential for abuse) to C-V (least potential for abuse).

320. **d**

321. **b** Diluting the agent is most important. Sometimes lidocaine is added to the infiltrate. Massaging the area and applying heat are also sometimes suggested.

322. **c**

Surgical Nursing

Joann Colville

QUESTIONS

1. If during surgery you notice an item at the edge of a sterile field, you should
   a. Ask others to find out whether it was contaminated.
   b. Consider it unsterile if you are not absolutely certain.
   c. Consider it sterile.
   d. Move it further into the sterile field.

2. Preparing a patient's skin for surgery
   a. Renders the skin sterile
   b. Does nothing to affect the outcome of the surgery
   c. Reduces the bacterial flora to a level that can be controlled by the patient's immune system
   d. Is not necessary if antibiotics are given

3. Ovariohysterectomy is most commonly performed
   a. In excitable dogs that need immediate calming
   b. In young female dogs
   c. In male dogs with female characteristics
   d. Exclusively in female dogs who have already had litters of puppies

4. Which of the following do/does *not* have to be sterile during a surgical procedure to maintain aseptic technique?
   a. Mask
   b. Drapes
   c. Instruments
   d. Gloves

5. The effectiveness of a surgical scrub of the hands and arms with an antibacterial soap depends on the
   a. Combination of contact time and scrubbing action
   b. Amount of soap used throughout the scrub
   c. Scrubbing action of the brush
   d. Temperature of the water

6. Which statement regarding first-intention wound healing is false?
   a. It occurs without infection.
   b. It occurs when the skin edges are held together in apposition.
   c. It usually has some degree of suppuration.
   d. It occurs with minimal scar formation.

7. Which of the following statements about electrocautery is false?
   a. If the patient is not properly grounded, the surgeon may get shocked.
   b. The intensity of the current passed through the unit is adjustable.
   c. Small bleeding blood vessels are sealed with a controlled electrical current that burns the bleeding end.
   d. All portions of the electrocautery unit can and should be sterilized.

8. Before starting the surgical procedure, the technician who has scrubbed in with the surgeon should do all of the following except
   a. Count the gauze sponges in the pack.
   b. Arrange the instruments to be quickly and easily located.
   c. Place the scalpel blade on the handle.
   d. Open the suture material.

9. An ovariohysterectomy may be performed for all of the following reasons except
   a. Prevention of prostate cancer
   b. Prevention of pyometra
   c. Sterilization of the animal
   d. Prevention of estrus

161

Correct answers are on pages 190-201.

10. Which of the following statements is true?
    a. Female cats over age 3 are too old to be spayed.
    b. Female ferrets that are not bred or spayed are likely to develop a life-threatening anemia.
    c. All female animals become fat after spaying.
    d. It is beneficial to allow a female dog to have one litter before spaying.

11. If an animal goes home with a bandage, the client should observe the bandage daily and remove it if any of the following are observed except
    a. Skin irritation at the edge of the bandage
    b. All bandages should be removed 24 hours after being applied.
    c. The bandage is wet
    d. The position of the bandage has shifted

12. Which of the following is not true about dogs being spayed before their first estrus cycle?
    a. The hair coat will change and become easier to manage with less shedding.
    b. The surgery is generally considered easier to perform if the bitch has not been through an estrus cycle.
    c. Mammary cancer is less likely to occur in a bitch that has been spayed before her first estrus cycle.
    d. The uterus and ovaries enlarge after the first estrus cycle. This necessitates a larger abdominal incision when the bitch is spayed.

13. Which one of the following statements regarding pyometra is false?
    a. The bitch that goes to surgery will have the ovaries and uterus removed.
    b. The bitch that goes to surgery will have only her uterus removed.
    c. The uterus may have ruptured before surgery begins.
    d. The patient represents a high-risk anesthesia case, because other organs in the body may be compromised.

14. All of the following statements regarding cesarean sections are true except
    a. Once the newborns are removed, the mother is out of danger, and most of the technician's attention should be on the newborns.
    b. A cesarean section is also known as a *hysterotomy*
    c. For some breeds of dogs, such as the English bulldog, it is expected that a cesarean section will need to be performed.
    d. Wait to put the mother with the newborns until after she has adequately recovered from anesthesia.

15. Which one of the following statements regarding cesarean sections is false?
    a. Bloody vaginal discharge is to be expected following surgery.
    b. The newborns delivered by cesarean section are under the effects of anesthesia.
    c. The surgical incision should be observed by the client after 1 week, because it is best not to disturb the nursing newborns.
    d. The newborn should be immediately removed from the membranous sac that covers its body when it is removed from the uterus.

16. When a male dog is presented to the hospital for a castration procedure, the technician should do all of the following except
    a. Make sure that the dog is a male.
    b. Make sure that there are two testicles in the scrotum.
    c. Make sure that he is not in heat.
    d. Make sure that there is a telephone number to reach the client.

17. When a tomcat is presented to the hospital for a castration procedure, the technician should do all of the following except
    a. Make sure that the cat is a male.
    b. Make sure that he has not been previously castrated.
    c. Make sure that there are two testicles in the scrotum.
    d. Make sure that he is not in heat.

18. When a bitch is presented to the hospital for an ovariohysterectomy, the technician should do all the following except
    a. Make sure the dog is a female.
    b. Get a telephone number where the client can be reached that day.
    c. Make sure that she is not in heat, because it would significantly complicate the surgery.
    d. Give the dog aspirin, because the surgical procedure will be painful.

19. When a queen is presented to the hospital for an ovariohysterectomy, the technician should do all the following except
    a. Make sure that the cat is a female.
    b. Get a telephone number where the client can be reached that day.
    c. Make sure that the cat is not in heat, because it would significantly complicate the surgery.
    d. Get the client or guardian's signature on the consent form.

20. When a dog is to be castrated, the veterinary technician should prepare the surgical site. The incision is most commonly made in what location?
   a. Flank
   b. Scrotum
   c. Prescrotal prepuce
   d. Mid abdomen

21. When a cat is to be castrated, the veterinary technician should prepare the surgical site. The incision is most commonly made in what location?
   a. Flank
   b. Scrotum
   c. Prescrotal prepuce
   d. Mid abdomen

22. When a dog is to be spayed, the veterinary technician should prepare the surgical site. The incision is most commonly made in what location?
   a. Inguinal
   b. Scrotum
   c. Prescrotal prepuce
   d. Abdominal ventral midline

23. The hair coat can be most efficiently and gently removed when preparing a dog to be spayed by which of the following methods?
   a. Plucking
   b. Clipping with sharp scissors
   c. Clipping against the grain of the hair with electrical clippers using a No. 40 blade
   d. Clipping against the grain of the hair with electrical clippers using a No. 10 blade

24. Which of the following statements would be false after serious oral surgery, such as mandibular fracture repair or oral-nasal tumor resection?
   a. The patient may refuse to eat.
   b. The patient may need a gastrotomy tube.
   c. The patient may refuse to drink.
   d. The patient will no longer be in pain.

25. When feeding the patient through a tube, the technician should
   a. Rapidly inject the fluids and food.
   b. Flush the tube with water.
   c. Flush the tube with air.
   d. Warm the food and fluids to 50° C before administering to the patient.

26. Which of the following statements about gastrointestinal (GI) surgery is false?
   a. The patient should be fed immediately upon recovery from anesthesia.
   b. Before closing the abdomen, the surgical team should check for sponges, instruments, strands of suture material, needles, and other possible foreign objects.
   c. During surgery additional sterile instruments, drapes, and gloves should be immediately available for the surgeon to exchange if contamination occurs.
   d. GI surgery comes with a high risk of bacterial contamination of the abdomen.

27. A semipermanent feeding tube may be placed in all of the following ways except
   a. Through the nose
   b. Through a pharyngostomy site
   c. Through a gastrostomy site
   d. Through the mouth

28. All of the following statements are true about GI surgery except
   a. It is absolutely essential to fast all patients before GI surgery. The GI tract must be empty before surgery.
   b. At no point is the GI tract sterile, therefore it is important to guard against contamination.
   c. Irrigation of the peritoneal cavity with a sterile isotonic solution after GI surgery helps reduce the number of microorganisms that remain free in the peritoneum following the procedure.
   d. The surgical assistant must be alert to the possibility of intestinal contents contaminating the abdominal cavity and must help the surgeon prevent this from happening.

29. It is important that the nursing care provided to paralyzed patients focuses on patient comfort. The prevention of decubital ulcers can be accomplished by all of the following procedures except
   a. Frequent turning or repositioning of the patient's position
   b. Adequate padding in the cage or bed
   c. Appropriate analgesic therapy
   d. Whirlpool bath hydrotherapy

30. Proptosis of the globe
   a. Can be caused by overzealous restraint of the animal
   b. Is not considered an emergency
   c. Can most easily occur in dolicocephalic breeds, such as collies
   d. Is commonly a consequence of conjunctivitis

Correct answers are on pages 190-201.

31. An abscess
    a. Is usually lanced, drained, flushed, and sutured shut
    b. Is a solid infiltration of inflammatory cells
    c. Is a rare consequence of bite wounds
    d. Is a "walled-off" or circumscribed accumulation of pus

32. All of the following are instructions to give to clients of animals that have Penrose drains placed except
    a. An Elizabethan collar may be needed.
    b. Clean the skin around the drain with warm water or dilute chlorhexidine.
    c. The drain will fall out, and there is no need to return for removal.
    d. Carefully watch the animal and prevent it from licking or chewing at the drain.

33. The client should be instructed to contact the veterinary hospital if any of the following occur with a splint or cast except
    a. The animal chews at the splint or cast
    b. The splint or cast is wet.
    c. The leg looks swollen above or below the cast.
    d. The animal is walking on or using the splinted or casted leg.

34. Proper splint and bandage care includes all of the following except
    a. Washing the splint or bandage daily
    b. Preventing the bandage or splint from becoming wet
    c. Inspecting the bandage or splint daily for any change, such as swelling above or below the splint or bandage
    d. Inspecting the bandage or splint for any shifting or change in position on the limb

35. Which of the following is *not* true of an aural hematoma?
    a. Must be drained
    b. Is repaired by trimming back the pinna
    c. Is painful and bothersome to the animal
    d. May be drained and bandaged by wrapping the head with the ear folded back across the top of the head

36. When a dog or cat is spayed, the surgical incision is most commonly made
    a. Midline, cranial to the umbilicus
    b. In the left inguinal region
    c. In the right inguinal region
    d. Midline, caudal to the umbilicus

37. Suture materials
    a. Are all absorbable
    b. Are nonabsorbable only
    c. Can be braided or monofilament
    d. Are only supplied with a needle attached

38. When passing surgical instruments to the surgeon, the technician should do all of the following except
    a. Gently but firmly slap the palm of the surgeon with the instrument.
    b. Pass the instrument in the open position.
    c. Pass the instrument with the handle placed into the surgeon's hand.
    d. Pass the curved instrument so that it is oriented in the surgeon's hand with the concave side up.

39. When assisting the surgeon, the technician should
    a. Always cut sutures on top of the knot.
    b. Cut sutures with the middle part of the scissors blade.
    c. Wipe the surgical site with a gauze square to clear the site of blood.
    d. Attach the scalpel blade using a pair of hemostats or needle holders to hold the blade.

40. Staples and other metal clips
    a. Can be used in infected wounds
    b. Cause little scarring
    c. Can be removed easily using scissors
    d. Can be applied by hand without any special application device

41. Surgical instruments should be
    a. Lubricated with oil between uses
    b. Cleaned without water to avoid the possibility of rusting
    c. Placed on surfaces, never dropped or thrown
    d. Cleaned with abrasive cleaners

42. External fixation devices include all of the following except
    a. Cast
    b. Splint
    c. Bone plate
    d. Kirschner-Ehmer (K-E) apparatus

43. Overinflation or underinflation of the endotracheal tube cuff can result in all of the following except
    a. Prevention of fluid aspiration into the lungs
    b. Pressure necrosis of the cells lining the trachea
    c. Inability to keep the patient under anesthesia with the expected concentration of gas anesthetic
    d. Increased levels of waste gas anesthesia in the surgical room

44. A chest tube is placed when an animal has
    a. Subcutaneous emphysema
    b. Pulmonary edema
    c. Ascites
    d. Pneumothorax

45. There is more concern about pulling out the endotracheal tube too soon in what breed of dog?
    a. English bulldog
    b. German shepherd
    c. Jack Russell terrier
    d. Greyhound

46. Dystocia is
    a. Difficult breathing
    b. Due to a side effect of opioid drugs
    c. Difficult or abnormal birth
    d. Always a surgical emergency

47. Surgical procedures of the ear include all of the following except
    a. Otoplasty
    b. Bulla osteotomy
    c. Aural hematoma drainage
    d. Enucleation

48. Surgical procedures of the eye and adnexal structures include all of the following except
    a. Entropion repair
    b. Keratectomy
    c. Onychectomy
    d. Enucleation

49. The animal is to be prepared for a cystotomy. What part of the body is prepped?
    a. Ventral abdomen
    b. Lumbar spine
    c. Ventral cervical area
    d. Top of the head

50. The animal is to be prepared for an ovariohysterectomy. What part of the body is prepped?
    a. Paw
    b. Ventral chest wall
    c. Ventral abdomen
    d. Ear

51. The animal is to be prepared for a femoral head ostectomy. What part of the body is prepped?
    a. Top of the head
    b. Hip
    c. Shoulder
    d. Lumbar spine

52. The animal is to be prepared for an orchidectomy. What part of the body is prepped?
    a. Ventral abdomen
    b. Scrotal/prescrotal area
    c. Paw
    d. Ear

53. The animal is to be prepared for a popliteal lymph node biopsy. What part of the body is prepped?
    a. Caudal aspect of the stifle
    b. Cranial aspect of the elbow
    c. Medial aspect of the thigh
    d. Cranial to the shoulder

54. A declaw is also known as an
    a. Orchidectomy
    b. Onychectomy
    c. Ovariohysterectomy
    d. Onychotomy

55. Which of the following is not part of the spermatic cord?
    a. Pampiniform plexus
    b. Vas deferens
    c. Testicular artery
    d. Epididymis

56. Which of the following is not completely removed in an ovariohysterectomy?
    a. Broad ligament
    b. Ovaries
    c. Uterine horns
    d. Oviducts

57. Enucleation may be required to correct
    a. Third eyelid prolapse
    b. Penile prolapse
    c. Proptosis of the eye
    d. Aural hematoma

58. Which of the following is a needle driver that is also able to cut sutures?
    a. Hegar-Olsen
    b. Mayo-Hegar
    c. Brown-Adson
    d. Rochester-Pean

59. Which of the following forceps has the best crushing action?
    a. Rochester-Carmalt
    b. Rochester-Pean
    c. Ochsner
    d. Crile

Correct answers are on pages 190-201.

60. Which of the following does not describe a characteristic of ethylene oxide?
    a. Carcinogenic
    b. Teratogenic
    c. Mutagenic
    d. Mitogenic

61. Which of the following suture materials persists in the body for the longest period?
    a. Polydioxanone
    b. Prolene
    c. Chromic catgut
    d. Vicryl

62. Scrotal swelling after orchidectomy is most likely due to a
    a. Hematoma
    b. Seroma
    c. Hemangioma
    d. Lipoma

63. Which of the following instruments is the only one appropriate for handling tissues during surgery?
    a. Dressing forceps
    b. Standard surgical scissors
    c. Sponge forceps
    d. Rat-tooth forceps

64. What suture pattern is commonly used to close the skin of cattle following a rumenotomy?
    a. Simple interrupted
    b. Simple continuous
    c. Interrupted horizontal mattress
    d. Continuous horizontal mattress

65. Which of the following suture materials is most appropriate to close the muscle layers of a cow following a left-displaced abomasum surgery?
    a. 3-0 catgut
    b. 3-0 polydioxanone
    c. 3 chromic catgut
    d. 3 polydioxanone

66. Which of the following statements regarding pyometra is incorrect?
    a. Ovariohysterectomy is usually curative.
    b. A purulent vaginal discharge is always present.
    c. Affected females usually have polyuria and polydipsia.
    d. It often occurs soon after a heat cycle.

67. Which of the following is not considered an elective procedure?
    a. Orchidectomy
    b. Ovariohysterectomy
    c. Onychectomy
    d. Enucleation of a proptosed eye

68. Nephrectomy refers to
    a. An incision into the kidney
    b. The removal of a kidney
    c. The removal of a tumor from the kidney
    d. The biopsy of a kidney

69. When preparing for an orthopedic surgery, shaving the surgical site should be done
    a. The night before to shorten the anesthesia time
    b. First thing in the morning to help things run more smoothly
    c. Immediately before induction of anesthesia
    d. Just after induction of anesthesia

70. Fracture apposition refers to
    a. Placing the bones back in to their normal position
    b. Keeping the bones very still until healing has taken place
    c. Removing small fragments from around the fracture
    d. Placing pins through the marrow cavity

71. A Caslick operation is done in horses to
    a. Stop roaring
    b. Improve fertility
    c. Treat navicular disease
    d. Clean out the guttural pouches

72. Which of the following agents can be used as both an antiseptic as well as a disinfectant?
    a. Quaternary ammonium compounds
    b. Mercurial compounds
    c. Isopropyl alcohol
    d. Formaldehyde

73. For which of the following surgeries are stay sutures not normally necessary?
    a. Cystotomy
    b. Gastrotomy
    c. Intestinal anastomosis
    d. Hepatic biopsy

74. What is the minimum number of throws required when making a surgical knot?
    a. One
    b. Two
    c. Three
    d. Four

75. When is it appropriate to use a hand tie instead of an instrument tie?
    a. When suturing very tough tissue
    b. When suturing the linea alba
    c. When suturing the skin
    d. A hand tie can be used any time an instrument can.

76. What technique can be used to help prevent a suture from slipping off the uterine stump?
    a. Stay sutures
    b. Transfiguration
    c. Transfixation
    d. Transitional sutures

77. Which of the following is an advantage of monofilament material over multifilament material?
    a. Greater knot security
    b. Greater suture strength
    c. Less likely to cause suture reactions
    d. Passes through tissue more easily

78. Which of the following suture sizes is most appropriate for eye surgeries?
    a. 0
    b. 3-0
    c. 6-0
    d. 10-0

79. Why is it important to minimize the amount of dead space when suturing?
    a. To decrease the chance of infection
    b. To decrease the chance of seroma formation
    c. To improve hemostasis
    d. To minimize necrosis

80. Which of the following is an absorbable suture material?
    a. Polydioxanone
    b. Prolene
    c. Silk
    d. Cotton

81. What factor will not influence how rapidly suture materials are absorbed by the body?
    a. Age of the patient
    b. Presence of infection
    c. The location of the suture
    d. The composition of the suture material

82. Which of the following is not considered a contaminated surgery?
    a. Anal sac removal
    b. Dental extractions
    c. Intestinal anastomosis
    d. Gastrotomy

83. Which of the following forceps should not be used to hold the edges of the incision open?
    a. Rat tooth
    b. Brown-Adson
    c. Crile
    d. Allis tissue

84. Which of the following does not describe a type of surgical scissors?
    a. Mayo
    b. Metzenbaum
    c. Iris
    d. Lembert

85. A sponge count should be done
    a. At the beginning of the surgery and before closure
    b. Several times during the surgery
    c. Before surgery only
    d. Before closure only

86. When performing a canine orchidectomy, the location of the incision is usually
    a. Around the umbilicus
    b. Prescrotal
    c. Intercostal
    d. Perineal

87. Which of the following clinical signs would not normally be seen if a dog were suffering from hemorrhage after an ovariohysterectomy?
    a. Decreased heart rate
    b. Pale mucous membranes
    c. Slow recovery from anesthesia
    d. Slow capillary refill time

88. You are monitoring a cat during an exploratory surgery and notice the pupils are central and dilated. The cat is
    a. Too light
    b. Too deep
    c. Under the influence of atropine
    d. Impossible to determine without more information

89. Which of the following does not cause an increase in respiratory rate in an anesthetized animal?
    a. Increased blood CO_2
    b. Anesthesia is too light
    c. Increased PaO_2
    d. Hyperthermia

90. What is the proper term for trimming the edges of a jagged tear before suturing?
    a. Debridement
    b. Decoupage
    c. Curettage
    d. Cauterization

91. Which of the following is not a factor influencing the formation of exuberant granulation tissue?
    a. Presence of infection
    b. Amount of missing tissue
    c. Depth of the wound
    d. Location of the wound

Correct answers are on pages 190-201.

92. If a surgical incision is dehiscing, the discharge, if present, is most likely to be
    a. Mucopurulent
    b. Serosanguineous
    c. Serous
    d. Purulent

93. Which of the following agents has been associated with causing neurologic disorders in cats?
    a. Chlorhexidine
    b. Povidone iodine
    c. Quaternary ammonium compounds
    d. Hexachlorophene

94. If a nonsterile person must move to the other side of a sterile person, the nonsterile person should pass
    a. Back to back
    b. Front to front
    c. Facing the back of the surgeon
    d. With his or her side facing the back of the surgeon

95. When opening a double-wrapped gown pack, nonscrubbed surgical personnel may touch the
    a. Autoclave tape
    b. Indicator
    c. Towel
    d. Gown

96. Which of the following suture materials is most likely to cause stitch granulomas if left in too long?
    a. Silk
    b. Cotton
    c. Nylon
    d. Prolene

97. When scrubbing, the hands should be held
    a. Below the elbows
    b. Parallel to the elbows
    c. Above the elbows
    d. Above the head

98. When cleaning instruments, the instruments should first be soaked in a surgical soap solution (e.g., ASEPTI-zyme) to
    a. Remove bacteria
    b. Remove blood
    c. Sterilize them
    d. Enhance the effect of the ultrasonic cleaner

99. Which of the following patterns is not suitable for the closure of an intestinal biopsy incision?
    a. Simple continuous
    b. Simple interrupted
    c. Everting
    d. Inverting

100. Which of the following does not need to be included when labeling a surgical pack?
    a. Contents of the pack
    b. Date the pack was made up
    c. Initials or name of the person making up the pack
    d. Date the pack must be used by

101. Which of the following hemostatic forceps has striations different from the others?
    a. Halstead mosquitoes
    b. Crile
    c. Rochester-Pean
    d. Rochester-Carmalt

102. Which of the following is not the formal name of a retractor?
    a. Finochietto
    b. Gelpi
    c. Lembert
    d. Balfour

103. Which of the following is not a requirement for fracture healing?
    a. Apposition
    b. Shearing
    c. Fixation
    d. Reduction

104. Using the dissection method, which parts of the distal forelimb are removed in an onychectomy?
    a. Nail and proximal phalanx
    b. Proximal and distal phalanges
    c. Middle and distal phalanges
    d. Distal phalanx and nail

105. Anterior drawer movement detects a problem with the
    a. Elbow
    b. Stifle
    c. Hip
    d. Hock

106. An incision into the bladder is known as a
    a. Cystotomy
    b. Cystectomy
    c. Cystocentesis
    d. Cystostomy

107. Which of the following conditions does not require surgical repair?
    a. Gastric dilatation and volvulus
    b. Intussusception
    c. Mesenteric torsion
    d. Ileus

108. A laminectomy is used to treat
    a. Intervertebral disk disease
    b. Fractures of spinous processes
    c. Hip dysplasia
    d. Foot disorders in horses

109. If a fracture is found on the proximal part of the tibia, it is
    a. Distal to the femur
    b. Proximal to the femur
    c. In the middle of the bone
    d. Distal to the metatarsals

110. If the testicles are not palpable, and a cryptorchidectomy is performed, the incision would most likely be
    a. Prescrotal
    b. Inguinal
    c. Ventral midline
    d. Perineal

111. In dogs, the most common location for a thoracotomy incision is
    a. Through the sternum
    b. Through the diaphragm
    c. Along the linea alba
    d. Between the ribs

112. What is the minimum number of air changes per hour required for adequate ventilation in a surgical suite?
    a. 2
    b. 5
    c. 10
    d. 15

113. Which of the following disinfectants has the weakest virucidal activity?
    a. Glutaraldehyde (2%)
    b. Quaternary ammonium compounds at standard concentrations
    c. Formalin (37%)
    d. Isopropyl alcohol (70%)

114. Which of the following does not describe a type of surgical scissors?
    a. Iris
    b. Metzenbaum
    c. Wire-cutting
    d. Mayo-Hegar

115. Which of the following instruments is most suitable for the removal of bone to perform spinal surgery?
    a. Rongeurs
    b. Curette
    c. Periosteal elevator
    d. Trephine

116. Clear fluid removed from thoracic cavity is known as
    a. Pleural effusion
    b. Pulmonary edema
    c. Ascites
    d. Pyothorax

117. Where is the most likely place for a rumenotomy incision in a dairy cow?
    a. Right paralumbar fossa
    b. Left paralumbar fossa
    c. Linea alba
    d. Paramedian

118. What does a change in color in autoclave tape indicate to a surgical nurse?
    a. The surgical instruments in the pack have been adequately sterilized.
    b. During the autoclaving process, steam has reached the tape.
    c. Adequate temperature and pressures have been achieved.
    d. The pack has been exposed to adequate pressures.

119. Assuming 15 psi, the minimum conditions that must be met to ensure that a pack has been adequately sterilized by autoclaving are
    a. 121° C for 15 minutes
    b. 131° F for 15 minutes
    c. 121° C for 25 minutes
    d. 131° F for 30 minutes

120. Which of the following is *not* a concern when assisting a surgeon in a canine cesarean section surgery?
    a. Minimizing anesthetic drugs that may pass on to the puppies
    b. Minimizing the time the bitch is in dorsal recumbency because of the weight of the uterus on the aorta
    c. Suctioning fluid from the puppies' nasal cavities and mouths to stimulate breathing
    d. Intubating the puppies

121. Which of the following is *not* a primary concern when assisting a surgeon performing a pyometra surgery?
    a. Providing preoperative and intraoperative antibiotics for the patient
    b. Gentle handling of the friable tissue to prevent rupture and drainage of the contents of the uterus into the abdominal cavity
    c. Fluid therapy to diurese the kidneys
    d. Lidocaine infusion to prevent ventricular arrhythmias

Correct answers are on pages 190-201.

122. When assisting a surgeon in a gastric dilatation and volvulus surgery, your immediate concern is not with which of the following?
    a. Establish intravenous access to deliver shock doses of fluids.
    b. Calculate lidocaine dose for constant rate infusion.
    c. Monitor for cardiac arrhythmias intraoperatively and postoperatively.
    d. Prepare ultrasound unit to confirm gastric dilatation and volvulus status of animal.

123. What size scalpel blade fits on a No. 3 scalpel handle?
    a. No. 10
    b. No. 20
    c. No. 21
    d. No. 30

124. What size scalpel blade fits on a No. 4 scalpel handle?
    a. No. 10
    b. No. 12
    c. No. 15
    d. No. 20

125. What is meant by the term *pathogenic bacteria*?
    a. Bacteria that produce toxins
    b. Bacteria that cause disease
    c. Bacteria that live off and gain nutrients from the host
    d. Bacteria that multiply in the host

126. Which of the following need *not* be considered in the timing of the autoclave cycle?
    a. Time required to heat up the interior of the chamber
    b. Time required to allow the steam to penetrate the interior of the packs
    c. Time required to seal the chamber
    d. Time required to sterilize those items in contact with the steam

127. The definition of *sterile* is
    a. Without microbes or living spores
    b. Without pathogenic microbes
    c. With the presence of commensal organisms only
    d. Without bacteria or their by-products

128. What items should personnel wear when entering the operating room?
    a. Cap and mask
    b. Cap, mask, and booties
    c. Cap, mask, booties, and clean scrubs or gown
    d. Cap, mask, and sterile gown

129. Which of the following surgical packs would *not* be considered contaminated and would not need to be reautoclaved?
    a. Single-wrapped paper pack stored on an open shelf for 8 weeks
    b. Pack that was opened for a procedure but not used and needed for the next day's procedure
    c. Double-wrapped paper pack stored in a closed cabinet for 6 weeks
    d. Instrument in an autoclave pouch that has a very small tear near the top of the pack

130. Instruments are autoclaved
    a. With the ratchets closed to prevent tearing the wrap material
    b. With the ratchets open to allow steam exposure to the entire surface
    c. Always in a surgical tray to prevent the instruments from shifting
    d. Without touching any other instruments to prevent corrosion

131. An advantage of using a Gelpi retractor over a Senn retractor is
    a. The Gelpi is much less expensive to purchase.
    b. The Gelpi is smaller overall than the Senn.
    c. The Senn must be molded to fit the position required.
    d. The Gelpi is self-retaining.

132. What three factors determine whether a microbe will cause disease?
    a. Number of pathogens, host resistance, and proper use of aseptic technique
    b. Number of pathogens, host resistance, and virulence of the pathogen
    c. Type of suture involved, host resistance, and proper use of aseptic technique
    d. Host resistance, virulence of the pathogen, and proper use of aseptic technique

133. What specifically does the strip on the autoclave tape indicate when it turns dark?
    a. The correct temperature has been reached.
    b. The correct pressure has been reached.
    c. The correct temperature for the proper amount of time has been reached.
    d. The correct temperature, pressure, and time have been reached.

134. Metzenbaum scissors are used only for
    a. Cutting suture
    b. Cutting paper drape
    c. Ophthalmic surgery
    d. Cutting tissue

135. Where is the sterile zone located on scrubbed personnel?
    a. Front and sides, from the neck to the bottom of the gown, including the arms
    b. Front, from the neck to the bottom of the gown, including the arms
    c. Front, sides, and back, from the neck to the waist
    d. Front, from the neck to the waist, including the arms

136. Rank the following from greatest tensile strength to least.
    a. 00 gut, 3-0 Vicryl, 1 chromic gut, 6-0 silk
    b. 1 chromic gut, 00 gut, 3-0 Vicryl, 6-0 silk
    c. 6-0 silk, 3-0 Vicryl, 00 gut, 1 chromic gut
    d. 6-0 silk, 3-0 Vicryl, 1 chromic gut, 00 gut

137. Why must instrument milk be used after ultrasonic cleaning?
    a. To complete the sterilization process
    b. To provide further cleaning and sanitizing of the instruments
    c. To replace lubrication removed by the ultrasonic cleaner
    d. To prevent rust from forming on the instruments

138. What needle type is reusable?
    a. Swaged-on
    b. Taper point
    c. Trocar tip
    d. Eyed

139. Which of the following operating room personnel should face the sterile field during a procedure?
    a. The surgeon only
    b. The scrubbed-in technicians and surgeon only
    c. All personnel, both scrubbed in and nonsterile
    d. Only the surgeon and nonsterile personnel; the scrubbed-in technician should face the instrument field.

140. Which of the following is not a major criterion used to classify suture material?
    a. Absorbable versus nonabsorbable
    b. Tensile strength versus size
    c. Synthetic versus natural
    d. Braided versus monofilament

141. An advantage of braided suture over monofilament is
    a. Knot security
    b. Tensile strength
    c. Does not hide bacteria in contaminated wounds
    d. Tissue reactivity

142. When attaching an animal to an ECG, which lead is hooked up to the right foreleg?
    a. Red
    b. Black
    c. White
    d. Green

143. When attaching an ECG, which leg should have the red lead attached to it?
    a. Right foreleg
    b. Left foreleg
    c. Right hind leg
    d. Left hind leg

144. A disinfectant labeled to be virucidal
    a. Prevents bacteria from growing
    b. Kills all microbes
    c. Kills viruses
    d. Prevents viruses from growing

145. How often should instrument milk be changed?
    a. Every day
    b. Once a week
    c. Every 18 days
    d. Monthly

146. When autoclaving, the minimum temperature and exposure time for the center of the surgical packs is
    a. 121.5° F for 10 minutes
    b. 250° F for 15 minutes
    c. 250° F for 20 minutes
    d. 300° F for 30 minutes

147. What is the significance of an autoclave that will not properly seal, but steam still rises from it?
    a. Because it is the sterilizing agent, it will work fine, but you must be more cautious to prevent burns to personnel.
    b. The pressure is what kills the microbes, and thus the autoclave will not work.
    c. It will continue to sterilize but will require more water as the steam escapes.
    d. The pressure will not increase, which is required to meet the minimum temperature for sterilization.

148. In general, the difference between a disinfectant and an antiseptic is
    a. Disinfectants are agents used on inanimate objects, and antiseptic agents are used on living tissue.
    b. Disinfectants are used on living tissues, and antiseptics are used on inanimate objects.
    c. Disinfectants are bacteriostatic, and antiseptics are bacteriocidal.
    d. Disinfectants kill microbes, whereas antiseptics inhibit their growth only.

Correct answers are on pages 190-201.

149. How can you help prevent "strike through" during surgery?
    a. Make sure sharp instruments are protected so they do not puncture the wrap and cause contamination.
    b. Assist in keeping the surgical drapes and gown from getting wet during surgery.
    c. Make sure the drape is properly placed and opened so the fenestration is not over a contaminated area.
    d. Have reverse cutting needles available so the suture does not pull through the tissue.

150. Why is a typical autoclave cycle set for 20 minutes on an instrument pack?
    a. This is the minimum time for sterilization in a steam autoclave.
    b. This is the minimum time required to turn the autoclave tape dark.
    c. This allows enough time for the pressure to sterilize the pack.
    d. This allows time for steam penetration to the center of the pack and still provides the minimum time of steam exposure.

151. The agent used in gas sterilization is
    a. Glutaraldehyde
    b. Chlorhexidine
    c. Ethylene oxide
    d. Formaldehyde

152. Needle holders that have a scissors, as well as a needle-holding surface, are named
    a. Mayo-Hegar
    b. Olsen-Hegar
    c. Metzenbaum
    d. Crile-Wood

153. Rochester-Carmalt forceps
    a. Are generally smaller than a Kelly forceps
    b. Have longitudinal serrations with interdigitating teeth at the tips
    c. Have longitudinal serrations with a crosshatched pattern at the tips
    d. Have transverse serrations along the entire length

154. A Buhner needle is used
    a. In repair of bovine vaginal and uterine prolapses
    b. In enucleations on dogs
    c. In intestinal anastomosis surgeries
    d. In orthopedic surgeries

155. A Snook hook is typically used during
    a. A castration
    b. An ovariohysterectomy
    c. A diaphragmatic hernia repair
    d. Declawing

156. What does the medical term *ovariohysterectomy* mean?
    a. Removal of the ovaries only
    b. Removal of the uterus only
    c. Removal of the ovaries and uterus only
    d. Removal of the entire reproductive tract, including ovaries, uterus, cervix, and vagina

157. An accumulation of purulent discharge within the uterus is called
    a. Pyometritis
    b. Mastitis
    c. Peritonitis
    d. Vaginitis

158. A pack double wrapped in muslin and kept in a closed cabinet is good for how long?
    a. 1 week
    b. 3 to 4 weeks
    c. 6 to 7 weeks
    d. 6 months

159. Instruments suitable for cutting suture include
    a. Scissors on Mayo-Hegar needle holders, operating scissors, and Mayo scissors
    b. Operating scissors, scissors on Olsen-Hegar needle holders, and Metzenbaum scissors
    c. Operating scissors, scissors on Olsen-Hegar needle holders, and Mayo scissors
    d. Suture (stitch) scissors, Mayo scissors, and Metzenbaum scissors

160. What is a Steinmann IM pin?
    a. An intramedullary pin used in orthopedics
    b. An intramuscular pin used in orthopedics
    c. A type of screw used in orthopedics
    d. A staple used to hold muscle or bone fragments together

161. You are checking on a recent surgical wound and find that the tissue is slightly warmer and redder than the surrounding tissue. What is the significance of this?
    a. It is an indication that the wound is contaminated and requires an emergency intervention.
    b. The wound will likely dehisce and should be checked immediately by the veterinarian.
    c. It is normal, because the first stage of wound healing is inflammation.
    d. It is an indication that the sutures are interfering with blood flow, and necrosis is likely.

162. What should you wear when cleaning the surgical suite before and after surgeries?
    a. Cap
    b. Cap, mask, booties, and clean scrubs
    c. Cap, mask, booties, and sterile gown
    d. Mask, sterile cap, and gown

163. What should you be wearing when performing as a nonsterile surgical assistant?
    a. Mask and clean scrubs
    b. Mask, cap, and clean scrubs
    c. Mask, cap, shoe covers, and clean scrubs
    d. Mask, cap, shoe covers, and sterile gown

164. While you are performing as a sterile surgical assistant, your mask slips down below your nose. What should you do?
    a. The nonsterile assistant may stand in front of you and secure the mask in its proper position.
    b. The nonsterile assistant may secure the mask in position while standing behind you.
    c. You may take a nonsterile piece of gauze and place it over the mask to allow you to adjust it into position.
    d. You are completely contaminated and must leave surgery.

165. Which of the following is *not* an advantage to spaying a bitch?
    a. Eliminates the hemorrhagic discharge associated with the estrus stage of the cycle
    b. Decreases the risk of mammary cancer
    c. Eliminates estrus behavior
    d. Eliminates the risk of pyometra associated with multiple nonpregnant estrus cycles

166. Which of the following is not a recommended agent for patient surgical preparation?
    a. Chlorhexidine
    b. Roccal
    c. Alcohol
    d. Povidone iodine

167. Abscesses are generally allowed to heal open to provide continuous drainage. This type of wound healing is considered
    a. First intention
    b. Second intention
    c. Third intention
    d. Fourth intention

168. Which of the following best describes the location of an incision through the skin and linea alba, extending from the xiphoid process to the umbilicus?
    a. Flank
    b. Paracostal
    c. Paramedian
    d. Ventral midline

169. Cesarean sections in cattle are most commonly performed via what surgical approach?
    a. Through a right paracostal incision
    b. Through a right paravertebral approach
    c. Through the left paralumbar fossa
    d. Through the ventral midline approach

170. Emasculators are used
    a. In large animal castrations
    b. During surgical ovariectomies in heifers and mares
    c. During enucleations in large-breed dogs
    d. To perform tail docking in lambs

171. You are to assist with a rumenotomy. Where do you prep for the surgery?
    a. Ventral midline from xiphoid to pubic bone
    b. Left paralumbar fossa
    c. Right paralumbar fossa
    d. Right paramedian region

172. A disadvantage of tilting the surgical table so the patient's head is lower than its tail is
    a. The increased pressure on the diaphragm interferes with respiration.
    b. The tension on the large bowel may initiate defecation.
    c. It interferes with visualization of the caudal abdomen.
    d. It can cause a gastric volvulus.

173. A visiting relief veterinarian whom you are assisting in surgery asks you to provide a nonabsorbable suture, less than 2-0 in size. Which of the following would meet the request?
    a. 3-0 chromic gut
    b. 4-0 silk
    c. 00 Dermalon nylon
    d. 0 polydioxanone

174. *Hanging preps*
    a. Are preps used on the perineal region of mares, in which the tail is "hanged" out of the way
    b. Are often used for orthopedic procedures that involve a limb
    c. Is a term used when referring to surgical preps of the neck
    d. Refers to preparations for ear surgeries, because the ear is "hanged up" for preparations

175. A surgical prep for feline castration
    a. Involves clipping the prescrotal region from the umbilicus to the scrotum
    b. Involves clipping the scrotum with a No. 40 clipper blade
    c. Does not involve hair removal, because the entire scrotal area is prepped with Nolvasan and alcohol
    d. Includes plucking or pulling the hair from the scrotum before the surgical scrub

Correct answers are on pages 190-201.

176. Which of these is *not* a common surgical site for correction of a left-displaced abomasum in cattle?
    a. Right paralumbar
    b. Left paralumbar
    c. Ventral midline
    d. Right paramedian

177. Postoperative care for horses following castration
    a. Includes strict confinement to the stall for at least 1 week to prevent hemorrhage
    b. Includes suture removal at 10 to 14 days
    c. Involves antibiotic administration for 5 days following surgery
    d. Involves exercise twice daily to promote drainage

178. The term that means "surgically opening the abdominal cavity" is
    a. Laparotomy
    b. Pleurotomy
    c. Thoracotomy
    d. Cystotomy

179. What parameter(s) does the pulse oximeter measure?
    a. Heart rate only
    b. Respiration rate and depth
    c. Oxygen saturation of hemoglobin and heart rate
    d. Respiration rate and heart rate

180. Which of the following is false regarding the ECG?
    a. It measures the electrical impulses of the heart.
    b. There can be a normal ECG tracing when there is no cardiac output.
    c. There is always a pulse beat with each QRS complex.
    d. Alcohol and sterile lubricant will enhance the connection of the skin leads.

181. What orthopedic fixation consists of pins that penetrate fractured bones and skin from the outside and are held in place externally by bolts attached to another cross pin?
    a. Rush pinning
    b. External fixators
    c. Steinmann fixation
    d. Bone plating

182. What is a nosocomial infection?
    a. Infection arising from bacteria in the gastrointestinal tract
    b. Infection originating from the respiratory tract, especially the nose
    c. Hospital-acquired infection
    d. Resistant infection

183. Which of the following should *not* be used to help prevent hypothermia in surgical patients?
    a. Electric heating pad set on low
    b. Warm-water circulating pad
    c. Warm rice pads
    d. Towel placed between the surgery table and patient

184. While preparing for what type of surgical procedure would you make sure the Jacob's bone chuck is sterilized and available?
    a. Onychectomy
    b. Celiotomy
    c. Thoracotomy
    d. Orthopedic

185. Which of the following is *not* an advantage to neutering a male dog?
    a. Decreased risk for perineal hernias
    b. Decreased roaming
    c. It will prevent it from lifting its leg to urinate
    d. Decreased aggression toward other dogs

186. Which of the following can be used as a surgical scrub on a patient?
    a. Povidone iodine solution
    b. Chlorhexidine scrub
    c. Alcohol
    d. Nolvasan solution

187. Which of the following need *not* be done before moving a horse into surgery for a general anesthesia procedure?
    a. Remove the shoes
    b. Rinse out the mouth
    c. Clip as much of the surgical area as possible
    d. Perform a complete tail wrap

188. What is an important measure that can help prevent myositis during equine surgery?
    a. Providing proper padding
    b. Ensuring that the horse does not get hypothermia
    c. Not overinflating the endotracheal tube cuff
    d. Withholding food for 12 hours

189. Which of the following is *not* true regarding cryptorchidism in horses?
    a. One or both of the testicles have not descended into the prepuce.
    b. Surgery for removal of the undescended testicle is more involved than a normal castration.
    c. It is an inheritable condition.
    d. Stallions affected with unilateral cryptorchidism will breed mares.

190. What nerve in the horse's head should be protected from injury during prolonged surgical procedures?
    a. Corneal nerve
    b. Facial nerve
    c. Mandibular nerve
    d. Optic nerve

191. A gastrotomy refers to
    a. A surgical incision into the gastrocnemius muscle
    b. A surgical incision into the peritoneal wall
    c. A surgical incision into the stomach
    d. A surgical incision into the small intestines

192. During a surgical scrub, you bump your hand on the faucet. What should you do?
    a. Continue the scrub, giving the bumped area double the number of brush strokes to compensate
    b. You have contaminated yourself and must start the entire scrub over
    c. Rescrub the area immediately, rinse the brush, and then continue the scrub
    d. Continue the scrub and add one more cycle on the bumped hand, because you cannot make your hands truly sterile anyway

193. Why are such elaborate measures taken to maintain aseptic technique during surgery?
    a. To protect personnel from pathogenic microbes encountered in the animals
    b. To decrease the risk of nosocomial infections spread among patients
    c. To decrease the risk of contamination into the surgical site and interference with wound healing
    d. To decrease the virulence of the microbes in the hospital

194. What is meant by the term *iatrogenic*?
    a. Wounds induced by the animal itself
    b. Patient-caused additional trauma to an existing wound
    c. Patient-caused additional trauma to a surgical incision, generally licking
    d. Induced or caused by the veterinary surgeon or staff

195. A fenestrated drape
    a. Has a window opening in middle for the surgery to be performed through
    b. Is folded or plicated in accordion style for ease of opening
    c. Is folded such that the middle of the drape can easily be found
    d. Is a cloth drape made of doubled muslin

196. What is the pressure that must be reached in a steam autoclave for the temperature to reach 121.5° C?
    a. 1 psi
    b. 10 psi
    c. 15 psi
    d. 45 psi

197. Healing of a properly sutured surgical wound is most appropriately termed
    a. First-intention healing
    b. Granulation
    c. Secondary union
    d. Second-intention healing

198. Which of the following has the poorest potential for healing and return to normal function after damage and effective surgical repair?
    a. Bone
    b. Gastrointestinal tract
    c. Liver
    d. Nervous tissue

199. Which of the following best describes the location of an incision extending from the xiphoid process to the umbilicus of an animal?
    a. Flank
    b. Paracostal
    c. Paramedian
    d. Ventral midline

200. What agent, method, or device is most appropriate for sterilizing an electric drill to be used in an orthopedic surgical procedure?
    a. Autoclave
    b. Dry heat
    c. Ethylene oxide gas
    d. Liquid chemical disinfectant

201. What agent, method, or device is most appropriate for sterilizing a needle holder to be used in a surgical procedure?
    a. Autoclave
    b. Dry heat
    c. Ethylene oxide gas
    d. Liquid chemical disinfectant

202. What agent, method, or device is most appropriate for sterilizing a pair of dissecting scissors to be used in a surgical procedure?
    a. Autoclave
    b. Dry heat
    c. Ethylene oxide gas
    d. Liquid chemical disinfectant

Correct answers are on pages 190-201.

203. Which of the following describes the minimum exposure time and temperature to which all parts of an autoclaved surgical pack should be exposed to achieve sterility?
    a. 121° C for 15 minutes
    b. 121° F for 15 minutes
    c. 250° C for 20 minutes
    d. 250° F for 20 minutes

204. Which of the following is the most effective and timely indicator that sterilization conditions have been met in an autoclaved surgery pack?
    a. Autoclave tape
    b. Chemical indicator
    c. Culture test
    d. Melting pellet

205. What is the proper term for microorganisms that gain entrance into an incision during a surgical procedure?
    a. Contamination
    b. Debridement
    c. Infection
    d. Septicemia

206. Which of the following do/does *not* have to be sterile during a surgical procedure to maintain aseptic technique?
    a. Drapes
    b. Gloves
    c. Gown
    d. Mask

207. Which of the following is the agent for autoclave sterilization?
    a. Chemical disinfectant solution
    b. Dry heat
    c. Ethylene oxide gas
    d. Steam

208. What size of electrical clipper blade is most commonly used for removing the hair from a surgical site?
    a. No. 10
    b. No. 20
    c. No. 30
    d. No. 40

209. Which of the following is not an effective form of surgical hemostasis?
    a. Crushing
    b. Curettage
    c. Ligation
    d. Pressure

210. Which of the following is not a likely cause of dehiscence of an abdominal incision?
    a. Excessive physical activity
    b. Stormy recovery from anesthesia
    c. Surgical wound infection
    d. Suture material larger than needed

211. Which of the following is not an effective aseptic surgical technique?
    a. Consider a sterile item to be nonsterile if it touches a nonsterile item.
    b. If the sterility of an item is in doubt, consider it sterile.
    c. Nonscrubbed personnel can touch nonsterile items only.
    d. Only sterile items can touch other sterile items.

212. Which of the following does not enhance the healing of an open wound?
    a. Debridement
    b. Exuberant granulation tissue
    c. Granulation tissue
    d. Wound flushing

213. Which of the following is not a characteristic of first-intention wound healing?
    a. Minimal contamination
    b. Minimal tissue damage
    c. No continuous movement of wound edges from body movement
    d. Wound edges not approximated

214. What incision is most appropriate for exploratory surgery of the abdomen of a dog in which the precise location of the problem is not known?
    a. Flank
    b. Paracostal
    c. Paramedian
    d. Ventral midline

215. Which of the following is not an early sign of wound dehiscence during the first 24 hours after abdominal surgery?
    a. Body temperature elevation of 1 degree to 2 degrees
    b. Serosanguineous discharge from the incision
    c. Swollen incision
    d. Very warm incision

216. The main goal of aseptic surgical technique is to prevent contamination of the
    a. Sterile fields
    b. Sterile zones
    c. Surgical instruments
    d. Surgical wound

217. What factor relating to infection of a surgical wound can aseptic technique reasonably expect to significantly influence?
  a. Number of microorganisms entering the wound
  b. Pathogenicity of microorganisms entering the wound
  c. Route of exposure to infectious microorganisms
  d. Susceptibility of the patient

218. The effectiveness of a surgical scrub of the hands and arms with a bactericidal soap depends on the
  a. Combination of contact time and scrubbing action
  b. Time the soap is in contact with the skin
  c. Scrubbing action of the brush
  d. Temperature of the water

219. Which of the following is a surgical scrub soap that forms a bacteriostatic film over the skin when it is used exclusively?
  a. Chlorhexidine
  b. Chlorpheniramine
  c. Hexachlorophene
  d. Povidone-iodine

220. Which of the following does not normally need to be sterilized as a part of good aseptic surgical technique?
  a. Cap
  b. Drapes
  c. Gown
  d. Scrub brush

221. Liquid chemical sterilization is used primarily for
  a. Electrical equipment
  b. Instruments with sharp edges
  c. Orthopedic equipment
  d. Surgical drapes

222. The time necessary to disinfect surgical instruments with liquid chemicals can be shortened by
  a. Cooling the solution
  b. Making the solution less concentrated than recommended
  c. Making the solution more concentrated than recommended
  d. Warming the solution

223. What surgical drape material prevents bacteria from penetrating the drape by capillary action when the top surface of the drape becomes wet?
  a. Polyester
  b. Muslin
  c. Paper
  d. Plastic

224. What surgical instrument should not be routinely steam sterilized?
  a. Backhaus towel clamp
  b. Halstead mosquito forceps
  c. Mayo-Hegar needle holder
  d. Metzenbaum scissors

225. What is the most appropriate wound-flushing solution?
  a. Hydrogen peroxide
  b. Isotonic saline
  c. Povidone-iodine solution
  d. Tap water

226. What incision is the most appropriate for a rumenotomy in a standing cow?
  a. Left flank
  b. Right ventral paramedian
  c. Left ventral paramedian
  d. Ventral midline

227. What, if any, operating room personnel should always face away from sterile fields during a surgical procedure?
  a. Nonscrubbed personnel only
  b. Scrubbed personnel only
  c. Both nonscrubbed and scrubbed personnel
  d. Neither nonscrubbed nor scrubbed personnel

228. What is the significance of ventral midline surgical wound dehiscence of the muscle, subcutaneous tissue, and skin layers?
  a. Emergency
  b. Cosmetic only
  c. Minor significance
  d. Serious but not an emergency

229. Why is a recent surgical wound usually slightly warmer than surrounding normal tissues?
  a. Contamination
  b. Debridement
  c. Infection
  d. Inflammation

230. When does a sutured surgical wound begin to gain significant strength from production of collagen strands, so that the wound edges are held together by not only the sutures?
  a. Immediately
  b. 5 days
  c. 14 days
  d. 35 days

231. Wound contraction is produced by
  a. Reproduction of the dermis
  b. Movement of the epidermis only
  c. Movement of the whole thickness of skin
  d. Reproduction of epidermal cells

Correct answers are on pages 190-201.

232. As a part of effective aseptic technique, surgical gowns
   a. Are commonly made of cloth or paper
   b. Are put on by touching the outside only
   c. Are routinely sterilized by ethylene oxide gas
   d. Do not need to be sterile, only clean

233. Which of the following is not a sign of hemorrhagic shock in a postsurgical patient?
   a. Deep, slow breathing
   b. Slow capillary refill
   c. Tachycardia
   d. Weakness

234. The usual significance of a small seroma beneath a skin suture line is
   a. Emergency
   b. Cosmetic only
   c. Major problem
   d. Serious but not an emergency

235. The healing potential for a fractured bone that is properly aligned and kept immobile is
   a. Excellent
   b. Fair
   c. Good
   d. Poor

236. What coloration indicates the best blood supply to the edges of a wound in nonpigmented skin?
   a. Bluish-purple
   b. Gray
   c. Pink
   d. White

237. What abdominal incision is most appropriate for a standing cesarean section on a heifer?
   a. Ventral midline
   b. Flank
   c. Paracostal
   d. Ventral paramedian

238. What portion of a surgical gown is considered sterile during surgery?
   a. Front and sides, from the neck to the bottom, including the arms
   b. Front, from the neck to the bottom, including the arms
   c. Front and sides, from the waist to the neck
   d. Front, from the waist up, including the arms

239. What bacterial form is most easily destroyed by common sterilization methods?
   a. Spores of aerobes
   b. Spores of anaerobes
   c. Dormant form
   d. Vegetative form

240. The first phase of the wound-healing process is the
   a. Epithelial
   b. Fibroblast
   c. Inflammatory
   d. Maturation

241. In the first 24 hours of primary union wound healing, most of the resistance to opening of the wound is provided by
   a. Collagen strands
   b. Fibrin strands
   c. Granulation tissue
   d. Sutures

242. In what type of abdominal incision can the muscle wall be most effectively closed with one layer of sutures?
   a. Flank
   b. Paracostal
   c. Paramedian
   d. Ventral midline

243. Scrubbed surgical personnel become contaminated if they touch
   a. Objects in sterile fields
   b. Objects outside of the sterile zone
   c. Properly sterilized surgical instruments
   d. Freshly exposed tissues of the patient

244. Nonscrubbed surgical personnel may properly touch anything that is
   a. Contaminated
   b. Inside the patient's body
   c. Inside the sterile zone
   d. Part of a sterile field

245. How should a person scrubbed for surgery and the anesthetist pass each other in the operating room?
   a. Scrubbed person back to anesthetist back
   b. Scrubbed person back to anesthetist front
   c. Scrubbed person front to anesthetist back
   d. Scrubbed person front to anesthetist front

246. When not otherwise occupied, scrubbed surgical personnel should stand with their
   a. Arms folded
   b. Hands above shoulder level
   c. Hands clasped between waist and shoulder level
   d. Hands down at their sides

247. When is it permissible for nonscrubbed surgical personnel to pass between scrubbed personnel and the patient during surgery?
    a. Never
    b. When opening suture material
    c. When adjusting the anesthesia machine
    d. When adjusting the intravenous drip

248. When aseptically opening a sterile surgical pack on an instrument stand, it is not proper for nonscrubbed surgical personnel to touch the
    a. Autoclave tape
    b. Contents of the pack
    c. Corners of the wrap
    d. Instrument stand

249. What characteristic is true of ethylene oxide gas?
    a. Flammable
    b. Exposure is not considered a health hazard.
    c. Noncombustible
    d. Nontoxic to tissues

250. Which of the following is not a likely contributor to postoperative wound dehiscence?
    a. Chronic postoperative vomiting
    b. Internal suture ends cut too short
    c. Infection
    d. Skin sutures left in too long

251. What type of dressing best helps debride a wound with extensive tissue damage?
    a. Dry gauze
    b. Gauze dressing with an oily antiseptic
    c. Gauze dressing with a water-soluble antiseptic
    d. Wet saline dressing

252. Most of the clinical signs seen in an animal in shock from excessive blood loss are attributable to
    a. Acidosis
    b. Alkalosis
    c. Cell death
    d. Redistribution of blood flow

253. The main goal of surgery to remove a pus-filled uterus (pyometra) is
    a. As a prophylactic measure
    b. To make a diagnosis
    c. To restore the animal to a normal reproductive state
    d. To return the animal to health without restoring normal reproductive function

254. What tissue must form in a wound that is healing by second intention before wound contraction or epithelial regeneration can occur?
    a. Collagen fibers
    b. Fibrin clot
    c. Granulation tissue
    d. Scar tissue

255. When gloving for surgery, which of the following is not permitted?
    a. One gloved thumb touches the other gloved thumb.
    b. The outside of the glove is touched by the scrubbed fingers.
    c. The outside of the gown cuff is touched by inside of the glove cuff.
    d. The scrubbed fingers touch the inside of the glove cuff.

256. How should a pack be placed in an autoclave for sterilization?
    a. Diagonally
    b. Horizontally
    c. Upside down
    d. Vertically

257. Metzenbaum scissors are used for
    a. Cutting sutures
    b. Soft-tissue dissection
    c. Cutting the linea alba
    d. Cutting skin

258. What retractors are not handheld?
    a. Deaver
    b. Senn
    c. Rake
    d. Gelpi

259. What is the appropriate time to soak an instrument in a cold sterilization solution before adequate sterilization is achieved?
    a. 30 minutes
    b. 15 minutes
    c. 45 minutes
    d. 10 minutes

260. How long does an instrument that is sterilized and wrapped in paper remain sterile?
    a. 6 months
    b. 1 week
    c. 1 month
    d. 1 year

Correct answers are on pages 190-201.

261. A dust cover extends the sterility time of an instrument from 1 month to
   a. 6 months
   b. 2 months
   c. 12 months
   d. 2 years

262. Instrument milk is used for all of the following except
   a. Lubrication
   b. Rust inhibition
   c. Extending the life of the instrument
   d. Cleaning the instrument

263. For what bovine surgical procedure are obstetric (OB) chains used?
   a. Rumenotomy
   b. Abomasopexy
   c. Cesarean section
   d. Uterine torsion correction

264. To flash sterilize an instrument, the autoclave settings should be
   a. 250° F, 20-lb pressure, 30 min, fast exhaust and dry
   b. 270° F, 20-lb pressure, 30 min, fast exhaust and dry
   c. 250° F, 30-lb pressure, 4 min, fast exhaust
   d. 270° F, 30-lb pressure, 4 min, fast exhaust

265. Which of the following does not have to be gas sterilized?
   a. Arthroscope
   b. Plastic pipette tips
   c. Polyethylene tubing
   d. Plastic spray bottles

266. Ultrasonic cleaners are used for
   a. Removing small particles of blood and tissue from instruments
   b. Removing rust from instruments
   c. Disinfecting instruments
   d. Lubricating instruments

267. A laryngeal burr is used in
   a. Arthroscopy
   b. Abomasopexy
   c. Sigmoidoscopy
   d. Sacculectomy

268. Which of the following is not a consideration when evaluating a surgical pack for sterility?
   a. Sterilization date
   b. Indicator color change
   c. Holes or moisture damage
   d. Incorrect labeling

269. Mayo-Hegar scissors are used in all of the following situations except for cutting
   a. Sutures
   b. Delicate tissue
   c. Paper drapes
   d. Skin or muscle

270. When steam autoclaving bottles of solution, what two preparations should be made to prevent explosion of the bottles?
   a. Vent the bottles and set the autoclave to slow exhaust.
   b. Cap the bottles and set the autoclave to slow exhaust.
   c. Vent the bottles and set the autoclave to fast exhaust and dry.
   d. Cap the bottles and set the autoclave to flash.

271. How long must instruments be aerated after ethylene oxide gas sterilization before they can be used?
   a. 12 hours
   b. 1 to 7 days
   c. 7 to 14 days
   d. 1 hour

272. What size scalpel blade is generally used in an arthroscopy for making the stab incision into the joint because of its pointed, rather than rounded or hooked, end?
   a. No. 10
   b. No. 11
   c. No. 12
   d. No. 15

273. What size scalpel blade is used for making an abdominal skin incision?
   a. No. 10
   b. No. 11
   c. No. 12
   d. No. 15

274. What type of sterilization technique is not acceptable for instruments used in a canine castration?
   a. Gas sterilization
   b. Autoclaving
   c. Chemical sterilization
   d. Boiling

275. All of the following are objectives of the surgical hand scrub except
   a. To remove gross dirt and oil from the hands
   b. To sterilize the hands
   c. To reduce the microorganism count on the hands to as close to zero as possible
   d. To have a prolonged depressant effect on numbers of microflora on the hands and forearms

276. What type of surgical scrub solution is most effective in reducing numbers of bacteria on the skin?
     a. Hexachlorophene
     b. Povidone-iodine
     c. Chlorhexidine gluconate
     d. Polypropylene

277. When a surgeon encounters bleeding, all of the following can be used to control it except
     a. Electrocautery
     b. A hemostat
     c. Suction
     d. Rat-tooth forceps

278. How long does a sealed item remain sterilized after being sterilized by gamma radiation?
     a. 1 year
     b. 6 months
     c. Until it is opened
     d. 1 month

279. What instrument would be considered sterile on August 19, 2012?
     a. The instrument wrapped in double-layered muslin, with moisture on it, dated July 19, 2012
     b. The instrument sterilized with blood still on it dated August 18, 2012
     c. The instrument wrapped in a peel pouch dated August 20, 2011
     d. The instrument wrapped in paper and a dust cover dated August 20, 2011

280. What retractor is not self-retaining?
     a. Weitlaner
     b. Alms
     c. Sauerbruch
     d. Balfour

281. Sterilization is the process of killing microorganisms by physical or chemical means. What is the most reliable form of sterilization?
     a. Steam under pressure
     b. Gas
     c. Dry heat
     d. Radiation

282. Instruments wrapped in a single linen wrap can become contaminated with microbes within 2 to 3 days. How long does double wrapping an instrument extend the sterility period?
     a. 6 months
     b. 4 weeks
     c. 4 to 6 days
     d. 1 year

283. What is the best type of cleaner to use when hand washing surgical instruments?
     a. Ordinary hand soap
     b. Abrasive compounds
     c. Low-sudsing detergents
     d. Plain hot water

284. Which of the following is an absorbable suture?
     a. Prolene
     b. Vicryl
     c. Mersilene
     d. Silk

285. All of the following are considered benefits of using skin staples except
     a. Skin is more resistant to abscess formation than when sutures are used.
     b. Staples provide excellent wound healing.
     c. Staples are more cost effective.
     d. Staples save time.

286. If skin edges are under extreme tension (e.g., in a large skin wound), what is the suture pattern of choice?
     a. Simple continuous
     b. Simple interrupted
     c. Interrupted horizontal mattress
     d. Continuous horizontal mattress

287. What suture pattern is most commonly used in large-animal surgery?
     a. Simple continuous
     b. Simple interrupted
     c. Interrupted horizontal mattress
     d. Continuous horizontal mattress

288. What suture is not recommended for skin closure?
     a. Polydioxanone
     b. Nylon
     c. Chromic gut
     d. Stainless steel

289. What is the purpose of using a subcuticular suture pattern for final closure?
     a. To keep tissues apposed for quick healing
     b. To eliminate small scars produced around suture holes of the more common patterns
     c. To eliminate infection
     d. To be more cost effective

290. What suture pattern would *not* be used to close skin?
     a. Cushing
     b. Horizontal mattress
     c. Simple interrupted
     d. Ford interlocking

Correct answers are on pages 190-201.

291. Which one of the following suture patterns is an inverting stitch?
    a. Cruciate
    b. Cushing
    c. Horizontal mattress
    d. Vertical mattress

292. In what way is a surgeon's knot different from a square knot?
    a. A surgeon's knot has one throw on the first pass and two throws on the second pass; a square knot has two throws on each pass.
    b. A surgeon's knot has two throws on the first pass and one throw on the second pass; a square knot has one pass on each throw.
    c. A surgeon's knot has one throw on each pass; a square knot also has two throws on each pass.
    d. A surgeon's knot has two throws on the first pass and one throw on the second pass; a square knot has one throw on each pass.

293. Why is it better to ligate many small vessels rather than one mass ligation of tissues?
    a. Mass ligation of tissues is unsightly.
    b. Mass ligation of tissue may result in an infected area.
    c. Mass ligation of tissue is more likely to fail.
    d. Tissues included in a mass ligation may be too difficult for the body to resorb.

294. What is the purpose of a transfixation ligature?
    a. To make the ligature stronger
    b. To close a hollow organ
    c. To prevent breakage of the suture
    d. To prevent slippage of the suture

295. All of the following are good reasons for using an instrument tie (with the use of a needle holder) except
    a. It is economical; small pieces of suture can be used, and therefore suture material not wasted.
    b. It saves time.
    c. It is more accurate than a one- or two-handed tie.
    d. It is readily adaptable to any type of wound closure.

296. Which of the following is not a consideration when choosing a needle for use in a surgical procedure?
    a. Type of tissue to be sutured
    b. Location of the tissue to be sutured
    c. Size of suture material
    d. Strength of suture material

297. When suturing skin, the needle of choice is
    a. Blunt
    b. Reverse cutting
    c. Cutting
    d. Taper

298. What is the most significant advantage of using a swaged-on needle as opposed to a closed-eye needle?
    a. The needle never separates from the suture.
    b. The suture diameter is smaller than the needle diameter.
    c. Tissue is subjected to less trauma, because a single strand is pulled through the tissue.
    d. It saves time and money.

299. Suture patterns can be classified into three types: appositional, inverting, and tension. What tissue is most appropriately sutured in an appositional pattern?
    a. Tendon
    b. Hollow viscus
    c. Skin
    d. Nerve

300. Which of these sequences correctly lists suture material diameter, from largest to smallest?
    a. 3-0, 2-0, 0, 1, 2, 3
    b. 000, 00, 0, 1, 2, 3
    c. 3, 2, 1, 1-0, 2-0, 3-0
    d. 7-0, 5-0, 3-0, 1

301. For suturing a uterine incision in a cow, the proper suture size is
    a. 2-0
    b. 1
    c. 2
    d. 3-0

302. Which one of the following is a disadvantage of multifilament suture material?
    a. Less knot security than monofilament suture material
    b. Tears tissue more easily than monofilament suture material
    c. Has a greater tendency for wicking bacteria than monofilament suture material
    d. Has less strength than monofilament suture material

303. Which of the following is a monofilament suture material?
    a. Polyglactin 910 (Vicryl)
    b. Polyester (Mersilene)
    c. Polyethylene (Dermalene)
    d. Cotton

304. Which of the following has the poorest handling ease?
   a. Silk
   b. Braided polyglycolic acid (Dexon-Plus)
   c. Chromic catgut
   d. Monofilament stainless steel wire

305. Characteristics of an ideal suture material include all of the following except
   a. Minimal tissue reaction
   b. Favorable for bacterial growth
   c. Comfortable to work with
   d. Economical to use

306. An example of an inverting suture pattern is the
   a. Purse-string
   b. Simple interrupted
   c. Interrupted horizontal mattress
   d. Simple continuous

307. After what time does synthetic absorbable suture lose its tensile strength?
   a. 120 days
   b. 60 days
   c. 30 days
   d. 6 months

308. What suture material is absorbed most rapidly from an infected wound through increased local phagocytic activity?
   a. Vicryl (polyglactin 910)
   b. PDS (polydioxanone)
   c. Catgut
   d. Nylon

309. Which of the following is not a consideration in choosing a suture material?
   a. The surgeon's training and experience
   b. The part of the body where it will be used
   c. The size of the animal on which it will be used
   d. The age of the animal on which it will be used

310. In regard to wound healing, it is better to
   a. Increase the size of the suture material rather than the number of sutures.
   b. Increase the number of sutures rather than the size of the suture material.
   c. Decrease both the size of the suture material and number of the sutures.
   d. Increase both the size of the suture material and number of the sutures.

311. Which of these statements concerning surgical catgut is false?
   a. It can be used for ligating superficial blood vessels.
   b. It is recommended for epidermal use.
   c. It is recommended for internal use.
   d. It is fast absorbing.

312. Chromic catgut is produced by exposure to basic chromium salts. How does this process affect it?
   a. Increases intermolecular bonding
   b. Decreases its strength
   c. Increases tissue reaction to it
   d. Decreases absorption time

313. *Memory* is defined as a suture material's ability to resist bending forces and to return to its original configuration. This can cause what problem when suturing?
   a. The suture material is more easily tangled.
   b. The suture material is difficult to knot securely.
   c. The suture breaks more readily.
   d. The suture is more likely to cause infection.

314. *Strike through* refers to
   a. Making the first skin incision
   b. Incision of a sterile adhesive drape applied directly over the skin
   c. Rapping the table to arouse the patient
   d. Wicking of bacteria through a surgical drape that has become wet, allowing bacteria to contaminate the sterile area

315. Perioperative antibiotics
   a. Should never be used
   b. Should always be used
   c. Are indicated in surgical procedures longer than 1.5 hours
   d. Are questionable in their effectiveness

316. What type of instrument is an Adson?
   a. Retractor
   b. Rongeur
   c. Periosteal elevator
   d. Thumb forceps

317. What is the primary function of a Balfour?
   a. Retractor
   b. Rongeur
   c. Periosteal elevator
   d. Thumb forceps

318. What is the primary function of a Lempert?
   a. Retractor
   b. Rongeur
   c. Periosteal elevator
   d. Thumb forceps

Correct answers are on pages 190-201.

319. What is the primary function of a Brown-Adson?
    a. Retractor
    b. Rongeur
    c. Periosteal elevator
    d. Thumb forceps

320. Chlorhexidine gluconate surgical scrub
    a. Tends to stain the skin and hair coat
    b. Is effective against *Pseudomonas* species
    c. Is marketed as Nolvasan
    d. Should be rinsed with alcohol

321. A gauze sponge that is being used for the surgical scrub inadvertently touches the patient's hair. It
    a. Can continue to be used for the scrub because the antimicrobial agents in the scrub will kill any bacteria picked up in the hair
    b. Should be thrown out and replaced with a new sponge
    c. Should now be used for only the edges of the clipped site
    d. Should not be considered contaminated unless gross contamination is visible

322. Surgical scrubs are applied to the surgically prepared site
    a. In any pattern, just so the area is covered thoroughly
    b. In target fashion, starting with the incision site and spiraling outward to the edge of the clipped area
    c. Starting with the edges, because they are the dirtiest areas, and working in toward incision site
    d. Without subsequent rinsing, because dilution reduces the antimicrobial effect

323. Why is an anal purse-string suture placed before perianal surgery?
    a. To keep the tail out of the surgical field
    b. To prevent fecal contamination during surgery
    c. To close the urethra
    d. To tighten loose folds of perianal skin

324. In male dogs, the prepuce is
    a. Sutured closed before an abdominal surgical procedure to prevent contamination
    b. Considered an uncontaminated area and is not given special consideration
    c. Flushed with alcohol while the dog is awake
    d. Flushed with a weak povidone-iodine and saline solution before abdominal surgery

325. What structure is commonly emptied before abdominal surgery?
    a. Stomach
    b. Anal sac
    c. Urinary bladder
    d. Gallbladder

326. What type of instrument is a Metzenbaum?
    a. Needle holder
    b. Scissors
    c. Towel clamp
    d. Hemostatic forceps

327. What type of instrument is a Mayo-Hegar?
    a. Needle holder
    b. Scissors
    c. Towel clamp
    d. Hemostatic forceps

328. What type of instrument is a Kelly?
    a. Needle holder
    b. Scissors
    c. Towel clamp
    d. Hemostatic forceps

329. What type of instrument is a Backhaus?
    a. Needle holder
    b. Scissors
    c. Towel clamp
    d. Hemostatic forceps

330. The most effective use for a rongeur is to
    a. Pinch off a bleeding vessel
    b. Elevate soft tissue off a bony surface
    c. Remove small pieces of bone
    d. Retract soft tissue away from bone

331. Talking in the surgery room should be kept to a minimum
    a. To prevent unnecessary injection of bacteria into the operating theater
    b. To prevent distractions
    c. To expedite the surgery
    d. At all times except during draping

332. An instrument suitable for cutting a paper drape is a/an
    a. Mayo-Hegar scissors
    b. Metzenbaum scissors
    c. Scalpel blade
    d. Iris scissors

333. What instrument is not a self-retaining tissue retractor?
    a. Finochietto
    b. Army-Navy
    c. Balfour
    d. Gelpi

334. A surgical scrub with residual antibacterial activity is important because
   a. Bacteria below the superficial dermal area are constantly rising to the surface.
   b. It makes it unnecessary to worry about touching a scrubbed area with an ungloved hand.
   c. It makes it unnecessary to be as fastidious in the scrubbing technique.
   d. Surgical masks are basically ineffective.

335. The most effective sterilizing method for an object that could be damaged by heat is
   a. Autoclaving
   b. Gas sterilization
   c. Flash flaming
   d. Alcohol scrub

336. What term best describes freedom from infection as it applies to surgical technique?
   a. Uncontaminated
   b. Asepsis
   c. Healthy
   d. Clean

337. What surgical materials are sterilized by filtration?
   a. Nutrient solutions
   b. Irrigation solutions
   c. Surgical solutions
   d. Pharmaceutical solutions

338. What piece of equipment delivers saturated steam under pressure?
   a. Oven
   b. Crematorium
   c. Autoclave
   d. Microwave

339. A safeguard to ensure that a pack is sterilized adequately
   a. Does not exist; you can never really be certain
   b. Is a sterilization indicator strip
   c. Is to feel how hot the instrument is after the process is over
   d. Is to visually inspect the pack

340. An autoclave
   a. Is not a reliable way to sterilize instruments
   b. Must not be overloaded because this decreases its effectiveness
   c. Is a good appliance to freshen the air
   d. Is expensive and therefore not practical for most veterinary clinics

341. Electrocautery
   a. Is an effective way to sterilize skin
   b. Is used to coagulate blood flow from a cut vessel
   c. Cannot be used for most surgical procedures
   d. Is atraumatic and can be used liberally

342. After donning sterile latex surgical gloves and before beginning the procedure, powder is wiped from the gloves with a wet sponge to
   a. Make glove punctures more easily visible
   b. Prevent postoperative starch granulomas in the patient's tissues
   c. Reduce the likelihood of bacterial proliferation in the event the gloves become contaminated
   d. Improve the gloves' gripping ability

343. The main goal of aseptic surgical technique is to prevent contamination of the
   a. Operative personnel
   b. Surgical instruments
   c. Surgical wound
   d. Surgical drapes

344. When preparing a cat for a routine spay, administration of antibiotics prior to surgery
   a. Should be given if your employer does not wear a cap or mask
   b. Is not indicated for short, uncomplicated procedures
   c. Should always be given as a precaution to prevent infection
   d. Is never useful in conjunction with surgery

345. The main function of bactericidal disinfectants is to
   a. Slow bacterial proliferation
   b. Kill bacteria
   c. Remove organic debris from the site
   d. Flush bacteria from the site

346. Keeping the environment (floors, walls, counters) clean throughout your clinic is
   a. Not important if your surgery areas are separate from other areas of the clinic
   b. Advisable because it is good for public relations
   c. Mandated by the AVMA
   d. Mandatory to prevent cross-contamination into the surgery area

347. The type of disinfectant used in your clinic
   a. Depends on what is on sale at the moment
   b. Should have a pleasant odor
   c. Should be chosen for its broad spectrum of bacteriostatic or bactericidal properties
   d. Has no bearing on the outcome of your surgeries

Correct answers are on pages 190-201.

348. The sterile field in the surgery room
    a. Is difficult to define
    b. Consists of the shaved and prepared area on the animal's skin
    c. Is impossible to maintain in veterinary surgery
    d. Consists of the draped field and instrument table

349. The surgical nurse circulating for the scrubbed-in surgeons
    a. Has the task of keeping the animal anesthetized
    b. Does not need a cap and mask because he or she is not assisting with surgery
    c. Must constantly be concerned with maintaining aseptic technique
    d. Need not wear sterile surgical gloves to pass anything to the surgeon

350. Assuming that good aseptic technique is being followed, the most common source of contamination in a surgical wound is
    a. The patient's skin or internal organs
    b. Your own breath
    c. Dust falling from the ceiling
    d. Dust from the floor

351. The clothing worn in a surgical room
    a. Can be clothes worn on the street
    b. Should be clothes worn while in the clinic only
    c. Should be a scrub suit dedicated to surgery use
    d. Is required to be clean only and not torn

352. Surgical masks
    a. Prevent unpleasant odors from reaching the surgeon's nose
    b. Lose their effectiveness when saturated with moisture
    c. Are used for orthopedic procedures only
    d. Can be tied loosely so that they are not as confining

353. When folding surgical gowns for sterilization,
    a. Tie the arms together so they do not dangle when the surgeon is gowning.
    b. Have the ends of the sleeves on top for easy grasping.
    c. Make sure the ties are on top so they can be used to pick up the gown.
    d. Place the inside of the shoulder seams on top and fold all outer areas of the gown to the inside.

354. During surgery, the back outside aspect of a surgeon's gown should be considered
    a. Sterile
    b. Sterile as long as someone has not touched it
    c. Unsterile
    d. Neither sterile nor unsterile, because it is not likely to contact the patient

355. If a gowned and gloved person at the surgery table is not participating in the surgery at some point,
    a. His or her hands should be held quietly at the sides.
    b. His or her hands may be held behind the back if it is still sterile.
    c. His or her hands should be folded at chest level or placed on the instrument table.
    d. He or she must leave the room.

356. An anatomic scrub
    a. Is not practical on a routine basis
    b. Is quicker than a timed scrub
    c. Refers to scrubbing the arms and hands in a methodical, consistent manner
    d. Is more thorough than a timed scrub

357. A timed scrub should last at least
    a. 15 min
    b. 5 min
    c. 30 min
    d. 1 min

358. The preferred method for gloving is
    a. Open
    b. Closed
    c. Assisted
    d. Double

359. When scrubbing for a surgical procedure, the position of the arms
    a. Varies with the height of the scrub sink
    b. Should always be with the hands higher than the elbows
    c. Should always be with the elbows higher than the hands
    d. Varies with the height of the scrubbing personnel

360. Iodophors, such as povidone-iodine scrub,
    a. Are the ideal surgical preparation
    b. Have been replaced by newer, more effective scrubbing agents
    c. Are effective when used with alcohol only
    d. Are bactericidal against all common contaminants

361. The number of personnel in the operating theater
   a. Has no bearing on the outcome of the surgery
   b. Cannot be controlled in most situations
   c. Must be high to keep the temperature in the room high
   d. Should be kept to a minimum to keep air borne bacteria levels low

362. Cleaning instruments before sterilization
   a. Must be performed carefully by hand
   b. Is done only if there is time
   c. Can be done exclusively with ultrasonic cleaners
   d. Is not necessary if proper sterilization practices are followed

363. Ethyl and isopropyl alcohols
   a. Have characteristics that make them ideal for sterilizing instruments
   b. At lower concentrations are bacteriostatic rather than bactericidal
   c. Have an excellent residual effect because of their rapid evaporation
   d. Have no place in veterinary surgery

364. An effective disinfectant to clean a cage after an animal that has had a *Pseudomonas* contaminated wound is
   a. Chlorhexidine
   b. Isopropyl alcohol
   c. Quaternary ammonium
   d. Povidone-iodine

365. A good solution to instill in the conjunctival sac before surgery is
   a. 10% chlorhexidine gluconate
   b. 1:25 povidone-iodine solution
   c. 5% isopropyl alcohol
   d. Dilute soapy water

366. *Clean-contaminated surgery* refers to
   a. All surgeries
   b. Incisions in sterile areas that become contaminated during surgery
   c. Incisions made in contaminated areas
   d. Incisions in a previously contaminated area that has been rendered sterile

367. In terms of surgical contamination, endogenous organisms are those that
   a. Originate from the patient's own body
   b. Come from the external surgical environment
   c. Rarely cause any problem in surgical wounds
   d. Come from the surgeon

368. When a break in aseptic technique occurs,
   a. The surgery must be called off immediately.
   b. The break can be ignored and surgery can continue if the surgery is just about finished.
   c. The patient is unlikely to recover from the surgery because of infection.
   d. Steps must be taken to immediately remedy the situation to the best of everyone's ability.

369. A good time to clean the surgery room is
   a. On the night before surgery to allow air borne dust to settle before surgery
   b. Immediately before the surgery so things can be as clean as possible
   c. Once a week
   d. Once a month

370. If during surgery you notice an item close to the edge of the sterile field, you should
   a. Ask others to find out whether it was contaminated
   b. Consider it unsterile if you are not absolutely certain
   c. Consider it sterile
   d. Move it farther into the sterile field

371. Preparing a patient's skin for surgery
   a. Renders the skin completely sterile
   b. Does nothing to affect the outcome of the surgery
   c. Reduces the bacterial flora to a level that can be controlled by the patient's defense mechanisms
   d. Is not necessary if antibiotics are given

372. Lavaging (flushing) a body cavity with warm, sterile saline after a surgical procedure is completed and before closing the incision
   a. Is of minimal value in abdominal surgeries
   b. Decreases the amount of bacteria left behind and warms the patient
   c. Serves as a medium for bacteria to multiply in, and so it should be avoided
   d. Is necessary only if there has been a break in aseptic technique

373. An example of an elective procedure is
   a. Ovariohysterectomy
   b. Nephrotomy
   c. Exploratory laparotomy
   d. Thyroidectomy

374. A tapered suture needle is
   a. Best to use in skin
   b. The least traumatic and most often used in deep tissue layers
   c. Not used very often because of its relative inability to penetrate tissue
   d. Too expensive for routine surgical use

Correct answers are on pages 190-201.

375. A thoracotomy is an incision into the
    a. Abdomen
    b. Chest
    c. Skull
    d. Ear canal

376. The suffix -*ectomy* refers to
    a. Surgical removal
    b. Reduction
    c. Drainage
    d. Incision into

377. Which orthopedic fixation consists of pins that penetrate fractured bones and are held in place externally by bolts?
    a. Rush pinning
    b. Steinmann fixation
    c. Stack pinning
    d. Kirschner-Ehmer fixation

378. The term *arthrotomy* refers to an incision into a/an
    a. Artery
    b. Joint
    c. Muscle
    d. Long bone

379. Arresting the flow of blood from a vessel or to a part is called
    a. Aspiration
    b. Fibrinolysis
    c. Hemostasis
    d. Hemolysis

380. Peritonitis refers to
    a. Inflammation of the pericardial space
    b. Inflammation of the lining of the abdominal cavity
    c. Inflammation caused by parasite infection
    d. Inflammation of the perianal area

381. Cryptorchidectomy is performed on male dogs
    a. When one or both testicles have not descended into the scrotal sac
    b. When no other treatment for cryptosporidiosis is available
    c. And is similar to the vasectomy procedure done in people
    d. When complications from routine castration arise

382. Fenestration refers to
    a. Cutting a part exactly in half
    b. Creating a window in tissue
    c. The draping procedure
    d. Folding back the top skin layer

383. Ovariohysterectomy is routinely performed
    a. In excitable dogs that need immediate calming
    b. In young female dogs that the owners wish rendered sterile
    c. In male dogs with female characteristics
    d. Exclusively in female dogs who have already had litters of puppies

384. *Hepatic* refers to
    a. Heparin preparations
    b. Liver
    c. Hemoglobin
    d. Stomach

385. Blood vessels are ligated
    a. To remove them completely from the body
    b. When blood flow needs to be stopped
    c. Using trauma to coagulate the blood
    d. Rarely and in emergency situations only

386. Chemical cauterization
    a. Is an excellent method of stopping blood flow
    b. Is rarely used in veterinary medicine
    c. Is traumatic to adjacent tissues and therefore is not used in surgical cases
    d. Is a misnomer; chemicals cannot stop bleeding

387. Keeping tissues moist during a surgical procedure
    a. Is important because dry tissues are less resistant to bacterial infection
    b. Is undesirable because wet tissue is an ideal medium for bacterial regeneration
    c. Is of little value
    d. Should be accomplished with 70% isopropyl alcohol

388. Plating a fractured bone
    a. Refers to coating it with a rigid metallic substance to induce healing
    b. Is beyond the scope of most veterinary practices
    c. Is an internal method of fracture fixation involving stainless steel plates and screws
    d. Can be done without skin incision

389. The distal portion of a long bone is
    a. The one closest to the trunk of the body
    b. The one farthest away from the trunk of the body
    c. The inner portion of the bone
    d. The outer layer of the bone

390. Perineal urethrostomies are performed only on
    a. Pregnant cats
    b. Male cats with urethral obstruction
    c. Large-breed dogs with gastric torsion
    d. Small dogs with pyometra

391. *Torsion* of an organ or part refers to
    a. Swelling or expansion
    b. Inflation with fluid
    c. Inflation with gas
    d. Twisting or rotation

392. What surgical procedure is least likely to combat canine hip dysplasia's debilitating complications?
    a. Triple pelvic osteotomy
    b. Total hip replacement
    c. Intramedullary pinning
    d. Pectineal myotomy

393. *Ear canal ablation* refers to
    a. Irrigation of the ear canal
    b. Instilling antibiotics to correct otitis media
    c. Surgical removal and closure of the external ear canal
    d. Enlarging the external ear canal

394. *Perioperatively* refers to
    a. Before surgery
    b. After surgery
    c. Around the time of surgery
    d. During surgery

395. A proptosed eye is one that is
    a. Normally positioned
    b. Displaced rostrally from the socket
    c. Shrunken and shriveled
    d. Deviated in any direction other than normal

396. Onychectomy
    a. Is the procedure used to remove a cat's testicles and spermatic cord
    b. Is the procedure used to remove a cat's claws and associated phalanges
    c. Can be done without anesthesia
    d. Can be done on female cats only

397. Postoperative complications
    a. Do not occur if the surgeon is skilled
    b. Should never be discussed with a client
    c. Can occur even if the surgery went well
    d. Are almost always attributable to poor assistance in surgery

398. Fracture reduction
    a. Involves trimming the areas of bone adjacent to the fracture site
    b. Involves apposing (pulling together) the fractured bone ends
    c. Is rarely necessary for good healing
    d. Can usually be done without anesthesia

399. A diaphragmatic hernia
    a. Is a diaphragm that is in a continuous spasm
    b. Is displacement of the heart and part of the lungs into the abdomen
    c. Cannot be corrected and is considered fatal
    d. Should be suspected if the animal is dyspneic following a traumatic experience

400. When an animal is sent home after surgery,
    a. The wound should already be completely healed.
    b. The client should be given written detailed home care instructions.
    c. The animal is no longer legally your patient and no longer your concern.
    d. The technician should make daily visits to ensure that the patient is given the same care as in the hospital.

401. Absorbable gelatin sponges
    a. Are typically soaked or sutured into a bleeding site
    b. Should never be left in the body after surgery
    c. Are radiopaque
    d. Are not available for veterinary surgery

402. Exteriorizing a body part or organ during surgery
    a. Is a routine practice when the part or organ contains contaminants
    b. Is very hazardous to the patient and not routinely done
    c. Precludes the need for lavaging
    d. Is done only if that part or organ is to be resected (surgically removed)

Correct answers are on pages 190-201.

ANSWERS

1. **b** Successful surgery depends on careful attention to the rules of asepsis.

2. **c** Scrubbing the surgical site reduces, but does not completely eliminate, normal microbial flora on the patient's skin.

3. **b** An ovariohysterectomy is the surgical removal of the ovaries and uterus.

4. **a**

5. **a**

6. **c** First-intention wound healing occurs with no infection or suppuration (pus formation).

7. **d** The cautery unit is not sterilized. Only the handle and adapter ends are sterilized.

8. **d** The packs of suture material should not be opened until they are needed.

9. **a** Females do not have prostate glands.

10. **b** The other three statements are popular public misconceptions.

11. **b** Bandages can remain on an animal for variable amounts of time. The length of time that a bandage is kept on depends on the reason for which the bandage was applied.

12. **a** The hair coat of a puppy is always different than that of the adult. The quality of the coat will change no matter what the reproductive status of the dog. Shedding will always be an issue.

13. **b** Ovaries and the uterus will be removed.

14. **a** When the newborns are removed from the uterus, the circulation pattern in the body of the mother undergoes a drastic change, and she runs the risk of going into shock. The anesthesia-monitoring technician should be particularly vigilant during this time.

15. **c** The surgical incision should be observed closely by the client daily. The newborns can contribute to surgical-site problems by sucking on suture ends and kneading at the incision. Thus, it is very important that the incision be monitored.

16. **c** Male animals do not go through heat or estrus.

17. **d** Male animals do not go through heat or estrus.

18. **d** Aspirin is not given for preemptive analgesia before a surgery because of its effect on platelet function, which may diminish blood clotting during the procedure. Also, preemptive analgesics are generally given by injection before surgery, and aspirin comes in an oral form only.

19. **c** It is not important to know whether a cat is in heat. The surgery can be easily performed on a cat in estrus.

20. **c** Spay procedures may be performed through a mid-abdominal or flank incision. Dog castrations are usually performed through a prescrotal incision.

21. **b** Spay procedures may be performed through a mid-abdominal or flank incision. Cats are usually neutered through a scrotal incision.

22. **d** The ventral midline abdominal incision opens the abdomen at a location where the ovaries and the uterus can be removed through the one incision.

23. **c** Plucking and scissoring will take too long. No. 10 blades have fewer teeth than No. 40 blades and thus do not cut as closely.

24. **d** The patient will be in pain after the surgery as with all surgeries. Oral surgeries are no different in this regard.

25. **b** Water, not air, is used to flush all food through the tube. A temperature of 50° C will burn the patient. Injecting the food rapidly into the gastrotomy tube may induce vomiting.

26. **a** Patients are usually fed no sooner than 24 to 36 hours after recovering from GI surgery.

27. **d** Feeding tubes are not placed through the mouth. The patient would chew through a tube placed through the mouth, rendering it useless.

28. **a** Sometimes it is impossible to fast the patient before surgery; for example, surgery to correct a twisted stomach must be performed without taking time to fast the patient.

29. c Appropriate analgesic therapy is necessary for patient comfort; however, it will not prevent decubital ulcers.

30. a Brachycephalic breeds of cats and dogs run the risk of proptosis (dislocation of the eye globe from the socket) when held too tightly around the neck.

31. d Abscesses are drained by lancing but are left open to continue draining and are not sutured closed. Abscesses are fluid-filled and not solid infiltrates of inflammatory cells. The formation of an abscess is a common sequela of bite wounds, especially in cats.

32. c Sutures may be absorbable, not drains. Drains are usually removed when little to no fluid continues to flow from the site.

33. d One purpose of splints or casts is to make the injured limb usable while it is healing.

34. a It is important to keep a splint or bandage clean and *dry*.

35. b Trimming the pinna is done when tumors are removed from the pinna or when ears are cropped.

36. d The uterus and ovaries are best exposed through a midline incision made caudal to the umbilicus.

37. c Suture material can be absorbed by the body or not. It can be supplied with a needle attached or not. It can be braided or monofilament.

38. b Instruments should be passed with the ratchets or jaws in the closed position.

39. d The technician should cut the sutures to the length that the surgeon suggests. The tips of the scissors should be used to cut sutures. Blotting the surgical site to remove blood is preferred. Wiping may cause more bleeding and is irritating to the tissues.

40. a Metal clips and staples are inert and made of noncorrosive metal. They are easily and effectively sterilized.

41. c Instruments should be lubricated with instrument milk, not oil. Instruments need to be cleaned in water with nonabrasive cleansers and dried completely to avoid rusting.

42. c A bone plate is an example of an internal fixation device. A bone plate is a steel device that is screwed on to the bone to line up and stabilize the fracture site.

43. a Properly inflating the endotracheal tube and keeping it inflated while the patient's gag reflex is absent is the only way to guard against aspiration when the pet is under anesthesia.

44. d Pneumothorax is air trapped in the chest cavity between the lungs and the chest wall. The lungs collapse because of increased pressure within the chest cavity. A chest tube can help evacuate the air and allow the lungs to expand. Pulmonary edema is fluid within the lungs. Ascites is fluid within the abdominal cavity. Subcutaneous emphysema is air trapped under the skin. A chest tube is not a treatment for any of those three.

45. a The English bulldog has an elongated soft palate. If the endotracheal tube is pulled before the dog is awake, the soft palate may act as a respiratory obstruction. It is wise to keep the endotracheal tube in as long as possible in most brachycephalic breeds.

46. c Dyspnea is difficult breathing. Dysphoria is a side effect of opioid drugs. Dystocia may be managed medically or surgically.

47. d Enucleation is removal of the eye.

48. c Onychectomy is defined as "declawing or removal of the entire nail."

49. a A cystotomy is a surgical procedure to open the urinary bladder.

50. c An ovariohysterectomy is the removal of the uterus and ovaries. This is usually performed through a midabdominal incision.

51. b A femoral head ostectomy is the removal of the proximal end of the femur.

52. b An orchidectomy is the removal of the testes.

53. a The popliteal lymph nodes are located behind the knee.

54. b

55. d

56. a

57. c

58. a

59. a

60. d

61. **b** It is nonabsorbable.

62. a

63. d

64. d

65. **c** 3 PDS may be used but is too expensive for routine use in large animals.

66. b

67. d

68. b

69. **d** Contamination of the surgical site can occur because of microbial contamination of small abrasions if the area is shaved with the patient awake.

70. a

71. b

72. c

73. d

74. b

75. **d** However, because they are wasteful of suture material, hand ties have fallen into disuse.

76. **c** This involves passing the suture material through the stump before tying it.

77. **d** Suture reaction is due to the suture material rather than to whether the material is monofilament or multifilament.

78. c

79. b

80. a

81. **a** Although healing of the tissue will take place faster in a younger animal, the material will still absorb at a predictable rate. Presence of infection will increase the rate of absorption of most materials. Sutures placed in areas such as the pancreas will be absorbed more quickly than those placed in the fascia. Finally, natural materials, such as catgut, are absorbed much more rapidly than synthetic materials, such as polyglactin.

82. **a** If the anal sac is not incised, it is possible to remove it aseptically.

83. **c** These forceps are too traumatic to the edges of the incision.

84. d

85. a

86. b

87. **a** The heart rate increases in hemorrhagic shock.

88. **d** Other vital signs and reflexes must be assessed.

89. c

90. a

91. **c** The other factors may increase the likelihood of exuberant granulation tissue forming.

92. b

93. **d** It has now fallen into disfavor as an antiseptic.

94. **c** Although by passing back to back, asepsis is not broken, by facing the back of the surgeon, the nonsterile person can more easily watch for situations that may lead to contamination.

95. **a** The indicator should be touched by transfer forceps only, whereas the rest should be handled by scrubbed personnel.

96. **c** Most of these resolve on their own once the suture material is removed.

97. c

98. b

99. **c** Everting patterns are contraindicated, because the mucosa would then be exposed.

100. **d** By convention, only the date the pack was made up is required.

101. **d** Rochester-Carmalt is the only forceps in this group with longitudinal striations.

102. **c**

103. **b**

104. **d**

105. **b**

106. **a**

107. **d** The other conditions must be corrected by surgical intervention.

108. **a**

109. **a**

110. **c** This gives the best visualization of the retained testicles.

111. **d** Although incisions are commonly done through the sternum in people, lateral incisions are more common in dogs and appear to result in less postoperative pain.

112. **d**

113. **b** Quaternary ammonium compounds must often be used at more concentrated solutions to kill some resistant viruses.

114. **d** Mayo-Hegar is a type of needle driver.

115. **a**

116. **a**

117. **b**

118. **b** The only piece of information that the autoclave tape provides is that steam has reached the tape and resulted in a color change. It is by no means an indicator that adequate sterilization conditions have been achieved.

119. **a** If all parts of a surgical pack are exposed to 121° C for a minimum of 15 minutes (at 15 psi pressure), sterilization should be achieved.

120. **d** Puppies are not intubated following delivery; instead their nasal and oral passages are suctioned, and doxapram may be placed under the tongue to stimulate respiration. They can be physically stimulated to begin breathing with vigorous rubbing and a gentle swinging motion.

121. **d** Ventricular arrhythmias are not commonly associated with pyometra surgeries. However, sepsis and renal damage secondary to *Escherichia coli* toxins are a major concern.

122. **d** Gastric dilatation and volvulus status can usually be confirmed visually, by passing an orogastric tube, or via radiography. Hemodynamic shock, sepsis, and cardiac arrhythmias are possible sequelae. Fluids should be provided in shock doses, and lidocaine should be readily available to treat ventricular arrhythmias.

123. **a** Only the No. 10 of this list fits a No. 3 scalpel handle.

124. **d** No. 4 scalpel handles use blades in the 20s.

125. **b** *Pathogenic* means that it causes disease.

126. **c** The chamber is sealed before setting the timer for the cycle.

127. **a** Sterile implies that there are no living organisms of any type.

128. **c** All are required to enter the operating room, but the gown does not need to be sterile.

129. **c** A double-wrapped pack can be stored in this manner for 6 to 8 weeks.

130. **b**

131. **d** The Gelpi is a self-retaining retractor and does not require a surgical assistant to hold it in place.

132. **b** Aseptic technique is a method of reducing the number of organisms that may enter the surgical wound.

133. **a** The strip turns dark when the temperature of 121° C has been reached.

134. **d** These fine-edged scissors are used to cut tissue only.

135. **d**

136. **b**

137. **c** Ultrasonic cleaners remove all lubrication from the instruments.

138. **d** Eyed needles can be reautoclaved and reused, because they are not attached to any suture.

139. **c**

140. **b** Suture is not classified by tensile strength, but various sizes are graded according to strength, determining the "ought" sizing.

141. **a** Braided suture has more friction and better knot security than the same material in a monofilament.

142. **c** The white lead is attached to the right foreleg.

143. **d** The red lead is attached to the left hind leg.

144. **c** The suffix *-cidal* means "to kill."

145. **c**

146. **b** The minimum temperature and exposure time to the steam of an autoclave to provide sterility is 250° F or 121° C for 15 minutes.

147. **d** Without the pressure, water continues to boil at 100° C and will not increase in temperature.

148. **a**

149. **b** Moisture allows microbes to migrate up through the drapes and contaminate the upper surface.

150. **d** Time must be allowed for penetration to the center of the pack and then 15 minutes of exposure time.

151. **c** Ethylene oxide is the most commonly used agent in gas sterilization.

152. **b**

153. **c** Rochester-Carmalt forceps are generally a large forceps. Choice **b** describes an Allen clamp, and choice **d** is a Rochester-Pean forceps.

154. **a**

155. **b** A Snook hook is typically used to elevate the uterus during an ovariohysterectomy or spay.

156. **c** *Ovario,* "ovaries"; *hyster,* "uterus"; *ectomy,* "to remove"

157. **a** This is a serious condition that may have a closed cervix or open cervix.

158. **c** About 6 to 7 weeks, as long as the cabinet has doors and it is not open shelving. Open shelving shortens the lifespan to roughly half.

159. **c** Mayo-Hegar needle holders do not have scissors, and Metzenbaum scissors are never used to cut suture.

160. **a** The *IM* stands for "intramedullary," because these pins are often placed into the medullary cavity of long bones.

161. **c** Normal wound healing causes inflammation, which causes minor increases in skin temperature and erythema.

162. **b** It is not necessary to have a sterile gown, but clean scrubs or a gown should be worn.

163. **c** It is not necessary to have a sterile gown when performing as a nonsterile assistant.

164. **b** The nonsterile assistant must approach from the back so that the front of your gown will not be contaminated.

165. **a** The hemorrhagic discharge is associated with proestrus not estrus.

166. **b** Roccal is a disinfectant not intended for use on living tissue.

167. **b**

168. **d**

169. **c** This approach is often called a *left flank incision.*

170. **a** They are used to crush and cut the spermatic cord during castrations.

171. **b** The rumen is located on the left side of the body.

172. **a**

173. **b** The suture in choice **a**, chromic gut, is absorbable; the suture in choices **c** and **d** are too large.

174. **b**

175. **d** The hair is plucked until the scrotum is free of hair, then the surgical scrub is performed.

176. **c** All other approaches are used in left-displaced abomasum (LDA) surgeries.

177. **d** After 24 hours, exercise is required to promote drainage from the surgical site and prevent excessive swelling.

178. **a**

179. **c**

180. **c** The ECG indicates electrical activity only; it does not measure the contractility or perfusion of the heart. There may be a normal ECG with no heartbeat or pulse at all.

181. **b** Also called Kirschner-Ehmer Apparatus

182. **c**

183. **a** Electric heating pads can cause severe burns and should not be used.

184. **d** This piece of equipment is used to place IM pins.

185. **c** Although if performed at an early age, some dogs may not lift their legs to urinate, but many still develop this normal behavior.

186. **b** Solutions cannot be used as surgical scrubs.

187. **d** It is not necessary to have a complete tail wrap unless the tail will cause contamination because of proximity to the surgical site.

188. **a** Padding is one of the measures that helps prevent myositis, a severe inflammation of the muscles that can be life threatening.

189. **a** Testicles descend into the scrotum, not the prepuce.

190. **b**

191. **c**

192. **b**

193. **c** The main reason for aseptic technique is to protect the animal from microbes entering through the surgical site.

194. **d**

195. **a** A fenestration is a window.

196. **c**

197. **a** The basic requirements for first-intention healing are minimal tissue damage and apposition of the wound edges, usually with sutures.

198. **d** The basic functional unit of the nervous system, the neuron, is incapable of reproduction; consequently, damage to the nervous system is often repaired by scar tissue. The other organs and tissues listed have excellent healing potential.

199. **d** The xiphoid process and umbilicus are both on the animal's ventral midline.

200. **c** An electric drill would be damaged or inadequately sterilized by any of the other methods.

201. **a** Steam sterilization in an autoclave is used most often for instruments and equipment that would not be damaged by moisture or heat.

202. **d** The sharp edges of scissors are dulled by steam in an autoclave; boiling and dry heat are not sufficiently effective; and the expense and danger of ethylene oxide use are not warranted.

203. **a** The minimum standard for sterilization of surgical instruments in an autoclave is 121° C (250° F) for at least 15 minutes.

204. **b** Chemical autoclave indicators are the only type listed that can give immediate information on all three of the basic criteria for autoclave sterilization: (1) the presence of steam at the proper combination, (2) exposure time, and (3) temperature.

205. **a** Microorganisms in a wound during surgery are considered contaminants until, or unless, they multiply and cause damage.

206. **d** A surgical mask does not come in contact with anything sterile during a surgical procedure, so it has only to be clean.

207. **d** An autoclave sterilizes by exposing packs to high-temperature steam under pressure.

208. **d** A No. 40 clipper blade is a surgical blade. It clips the hair off at the skin surface.

209. **b** Curettage involves scraping of a tissue or cavity.

210. **d** Using overly large suture material would not cause a wound to break down. It would actually have greater holding power than a smaller size of suture material.

211. **b** Contaminated items look identical to sterile items; if there is any doubt about the sterility of an item, it must be considered contaminated.

212. **b** Exuberant granulation tissue (proud flesh) inhibits wound healing and epithelial regeneration. The other choices would likely enhance wound healing.

213. **d** One of the most important characteristics of wound healing by first intention is approximation of the wound edges.

214. **d** The ventral midline approach gives the most extensive access to the abdominal cavity.

215. **a** A slight elevation of body temperature that lasts for a day or two is normal after major surgery. The other choices are all early indicators of wound dehiscence.

216. **d** Prevention of surgical wound contamination is the whole purpose of aseptic technique in the operating room.

217. **a** This is the only choice that can be influenced by aseptic technique. The others are inherent in the patient, the surgical procedure being performed, or the microorganisms in the environment.

218. **a** The antimicrobial effect of a surgical scrub is dependent on sufficient exposure of the skin to the soap, as well as the scrubbing action that loosens dead skin and debris and works the soap into the cracks and crevices of the skin.

219. **c** Hexachlorophene forms a bacteriostatic film on the skin if used exclusively to wash the hands and arms. Other soaps remove the protective film.

220. **a** The surgical cap does not come in contact with the tissues of the patient either directly or indirectly. It therefore needs to be clean, not sterile.

221. **b** Liquid chemical sterilization does not dull sharp edges.

222. **d** Warming the solution speeds up the chemical reactions necessary to kill microorganisms.

223. **d** Cloth and paper drapes are subject to capillary action; plastic drapes are not.

224. **d** Steam dulls the sharp edges of scissors.

225. **b** The other solutions listed are either irritating to the tissues or not isotonic with the patient's tissue fluids.

226. **a** None of the other approaches can be used in a standing cow, and they do not provide good access to the rumen.

227. **d** All personnel in the operating room should face toward sterile fields so they are aware of their relationship to them.

228. **a** Dehiscence of all layers of the body wall exposes abdominal viscera. Repair must be immediate to prevent serious damage to the abdominal organs and structures.

229. **d** Inflammation results from any injury to the body, whether intentional (surgical) or unintentional (traumatic). The increased blood supply to an area of inflammation results in increased warmth to the area. Good surgical technique minimizes inflammation but does not eliminate it.

230. **b** It takes 4 to 6 days for production of collagen strands in a wound to reach a significant level. Until that time, the sutures are the main thing holding the suture line together.

231. **c** Wound contraction represents movement of the whole thickness of the skin toward the center of the wound.

232. **a**

233. **a** A patient in shock would be expected to show rapid, shallow breathing in an effort to oxygenate the blood as rapidly as possible.

234. **b** Unless very large or ruptured, postoperative seromas are unsightly but of little importance to the animal's health.

235. **a** Bones have excellent healing capacities, provided that the fragments are properly aligned and movement is minimized.

236. **a** Bluish-purple wound edges indicate that the blood vessels of and under the skin are congested with blood.

237. **b** None of the other approaches would be appropriate for a standing animal.

238. **d** This is the only portion of a surgical gown that is considered sterile during surgery.

239. **d** The vegetative form of bacteria is the actively feeding, growing, reproducing form and is most easily destroyed by common sterilization and disinfection methods.

240. **c** Inflammation is the first step in wound healing.

241. **d** Other than the sutures, a surgical wound has no appreciable strength until significant numbers of collagen fibers are produced in about 4 to 6 days.

242. **d** The linea alba, on the ventral midline of the abdominal wall, is the tendinous attachment of all of the ventral abdominal muscles. One layer of sutures in this area effectively closes the abdominal wall.

243. **b** Anything outside the sterile zone in an operating room is considered contaminated.

244. **a** Nonscrubbed personnel should touch only items that are not sterile.

245. **a** Passing back to back prevents accidental contamination.

246. **c** The hands of scrubbed personnel should always be held between waist level and shoulder level to help prevent inadvertent contamination. Clasping the hands when not otherwise occupied helps prevent fatigue from compromising the position of the hands and arms.

247. **a** Nonscrubbed personnel should never violate the sterile zone in which scrubbed personnel are working.

248. **b** Sterility is destroyed if pack contents are touched by a nonscrubbed person.

249. **a** Ethylene oxide gas is very flammable.

250. **d** Leaving skin sutures in too long increases scarring but does not directly contribute to breakdown of the surgical wound.

251. **d** Wet saline dressings are useful to help débride wounds with extensive tissue damage. They absorb and remove inflammatory products from the wound.

252. **d** Redistribution of blood flow results in pale mucous membranes, poor capillary refill, and cold extremities seen in an animal in shock.

253. **d** Removal of the uterus would restore the animal to health, but absence of the uterus, would preclude future breeding.

254. **c** Once the dead and damaged tissue has been removed from a wound by inflammation, a bed of granulation tissue, consisting primarily of collagen fibers and capillaries, must form on the floor of the wound before wound contraction can begin.

255. **b** If the outside of the glove is touched by anything that is not sterile, including the freshly scrubbed fingers, it becomes contaminated and must not be used for surgery.

256. **d** A pack placed vertically in the autoclave receives the best circulation of steam around its contents.

257. **b** These scissors are made for delicate tissue dissection only. They become dull or spring open if used on heavier material.

258. **d** These retractors have a ratchet device to hold them in place during use.

259. **d**

260. **d**

261. **a**

262. **d** There are no cleansing agents in instrument milk.

263. **c** A cesarean section is the surgical removal of the calf from the cow, and OB chains are used to slip over the calf's hocks to help pull it out.

264. **d**

265. **b** Plastic pipette tips can be sterilized effectively in an autoclave, whereas all of the others would be damaged by the high heat or moisture.

266. **a** All of the other answers are features of instrument milk, not ultrasonic cleaners.

267. **d** A laryngeal bur is used to remove the laryngeal saccule.

268. **d**

269. **b** These scissors are heavy and can cut thicker things. If used on delicate tissue, they might crush the tissue instead of cleanly cut it.

270. **a** Bottles must be vented to prevent pressure from building up. Slow exhaust is necessary to avoid evacuation of solution from the bottles.

271. **b**

272. **b** A No. 11 blade has a sharp point for making a small incision just large enough for the arthroscope or cannula to enter the joint.

273. **a** A No. 10 blade is a broad blade with the proper shape for a skin incision.

274. **d** Boiling does not sterilize instruments but is a disinfectant only. It is acceptable only for contaminated or clean-contaminated surgery. A laryngoplasty is sterile surgery.

275. **b** It is impossible to sterilize a surgeon's hands.

276. **c** Of those listed, chlorhexidine gluconate produces the greatest initial reduction of bacterial numbers.

277. **d** A rat-tooth forceps is used for grasping tissue; it cannot control bleeding.

278. **c** As long as an item remains sealed, it remains sterile indefinitely when subjected to gamma radiation.

279. **c** Any moisture on a cloth-wrapped item constitutes contamination, blood constitutes contamination, and a dust cover extends the sterility time to 6 months only, so this item is out of date.

280. **c** A Sauerbruch retractor has no ratchet and must be held in the hand to be functional.

281. **a** Steam under pressure can permeate rapidly and then condense; this kills the microorganisms most effectively.

282. **b**

283. **c** Ordinary hand soaps can leave behind insoluble alkaline residue, abrasive compounds can damage the surface of the instruments, and plain water is too slow and less thorough than a low-sudsing detergent.

284. **b**

285. **c** Skin staples are more expensive than skin sutures.

286. **c** The interrupted horizontal mattress provides more strength than any of the other suture patterns. It also is the one most easily used with rubber tubing for tension reduction.

287. **b** This is a fast and efficient way of closing most incisions.

288. **c** Gut is an absorbable suture that breaks down rapidly.

289. **b** Choice **a** is true of many patterns, and the others do not apply.

290. **a** A Cushing suture pattern is inverting; it is not used to close the skin.

291. **b**

292. **b**

293. **c** With mass ligation, the blood supply to the area may still be great enough to cause the suture to break.

294. **d**

295. **c**

296. **d** The strength of the suture is not affected by the type of needle and vice versa.

297. **c** A cutting needle penetrates the skin with the least amount of trauma.

298. **c** All of the answers are true; however, trauma to the tissues is the most important factor to consider.

299. **c** Tendons and nerves should be sutured with tension sutures, whereas viscera should be closed with inverting sutures; therefore the skin should be closed with appositional sutures.

300. **c**

301. **c** The No. 2 suture is the largest of these answers, and a cow's uterus, being large and heavy, requires larger suture material.

302. **c**

303. **c**

304. **d**

305. **b** A good suture material would not constitute a favorable environment for bacterial growth.

306. **a**

307. **b**

308. **c**

309. **d**

310. **b** With each suture placed, the stress on the other sutures is decreased; thus, more sutures are better than fewer.

311. **c** Surgical catgut is not recommended for internal use because of its rapid absorption and short duration of tensile strength.

312. **a** This chemical reaction increases strength, decreases absorption, and reduces tissue reaction.

313. **b** The suture is coiled and more difficult to tighten down; none of the other answers are direct results of memory.

314. **d**

315. **c** If proper aseptic technique is used, antibiotics should not be given for short, routine, uncomplicated procedures.

316. **c**

317. **a**

318. **b**

319. **d**

320. **b** It does not stain and has a broader antimicrobial spectrum than iodophors.

321. **b**

322. **b**

323. **b** The anal sacs and ducts should be avoided to prevent postoperative problems.

324. **d**

325. **c**

326. **b**

327. **a**

328. **d**

329. **c**

330. **c**

331. **a**

332. **a** Metzenbaums are for cutting fine tissue only.

333. **b**

334. **a**

335. **b** Gas processing is more effective, and indicator strips can be used to ensure complete processing.

336. **b**

337. **d**

338. **c**

339. **b**

340. **b**

341. **b** It is not atraumatic and must be used judiciously.

342. **b**

343. **c**

344. **b**

345. **b**

346. **d**

347. **c** Good records should be kept of nosocomial outbreaks in your clinic so that effective disinfectants can be selected.

348. **d**

349. **c**

350. **a**

351. **c**

352. **b** Masks should be changed every few hours for this reason.

353. **d**

354. **c** Surgeons should pass each other in the surgery room either back to back or front to front.

355. **c** Hands should not drop below waist or instrument-table level.

356. **c**

357. **b**

358. **b** Closed gloving provides the least chance for glove contamination.

359. **b** The dirtiest water is at the elbow; this should not be allowed to travel back down to the hands.

360. **b**

361. **d**

362. **a**

363. **b**

364. **c**

365. **b** Any of the others could severely damage the eye.

366. **c** Contaminated areas, such as the mouth and bladder, cannot be made sterile.

367. **a** Exogenous organisms are those from sources outside of the patient's body.

368. **d** Breaks will occur; it is important to have plans to remedy the situation.

369. **a**

370. **b**

371. **c**

372. **b**

373. **a** Elective procedures are not necessary to the patient's immediate health.

374. **b** Cutting needles are used in skin and other tough tissues.

375. **b**

376. **a**

377. **d** Often shortened to "K-E" apparatus

378. **b**

379. **c**

380. **b**

381. **a**

382. **b** Fenestrated drapes have a small window for the incision site; the surgeon fenestrates an intervertebral disk to remove disk material.

383. **b**

384. **b**

385. **b**

386. **c**

387. **a** "Moist tissues are happy tissues."

388. **c**

389. **b** Distal refers to the area farthest away from the trunk; proximal refers to the area of bone closest to the trunk. The inner portion of the bone is the medulla, and the outer layer of the bone is the cortex.

390. **b**

391. **d**

392. **c** Intramedullary pinning is performed on fractured long bones, such as the femur.

393. **c**

394. **c**

395. **b**

396. **b**

397. c The client should be well informed of surgical risks and possible complications.

398. b

399. d Displacement of abdominal contents into the thorax constitutes an emergency situation.

400. b

401. a

402. a Care must be taken to keep the exteriorized part moist.

Dentistry

Marianne Tear

QUESTIONS

1. *Apical* means "toward the ___."
   a. Root tip
   b. Crown
   c. Cheeks
   d. Tongue

2. Which of the following is a proper dental term for describing a tooth surface?
   a. Mesial—farthest from the midline
   b. Mesial—nearest the front
   c. Distal—nearest the midline
   d. Distal—farthest from the midline

3. Which of the following is a proper dental term for describing a tooth surface?
   a. Palatal—facing the cheek
   b. Labial—facing the tongue
   c. Buccal—facing the cheek
   d. Rostral—toward the back

4. The cat has which of the following numbers of maxillary and mandibular premolars in one half of the mouth?
   a. 3 and 2
   b. 3 and 3
   c. 2 and 3
   d. 2 and 2

5. The dental formula for the permanent teeth in the dog is 2 (I 3/3 and C 1/1) plus
   a. P 3/4 and M 3/2 = 40
   b. P 3/4 and M 3/3 = 42
   c. P 4/4 and M 2/3 = 42
   d. P 4/4 and M 3/2 = 42

6. What is the main purpose of premolar teeth?
   a. Holding and tearing
   b. Cutting and breaking
   c. Grinding
   d. Gnawing and grooming

7. What teeth on each side of the mouth in a dog have three roots?
   a. Maxillary third and fourth premolars and first molar
   b. Maxillary fourth premolars and first and second molars
   c. Mandibular fourth premolars and first and second molars
   d. Mandibular and maxillary fourth premolars and first and second molars

8. The permanent canine and premolar teeth in dogs generally erupt at about what age?
   a. 3 to 5 months
   b. 4 to 6 months
   c. 5 to 7 months
   d. 6 to 8 months

9. Using the Triadan system, the proper way of describing a dog's first upper left permanent premolar is
   a. 205
   b. 105
   c. 306
   d. 502

10. Using the Triadan system, the proper way of describing a cat's first lower right molar is
    a. 407
    b. 409
    c. 109
    d. 909

11. The pulp canal of a tooth contains
    a. Nerves
    b. Blood vessels
    c. Connective tissue and blood vessels
    d. Blood vessels, nerves, and connective tissues

Correct answers are on pages 214-220.

12. As part of normal tooth growth, what part of the tooth thickens?
    a. Enamel
    b. Pulp
    c. Dentin
    d. Gingiva

13. Enamel, which is the hardest body substance
    a. Contains living tissue
    b. Covers the tooth crown and root
    c. Continues production by the ameloblasts after eruption
    d. Is relatively nonporous and impervious

14. Dentin is covered by
    a. Enamel and bone
    b. Bone and pulp
    c. Cementum and enamel
    d. Pulp and cementum

15. Normal scissor occlusion is when the maxillary fourth premolars occlude
    a. Level with the mandibular fourth premolar
    b. Buccally to the mandibular first molar
    c. Buccally to the mandibular fourth premolar
    d. Lingually to the mandibular first molar

16. The heaviest calculus deposition in dogs and cats is typically located on the
    a. Lingual surfaces of the lower cheek teeth
    b. Lower canine teeth
    c. Incisor teeth
    d. Buccal surfaces of the upper cheek teeth

17. The carnassial teeth in dogs are
    a. P^4 and M_1
    b. P^4 and P_4
    c. M^1 and M_1
    d. C^1 and C_1

18. Free or marginal gingiva
    a. Occupies the space between the teeth
    b. Is the most apical portion of the gingiva
    c. Forms the gingival sulcus around the tooth
    d. Is tightly bound to the cementum

19. The periodontium includes the periodontal ligament and all of the following except
    a. Gingiva
    b. Cementum
    c. Alveolar bone
    d. Enamel

20. A bulldog would be described as having what type of head shape?
    a. Brachycephalic
    b. Dolichocephalic
    c. Mesaticephalic
    d. Prognacephalic

21. In veterinary dentistry, chlorhexidine solutions are used because they
    a. Prevent cementoenamel erosion
    b. Have antibacterial properties
    c. Remove enamel stains and whiten teeth
    d. Are used to treat gingival hyperplasia in brachycephalic breeds

22. When using hand instruments to clean teeth,
    a. Use a modified pen grasp with a back-and-forth-scraping motion.
    b. Use a modified pen grasp with overlapping pull strokes that are directed away from the gingival margin.
    c. Use the sickle scaler for subgingival curettage.
    d. The curette is best used supragingivally.

23. Pocket depth is measured from the
    a. Cementoenamel junction to the bottom of the pocket
    b. Current free gingival margin to the bottom of the gingival sulcus
    c. Cementoenamel junction to the current free gingival margin and then adding 1 to 2 mm
    d. Cementoenamel junction to the apical extent of the defect

24. Between patients, it is best to use the following order for maintaining instruments:
    a. Use, sharpen, wash, and sterilize
    b. Use, wash, sterilize, and sharpen
    c. Use, wash, sharpen, and sterilize
    d. Wash, sterilize, use, and sharpen

25. When performing dental prophylaxis, minimal safety equipment includes
    a. Gloves only
    b. Gloves and mask only
    c. Safety glasses only
    d. Safety glasses, mask, and gloves

26. You have an instrument in your hand that has two sharp sides, a rounded back, and a rounded point. You are holding a
    a. Sickle scaler
    b. Morris scaler
    c. Universal curette
    d. Sickle curette

27. When polishing teeth using an air-driven unit, the speed of the hand piece that should be used is the
    a. High
    b. Low
    c. Either high or low is acceptable
    d. Finishing

28. The term that best describes a dog with an abnormally short mandible is
    a. Prognathism
    b. Brachygnathism
    c. Mesaticephalic
    d. Dolichocephalic

For Questions 29 through 32, select the correct answer from the choices below.

    a. Posterior crossbite
    b. Base-narrow mandibular canines
    c. Wry mouth
    d. Anterior crossbite

29. Malocclusion in which one side of the mandible or maxilla is disproportionate to its other side

30. Malocclusion in which the upper fourth premolar lies palatal to the first molars

31. Malocclusion in which the canines erupt in an overly upright position, or the mandible is narrowed

32. Malocclusion in which one or more of the upper incisor teeth are caudal to the lower incisors

33. The most common benign soft tissue tumor of the oral cavity is
    a. Epulide tumor
    b. Fibrosarcoma
    c. Malignant melanoma
    d. Squamous cell carcinoma

34. Dry socket is more likely to occur when one
    a. Ensures there is an increased blood supply to the area
    b. Practices good surgical technique
    c. Allows a blood clot to form so that fibroblasts are formed
    d. Overirrigates the tooth socket so that no clot can form

35. Gingivoplasty is the
    a. Addition of more gingiva to the site
    b. Binding of the loose teeth together to stabilize them during a healing process
    c. Removal of hyperplastic gingival tissue
    d. Removal of a portion of the tooth structure

36. To protect the pulp tissue of teeth from thermal damage during ultrasonic scaling, one should
    a. Use constant irrigation.
    b. Change tips frequently.
    c. Use slow rotational speed.
    d. Use appropriate amounts of paste.

37. Another term for neck lesions on feline teeth is
    a. Odontogenic fibroma
    b. Feline internal odontoclastic resorptive lesions
    c. Feline external odontoclastic resorptive lesions
    d. Class 1 enamel fracture

38. The most common dental procedure performed on a horse is
    a. Quidding
    b. Curettage
    c. Scaling
    d. Floating

39. Stomatitis is the
    a. Bad breath evident when dental work must be completed
    b. Inflammation of the mouth's soft tissue
    c. Inflammation of the stomites found in bones
    d. Inflammation of lesions found in the gastrointestinal tract

40. A client wants to know what chew toy would be safest for her dog's teeth. You suggest that she is best to give Fido a
    a. Dried cow hoof
    b. Nylon rope toy
    c. Dense rubber exerciser
    d. Large knuckle bone

41. For dental radiography of the canine tooth, you should use what size of dental film to ensure that the whole tooth is included?
    a. 0
    b. 2
    c. 4
    d. 8 × 10 screen film

42. Dental film should be placed in the mouth with the dimple
    a. Up and pointing rostrally
    b. Up and pointing caudally
    c. Down and pointing rostrally
    d. Down and pointing caudally

43. The flap side of the dental film should be facing
    a. Any direction, because it does not matter
    b. Toward the tube head
    c. Away from the tube head
    d. The caudal side of the animal

44. The bisecting angle principle states that the plane of an x-ray beam should be 90 degrees to the
    a. Long axis of the tooth
    b. Plane of the film
    c. Imaginary line that bisects the angle formed by the tooth's long axis and the film plane
    d. Imaginary line that bisects the angle formed by the animal's head and the film plane

Correct answers are on pages 214-220.

45. You are looking at your dental radiograph and notice that the tooth is elongated. This happened because the beam was perpendicular to the
    a. Film
    b. Tooth
    c. Bisecting angle
    d. Wrong tooth

46. A curette is used to
    a. Check the tooth's surface for any irregularities
    b. Measure the depth of gingival recession
    c. Scale large amounts of calculus from the tooth's surface
    d. Scale calculus from the tooth surface located in the gingival sulcus

47. A scaler is used to
    a. Check the tooth's root surface for any irregularities
    b. Measure the depth of gingival recession
    c. Scale large amounts of calculus from the tooth's surface
    d. Scale calculus from the tooth surface located in the gingival sulcus

48. What mineralized tissue covers the root of the tooth?
    a. Calculus
    b. Enamel
    c. Cementum
    d. Dentin

49. The nerve and blood vessel of a tooth is located in the
    a. Sulcus
    b. Pulp cavity
    c. Marrow cavity
    d. Calculus

50. When scaling gross calculus from the teeth,
    a. Hold the scaler using a modified pen grasp
    b. Hold the scaler using a modified screw driver grasp
    c. Use long controlled strokes toward the gums
    d. Hold the curette using a modified pen grasp

51. Ultrasonic scaling
    a. Can substitute for hand scaling
    b. May cause thermal damage to the tooth if the tip is kept on a tooth for longer than 5 seconds
    c. Sprays the tooth with water to wash the tooth clean
    d. Sprays the tooth with water to cool the tooth and prevent pulp damage

52. The following statements are all true except
    a. Sulcus depth is measured using a probe.
    b. A sulcus depth up to 3 mm is normal in a cat.
    c. A sulcus depth greater than 3 mm indicates periodontal disease.
    d. The probe is inserted gently into the gingival sulcus parallel to the root of the tooth.

53. The purpose of polishing during the dental prophy is to
    a. Massage the gums
    b. Smooth out the rough areas and retard plaque formation
    c. Apply fluoride
    d. Disinfect the surface of the tooth

54. An older dog with dental disease is presented to the clinic with a draining tract below his right eye. What is the most likely cause?
    a. Right-sided maxillary carnassial tooth root abscess
    b. Left-sided maxillary carnassial tooth root abscess
    c. Right-sided mandibular carnassial tooth root abscess
    d. Maxillary incisor tooth root abscess

55. *Wry mouth* refers to which of the following types of oral malocclusions?
    a. Elongation of the head on either the left or right side
    b. Elongation of the maxilla in comparison to the mandible
    c. Elongation of the mandible in comparison to the maxilla
    d. Loss of maxillary incisors

56. The buccal surface of the mandibular molars in a dog refers to the
    a. Occlusal surface with the maxillary molars
    b. Most rostral surface
    c. Surface in contact with the tongue
    d. Surface in contact with the cheek tissue

57. Brachygnathism is a genetic defect best characterized as
    a. A maxilla that is longer than the mandible
    b. A mandible that is longer than the maxilla
    c. Lack of incisors
    d. Polydontia

58. Prognathism is a normal condition in brachycephalic breeds but is considered a genetic defect in other breeds. It is best characterized as
    a. A mandible that is longer than the maxilla
    b. A maxilla that is longer than the mandible
    c. One side of the head is longer than the other
    d. An overly long soft palate

59. Malocclusions can lead to dental disease for all of the following reasons except
    a. Soft tissue trauma from teeth that are abnormally positioned
    b. Accelerated development of periodontal disease resulting from lack of normal wear and the normal flushing of teeth with saliva
    c. Abnormal wear of teeth resulting from malposition leading to fracture and pulp exposure
    d. Presence of resorptive lesions leading to destruction of teeth

60. Which of the following teeth are not normally present in the adult cat?
    a. P^1 and P_1 and P_2
    b. P_1 and P^1 and P^2
    c. M^2 and M_1
    d. M_2 and M^2

61. The furcation is best described as
    a. The area between the cementum and enamel
    b. The space between two roots where they meet the crown
    c. The space between the root and the gingiva
    d. The space between two occlusal surfaces

62. Severe stomatitis is a clinical sign commonly associated with which of the following feline disorders?
    a. Feline infectious peritonitis
    b. Inflammatory bowel disease
    c. Feline immunodeficiency virus
    d. Toxoplasmosis

63. An oronasal fistula can often occur secondary to
    a. Abscess of the mandibular canine tooth
    b. Incisor root abscess
    c. Abscess of the maxillary canine tooth
    d. Retained deciduous incisors

64. Which of the following statements about canine toy breeds is true?
    a. Chronic impaction of incisor teeth with hair and debris often results in a chronic osteomyelitis.
    b. Malocclusions are rare in toy breeds in comparison with giant-breed dogs.
    c. Enamel hypoplasia is a common finding in toy breeds.
    d. Prognathism is considered a genetic defect in brachycephalic breeds.

65. A biopsy report confirms that an oral mass is an acanthomatous epulis; what can be said about this growth?
    a. It is a nonmalignant tumor.
    b. It is a malignant tumor.
    c. It is very likely to metastasize.
    d. It is related to the presence of a malocclusion.

66. While performing a routine prophylactic dentistry, the veterinary technician notes a large, red raised lesion on the lip of her feline patient. The client noted that the lesion "comes and goes." What is a reasonable differential for this lesion?
    a. Feline resorptive lesion
    b. Trauma-related lesion
    c. Eosinophilic ulcer
    d. Tumor

67. Feline cervical line lesions/feline neck lesions/feline resorptive lesions are of great concern to veterinarians. Which of the following statements regarding these lesions is false?
    a. Feline resorptive lesions are aggressive dental caries that result in resorption of roots and subsequent tooth loss.
    b. Feline resorptive lesions often present with a raspberry seed type sign at the base of the tooth where it meets the gingival margin.
    c. Feline resorptive lesions are effectively managed with steroid administration.
    d. It is common to find more than one feline cervical line lesion in the oral cavity.

68. Which of the following statements about eruption of permanent teeth is false?
    a. The permanent upper canines erupt mesial to the deciduous canines.
    b. The permanent lower canines erupt buccal to the deciduous canines.
    c. The permanent incisors erupt distal to the deciduous incisors.
    d. The permanent canine teeth erupt at 5 to 6 months of age in the dog.

69. The pulp of the tooth has which of the following functions?
    a. Anchors the tooth in the alveolar bone with a fibrous ligament
    b. Provides the tooth with a protective strong, hard surface
    c. Contains blood vessels and nerves that provide nutrition and sensation to the tooth.
    d. Develops roots to anchor the tooth into the alveolar bone

70. When the pulp cavity of a tooth is exposed, what is the appropriate procedure(s) that should be performed?
    a. Tooth extraction or pulp capping
    b. No procedure is required.
    c. Filing of the crown leaving roots behind
    d. Prophylactic dentistry to reduce tartar and plaque buildup on the tooth

Correct answers are on pages 214-220.

71. In patients with severe, chronic periodontal disease and possible osteomyelitis, antibiotics are often begun before a dentistry is performed. What is the most common antibiotic chosen for these animals?
    a. Clindamycin
    b. Amoxicillin
    c. Trimethoprim sulfa
    d. Cephalexin

72. Which of the following cardiac diseases is often associated with severe dental disease?
    a. Vegetative endocarditis
    b. Hypertrophic cardiomyopathy
    c. Dilative cardiomyopathy
    d. Ventricular arrhythmias

73. Perioceutics refer to which of the following?
    a. Procedure to restore the periodontal ligament
    b. Application of time-released antibiotics directly within the oral cavity
    c. Use of antibiotics before dental procedure
    d. Procedure to cap the pulp cavity of the tooth

74. The bisecting angle technique is a method for radiographing the oral cavity. The description that adequately describes this technique is
    a. The central radiation beam is directed perpendicular to the line that bisects the angle formed by the film and the long axis of the tooth.
    b. The central radiation beam is directed parallel to the line that bisects the angle formed by the film and the perpendicular axis of the tooth.
    c. The central radiation beam is directed perpendicular to the tooth root.
    d. The central radiation beam is directed parallel to the occlusal surface of the tooth.

75. Fluoride acts to accomplish all but which of the following?
    a. Desensitize the tooth
    b. Provide antibacterial activity
    c. Strengthen the enamel
    d. Strengthen the periodontal ligament

76. Which of the following statements is false when performing an ultrasonic scaling during routine dental prophylaxis?
    a. The ultrasonic scaler should not be on the tooth for longer than 20 seconds at a time to prevent thermal damage to the pulp cavity.
    b. The ultrasonic scaler should be grasped like a pencil.
    c. The side of the instrument should be used rather than the tip against the tooth.
    d. The ultrasonic scaler can be used for supragingival and subgingival scaling.

77. Which of the following statements is false regarding patient safety during a dentistry?
    a. An appropriately sized mouth gag is essential to prevent temporomandibular joint damage.
    b. The endotracheal tube should be uncuffed so that the tube can be easily manipulated when performing a dentistry.
    c. Large-breed dogs should be rolled with their legs under to prevent a gastric dilatation and volvulus crisis.
    d. One must monitor the patient to ensure that fluids and debris from the dentistry do not gain access to the trachea.

78. A dog that was exposed to distemper perinatally may develop which of the following oral pathologic conditions?
    a. Adontia
    b. Polydontia
    c. Enamel hypoplasia
    d. Enamel staining

79. Sometimes a 0.12% chlorhexidine solution is sprayed in the patient's mouth before beginning dental prophylaxis. What is the benefit of this activity?
    a. Sterilizes the patient's mouth before the procedure
    b. Reduces the bacterial load in the mouth to reduce exposure to the technician who performs the procedure
    c. Substitutes for prophylactic antibiotic therapy
    d. Provides topical anesthetic activity

80. Which of the following statements is false with respect to polishing an animal's teeth following scaling?
    a. The polishing paste used should be of medium or fine granularity.
    b. Polishing acts to remove microscopic grooves left by the scaling process.
    c. The polishing instrument should be moved from tooth to tooth to prevent thermal damage to the pulp.
    d. Polishing is a means for removing stubborn plaque that occurs below the gumline.

81. The Triadan system is a
    a. Tooth identification system designed to aid in dental charting
    b. Complete system that includes an ultrasonic scaler and polisher
    c. Method for performing radiographs of molars
    d. Complete home care dental system for use by clients

82. In which of the following species do the teeth fail to continue growing?
    a. Equine
    b. Rabbit
    c. Rat
    d. Cat

83. The root length of an upper canine is how long compared with the length of the exposed portion of that tooth?
    a. One half the length
    b. Same length
    c. Three times the length
    d. One and a half times the length

84. The upper fourth premolar communicates with what sinus?
    a. Mandibular
    b. Occipital
    c. Maxillary
    d. Orbital

85. The crown of a tooth is defined as
    a. That portion above the gum line and covered by enamel
    b. The most terminal portion of the root
    c. That portion below the gum line
    d. The layer of bony tissue that attaches to the alveolar bone

86. The range for acceptable gingival sulcal measurements in cats is
    a. 1 to 3 mm
    b. 0.5 to 1 mm
    c. 1.5 to 4.5 mm
    d. 0.005 to 0.007 mm

87. When performing dental prophylaxis, you should be sure to wear
    a. Cap, mask, gloves
    b. Gown, gloves, mask
    c. Cap, eye protection, gloves
    d. Mask, eye protection, gloves

88. In what grade of periodontal disease does early pocket formation occur without initial bone loss?
    a. Grade I
    b. Grade II
    c. Grade III
    d. Grade IV

89. A curette
    a. Is used strictly as a supragingival instrument
    b. Can be used either supragingivally or subgingivally
    c. Is the most important dental instrument
    d. Is used to irrigate the teeth with air or water

90. What drug should not be given to pregnant dogs because it may cause discoloration of the puppies' teeth?
    a. Amoxicillin
    b. Tetracycline
    c. Chloramphenicol
    d. Penicillin

91. The occlusal surface of a caudal tooth is defined as the
    a. Surface facing the hard palate
    b. Surface nearer the cheek
    c. Chewing surface of the tooth
    d. Surface nearer the tongue

92. The normal adult canine mouth has how many permanent teeth?
    a. 40
    b. 42
    c. 48
    d. 52

93. The instrument used to measure pocket depth is a periodontal
    a. Explorer
    b. Scaler
    c. Curette
    d. Probe

94. A complication that may develop if subgingival plaque is improperly removed is
    a. Etched tooth enamel
    b. Torn epithelial attachment
    c. Overheated tooth
    d. Bitten technician

95. What tooth has three roots?
    a. Upper canine
    b. Lower first premolar
    c. Lower first molar
    d. Upper fourth premolar

96. Which statement concerning the polishing aspect of dental prophylaxis is least accurate?
    a. A slow speed should be used.
    b. Adequate prophy paste is needed for lubrication and polishing.
    c. The polisher should remain on the tooth for as long as is needed to polish the tooth.
    d. If teeth are not polished, the rough enamel will promote bacterial plaque formation.

97. What term identifies the wearing away of teeth by tooth-against-tooth contact during mastication?
    a. Plaque
    b. Attrition
    c. Calculus
    d. Erosion

Correct answers are on pages 214-220.

98. What term identifies the hard, mineralized substance on the tooth surface?
    a. Plaque
    b. Attrition
    c. Calculus
    d. Erosion

99. What term identifies the loss of tooth structure by chemical means?
    a. Plaque
    b. Attrition
    c. Calculus
    d. Erosion

100. The thin film covering a tooth that comprises bacteria, saliva, and food particles is
    a. Plaque
    b. Attrition
    c. Calculus
    d. Erosion

101. What is the minimum age for a cat to have all of its permanent teeth?
    a. 6 months
    b. 8 months
    c. 10 months
    d. 1 year

102. Generally speaking, most dental instruments should be held as you would a
    a. Knife
    b. Pencil
    c. Hammer
    d. Toothbrush

103. Of cats and dogs ages 6 years and older, approximately what percentage has periodontal disease?
    a. 20%
    b. 35%
    c. 50%
    d. 85%

104. Removal of calculus and necrotic cementum from the tooth roots is called
    a. Curettage
    b. Splinting
    c. Root planing
    d. Scaling

105. Prevention of periodontal disease involves all of the following except
    a. Daily teeth brushing or mouth rinsing
    b. Regular exercise
    c. Routine professional scaling and polishing
    d. Proper diet

106. To prevent the pulp tissue from thermal damage during ultrasonic scaling, which of the following should be done?
    a. Use constant irrigation.
    b. Change tips frequently.
    c. Use slow rotational speed.
    d. Use appropriate amounts of paste.

107. Ideally, the cutting edge of the scaler should be held at what angle to the tooth surface?
    a. 5 to 10 degrees
    b. 35 to 45 degrees
    c. 15 to 30 degrees
    d. 45 to 90 degrees

108. The purpose of fluoride treatment is to
    a. Prevent thermal damage and lubrication
    b. Strengthen enamel and help desensitize teeth
    c. Remove plaque and strengthen the enamel
    d. Irrigate and lubricate

109. Mrs. Walker comes to pick up her dog after dental prophylaxis has been performed. Which of the following topics would be least helpful to be discussed as a part of the discharge instructions?
    a. Chewing exercises
    b. Home care
    c. How to give injections
    d. Dietary concerns

110. Once plaque has formed on a tooth, how long does it take to mineralize into calculus?
    a. About 7 days
    b. 2 weeks
    c. 4 weeks
    d. 2 months

111. The most common dental procedure performed on horses is
    a. Quidding
    b. Floating
    c. Repelling
    d. Scaling

112. What tissue is not part of the periodontium?
    a. Periodontal ligament
    b. Alveolar bone
    c. Root
    d. Gingiva

113. The correct dental formula for an adult dog is
    a. 2(I 3/3 C 1/1 P 3/4 M 3/3) = 42
    b. 2(I 3/3 C 1/1 P 4/4 M 3/2) = 42
    c. 2(I 3/3 C 1/1 P 4/4 M 2/3) = 42
    d. 2(I 4/4 C 1/1 P 3/4 M 3/3) = 46

114. The correct dental formula for an adult cat is
    a. 2(I 3/3 C 1/1 P 3/2 M 1/1) = 30
    b. 2(I 4/4 C 1/1 P 2/3 M 1/1) = 34
    c. 2(I 3/3 C 1/1 P 2/3 M 1/1) = 30
    d. 2(I 3/3 C 1/1 P 3/2 M 2/1) = 32

115. What term identifies the space between the roots of the same tooth?
    a. Apical
    b. Rostral
    c. Furcation
    d. Buccal

116. What term identifies the tooth surface facing the cheeks?
    a. Apical
    b. Rostral
    c. Furcation
    d. Buccal

117. What is the directional term for "toward the root"?
    a. Apical
    b. Rostral
    c. Furcation
    d. Buccal

118. What is the directional term for "toward the front of the head"?
    a. Apical
    b. Rostral
    c. Furcation
    d. Buccal

119. Chlorhexidine contributes to dental prophylaxis by
    a. Slowly dissolving calculus
    b. Bonding to the cell membrane and inhibiting bacterial growth
    c. Bleaching stained teeth
    d. Decreasing tooth sensitivity

120. In normal occlusion, the bite is termed
    a. Scissor bite
    b. Straight bite
    c. Occlusal bite
    d. Razor bite

121. What is the proper dilution of chlorhexidine solution for use in the mouth?
    a. 20%
    b. 2.0%
    c. 0.2%
    d. 10%

122. Topical fluoride
    a. Will stain remaining calculus red
    b. Helps desensitize teeth and slows the rate of plaque formation
    c. Should never be used on feline teeth
    d. Enhances osteoclastic activity and helps desensitize teeth

123. What term identifies the instrument used for root planing?
    a. Periodontal probe
    b. Explorer
    c. Scaler
    d. Curette

124. What term identifies the instrument used to detect subgingival calculus?
    a. Periodontal probe
    b. Explorer
    c. Scaler
    d. Curette

125. What term identifies the instrument used for removal of supragingival calculus?
    a. Periodontal probe
    b. Explorer
    c. Scaler
    d. Curette

126. An elongation of one side of the animal's head results in
    a. Anterior crossbite
    b. Wry mouth
    c. Brachygnathism
    d. Prognathism

127. The bulk of a tooth is composed of
    a. Enamel
    b. Pulp
    c. Dentin
    d. Cementum

128. The most common mistake made in treating periodontal disease is
    a. Inadequate removal of supragingival calculus
    b. Inadequate root planing
    c. Insufficient polishing
    d. Iatrogenic trauma to subgingival tissues

129. As a dentifrice for use in small animals, baking soda
    a. Is an excellent choice
    b. Should be mixed with salt and water to form a paste
    c. Should be mixed with fluoride gel to form a paste
    d. Should not be used as a dentifrice for animals

Correct answers are on pages 214-220.

130. After polishing with a prophylactic paste that contains fluoride, rinsing with diluted chlorhexidine
    a. Is less effective, because the fluoride interferes with bonding of chlorhexidine to tissues
    b. Results in temporary blue staining of the teeth
    c. Enhances the activity of both fluoride and chlorhexidine
    d. May be toxic to the patient

131. If the lower incisors seem to be excessively loose in a brachycephalic or miniature-breed dog,
    a. The teeth should be extracted.
    b. The depth of the gingival sulcus should be tested.
    c. The dog is calcium deficient.
    d. The dog has advanced periodontal disease.

132. Fractured deciduous teeth
    a. Should be left in place until they are normally shed
    b. Should be repaired
    c. Are insignificant
    d. Should be extracted

133. The first dental examination should occur when
    a. The animal is 2 to 3 years old
    b. The client requests it
    c. A problem such as drooling or bad breath is noticed
    d. The animal is 6 to 8 weeks old

134. The deciduous incisors
    a. Erupt at 3 1/2 to 4 weeks of age
    b. Have roots that are proportionately longer than the roots of permanent incisors
    c. Are the most frequently retained teeth
    d. Are not usually replaced with permanent incisors until the dog is 6 months old

135. Nerves and blood vessels enter the tooth through the
    a. Apical delta
    b. Crown
    c. Pulp
    d. Sulcus

136. When one or more of the upper incisors rest caudally to the lower incisors and the rest of the occlusion is normal, it is called
    a. Level bite
    b. Wry mouth
    c. Anterior crossbite
    d. Anodontia

137. The term *polyodontia* refers to
    a. Retained deciduous teeth
    b. Supernumerary teeth
    c. Supernumerary teeth and retained deciduous teeth
    d. Tooth loss as a result of periodontal disease

138. The normal periodontal pocket depth in the dog is
    a. < 3 mm
    b. < 7 mm
    c. > 3 mm
    d. 5 mm

139. Excessive growth of gingival tissue is termed
    a. Gingivitis
    b. Gingival hyperplasia
    c. Gingival hypoplasia
    d. Gingivectomy

140. The shrinkage of free gingiva in the presence of bacteria, plaque, and/or dental calculus is termed
    a. Recessional gum disease
    b. Gingival intussusception
    c. Gingival reduction
    d. Gingival recession

141. Two tooth buds that grow together to form one larger tooth is referred to as
    a. Gemini
    b. Fusion
    c. Polydontia
    d. Oligodontia

142. The space between two roots, where they meet the crown, is called
    a. Crook
    b. Furcation
    c. Apex
    d. Fissure

143. The term for a tooth that has one root but two crowns is
    a. Gemini
    b. Fusion
    c. Polydontia
    d. Oligodontia

144. Surface of the tooth toward the lips is
    a. Occlusal
    b. Labial
    c. Buccal
    d. Mesial

145. Fewer teeth than normal is
    a. Polydontia
    b. Oligodontia
    c. Anodontia
    d. Wry mouth

146. Surface of the tooth toward the cheek is
    a. Occlusal
    b. Labial
    c. Buccal
    d. Mesial

147. More teeth than normal is
    a. Polydontia
    b. Oligodontia
    c. Anodontia
    d. Wry mouth

148. Surface of the tooth toward the tongue is
    a. Lingual
    b. Labial
    c. Buccal
    d. Mesial

149. Also called *distemper teeth,* the name for a condition where sections of the tooth enamel are reduced or missing is
    a. Prognathic
    b. Enamel hypoplasia
    c. Erosion
    d. Jaundice enamel

150. Class II malocclusions in which the teeth in the mandible are distal to their maxillary equivalents is termed
    a. Mesioclusions
    b. Distoclusions
    c. Neutroclusions
    d. Oroclusions

151. Class III malocclusions in which the mandibular teeth are occluded mesial to their maxillary equivalents is termed
    a. Mesioclusions
    b. Distoclusions
    c. Neutroclusions
    d. Oroclusions

152. The carnassial tooth in the cat is also known as
    a. Upper first premolar
    b. Upper first molar
    c. Upper last premolar
    d. Upper canine

153. Using the modified Triadan system, the right maxillary teeth would be in the ___ series.
    a. 100
    b. 200
    c. 300
    d. 400

154. A dorsal-ventral view in which the x-ray beam passes from the top of the nose through the teeth is
    a. Rostral maxillary
    b. Distal mandibular view
    c. Rostral mandibular view
    d. Rostral oblique view

155. A ventral-dorsal view in which the x-ray beam passes from the bottom of the jaw through the teeth is
    a. Rostral maxillary
    b. Distal mandibular view
    c. Rostral mandibular view
    d. Rostral oblique view

156. The only radiographic view that can be made with a true parallel technique is
    a. Rostral maxillary
    b. Distal mandibular view
    c. Rostral mandibular view
    d. Rostral oblique view

157. In radiographs, an apical abscess appears as a
    a. Radiopaque area around the apex of the tooth
    b. Radiolucent area around the apex of the tooth
    c. Radiopaque area inside the tooth pulp
    d. Radiolucent area inside the tooth pulp

Correct answers are on pages 214-220.

ANSWERS

1. **a** *Apical* refers to the apex of the tooth, which is toward the root. *Coronal* is the term that means "toward the crown" of the tooth.

2. **d** Mesial surface is the part closest to the midline of the arch, whereas distal is the part farthest away from the midline.

3. **c** Buccal is the surface facing the cheek, whereas palatal is toward the upper palate. Lingual is the surface facing the tongue, is used in reference to the mandibular teeth. *Labial* means "toward the lips." *Rostral* is the term meaning "toward the front" of the head, and *caudal* is "toward the back."

4. **a** Cats have three maxillary premolars and two mandibular premolars per side.

5. **c** Adult dogs have a total of 42 teeth with each mandibular and maxillary side having four premolars. There are two maxillary and three mandibular molars per side.

6. **b** The canine teeth are used for holding and tearing, incisors for gnawing and grooming, and molars for grinding.

7. **b** The three-rooted teeth are the maxillary fourth premolar and first and second molars. Two-rooted teeth in the dog are maxillary second and third premolars and the mandibular second, third, and fourth premolars and first and second molars. The rest of the teeth have single roots. There are no three-rooted mandibular teeth in either the dog or the cat.

8. **b** Permanent canines and premolars erupt at about 4 to 6 months, adult incisors appear at 3 to 5 months, and molars at 5 to 7 months.

9. **a** The Triadan system uses three numbers. The first number identifies one of the four quadrants of the mouth. The order is sequential, beginning with the upper right maxillary that is assigned 1; 2 is the left maxillary, 3 the left mandibular, and 4 the right mandibular. The same format is followed for the deciduous teeth, starting with 5 for the deciduous maxillary right teeth. The second and third numbers identify the teeth. There are always two numbers to represent the teeth. The tooth numbering begins in the front of the mouth with the central incisor being 01, the intermediate incisor 02, and the lateral or corner incisor 03. The canine is always 04, and the molar is always 09. Thus 205 refers to the left maxillary quadrant and the fifth tooth, which is the first premolar. Once memorized this system is simple.

10. **b** The rule of 4 and 9 in the Triadan system helps standardize the nomenclature for species that have fewer teeth. The cat has only three upper premolars and two lower premolars per side. The canine is always designated as 04 and the first molar is always 09. The count begins backward from the first molar so that for the maxillary teeth, the fourth premolar is 08, the third premolar is 07, and the second premolar is 06, just as in the dog. The first lower right molar then is designated as 409. (**Note:** Cats, then, do not have a 405, 406, 305, 306, 205, or 105.)

11. **d** These are all part of the pulp tissue that helps support odontoblastic cells that line the pulp chamber and root canal.

12. **c** The odontoblasts that line the pulp chamber and root canal produce secondary dentin throughout life and fill in the canal, causing the dentin to thicken with age.

13. **d** Enamel is thus relatively easy to clean and slow to stain. It is acellular and is considered nonliving. Cementum covers the root of the tooth. Ameloblasts do form enamel during tooth development, but enamel production (amelogenesis) stops just before tooth eruption and no more enamel is produced.

14. **c** Dentin, which makes up the bulk of the tooth, is about as hard as bone but softer than enamel. It is covered by enamel on the crown surface and cementum over the roots.

15. **b** In normal scissor bite, the upper fourth premolar should be buccal to the mandibular first molar. The upper incisors should slightly overlap the lower ones, and the lower canine teeth should fit comfortably in the interdental space between the upper third incisor and lower canine so that no tooth surfaces touch. The first tooth behind the upper canine is the first lower premolar. In the normal bite, each cusp points between the interdental space of the opposite premolar so that a zigzag or pinking-shear effect is seen.

16. **d** The heaviest calculus usually is found here because of the adjacent parotid salivary duct opening.

17. **a** Carnassial teeth in dogs are the upper fourth premolars and lower first molars.

18. **c** This is the most coronal portion of the gingiva and in healthy patients lies passively against the tooth, so that a potential space is formed around the tooth. This sulcar depth can be measured and should normally be between 0.5 and 1.0 mm in cats and between 1.0 and 3.0 mm in dogs, depending on the teeth.

19. **d** The periodontium is the supporting structure of the teeth and includes the periodontal ligament, gingiva, cementum, and alveolar and supporting bone.

20. **a** *Brachy* means "short" and *cephalic* is "head." Collies are described as being dolichocephalic (long head), whereas a retriever is a typical example of a mesaticephalic breed (medium head).

21. **b** Chlorhexidine has antibacterial properties.

22. **b** A modified pen grasp should be used. One should never direct the instruments toward the gum surface. Scalers should not be used subgingivally, but curettes are best used subgingivally.

23. **b** Pocket depth is from the gingival margin to the pocket's bottom; choice **a** describes how to measure attachment loss; **c** notes gingival recession, and **d** is the periodontal index that determines the amount of periodontal attachment loss.

24. **c** To minimize the danger of infection to the operator and maintain sterility, it is best to sharpen the instruments after washing but before sterilization.

25. **d** These should be worn at all times when performing dentistry.

26. **c** Curettes have two sharp edges and a rounded toe and are most effective for removing calculus subgingivally. They are designed so that each end is a mirror image of the opposite end. The universal curette can be adapted to almost all dental surfaces.

27. **b** A prophy angle used for polishing is used on low speed. Low-speed hand pieces have a high torque and speeds of 5000 to 20,000 RPM.

28. **b** *Brachy* refers to "short," and *gnath* means "jaw."

29. **c** Wry bite, or wry mouth, is a skeletal defect in which the affected animal has a nonsymmetrical head. The upper and lower incisors do not align.

30. **a** With posterior crossbite, the incisors are in the normal relationship, but the posterior teeth are not. The upper fourth premolars are either palatally displaced or the mandible is wider than the maxilla in the premolar area.

31. **b** The mandibular canines are lingually displaced. This is often seen in conjunction with retained lower deciduous teeth that push the mandibular canines inward. These base-narrow teeth then occlude with and cause trauma to the hard palate.

32. **d** Anterior crossbite is the most common orthodontic abnormality. The premolar relationship is a normal scissor occlusion, but one or more of the incisors are misaligned.

33. **a** The most common soft tissue tumor seen in the oral cavity is benign epulides. The origin is the gingiva. There are three classifications: fibromatous epulis, ossifying epulis, and acanthomatous epulis. The other three options are all malignant oral tumors.

34. **d** Dry socket has multifactorial causes and is a painful postoperative complication of extraction. One local factor seems to be a deficiency in blood supply to the alveolus so that a good clot does not develop. This alone will not cause dry socket, however.

35. **c** The suffix *-plasty* means "formation" or "plastic repair of." The diseased gingiva is removed to eliminate suprabony pockets.

36. **a** Constant irrigation is essential to prevent overheating of the teeth.

37. **c** FEORL is the acronym given to this condition, although there are many names used to describe this.

38. **d** Floating is the filing or rasping of a horse's premolar and molar teeth to remove the sharp edges. Quidding is the dropping of food while chewing it, often a sign that teeth need to be examined.

39. **b** *Stoma* is Greek for a "mouth like opening" and *-itis* means "inflammation." Halitosis is bad breath.

40. **c** These are the safest and work the jaws well. Dried cow hooves and knuckle bones are hard and could cause slab fractures and periodontal ankylosis (ligament shock-absorbing capacity is lost) among other problems. Nylon ropes are abrasive and can cause gingival trauma and wear of the crowns of the teeth.

41. **c** Size 4 dental film is the largest of the detail intraoral films. It is also referred to as *occlusal film* and is best used to ensure that the whole root is included.

42. **a** Most dental radiographic film has a small raised dot on one corner. This will be on the side that should be facing the tube head and for easy orientation is best placed pointing rostrally. Most film will also have a comment stating "opposite side toward the radiographic unit."

43. **c** Most of the dental film has a flap for easy grasping when processing. This side of the multilayered film package contains the foil or lead, which you do not want facing the tube head.

44. **c** If the beam is 90 degrees to the bisecting angle, minimal distortion will occur.

45. **b** If the x-ray beam is aimed more perpendicular to the tooth, rather than to the bisecting angle, the tooth will appear more elongated. Foreshortening will occur if the beam is more perpendicular to the film. You want the beam perpendicular to the bisecting angle to minimize distortion.

46. **d** Choices **a**, **b**, and **c** are wrong, because other instruments are used for those purposes.

47. **c** Choices **a**, **b**, and **d** are wrong, because other instruments are used for those purposes.

48. **c** Calculus is mineralized debris on teeth. Enamel covers the crown of the tooth. Dentin is the mineralized layer beneath the enamel and the cementum.

49. **b** The sulcus is the space between the gum and the root of the tooth. Teeth do not have marrow cavities. Calculus is the mineralized debris on teeth.

50. **a** The scaler is used by making strokes across the tooth away from the gums. The scaler is held like a pen.

51. **d** The spray from the ultrasonic scaler is for cooling purposes. Hand scaling should always be done to get the surfaces that the ultrasonic scaler cannot reach. Thermal damage to the tooth can happen if the scaler is kept on the tooth longer than 15 seconds.

52. **b** The normal sulcus depth in a cat is 0 to 1 mm.

53. **b** Polishing paste is applied to smooth the surface of the tooth so that plaque will not form so quickly. Fluoride is not applied at the polishing step. The polishing cup runs over only the surface of the teeth, not the gums. The polish does not disinfect anything.

54. **a** Carnassial tooth root abscesses often present as a draining tract in the sinus area of the affected side (below the eye). Clients often do not associate the tract with a dental problem.

55. **a** When one half of the head is longer than the other, the resulting outcome is a malocclusion on both sides (left and right) between the maxillary and mandibular teeth.

56. **d** The buccal surface is the side of the tooth that comes into contact with the cheek mucosa. The lingual surface is that side of the tooth that contacts the tongue.

57. **a** Brachygnathism is a common defect in a number of breeds, resulting from an overshot jaw or what is also called "parrot mouth." This malocclusion can lead to accelerated development of dental disease because of improper wearing of the teeth.

58. **a** Prognathism, also called an *undershot jaw,* is commonly seen in breeds such as the boxer, Pekingese, and bulldogs. This malocclusion can lead to accelerated development of dental disease because of improper wearing of the teeth.

59. **d** Choices **a** to **c** describe the manner in which malocclusions result in dental disease. Resorptive lesions are aggressive feline caries that result in tooth loss; however, these are not related to malocclusion pathology.

60. **a** Adult cats are missing their upper PM1 and lower PM1 and PM2. This information should be memorized so as not to result in faulty charting. The upper premolars are numbered PM 2, 3, and 4, and the lower premolars are numbered PM 3 and 4.

61. **b** Furcation scores are assigned to teeth in an effort to determine whether a tooth should be extracted. When much of the root is exposed, a tooth is normally extracted.

62. **c** Feline immunodeficiency virus (FIV)–positive cats often suffer from severe oral stomatitis. When a veterinary technician performs dental prophylaxis and notes stomatitis, especially when it is not associated with dental plaque, an FELV/FIV test should be performed on the patient to rule out infectious causes for the stomatitis.

63. **c** Maxillary canine tooth root abscessation often results in the development of an oronasal fistula, because the root is so long and can penetrate well into the maxilla.

64. **a** Dogs with chronic allergies that engage in chewing and self-excoriation in combination with malocclusions have impaction of hair between the incisor teeth. The subsequent infection spreads from the soft tissue to the alveolar bone, resulting in a chronic osteomyelitis. The animals often lose their teeth and experience pain secondary to the infection.

65. **a** An epulis is a nonmalignant tumor that can be locally invasive into bone. It is essential that a biopsy be performed to differentiate it from other tumors and to classify its type (fibromatous, ossifying, or acanthomatous).

66. **c** Eosinophilic ulcers, also known as *eosinophilic granuloma complex* and *rodent ulcers,* are allergy-related lesions that occur in cats. The inciting cause has not been well defined. They will resolve without treatment but are often responsive to corticosteroid administration. They often recur. These are not malignancies, but they should be distinguished from squamous cell carcinoma lesions via biopsy.

67. **c** Statements made in **a, b,** and **d** are all true; however, steroid administration does not appear to diminish or prevent the development of feline neck lesions. The cause of these lesions has not been determined.

68. **b** The permanent lower canines usually erupt lingual to the deciduous canines. The other statements are correct.

69. **c** The pulp of the tooth is located in the center cavity of a tooth. It contains blood vessels (nutritive function) and nerves (providing sensation). Odontoblasts line the wall of the chamber and produce dentin.

70. **a** A tooth in which the pulp is exposed should be extracted or a pulp capping procedure performed. This is a tooth in which the nerves are exposed, causing the animal discomfort. With respect to choice **c,** the only time that a crown is filed away leaving roots behind would be in the case of a resorptive lesion in a cat patient.

71. **a** For chronic, severe periodontal disease, the antibiotic spectrum should include anaerobes. Drugs such as clindamycin are effective against anaerobic species such as *Bacteroides* and *Fusobacterium* species and have been proven useful in treating osteomyelitis.

72. **a** Vegetative endocarditis is a clinical condition in which there is a buildup of bacteria on the atrioventricular valve leaflet. It is hypothesized that bacteria from the mouth gain access to the bloodstream because of periodontal disease and subsequent oral bleeding. The bacteria then colonize the valve leaflets, resulting in valvular incompetence that can lead to heart failure.

73. **b** Perioceuticals are drugs compounded such that they can be directly placed in the mouth, where the disease is occurring, and release the medication over time.

74. **a**

75. **d** Fluoride performs the functions described in choices **a** to **c** but does not directly affect the periodontal ligament over time.

76. **d** The statements made in choices **a** to **c** are all true; **d** is false because the ultrasonic scaler can be used for supragingival scaling only. Subgingival scaling can be accomplished with the handheld instrument called the *curette.*

77. **b** It is advisable to use a cuffed endotracheal tube to prevent fluid and debris from gaining access to the lungs around the endotracheal tube. It is also a common practice to keep the endotracheal tube partially inflated when extubating to ensure that accumulated debris does not progress down the trachea.

78. **c** Distemper virus can result in abnormal formation of enamel (reduced deposition or absence of enamel). Enamel staining usually occurs secondary to tetracycline exposure of animals at a young age.

79. **b** There is no means for sterilizing the oral cavity in any patient. Flushing with a dilute chlorhexidine solution may reduce the bacterial load that may potentially get aerosolized during the procedure. Veterinary technicians should wear surgical masks, shields or goggles, and gloves when performing a dental prophylaxis to further decrease their exposure to harmful pathogens.

80. **d** Polishing is not a means for removing plaque; rather it is an effort to smooth the tooth surface to eliminate any grooves or divots that would potentially allow tartar and plaque to gain purchase on a tooth. One must be cautious not to overheat the tooth with this instrument.

81. **a** The Triadan system is a charting system in which each tooth is identified with a specific number describing the quadrant in which it is located and the type of tooth it is.

82. **d** Equids should have their teeth floated on a regular basis to prevent the formation of points on their molars that interfere with their ability to grind their food. Rabbits and rats often require their teeth to be clipped to prevent overgrowth and damage to the palate. Cats' teeth do not continue to grow.

83. **d** None of the other lengths is appropriate.

84. **c** The upper fourth premolar communicates directly with the maxillary sinus.

85. **a** The other answer choices describe other portions of a tooth.

86. **b** The other answer choices are inappropriate ranges.

87. **d**

88. **c** Early bone loss in the late stage of Grade III can be verified by radiographic examination.

89. **b**

90. **b** None of the other drugs has this effect on neonatal dentition.

91. **c** The other answer choices describe other surfaces of a tooth.

92. **b**

93. **d** This is the only instrument that can be used for measurement.

94. **b** Excessive force may degrade epithelial attachment.

95. **d** The other teeth listed have one or two roots.

96. **c** Prolonged application creates overheating and damage to the tooth.

97. **b**

98. **c**

99. **d**

100. **a**

101. **a** Complete eruption of permanent dentition can occur as early as 6 months.

102. **b** A modified pen grip is the preferred method of holding dental instruments.

103. **d**

104. **c** This best describes the action.

105. **b** Exercise does not contribute to the prevention of periodontal disease.

106. **a** Constant irrigation helps prevent temperatures from rising too high.

107. **d** This is the most effective angle.

108. **b**

109. **c** Injections are generally not necessary after dental prophylaxis.

110. **a** Mineralization of plaque occurs fairly rapidly.

111. **b** Floating is the process of filing sharp edges off cheek teeth.

112. **c**

113. **c**

114. **a**

115. **c**

116. **d**

117. a

118. b

119. b Chlorhexidine bonds to the cell membrane and inhibits bacterial growth for up to 24 hours. The other choices do not describe actions of chlorhexidine. Fluoride decreases tooth sensitivity.

120. a

121. c All other answer choices are too concentrated.

122. b Fluoride does not stain the remaining calculus red, it is beneficial to feline teeth, and it inhibits, it does not enhance, osteoclastic activity.

123. d

124. b

125. c

126. b *Brachygnathism* refers to elongation of the maxilla (on both sides of the dog's head); *prognathism* refers to elongation of the mandible (on both sides of the head); *anterior crossbite* refers to malocclusion of the incisors.

127. c

128. b Both **a** and **c** refer to surfaces above the gingival sulcus, and it is in the sulcus that most of the damage from periodontal disease occurs. Proper removal of all calculus from the subgingival tooth surfaces is essential for proper treatment of periodontal disease. Although iatrogenic trauma to subgingival tissues may be a problem, it would not be considered the most common mistake in the treatment of periodontal disease.

129. d Baking soda contains large amounts of sodium that can be absorbed into the pet's system. Remember, dogs and cats swallow their "toothpaste." Because many pets that require frequent brushing may also have heart disease, this extra sodium could be life threatening.

130. a If chlorhexidine is used, the prophylactic paste should not contain fluoride. After the teeth are polished, the teeth and subgingival surfaces can be flushed with dilute chlorhexidine, and then fluoride gel can be applied to the teeth.

131. b In many of these types of dogs, the incisor teeth may not be in individual bony sockets but suspended in connective tissue, which allows them to be quite mobile. These may be healthy teeth.

132. d The permanent tooth bud lies very close to the deciduous tooth and could become infected if the deciduous tooth is fractured and left in place.

133. d The animal should have its first dental examination when it comes in for its first vaccinations and should have a dental examination on every visit after that. Waiting for problems such as drooling or bad breath to occur allows dental disease to progress to a point where it may be more difficult to treat successfully.

134. b

135. a

136. c

137. b

138. a

139. b Answer choice **a** means gingival inflammation, **c** refers to gingival shrinkage, and **d** refers to the removal of gingiva.

140. d

141. b *Fusion* is the term used to describe two tooth buds growing together to form one larger tooth. Polydontia and oligodontia refer to the number of teeth.

142. b

143. a *Gemini* refers to a tooth that has two crowns but only one root. Polydontia and oligodontia refer to the number of teeth.

144. b

145. b

146. c

147. a

148. a

149. b

150. **b** *Mesioclusions* and *neutroclusions* refer to Class III and Class I malocclusions, respectively; *oroclusion* is not a real condition.

151. **a** *Distoclusion* and *neutroclusions* refer to Class II and Class I malocclusions, respectively. *Oroclusion* is not a real condition.

152. **c**

153. **a** Rationale: In the modified Triadan system, the right maxillary is designated by 100, left maxillary is designated by 200, left mandible is designated 300, and right mandible is designated 400.

154. **a**

155. **c**

156. **b**

157. **b** The area will appear dark or radiolucent because the infection has eaten away at the radiopaque bone.

Clinical Laboratory

Eloyes Hill • Joann Colville

QUESTIONS

1. What is the morphology of *Vibrio* sp. bacteria?
   a. Bacillus
   b. Coccus
   c. Spirochete
   d. Coccobacillus

2. Which of the following is an important function of bacterial fimbriae?
   a. Attachment
   b. Locomotion
   c. Ion transport
   d. Antibiotic resistance

3. Bacterial endospores
   a. Are resistant to heat and desiccation
   b. Are a form of asexual reproduction
   c. Are a consequence of mating
   d. Are highly susceptible to antiseptics

4. Sarcinae morphology refers to what kind of bacterial arrangement?
   a. Pairs
   b. Grape like clusters
   c. Groups of four
   d. Cubes of eight

5. In the Gram stain procedure, the mordant is
   a. Crystal violet
   b. Iodine
   c. Alcohol
   d. Safranin

6. A bacterial genus can best be described as
   a. Composed of one or more species
   b. Composed of classes
   c. Composed of families
   d. Belonging to a species

7. An iodine scrub on skin would result in
   a. Antisepsis
   b. Disinfection
   c. Fumigation
   d. Sterilization

8. Lyophilization is
   a. Holding at 72° C for 15 seconds
   b. Competitive inhibition
   c. Freeze-drying
   d. Sterility testing

9. Compared to bacteria, fungi
   a. Grow better at alkaline pH
   b. Need less moisture to survive
   c. Are less resistant to osmotic pressure
   d. Are smaller

10. In the bacterial name *Borrelia burgdorferi,* what does *burgdorferi* represent?
    a. Species
    b. Genus
    c. Family
    d. Class

11. The temperature that must be reached in an autoclave to destroy microorganisms is ___.
    a. 110° C
    b. 121° C
    c. 170° C
    d. 240° C

12. The humoral immune system involves
    a. Monocytes
    b. B cells
    c. T cells
    d. Erythrocytes

Correct answers are on pages 293-323.

13. Which is a lentivirus?
    a. Coronavirus
    b. Feline immunodeficiency virus (FIV)
    c. Herpes virus
    d. Parvovirus

14. A prodromal period
    a. Is the time before signs and symptoms appear
    b. Immediately precedes convalescence
    c. Involves early signs and symptoms
    d. Involves acute signs and symptoms

15. A non–Gram-staining bacterium is
    a. *Clostridium*
    b. *Leptospira*
    c. *Pseudomonas*
    d. *Staphylococcus*

16. A hospital-acquired disease is
    a. Endemic
    b. Nosocomial
    c. Ergasteric
    d. Iatrogenic

17. Tetanus is considered
    a. Endemic
    b. Contagious
    c. Noncommunicable
    d. Epizootic

18. Hemolysins
    a. Coagulate blood
    b. Break down fibrin
    c. Destroy red blood cells
    d. Indicate a viral infection

19. Phagocytosis does not involve
    a. Chemotaxis
    b. Adherence
    c. Ingestion
    d. Antibiosis

20. Which statement is true regarding circulating leukocytes in a healthy adult cow?
    a. Always decrease in number during infections
    b. Always decrease in number during inflammations
    c. Always include more than one cell type
    d. Always are phagocytic

21. What is the function of interferon?
    a. Destroys toxins
    b. Inhibits viruses
    c. Kills bacteria
    d. Inactivates protozoa

22. Types of effector T cells include
    a. B cells
    b. Helper T cells
    c. Monocytes
    d. Erythrocytes

23. Which of the following is a gram-positive bacterium?
    a. *Clostridium*
    b. *Pasteurella*
    c. *Pseudomonas*
    d. *Salmonella*

24. Which of the following is a gram-negative bacterium?
    a. *Clostridium*
    b. *Pasteurella*
    c. *Staphylococcus*
    d. *Leptospira*

25. It is most difficult to find antimicrobials for
    a. Molds
    b. Bacteria
    c. Rickettsia
    d. Viruses

26. Rocky Mountain spotted fever is more prevalent in
    a. The Northeastern United States
    b. The Southeastern United States
    c. The Pacific Northwest
    d. The Rocky Mountains

27. The etiologic agent of Lyme disease is
    a. *Borrelia burgdorferi*
    b. Coronavirus
    c. Lentivirus
    d. *Pasteurella multocida*

28. In the name *Staphylococcus aureus*, *Staphylococcus* is the
    a. Order
    b. Family
    c. Genus
    d. Species

29. The counterstain in the Gram stain is
    a. Crystal violet
    b. Methylene blue
    c. Iodine
    d. Safranin

30. Most bacteria grow best at pH
    a. 1
    b. 3
    c. 9
    d. 7

31. Which of the following is an important function of bacterial flagella?
    a. Attachment
    b. Locomotion
    c. DNA replication
    d. Ion transport

32. What parasite has only the cat as its definitive host?
    a. *Toxoplasma gondii*
    b. *Giardia lamblia*
    c. *Isospora rivolta*
    d. *Balantidium coli*

33. What is not a method of culturing animal viruses?
    a. Laboratory animal inoculation
    b. Cell culture
    c. Agar plate inoculation
    d. Embryonated egg inoculation

34. What immunoglobulin is usually present in greatest quantity?
    a. IgA
    b. IgD
    c. IgE
    d. IgG

35. The most common portal of entry for microorganisms into the body is
    a. Skin
    b. Gastrointestinal tract
    c. Respiratory tract
    d. Genitourinary tract

36. Which of the following would be a parenteral route of pathogen transmission?
    a. Transfusion
    b. Contaminated food
    c. Droplet infection
    d. Direct contact

37. Phagocytes are a type of
    a. Red blood cell
    b. White blood cell
    c. Platelet
    d. Antibody

38. Leukopenia is
    a. A decrease in white blood cells
    b. An increase in white blood cells
    c. A bone marrow disease
    d. A type of blood cancer

39. Undulating fever is a zoonotic disease caused by
    a. *Listeria* species
    b. *Toxoplasma* species
    c. *Brucella* species
    d. *Hemophilus* species

40. Warts are caused by __.
    a. Bacteria
    b. Fungi
    c. Viruses
    d. Protozoa

41. What percentage of the glomeruli in both kidneys must be nonfunctional before serum chemistry changes indicate renal disease?
    a. 10%
    b. 20%
    c. 50%
    d. 70%

42. What laboratory test evaluates kidney function and is a breakdown product of protein?
    a. Glucose
    b. SGTP (ALT)
    c. Creatinine
    d. BUN

43. Creatinine concentrations in serum are influenced by
    a. Hydration level
    b. Amylase concentration
    c. Liver disease
    d. Insulin production

44. Nonrenal causes of increased levels of urea might include
    a. The amount of carbohydrate ingested
    b. The amount of protein ingested
    c. Insufficient insulin
    d. Insufficient ADH

45. Decrease in albumin may occur in
    a. Chronic liver disease
    b. A carnivorous diet
    c. Gastroenteritis
    d. A vegetarian diet

46. Fibrinogen is considered a part of
    a. Total plasma albumin
    b. Total plasma protein
    c. Total serum protein
    d. Total serum globulin

47. When evaluating the liver of dogs and cats, AST should be evaluated in conjunction with
    a. ALT
    b. Lipase
    c. LDH
    d. Glucose

Correct answers are on pages 293-323.

48. Plasma is composed of
    a. 90% water and 10% dissolved substances
    b. 80% water and 20% dissolved substances
    c. 70% water and 30% dissolved substances
    d. 60% water and 40% dissolved substances

49. To separate plasma from the cellular components, blood tubes should be counterbalanced and centrifuged for ___ minutes at ___ rpm.
    a. 2; 1000
    b. 5; 1000
    c. 10; 2000
    d. 15; 2000

50. Icteric serum is what color?
    a. Yellow
    b. Red
    c. Brown
    d. Green

51. What color blood collection tube top indicates that heparin is the anticoagulant?
    a. Purple
    b. Green
    c. Blue
    d. Gray

52. Which of the following substances is a by-product of muscle metabolism, produced at a constant rate, and filtered out by the renal glomeruli?
    a. Urea
    b. Creatinine
    c. Glucose
    d. Sodium

53. Which of the following substances used to evaluate kidney filtration and function is excreted by the kidneys and up to 40% reabsorbed by the tubules?
    a. Urea
    b. Creatinine
    c. Glucose
    d. Sodium

54. With significant dehydration in an otherwise healthy patient which of the following would likely be seen on a urinalysis and CBC?
    a. Increased urine SG and increased PCV
    b. Increased urine SG and decreased PCV
    c. Decreased urine SG and decreased PCV
    d. Decreased urine SG and increased PCV

55. Water deprivation tests should never be performed on patients with
    a. High MCV
    b. Suspected sufficient ADH
    c. Dehydration
    d. Suspected tubular malfunction

56. Glycosuria exists
    a. When blood glucose levels exceed the renal threshold for absorption of glucose
    b. When blood glucose levels are lower than the renal threshold for absorption of glucose
    c. When urine glucose levels are lower than the renal threshold for absorption of glucose
    d. When urine glucose levels are higher than the serum threshold for absorption of glucose

57. A false positive urine glucose reading may result from administration of
    a. Acetaminophen
    b. Morphine
    c. NaCl
    d. NaOH

58. Hypoglycemia may result from
    a. Insufficient insulin
    b. Serum remaining on the RBCs too long
    c. Cushing disease
    d. Heavy lactation after giving birth

59. Blood cells continue to utilize glucose at a rate of ___% to ___% per hour if allowed to remain in contact with the serum.
    a. 3; 5
    b. 5; 7
    c. 7; 10
    d. 10; 12

60. Amylase acts to break down
    a. Starches and glycogen
    b. Fats and carbohydrates
    c. Fats and starches
    d. Protein and amino acids

61. An increase in unconjugated bilirubin may be the result of
    a. Either hepatic or posthepatic failure
    b. Either hepatic or biliary failure
    c. Either prehepatic or posthepatic failure
    d. Either hepatic or prehepatic failure

62. ALT is also known as
    a. AST
    b. SGPT
    c. SGOT
    d. GGT

63. Horses typically have higher ___ values than other species.
    a. AST
    b. ALP
    c. ALT
    d. GGT

64. What blood chemistry test is not a test for liver damage?
    a. ALT
    b. GGT
    c. Lipase
    d. Bile acids

65. Which of the following ions is a cation?
    a. Bicarbonate
    b. Hydroxide
    c. Chloride
    d. Potassium

66. What percentage of the body's calcium is in bone?
    a. 49%
    b. 59%
    c. 79%
    d. 99%

67. Electrolytes are commonly measured by what method?
    a. Ion-specific electrodes
    b. Refractometry
    c. Adsorption
    d. Enzymatic digestion

68. When referring to the alteration of bilirubin in the liver, the verb *conjugation* means
    a. To break apart in equal parts
    b. To precipitate
    c. To become pigmented
    d. To join together

69. Which of the following is not an electrolyte?
    a. Calcium
    b. Glucose
    c. Phosphorous
    d. Potassium

70. A test done to help diagnose hyperthyroidism is
    a. LH
    b. Cortisol
    c. Bile acids
    d. T4

71. When performing urinalysis testing, the sample should be analyzed within ___ minutes or refrigeration is required.
    a. 10
    b. 20
    c. 30
    d. 40

72. For cytologic evaluation of urine, which of the following conditions should be observed?
    a. The specimen should be refrigerated as soon as possible.
    b. The specimen should be centrifuged as soon as possible.
    c. The specimen may sit at room temperature for up to 6 hours.
    d. The specimen may be frozen for later analysis.

73. Brown urine most likely contains
    a. Hemoglobin
    b. Bilirubin
    c. Bile pigments
    d. Myoglobin

74. Normal voided urine is clear, except in which of the following species?
    a. Dogs
    b. Cats
    c. Horses
    d. Cows

75. The average urine specific gravity for a healthy adult dog is
    a. 1.025
    b. 1.035
    c. 1.040
    d. 1.045

76. The average urine specific gravity for a healthy adult cat is
    a. 1.025
    b. 1.030
    c. 1.035
    d. 1.040

77. Urine crystals are estimated as the average per
    a. High-power field
    b. Low-power field
    c. Medium-power field
    d. Oil-immersion field

78. Epithelial cells in urine are estimated as the average number per
    a. High-power field
    b. Low-power field
    c. Medium-power field
    d. Oil-immersion field

79. Hyaline casts
    a. Are granular and contain white blood cells
    b. Are clear and red
    c. Are granular and contain fat
    d. Are clear and colorless

Correct answers are on pages 293-323.

80. Calcium oxalate crystals
    a. Are seen with ethylene glycol toxicity
    b. Have a characteristic coffin-lid appearance
    c. Are seen with hepatic disease
    d. Have three to six sides

81. Which of the following tests is not included in a routine CBC?
    a. Total WBC count
    b. Differential WBC count
    c. Total protein
    d. Reticulocyte count

82. MCHC is expressed in
    a. percent
    b. g/dl
    c. mg/dl
    d. mg/L

83. Toxic neutrophils may show large
    a. Blue granules
    b. Black granules
    c. Red granules
    d. Purple granules

84. Which of the following cells has a high nuclear-cytoplasmic ratio; coarse, clumped, dark-staining chromatin; and a sky blue cytoplasm?
    a. Neutrophil
    b. Small lymphocyte
    c. Basophil
    d. Eosinophil

85. Which of the following cells has cytoplasmic granules that stain blue to blue-black and gray-blue cytoplasm, often with small vacuoles?
    a. Neutrophil
    b. Small lymphocyte
    c. Basophil
    d. Eosinophil

86. Papanicolaou stains are specialized stains used in which of the following procedures?
    a. Red blood cell evaluation
    b. Platelet evaluation
    c. Cytologic evaluation
    d. Parasitic evaluation

87. Mesothelial cells are cells that
    a. Line the pleural, peritoneal, and visceral surfaces
    b. Are square with usually one round to oval nucleus
    c. Line blood and lymph vessels
    d. Are squamous with blue to purple oval inclusions

88. Supravital staining is
    a. Use of a stain that has extreme toxicity so that vital processes can be stopped abruptly
    b. Use of a stain that has low toxicity so that vital processes can be studied in live cells
    c. Use of a stain for nuclear material only
    d. Use of a stain for phase contrast microscopy only

89. Smudge cells are
    a. Created while spreading blood for making a blood smear
    b. Seen with Papanicolaou stains only
    c. Created during the blood smear staining process
    d. Specific to species with nucleated RBCs only

90. Megakaryocytes are the precursor cell to
    a. Metarubricytes
    b. Polychromatic cells
    c. Thrombocytes
    d. Monocytes

91. Amino acids, iron, vitamin B_{12}, folic acid, vitamin B_6, and the trace metals cobalt and nickel are all required to produce what cell?
    a. Leukocytes
    b. Erythrocytes
    c. Thrombocytes
    d. Plasma cells

92. Approximately what percentage of the total erythrocyte mass is replaced every day in healthy mammals under normal circumstances?
    a. 1%
    b. 10%
    c. 20%
    d. 30%

93. Basophilic stippling may be seen in erythrocytes of patients with which of the following pathologic conditions?
    a. Hypersegmented neutrophils
    b. Iron deficiency
    c. Lead poisoning
    d. Vitamin C toxicity

94. Polychromasia in an immature RBC will appear as a ___ on a blood smear stained with new methylene blue stain.
    a. Reticulocyte
    b. Döhle body
    c. Barr body
    d. Schistocyte

95. Adaptive or specific immunity includes
    a. Naturally occurring stomach acids
    b. Antibodies that an organism is born with that will respond to a variety of substances
    c. The response of the defenses of the body to a specific substance
    d. Lysozyme in tears

96. Platelet clumping could possibly affect the
    a. RDW
    b. PCV
    c. RBC morphology
    d. Manual WBC count

97. The first phagocytes to respond to an infection are
    a. Lymphocytes
    b. Neutrophils
    c. Monocytes
    d. Eosinophils

98. Which of the following cells is usually associated with a chronic infection or inflammation?
    a. Lymphocytes
    b. Neutrophils
    c. Monocytes
    d. Eosinophils

99. The chemical regulator of the cellular immune response is
    a. Vasopressin
    b. Mucin
    c. Interleukin
    d. Mucopolysaccharide

100. Which of the following combinations of objective lenses is the best for hematology work?
    a. 10×, 40×, 50×
    b. 10×, 40×, 100×
    c. 40×, 50×, 100×
    d. 40×, 100×, 150×

101. Allergy shots cause
    a. The suppressor T-ell population to increase
    b. A reduction in the formation of IgG antibodies
    c. A reduction in the formation of IgE antibodies
    d. An increase in the B-cell population

102. IgA
    a. Is a class of antibody that possesses 10 antigen-binding sites
    b. Makes up approximately 80% of the antibody pool in plasma
    c. Is found in body secretions
    d. Is found on lymphocyte membranes

103. IgD
    a. Is a class of antibody that possesses 10 antigen-binding sites
    b. Makes up approximately 80% of the antibody pool in plasma
    c. Is found in body secretions
    d. Is found on lymphocyte membranes

104. IgE
    a. Is a class of antibody that possesses 10 antigen-binding sites
    b. Makes up approximately 80% of the antibody pool in plasma
    c. Is found on lymphocyte membranes
    d. Functions to boost local inflammation reactions

105. Antibody titer is a test that measures
    a. The level of antibody in serum
    b. The level of antigenic response
    c. The level of antibody in a virus
    d. The level of antigen in a virus

106. By definition, an *allergen* is
    a. Produced in response to an antigen
    b. A material that invokes an allergic response
    c. A process of mutation
    d. Serum that contains antibodies

107. With respect to immunology, *tolerance* means
    a. The number of white blood cells that respond, expressed as a percentage
    b. A blistering of the skin
    c. Inflammation on the upper respiratory tract
    d. The lack of responsiveness by the immune system

108. A plasmid is a
    a. Nonchromosomal, circular strand of bacterial genome
    b. Chromosomal, circular strand of bacterial genome
    c. Nonchromosomal, circular strand viral particle
    d. Chromosomal, circular strand viral particle

109. According to the Punnett square, in a cross of Bb × Bb, the F1 generations will be made up of
    a. 25% and 75%, or 1:3
    b. 25%, 50%, and 25%, or 1:2:1
    c. 25%, 25%, 25%, and 25%, or 1:1:1:1
    d. 20%, 30%, and 50%, or 1:1:2

110. The type of immunity that is the function of B cells that transform into plasma cells and produce protective proteins, called *antibodies*, against antigens is
    a. Cell mediated
    b. Autoimmunity
    c. Humoral
    d. Anaphylaxis

Correct answers are on pages 293-323.

111. When T cells are processed in the ___, they develop specific antigen receptors on their cell membranes.
    a. Transitional epithelium
    b. Thymus
    c. Terminal ileum
    d. Thyroid

112. The third line of defense against foreign invaders in the body is
    a. Agglutination
    b. Inflammation
    c. Specific immunity
    d. Interferon production

113. Epistasis is
    a. The masking of a trait by another trait
    b. Traits that are due to the interaction of several pairs of alleles
    c. A cross in which each allele makes a comparable contribution to the trait
    d. A cross of three alleles over two alternate alleles

114. Females have which of the following sex chromosome designations?
    a. XX
    b. YY
    c. YZ
    d. XY

115. Cell-mediated immunity is the function of ___ that attach to antigenic sites on the surfaces of foreign cells.
    a. B cells
    b. Small lymphocytes
    c. Plasma cells
    d. T cells

116. A pedigree chart is a
    a. Chart that shows the ancestry of a particular family
    b. Chart that shows the crossing of two independent alleles
    c. Square to show a monohybrid cross
    d. Square to show a dihybrid cross

117. *Translocation* can be defined as
    a. A duplication of an allele (for example, in trisomy 21)
    b. The breakage of two chromosomes, resulting in the exact duplicate of the originals after repair
    c. The breakage of two chromosomes, resulting in repair in an abnormal arrangement
    d. A part or all of a chromosome is missing

118. An *anomaly* may be defined as
    a. The breakage of two chromosomes, resulting in repair in an abnormal arrangement
    b. All or part of a chromosome is missing
    c. Any deviation from normal
    d. An alternate form of a gene

119. If a homozygous polled bull were mated to a heterozygous polled cow, and the gene for horns was an X-linked dominant gene, the expected results would be which of the following?
    a. 1:2:1, or 25%, 50%, and 25%
    b. 2:2, or 50% and 50%
    c. 1:3, or 25% and 75%
    d. 1:1:1:1, or 25%, 25%, 25%, and 25%

120. Outbreeding may be described as which of the following?
    a. Mating of closely related individuals to produce ever-increasing similarities in the offspring
    b. A mating that is performed to determine the genotype of a particular phenotype
    c. The crossing of two traits
    d. Matings to other strains to increase the number of heterozygous genes

121. An attenuated antigen is a ___ antigen.
    a. Dead
    b. Multivalent
    c. Modified
    d. Transferred

122. Nutritive media will
    a. Grow almost all types of bacteria
    b. Grow only some types of bacteria
    c. Differentiate certain types of bacteria
    d. Grow gram-negative bacteria only

123. Selective media grow
    a. All types of bacteria
    b. Some types of bacteria only
    c. And differentiate certain types of bacteria
    d. Gram-negative bacteria only

124. Triplicate soy agar
    a. Contains 25% sheep blood
    b. Is a nutritive media
    c. Is used for observation of bacterial fermentation reactions
    d. Is also called *chocolate agar plate*

125. MacConkey agar
    a. Selects for gram-positive organisms
    b. Uses crystal blue as a gram-negative inhibitor
    c. Differentiates between dextrose and nondextrose fermenter
    d. Selects for gram-negative organisms

126. The most important laboratory procedure for microbiologic diagnosis is
    a. Inoculation of blood agar
    b. Antimicrobial susceptibility testing
    c. Direct microscopic examination of the specimen
    d. Serologic testing

127. Dermatophyte test medium
    a. Is used to identify organisms that produce hemolysis
    b. Will grow gram-positive organisms only
    c. Is used to identify fungal pathogens
    d. Will grow gram-negative organisms only

128. Which of the following is considered sterile?
    a. Hair
    b. Skin
    c. Saliva
    d. Lower respiratory tract

129. When culturing a swab for bacterial identification, which of the following media should be used?
    a. TSI, BAP, CAMPY
    b. EMB, BAP, MAC
    c. BAP, CNA, MAC
    d. CNA, TSI, MSA

130. The nonpathogenic gram-positive rods found on skin are
    a. Diphtheroids
    b. Coliforms
    c. Anaerobes
    d. Dermatophytes

131. To get the best results, all fecal cultures are
    a. Inoculated onto BAP, CNA, and TSB
    b. Inoculated onto MAC, SS, and GN
    c. Inoculated onto MH, SS, and THIO
    d. Inoculated onto BAP, MAC, and SS

132. Fungal cultures are
    a. Incubated at room temperature
    b. Incubated in a microaerophilic environment
    c. Incubated at body temperature
    d. Incubated in anaerobic environment

133. *Staphylococcus aureus*
    a. Is catalase-positive
    b. Is coagulase-negative
    c. Grows in an anaerobic environment only
    d. Is gram-negative

134. Streptococci
    a. Are catalase-positive
    b. Are catalase-negative
    c. Resemble shooting stars when grown in tube media
    d. Are never hemolytic like *Staphylococcus*

135. Enterobacteriaceae are found in what part of the body?
    a. Lungs
    b. Intestines
    c. Skin
    d. Stomach

136. Which of the following is a spreading organism when grown on agar plates?
    a. *Staphylococcus*
    b. *Streptococcus*
    c. *Shigella*
    d. *Proteus*

137. Which of the following is considered a serious primary pathogen in birds, reptiles, and amphibians?
    a. *Pseudomonas*
    b. *Shigella*
    c. *Staphylococcus*
    d. *Micrococcus*

138. Which of the following bacteria is a gram-negative spirochete?
    a. *Staphylococcus*
    b. *Streptococcus*
    c. *Micrococcus*
    d. *Campylobacter*

139. *Candida albicans* may cause many different diseases, especially when there is a predisposing condition such as
    a. Vegetarian diet
    b. Primary bacterial infection
    c. Prolonged analgesic use
    d. Carnivorous diet

140. An increased amount of ___ seen on a stained peripheral blood smear is a sign of RBC regeneration.
    a. Hypochromasia
    b. Crenation
    c. Howell-Jolly bodies
    d. Döhle bodies

Correct answers are on pages 293-323.

141. To make a smear with anemic blood,
    a. Increase the angle of the pusher slide
    b. Decrease the angle of the pusher slide
    c. Use a larger drop of blood
    d. Wait for the drop of blood to partially dry

142. Which of the RBC indices indicates cell size?
    a. MCH
    b. MCHC
    c. MCV
    d. MPV

143. A correction for nucleated red blood cells is done to avoid a falsely
    a. Elevated PCV
    b. Elevated WBC count
    c. Decreased PCV
    d. Decreased WBC count

144. Avian WBC counts can be determined indirectly by using what Unopette?
    a. WBC
    b. Platelet
    c. RBC
    d. Eosinophil

145. The platelets of what species tend to clump easily?
    a. Dogs
    b. Horses
    c. Cats
    d. Cows

146. RBCs with multiple, irregularly spaced projections are
    a. Crenated cells
    b. Schistocytes
    c. Acanthocytes
    d. Anisocytes

147. Reticulocytes on a modified Wright stain (e.g., Diff-Quik) appear
    a. Polychromatic
    b. Hypochromic
    c. Hyperchromic
    d. Crenated

148. What way of reporting WBC differential results is most useful?
    a. As percentages
    b. As relative numbers
    c. As absolute numbers
    d. As decimal numbers

149. Determination of which one of these is useful in the detection of inflammatory processes?
    a. Total protein
    b. Hematocrit
    c. RBC morphology
    d. Fibrinogen

150. The buffy coat in a spun hematocrit tube consists of
    a. WBCs
    b. WBCs and platelets
    c. WBCs and NRBCs
    d. Platelets and NRBCs

151. What cells are phagocytic?
    a. Granulocytes
    b. Lymphocytes
    c. Neutrophils and macrophages
    d. Macrophages and lymphocytes

152. Monocytes typically have
    a. Segmented nuclei
    b. Band-shaped nuclei
    c. Lobular nuclei
    d. No nuclei

153. Which one of these would not affect a manual WBC count?
    a. Condenser in the farthest "up" position
    b. Length of time that the hemocytometer has been loaded
    c. Objective lens used
    d. Mini clots in the blood

154. Which of these is not a sign of RBC regeneration?
    a. Polychromasia
    b. Nuclear remnants
    c. Spherocytes
    d. Anisocytosis with macrocytosis

155. A left shift refers to increased numbers of
    a. Immature neutrophils
    b. Immature RBCs
    c. Immature platelets
    d. Immature lymphocytes

156. What special stain would be used in assessing anemia?
    a. Lactophenol cotton blue
    b. New methylene blue
    c. Gram
    d. Acridine orange

157. What order of maturation is correct?
    a. Myeloblast, myelocyte, promyelocyte, metamyelocyte
    b. Myeloblast, promyelocyte, myelocyte, metamyelocyte
    c. Promyelocyte, metamyelocyte, myelocyte, band
    d. Promyelocyte, myelocyte, band, segmented neutrophil

158. What is the most immature erythrocyte?
    a. Rubricyte
    b. Metarubricyte
    c. Rubriblast
    d. Reticulocyte

159. Kittens are most likely to get roundworms (*Toxocara*) by what route?
    a. Fecal–oral
    b. Transplacental
    c. Transmammary
    d. Skin penetration

160. A route of infection by hookworms that is not shared by roundworms is
    a. Ingestion of infective stage
    b. Transplacental
    c. Transmammary
    d. Skin penetration

161. In appearance, hookworm ova resemble ___ ova.
    a. Strongyle
    b. Whipworm
    c. Roundworm
    d. Pinworm

162. Finding proglottids around a dog's anus indicates infection with
    a. Flukes
    b. Tapeworms
    c. Pinworms
    d. Hookworms

163. The intermediate host for heartworms is the
    a. Flea
    b. Rodent
    c. Mosquito
    d. Snail

164. Serology tests can detect heartworms in a dog's blood
    a. Immediately after becoming infected
    b. Several days after becoming infected
    c. Several weeks after becoming infected
    d. Several months after becoming infected

165. Heartworm treatment begins with killing the
    a. Eggs
    b. Infective L3 larvae
    c. Microfilariae
    d. Adult worms

166. What is not a type of coccidia?
    a. *Isospora*
    b. *Cryptosporidium*
    c. *Toxoplasma*
    d. *Giardia*

167. What are the two diagnostic forms of *Giardia*?
    a. Cysts and trophozoites
    b. Merozoites and schizonts
    c. Oocysts and sporocysts
    d. Ova and L3 larvae

168. Compared to a roundworm ova, coccidia appear
    a. Smaller
    b. The same size
    c. Twice as large
    d. Three times as large

169. The roundworm of horses is
    a. *Strongylus* sp.
    b. *Oxyuris* sp.
    c. *Anoplocephala* sp.
    d. *Parascaris* sp.

170. The difference in appearance between small and large strongyle ova in horses is
    a. Size
    b. Shape
    c. Color
    d. None; they look alike

171. Ruminant ova such as *Haemonchus, Ostertagia, Trichostrongylus,* and *Cooperia* resemble canine
    a. Roundworms
    b. Hookworms
    c. Tapeworms
    d. Whipworms

172. Which of the following protozoan parasites of cattle causes abortion or fetal resorption?
    a. *Tritrichomonas*
    b. *Eimeria*
    c. *Giardia*
    d. *Cryptosporidium*

173. In a healthy animal, diminished water intake or loss of water would result in ___ urine specific gravity.
    a. Increased
    b. Decreased
    c. Isosthenuric
    d. Isotonic

Correct answers are on pages 293-323.

174. What urine sediment component would be most significant?
    a. Sperm
    b. Fat droplets
    c. Squamous epithelial cells
    d. Blood cells

175. *Struvite crystals* is another name for
    a. Calcium carbonate crystals
    b. Calcium oxalate crystals
    c. Triple phosphate crystals
    d. Amorphous phosphate crystals

176. Crystals in urine sediment often indicate
    a. Uroliths
    b. Nothing
    c. Inflammation
    d. Urethral blockage

177. Which of the following would not be on a urine dipstick?
    a. Glucose
    b. Blood
    c. Total protein
    d. BUN

178. WBCs in urine sediment may be confused with
    a. Renal epithelial cells
    b. Transitional epithelial cells
    c. Squamous epithelial cells
    d. Caudate epithelial cells

179. A drop of ___ added to the urine sediment lyses RBCs but not fat droplets.
    a. Physiologic saline
    b. Sedi-Stain
    c. 3% potassium hydroxide
    d. Dilute acetic acid

180. Bacteria in urine sediment may be confused with
    a. Fat droplets
    b. Sperm
    c. Amorphous phosphates or urates
    d. Calcium carbonate crystals

181. Casts seen in urine sediment are
    a. Mucous threads filled with amorphous sediment
    b. Always significant
    c. Formed in the renal tubules
    d. Artifacts

182. The presence of protein in the urine may indicate
    a. Acid-base imbalance
    b. Hemolytic anemia
    c. Kidney disease
    d. Diabetes mellitus

183. Which of these would not be associated with ketones in the urine?
    a. Diabetes mellitus
    b. Lactating cows
    c. Starvation
    d. Hemolysis

184. Mucus is normally often seen in ___ urine.
    a. Dog
    b. Horse
    c. Cat
    d. Cow

185. Calcium oxalate crystals are
    a. Hexagonal
    b. Dark, needle like rods
    c. Brown spheres with long spicules
    d. Small squares that contain an X

186. The best urine sample for culture is a
    a. Bladder expression sample
    b. Metabolism cage collection
    c. Cystocentesis sample
    d. Voided sample

187. Fat droplets in urine samples are most commonly seen in
    a. Dogs
    b. Cats
    c. Horses
    d. Cows

188. Gram-negative bacteria retain what component of the Gram stain?
    a. Crystal violet
    b. Iodine solution
    c. Decolorizer
    d. Safranin

189. Which of these is a primary medium and would be used for initial inoculation of a sample?
    a. Triple-sugar iron
    b. Trypticase soy agar with 5% sheep blood
    c. Citrate
    d. Urea

190. What media is selective for gram-negative bacteria?
    a. MacConkey
    b. BAP (blood agar plate)
    c. Mannitol salt agar
    d. Mueller-Hinton agar

191. The catalase and coagulase tests are used in the presumptive identification of
    a. Gram-negative bacteria
    b. Gram-positive bacteria
    c. Saprophytes
    d. Dermatophytes

192. What gram-negative bacteria may "swarm" a blood agar plate, leaving a film over the entire surface?
    a. *Pseudomonas* sp.
    b. *Staphylococcus* sp.
    c. *Proteus* sp.
    d. *Escherichia coli*

193. What microorganism is frequently recovered from the ears of dogs with chronic otitis externa?
    a. *Candida* sp.
    b. *Cryptococcus* sp.
    c. *Microsporum* sp.
    d. *Malassezia* sp.

194. What microorganism is an etiologic agent of ringworm?
    a. *Microsporum* sp.
    b. *Mycobacterium* sp.
    c. *Micrococcus* sp.
    d. *Moraxella* sp.

195. The species of this genus are common contaminants and the causative agent of anthrax.
    a. *Escherichia*
    b. *Corynebacterium*
    c. *Bacillus*
    d. *Enterobacter*

196. What is a common pathogen in mastitis, skin wounds, and abscesses that is also found in the environment?
    a. *Proteus vulgaris*
    b. *Escherichia coli*
    c. *Streptococcus* spp.
    d. *Staphylococcus aureus*

197. The species of this genus can cause strangles in horses.
    a. *Streptococcus*
    b. *Clostridium*
    c. *Pseudomonas*
    d. *Malassezia*

198. A normal gastrointestinal inhabitant in turkeys, chickens, and humans that can cause serious urinary tract infections, diarrhea, and tissue infections is
    a. *Leptospira* sp.
    b. *Escherichia coli*
    c. *Pasteurella multocida*
    d. *Staphylococcus intermedius*

199. What family of bacteria is the largest group of potential pathogens and the most frequently isolated bacteria?
    a. Actinomycetaceae
    b. Bacteroidaceae
    c. Enterobacteriaceae
    d. Micrococcaceae

200. Skin scales and infected hair samples are mixed with ___ to dissolve the debris and aid in microscopic examination for fungal elements.
    a. Hydrogen peroxide
    b. Acetic acid
    c. Physiologic saline
    d. Potassium hydroxide

201. The temperature of a bacterial incubator would most likely be
    a. 4° C
    b. 25° C
    c. 37° C
    d. 56° C

202. What agar is used for antimicrobial susceptibility testing?
    a. Sabouraud agar
    b. Mueller-Hinton agar
    c. MacConkey agar
    d. Kligler iron agar

203. Stress and epinephrine release in cats may cause an increase in
    a. BUN
    b. Total protein
    c. ALT
    d. Glucose

204. A kidney function test that is useful in birds and Dalmatians is
    a. BUN
    b. Creatinine
    c. Uric acid
    d. AST

Correct answers are on pages 293-323.

205. What serum component can be used as a screening test for hypothyroidism?
    a. ALT
    b. Cholesterol
    c. Total protein
    d. Creatine kinase

206. During a glucose tolerance test, glucose levels in a diabetic animal will
    a. Show an initial peak then diminish to normal
    b. Remain high throughout the test
    c. Show a delayed peak at the end of the test period
    d. Show below normal levels throughout the test

207. Total protein levels are ___ in a dehydrated animal.
    a. Unaffected
    b. Decreased
    c. Increased
    d. Variable

208. What organ conserves nutrients, removes waste products, maintains blood pH, and controls blood pressure?
    a. Kidney
    b. Liver
    c. Pancreas
    d. Spleen

209. The small intestine receives digestive enzymes from the
    a. Kidney
    b. Pancreas
    c. Liver
    d. Spleen

210. Bile acids aid in the digestion of
    a. Proteins
    b. Carbohydrates
    c. Fats
    d. Globulins

211. Fibrinogen is produced in the
    a. Pancreas
    b. Bone marrow
    c. Liver
    d. Spleen

212. Gamma globulins can be estimated by subtracting
    a. Total protein from fibrinogen
    b. Heated total protein value from unheated total protein value
    c. Albumin from serum total protein
    d. Alpha globulins from beta globulins

213. What ion is important in regulating blood pH and in transporting carbon dioxide from the tissue to the lungs?
    a. Sodium
    b. Potassium
    c. Chloride
    d. Bicarbonate

214. It is useful to measure electrolyte values when an animal has
    a. Suspected pancreatitis
    b. Suspected liver disease
    c. Lost fluids
    d. Broken bones

215. Albumin is measured to help diagnose
    a. Heart disease
    b. Pancreatitis
    c. Hypothyroidism
    d. Liver disease

216. What ion increases with malignancy, particularly with lymphosarcoma?
    a. Calcium
    b. Phosphorus
    c. Magnesium
    d. Potassium

217. EDTA plasma cannot be used for testing ___ plasma levels because EDTA forms a complex with it.
    a. Magnesium
    b. Phosphorus
    c. Calcium
    d. Potassium

218. A 95% sensitivity in reference to a serology test kit refers to
    a. Effects of other influences on test results
    b. Ability of the test to properly identify a diseased patient's serum
    c. Ability of the test to give accurate results if stored properly
    d. How easily a test can be run

219. Veterinary reference ranges for blood chemistry values
    a. Are generally established by each individual veterinary clinic
    b. Include values from diseased and normal animals
    c. Often come with an analyzer and have been established by the company
    d. Are helpful to refer to but are not necessary

220. If a test result is a false positive, it means that the result is
    a. Within the reference range and the disease is absent
    b. Within the reference range and the disease is present
    c. Outside the reference range and the disease is absent
    d. Outside the reference range and the disease is present

221. Which of the following would not be an acceptable action if a control value is out of range?
    a. Ignore the result; it is a simple outlier (sporadic result)
    b. Call the technical representative from the company
    c. Repeat the test using the same reagent
    d. Repeat the test using a new reagent

222. Calibration standards for chemistry analyzers are
    a. Not used anymore
    b. Used in the same way as control sera
    c. Used by the manufacturer
    d. Used routinely at the veterinary clinic

223. The term *normal* is referring to
    a. Calibration standard values
    b. Reference ranges
    c. Control values
    d. Positive values

224. Which of the samples can be frozen and successfully thawed for performing an analytic test at a later time?
    a. Feces for a fecal float test
    b. Whole blood for chemistry testing
    c. Serum for chemistry testing
    d. Whole blood for a CBC

225. If there is only a small amount of serum separated after centrifuging a tube of whole blood, you should
    a. Invert the tube several times and respin it
    b. Assume the patient is dehydrated and draw off all of the serum you can
    c. Spin the tube again at a faster speed and longer time
    d. Rim/ring the clot and spin again at normal speed and time

226. To dilute a serum sample for retesting when the value is out of the instrument's linearity range, use
    a. Physiologic saline
    b. 5% saline
    c. 5% dextrose
    d. Sterile water

227. Samples used for serology test kits are
    a. Serum and plasma
    b. Plasma and whole EDTA blood
    c. Whole EDTA blood and serum
    d. Plasma, serum, and whole EDTA blood

228. For hematology tests, clots in EDTA blood are
    a. Acceptable if they are microscopic
    b. Acceptable if they are detected on a wooden stick only
    c. Acceptable if they are run through an automatic analyzer
    d. Never acceptable

229. Most newborn animals are
    a. Hypogammaglobulinemic
    b. Hypergammaglobulinemic
    c. Hypobetaglobulinemic
    d. Hyperbetaglobulinemic

230. Which of the following is not a serology test?
    a. Latex agglutination
    b. Kinetic reaction
    c. Rapid immunomigration (RIM)
    d. ELISA

231. Which of these immune responses refers to the production of antibodies?
    a. Innate
    b. Cell-mediated
    c. Humoral
    d. Cytotoxic

232. What type of antibodies are used in serology test kits?
    a. Autoantibodies
    b. Monoclonal antibodies
    c. Neutralizing antibodies
    d. Sensitizing antibodies

233. Food allergies are best treated with
    a. Hyposensitization
    b. Allergy shots
    c. Long-term steroid treatment
    d. Elimination diets

234. Which is *least* likely to be a sign of allergy?
    a. Face rubbing
    b. Ear problems
    c. Loss of appetite
    d. Skin rashes

235. Cornified epithelial cells are synonymous with ___ epithelial cells.
    a. Basal
    b. Parabasal
    c. Intermediate
    d. Superficial

236. What type of epithelial cell is most prominent during estrus in a bitch?
    a. Basal
    b. Parabasal
    c. Intermediate
    d. Superficial

237. Transudates and exudates are usually not examined for
    a. Cells
    b. Protein
    c. Color and turbidity
    d. Hematocrit

238. In which of the following sample preparation techniques is a small amount of aspirate placed on a slide, a second slide placed on top of the aspirate, and, finally, the top slide slid across the bottom slide and pulled apart?
    a. Starfish preparation
    b. Blood smear technique
    c. Squash preparation technique
    d. Line smear concentration technique

239. An impression smear is the technique to use for ___ analysis.
    a. Vaginal cytology
    b. Tissue sample
    c. Semen
    d. Fine-needle aspirate

240. Regarding the disadvantages of using commercial laboratories, which statement is false?
    a. They are not practical to use for a single laboratory test.
    b. The samples are not as fresh as those tested in-house.
    c. They often do not adhere to quality control standards.
    d. There is a long turnaround time for results.

241. A site of blood collection that is not frequently used, primarily because it is considered painful to the animal, is
    a. Facial vein
    b. Tail vein
    c. Jugular vein
    d. Toenail clip

242. Excess anticoagulant in a blood tube will
    a. Affect red blood cells only
    b. Affect white blood cells only
    c. Affect red blood cells and white blood cells
    d. Not affect the cellular components of blood

243. What is the difference between a red-top Vacutainer and one with a mottled red-and-black top?
    a. One contains diatomaceous earth and the other does not.
    b. One contains silicone and the other does not.
    c. One contains serum separator gel and the other does not.
    d. One contains anticoagulant and the other does not.

244. Which statement concerning EDTA is false?
    a. It is the anticoagulant of choice for hematology.
    b. It is the anticoagulant of choice for blood gas analysis.
    c. It is the anticoagulant found in a lavender-top Vacutainer.
    d. EDTA binds calcium in the plasma.

245. In which group of animals would you normally expect to find nucleated RBCs?
    a. Goat, chicken, snake
    b. Parrot, turkey, iguana
    c. Snake, goose, lamb
    d. Parakeet, calf, turtle

246. Common blood collection sites in the avian patient are the
    a. Saphenous and cephalic veins
    b. Retro orbital and toenail clip
    c. Jugular and cutaneous ulnar veins
    d. Tail and cephalic veins

247. Arterial blood is most commonly used for
    a. Hematology
    b. Blood gases
    c. Blood chemistry
    d. Organ function tests

248. When you view a specimen under a compound microscope using the 40× objective and a 10× ocular, the total magnification of the specimen being viewed is
    a. 4×
    b. 40×
    c. 400×
    d. 4000×

249. Which Vacutainer tube does not need to be inverted after collection of a blood sample?
    a. Lavender top
    b. Green top
    c. Red top
    d. Blue top

250. Nucleated erythrocytes are normally not found in which species?
    a. Avian
    b. Reptilian
    c. Amphibian
    d. Ovine

251. Which pair are both agranulocytes?
    a. Monocytes and neutrophils
    b. Lymphocytes and monocytes
    c. Eosinophils and basophils
    d. Lymphocytes and eosinophils

252. The least common leukocyte found on a normal bovine differential count is a(n)
    a. Neutrophil
    b. Monocyte
    c. Eosinophil
    d. Basophil

253. Macrocytic anemia suggests
    a. Regeneration
    b. Lack of hemoglobin
    c. Iron deficiency
    d. Bone marrow pathology

254. The bone marrow is not a major site of production for what cell type?
    a. Erythrocytes
    b. Lymphocytes
    c. Neutrophils
    d. Eosinophils

255. Looking under a microscope at a blood smear, you see erythrocytes that are elliptical, not nucleated, and lacking central pallor. This blood was most likely collected from a healthy adult
    a. Bird
    b. Horse
    c. Llama
    d. Snake

256. Erythrocyte life spans vary from species to species, but the average is generally considered to be
    a. 60 days
    b. 75 days
    c. 120 days
    d. 180 days

257. The total white blood cell count of a healthy adult dog ranges from
    a. 1000 to 3000/μL
    b. 30,000 to 50,000/μL
    c. 4000 to 8000/μL
    d. 6000 to 17,000/μL

258. Under the microscope you observe a leukocyte that you identify as an eosinophil. The eosinophil cytoplasm contains numerous rod-shaped granules. This blood sample is most likely from a healthy adult
    a. Dog
    b. Cat
    c. Horse
    d. Cow

259. The leukocyte most commonly associated with parasitic and allergic conditions is the
    a. Neutrophil
    b. Monocyte
    c. Lymphocyte
    d. Eosinophil

260. A common finding on a blood smear from an animal with autoimmune hemolytic anemia is
    a. Heinz bodies
    b. Howell-Jolly bodies
    c. Spherocytes
    d. Target cells

261. What test is usually considered of little diagnostic value?
    a. MCV
    b. MCH
    c. MCHC
    d. RDW

262. On a complete blood count (CBC), all of the following findings could be expected in a patient with an infection, except
    a. Neutrophilia
    b. Leukocytosis
    c. Narrow buffy coat
    d. A left shift

Correct answers are on pages 293-323.

263. An elevated hematocrit is most commonly associated with
    a. Polycythemia
    b. Anemia
    c. Dehydration
    d. Leukocytosis

264. The hematology analyzer is not functioning properly. A good mathematical method to estimate hemoglobin is
    a. Two times the PCV
    b. One half the PCV
    c. One third the PCV
    d. Three times the PCV

265. Which erythrocyte count is within the normal reference range for a healthy adult cat?
    a. 35,000/μL
    b. 6,250,000/μL
    c. 7500/μL
    d. 275,000/μL

266. RBC fragments, resulting from shearing of the red blood cells by intravascular trauma, are known as
    a. Acanthocytes
    b. Codocytes
    c. Leptocytes
    d. Schistocytes

267. For which of the following is low-power magnification not used?
    a. To detect the presence of rouleaux
    b. To detect RBC agglutination
    c. To detect clumping of platelets
    d. To estimate platelet numbers

268. Heinz bodies may be a normal finding in up to 5% of the erythrocytes in what species?
    a. Dogs
    b. Cats
    c. Horses
    d. Cows

269. What characteristic is not found in toxic neutrophils?
    a. Howell-Jolly bodies
    b. Vacuolated cytoplasm
    c. Döhle bodies
    d. Basophilic cytoplasm

270. What laboratory test evaluates primary hemostasis?
    a. Activated clotting time
    b. Activated partial thromboplastin time
    c. Buccal mucosal bleeding time
    d. One-step prothrombin time

271. The erythrocyte precursor that has a round, dense to completely pyknotic nucleus is a
    a. Rubricyte
    b. Metarubricyte
    c. Prorubricyte
    d. Rubriblast

272. The precursor cell of a thrombocyte is a
    a. Thromboblast
    b. Megakaryocyte
    c. Metakaryocyte
    d. Prothrombocyte

273. Secondary hemostasis refers to
    a. The coagulation cascade
    b. Vascular spasm
    c. Clot lysis
    d. Platelet plug formation

274. As an erythrocyte develops
    a. The cell size increases.
    b. The cytoplasm becomes bluer in color.
    c. The nucleus becomes larger.
    d. The nuclear chromatin becomes denser.

275. When collecting blood for a coagulation profile, it is especially important to
    a. Use a gray-top Vacutainer
    b. Analyze the sample immediately
    c. Use EDTA as the anticoagulant
    d. Minimize vascular trauma during venipuncture

276. A good presurgical screening test for von Willebrand disease is a(n)
    a. Total platelet count
    b. Buccal mucosal bleeding time
    c. Activated clotting time
    d. Activated partial thromboplastin time

277. The veterinarian must be careful not to injure the sciatic nerve when performing a bone marrow aspirate from which of the following sites?
    a. Wing of the ileum
    b. Proximal femur
    c. Proximal humerus
    d. Proximal tibia

278. Which intracellular parasite appears fairly large, paired, and teardrop-shaped when viewed microscopically?
    a. *Mycoplasma felis (Haemobartonella felis)*
    b. *Anaplasma marginale*
    c. *Babesia canis*
    d. *Ehrlichia canis*

279. An intracellular parasite, which appears as a structure called *morula,* found in the cytoplasm of leukocytes, is
    a. *Babesia*
    b. *Ehrlichia*
    c. *Anaplasma*
    d. *Theileria*

280. Physical signs of hypocoagulation include all of the following, except
    a. Petechiae or ecchymoses
    b. Epistaxis
    c. Hematuria
    d. Thromboembolism

281. The normal myeloid to erythroid ratio on a bone marrow smear is
    a. 1:1
    b. 1:2
    c. 3:1
    d. 2:1

282. What ectoparasite is barely visible to the naked eye?
    a. Ticks
    b. Fleas
    c. Lice
    d. Mites

283. Which of these is a nonburrowing mange mite?
    a. *Notoedres cati*
    b. *Sarcoptes scabiei*
    c. *Psoroptes cuniculi*
    d. *Demodex*

284. What ectoparasite has zoonotic potential?
    a. *Demodex*
    b. *Notoedres*
    c. *Sarcoptes*
    d. *Psoroptes*

285. Which statement regarding *Demodex* is false?
    a. Live mites and/or eggs may be found in skin scrapings.
    b. It is cigar-shaped.
    c. It resides in the hair follicles and sebaceous glands of certain mammals.
    d. It is highly contagious.

286. The genus that is commonly known as the *fur mite* is
    a. *Cheyletiella* spp.
    b. *Trixacarus* spp.
    c. *Psoroptes* spp.
    d. *Notoedres* spp.

287. The sarcoptic mange mite of the guinea pig is
    a. *Sarcoptes caviae*
    b. *Trixacarus caviae*
    c. *Notoedres caviae*
    d. *Psoroptes caviae*

288. What tick is a soft tick?
    a. *Amblyomma*
    b. *Dermacentor*
    c. *Ixodes*
    d. *Otobius*

289. Which of the following parasite ova is collected using a cellophane tape technique?
    a. *Ancylostoma*
    b. *Dirofilaria*
    c. *Dipylidium*
    d. *Oxyuris*

290. What tick is the vector for Lyme disease?
    a. *Argas persicus*
    b. *Ixodes scapularis*
    c. *Otobius megninii*
    d. *Rhipicephalus sanguineus*

291. It is possible to differentiate between sucking lice and chewing lice by which of the following features?
    a. Chewing lice have antennae, whereas sucking lice do not.
    b. Chewing lice are dorsoventrally flattened, whereas sucking lice are laterally flattened.
    c. Chewing lice have three pairs of legs, whereas sucking lice have four pairs of legs.
    d. Chewing lice have a head that is broader than the thorax, whereas sucking lice have a head that is narrower than the thorax.

292. An ectoparasite known both for its host specificity and site specificity is the
    a. Louse
    b. Mite
    c. Tick
    d. Flea

293. The parasite that is distinguished by white, operculated eggs that are cemented to the hairs of its host is the
    a. Tick
    b. Flea
    c. Mite
    d. Louse

Correct answers are on pages 293-323.

294. A buffy coat examination for microfilaria can be made in conjunction with what other hematologic procedure?
    a. Leukocyte count
    b. Packed cell volume
    c. Differential count
    d. Hemoglobin

295. What can the ELISA heartworm test detect that the Difil cannot?
    a. Dipetalonema
    b. Occult infection
    c. Microfilaria
    d. Anemia

296. A local dairy farmer has just acquired some livestock from Louisiana and is concerned that they may have *Fasciola hepatica*. What fecal examination method will give you the best chance of finding the eggs of this parasite?
    a. Sedimentation
    b. Centrifugal flotation
    c. Simple flotation
    d. Direct smear

297. In what host do the sexually mature adult parasites live?
    a. Definitive
    b. Intermediate
    c. Transport
    d. Secondary

298. Unlike a histologic section, a wet mount of parasite eggs is three-dimensional, therefore when examining the slide under the microscope, you must
    a. Lower the condenser all the way down to see all objects.
    b. Close the iris diaphragm to be able to view all objects.
    c. Continually adjust the focus to view all objects.
    d. Use the highest power objective to view all objects.

299. Occult heartworm infections occur in approximately 90% of
    a Dogs
    b Horses
    c Cats
    d Humans

300. What major disadvantage is common to both the direct smear and fecal sedimentation methods of fecal examination?
    a. Neither is a concentrating method.
    b. They both test a very small sample only.
    c. Fecal debris will make microscopic examination difficult.
    d. Both are more time consuming to perform than standard flotation methods.

301. The modified Knott technique for microfilaria has what two additives for ease of heartworm diagnosis?
    a. Alcohol and Gram stain
    b. Formalin and new methylene blue stain
    c. Wright stain and formalin
    d. New methylene blue and Wright stain

302. An animal that tested positive for heartworm infection might also have an elevation of which of the following blood cells?
    a. Leukocytes
    b. Lymphocytes
    c. Eosinophils
    d. Monocytes

303. Tapeworm infections are most often diagnosed in small animals by which of the following methods?
    a. Centrifugal fecal flotation
    b. Simple fecal flotation
    c. Direct smear
    d. Gross examination

304. The least sensitive diagnostic technique for finding microfilariae is
    a. Direct examination of blood
    b. Buffy coat method
    c. Modified Knott technique
    d. Difil test

305. What pair of parasites differs in morphology and size?
    a. *Trichuris* spp. versus *Capillaria* spp.
    b. *Dipetalonema* versus *Dirofilaria microfilaria*
    c. *Toxocara canis* versus *Toxocara cati*
    d. *Ancylostoma* versus *Toxascaris*

306. What is not a concentration method for parasite ova detection?
    a. Fecal flotation
    b. Centrifugation
    c. Sedimentation
    d. Direct smear

307. Fecal specimens should be examined routinely with what objective?
    a. 4×
    b. 10×
    c. 40×
    d. 100×

308. What is the minimum number of minutes a fecal flotation should stand before examination?
    a. 5 minutes
    b. 10 minutes
    c. 20 minutes
    d. 30 minutes

309. The instrument specifically designed to collect a fecal sample directly from the animal's rectum is a
    a. Fecal extractor
    b. Fecal spoon
    c. Fecal loop
    d. Fecal scoop

310. In what analysis could heartworm microfilariae appear as an incidental finding?
    a. Differential cell count
    b. Modified Knott test
    c. Difil test
    d. ELISA test

311. The fecal solution most likely to be successful in detecting *Giardia* cysts is
    a. Sodium chloride
    b. Sodium nitrate
    c. Zinc sulfate
    d. Physiologic saline

312. What is the main reason that flotation solutions with specific gravities over 1.300 are not commonly used?
    a. As very saturated solutions, they are difficult to make.
    b. They would distort ova.
    c. They would be prohibitively expensive.
    d. It is not necessary, because all ova have a specific gravity lower than 1.300.

313. A 4-year-old dog has a chronic cough and the veterinarian has included *Filaroides* on his list of possible diagnoses. What is the common name of this parasite?
    a. Tapeworm
    b. Roundworm
    c. Whipworm
    d. Lungworm

314. Which of the following nematodes are characterized by an ovoid egg with a thin shell and a morulated embryo?
    a. *Toxascaris leonine*
    b. *Toxocara canis*
    c. *Trichuris vulpis*
    d. *Ancylostoma caninum*

315. What is a proper lens cleaner to use for the care and maintenance of a compound microscope?
    a. Saline
    b. Xylene
    c. Hydrogen peroxide
    d. Sodium bicarbonate

316. A cytologic sample collected with a cotton swab should be applied to a microscope slide with a ___ action.
    a. Smearing
    b. Rolling
    c. Dabbing
    d. Rubbing

317. Fluid samples collected through fine-needle aspiration should be collected into
    a. An EDTA tube
    b. A heparinized syringe
    c. A clot tube
    d. A citrate tube

318. Preparation for fine-needle aspirate of a joint or body cavity would include
    a. Preparation as for venipuncture
    b. Washing the area with sterile water
    c. Preparation as for surgery
    d. Washing the area with physiologic saline

319. A method for diagnosing *Cheyletiella* is
    a. Tissue biopsy
    b. Fungal culture
    c. Fine-needle aspirate
    d. Cellophane tape method

320. A Wood's lamp is used to examine an animal for the presence of
    a. *Demodex*
    b. Scabies
    c. Ringworm
    d. Pinworm

321. When using Diff-Quik to stain bone marrow smears, it is especially important to
    a. Use freshly filtered stain
    b. Dip the smear twice as long as blood smears
    c. Rinse thoroughly with distilled water
    d. Let the smear dry for 30 minutes before staining

Correct answers are on pages 293-323.

322. The normal numbers of erythrocytes and leukocytes in urine sediment do not exceed
    a. 1 per high-power field
    b. 3 to 5 per high-power field
    c. 5 to 10 per high-power field
    d. More than 10 per high-power field

323. The ability of the renal tubules to concentrate or dilute a urine sample is assessed by what component of the urinalysis?
    a. pH
    b. Volume
    c. Specific gravity
    d. Examination of the sediment

324. The largest of the epithelial cells found in urine are the
    a. Squamous epithelial cells
    b. Caudate epithelial cells
    c. Transitional epithelial cells
    d. Renal epithelial cells

325. The most common uroliths found in feline and canine urine are
    a. Struvite
    b. Calcium oxalate
    c. Urate
    d. Cystine

326. The best method of urine collection to assess the patency of the urethra is
    a. Catheterization
    b. Manual expression
    c. Free catch
    d. Cystocentesis

327. Which of the following statements regarding casts is false?
    a. A few hyaline or granular casts may be seen in normal urine.
    b. All casts are cylindric with parallel sides.
    c. Casts dissolve in acidic urine.
    d. Casts may be disrupted with high-speed centrifugation and rough sample handling.

328. What change would not be seen in stale urine?
    a. Bacterial overgrowth
    b. Decrease in pH
    c. Cellular degeneration
    d. Cast degeneration

329. Puddin, a 2-year-old castrated male domestic shorthair cat, was missing for 5 days before coming home. His owners were very concerned that he appeared weak and tired, so they brought him to the clinic. You find on initial physical examination that he is significantly dehydrated. You are not at all surprised when you find that his urine specific gravity is
    a. 1.002
    b. 1.012
    c. 1.030
    d. 1.060

330. Lipuria is seen most commonly in what species?
    a. Dogs
    b. Cats
    c. Horses
    d. Cows

331. Bilirubinuria is considered a normal finding in what species?
    a. Dogs
    b. Cats
    c. Horses
    d. Sheep

332. Sadie, a 17-year-old spayed female domestic shorthair cat, is in the final stages of chronic renal failure. On presentation, you expect to find that her urine specific gravity will probably be
    a. 1.002
    b. 1.012
    c. 1.030
    d. 1.060

333. Which of the following tests is considered accurate when using colorimetric dip sticks for biochemical testing?
    a. Leukocytes
    b. Specific gravity
    c. pH
    d. Nitrites

334. What method of urine sample collection would not be associated with traumatic hematuria?
    a. Catheterization
    b. Manual expression
    c. Free catch
    d. Cystocentesis

335. Casts associated with chronic, severe degeneration of the renal tubules that appear smooth and refractile with squared ends are ___ casts.
    a. Hyaline
    b. Granular
    c. Fatty
    d. Waxy

336. A normal adult horse would most likely have a urinary pH of
    a. 5.5
    b. 6.5
    c. 7.0
    d. 7.5

337. Sasha, a 11-year-old spayed female domestic shorthair cat, was accidentally overhydrated with IV fluids. You would expect her urine specific gravity to be
    a. 1.002
    b. 1.012
    c. 1.030
    d. 1.060

338. Ketonuria is most commonly associated with what condition?
    a. Liver disease
    b. Urinary tract infection
    c. Renal failure
    d. Diabetes mellitus

339. Hoover was diagnosed with a urinary tract infection 2 weeks ago and was put on a course of amoxicillin. The veterinarian has asked that he return for a recheck to make sure the infection has resolved. The collection method of choice in this patient would be
    a. Catheterization
    b. Free catch
    c. Cystocentesis
    d. Manual expression

340. Leukocytes in the urine sediment and a positive nitrite reaction on the urinary colorimetric strip give presumptive evidence that the patient may have a
    a. Neoplasm
    b. Diabetic condition
    c. Renal failure
    d. Bacterial infection

341. Aged urine samples left at room temperature and exposed to UV light may cause a false negative result in which of the following biochemical tests?
    a. Ketones
    b. Protein
    c. Glucose
    d. Bilirubin

342. The best sample to examine for specific gravity of canine urine is the
    a. First morning sample
    b. Midday sample
    c. Late afternoon sample
    d. Last sample of the day

343. Mr. Downing has brought in a urine sample from Cleo, his 6-year-old female spayed Cocker spaniel. The color of the urine appears red. On centrifugation of the sample, you find that the supernatant is now clear. Most likely the red color was due to
    a. Hemoglobinuria
    b. Hematuria
    c. Myoglobinuria
    d. Uroglobinuria

344. Struvite crystals are composed of
    a. Calcium potassium carbonates
    b. Magnesium ammonium phosphates
    c. Oxalates
    d. Urates

345. Which statement regarding catheterization in female dogs is false?
    a. Catheterization is technically difficult in female dogs.
    b. Catheterization may introduce bacteria into the urinary tract.
    c. Catheterization may cause gross or microscopic hematuria.
    d. Catheterization is often better tolerated by the dog than cystocentesis.

346. Urinary pH is not affected by the
    a. Patient's diet
    b. Presence of bacteria in the urine
    c. Patient's acid–base status
    d. Presence of crystals in the urine

347. Squamous epithelial cells are not normally seen in urine samples obtained by
    a. Catheterization
    b. Manual expression
    c. Free catch
    d. Cystocentesis

348. The two most common problems encountered in samples to be evaluated for clinical chemistry are
    a. Coagulation and separation
    b. Dilution and concentration
    c. Hemolysis and lipemia
    d. EDTA and heparin

349. Uric acid is the major nitrogenous waste in
    a. Cattle
    b. Horses
    c. Birds
    d. Dogs

Correct answers are on pages 293-323.

350. Which of the following statements regarding creatinine is false?
    a. It is an indicator of the glomerular filtration rate.
    b. It is produced as a result of normal muscle metabolism.
    c. It is a less reliable indicator of renal function than BUN.
    d. It is usually evaluated in conjunction with the BUN and urine specific gravity.

351. A good initial urinary screening test for suspected Cushing disease is
    a. Endogenous ACTH
    b. Low-dose dexamethasone suppression test
    c. ACTH stimulation
    d. Cortisol/creatinine ratio

352. Proteins that induce chemical changes in other substances but are not changed themselves are called
    a. Activators
    b. Buffers
    c. Enzymes
    d. Substrates

353. What biochemical tests are not considered part of a primary hepatic profile?
    a. BUN and creatinine
    b. Cholestatic enzymes
    c. Hepatocellular leakage enzymes
    d. Total protein and albumin

354. The total serum protein is 7.3 g/dl and the albumin is 3.5 g/dl. What are the globulin value and the A/G ratio, respectively?
    a. 2.09 g/dl, 1.67
    b. 3.8 g/dl, 0.92
    c. 10.8 g/dl, 1.09
    d. 14.6 g/dl, 1.35

355. A fecal smear can be stained for fat. An increased amount of fat is indicative of
    a. Dyschezia
    b. Dysentery
    c. Steatorrhea
    d. Tenesmus

356. Which is the correct method to use when performing a serum bile acids assay?
    a. Draw a blood sample on a fasting animal.
    b. Draw a blood sample on an animal immediately after it eats a meal.
    c. Draw a blood sample on a fasting animal and another sample 2 hours later.
    d. Draw a blood sample on a fasting animal, feed the animal, and draw another sample 2 hours later.

357. The stain used to stain undigested fecal starch is
    a. New methylene blue
    b. Lugol iodine
    c. Sudan
    d. Gentian violet

358. The current test of choice for evaluating liver function is
    a. Ammonia assay
    b. Bile acids
    c. Bilirubin
    d. Alanine aminotransferase

359. The main function of bicarbonate is to
    a. Maintain the proper osmotic pressure of fluids in the body
    b. Maintain normal muscular function
    c. Maintain normal cardiac rhythm and contractility
    d. Maintain balanced body pH levels

360. A box of reagents for blood chemistry analysis labeled for storage at 8° C should be stored
    a. In the freezer
    b. At room temperature
    c. In the refrigerator
    d. In the incubator

361. Phosphorus concentrations in the body are usually inversely related to the concentration of what substance?
    a. Calcium
    b. Magnesium
    c. Potassium
    d. Sodium

362. Cholesterol and triglycerides are plasma
    a. Proteins
    b. Lipids
    c. Enzymes
    d. Electrolytes

363. It is importance for the body to maintain the blood pH at a constant level to maximize function of all body systems. Normal blood pH is
    a. 6.8
    b. 7.0
    c. 7.2
    d. 7.4

364. Which squares of the Neubauer hemocytometer are used to count leukocytes?
   a. All nine large squares
   b. All 25 small squares of the central primary square
   c. Four small corner squares and the small central square of the central primary square
   d. Four small squares of the central primary square

365. Which squares of the Neubauer hemocytometer are used to count platelets?
   a. All nine large squares
   b. All 25 small squares of the central primary square
   c. Four small corner squares and the small central square of the central primary square
   d. Four small squares of the central primary square

366. Heterophils in the avian species are the equivalent of the mammalian
   a. Monocytes
   b. Eosinophils
   c. Neutrophils
   d. Basophils

367. If eosinophil Unopettes are available, they can be used to indirectly determine the total count of avian
   a. White blood cells
   b. Red blood cells
   c. Platelets
   d. Heterophils

368. Kidney disease results in accumulation of metabolic waste in the blood, a condition known as
   a. Azotemia
   b. Bilirubinemia
   c. Hypernatremia
   d. Hyperkalemia

369. *Prerenal azotemia* refers to
   a. Increases in BUN resulting from severe renal disease
   b. Decreases in BUN resulting from severe renal disease
   c. Increases in BUN resulting from dehydration, shock, and/or decreased blood flow to the kidneys
   d. Increases in BUN resulting from inability to urinate

370. An example of specific immunity would be
   a. Mucociliary escalator
   b. Fine hairs in the trachea
   c. IgM antibodies to toxoplasmosis
   d. Nasal secretions

371. What blood cell is also known as a *PMN*?
   a. Basophil
   b. Eosinophil
   c. Neutrophil
   d. Monocyte

372. The most common urine crystal seen in horses and rabbits is
   a. Calcium oxalate
   b. Calcium carbonate
   c. Triple phosphate
   d. Ammonium biurate

373. For determining specific gravity values, what is the order, from most reliable to least reliable method?
   a. Urinometer, refractometer, reagent test strip
   b. Refractometer, reagent test strip, urinometer
   c. Reagent test strip, urinometer, refractometer
   d. Refractometer, urinometer, reagent test strip

374. Which of the following crystals is most likely to be found in the urine of an animal with ethylene glycol toxicity?
   a. Ammonium biurate
   b. Tyrosine
   c. Triple phosphate
   d. Calcium oxalate

375. What species has multiple forms of reticulocytes?
   a. Horse
   b. Cow
   c. Cat
   d. Dog

376. *Postrenal azotemia* refers to
   a. Increases in BUN resulting from severe renal disease
   b. Increases in BUN resulting from an inability to urinate
   c. Decreases in BUN resulting from severe renal disease
   d. Increases in BUN resulting from dehydration

377. A glucose tolerance test is used to help diagnose
   a. Cushing disease
   b. Hypothyroidism
   c. Addison disease
   d. Diabetes mellitus

378. Which white blood cell is known as "the first line of defense" after a microorganism has entered the body?
   a. Eosinophil
   b. Lymphocyte
   c. Monocyte
   d. Neutrophil

Correct answers are on pages 293-323.

379. A California mastitis test
     a. Measures leukocytes in the milk of each quarter
     b. Measures trypsin-like factor in the milk of each quarter
     c. Measures bacterial cells in the whole milk of the udder
     d. Measures cellular nuclear protein in the whole milk of the udder

380. What is the best method to obtain a sample when attempting to determine whether dermatophytes are present?
     a. Take hair from the periphery of the lesion.
     b. Make an impression smear of the entire lesion.
     c. Take hair from the center of the lesion.
     d. Perform a skin scrape from the center of the lesion.

381. The anticoagulant of choice for avian and reptile hematology is
     a. Potassium oxalate
     b. Lithium heparin
     c. Sodium citrate
     d. Sodium fluoride

382. The red-top Vacutainer tube should sit at room temperature for ___ before centrifugation, allowing the clot to form.
     a. 5 minutes
     b. 30 minutes
     c. 1 hour
     d. 0 minutes (No clot will form.)

383. Which of these tubes must never be placed on a blood rocker after being filled with blood?
     a. Blue top
     b. Green top
     c. Purple top
     d. Red top

384. Once blood has formed a clot, you can reverse this process by
     a. Adding anticoagulant
     b. Vigorous mixing
     c. There is no reversal
     d. Adding isotonic saline

385. If you are unable to perform a CBC within 1 hour of blood collection, which of the following is the best method of preservation?
     a. Freeze the sample
     b. Spin down the sample, refrigerate cells, and freeze serum
     c. Add formalin to the sample
     d. Refrigerate the sample

386. The mucin clot test is performed on
     a. Joint fluid
     b. Plasma
     c. Serum
     d. Urine

387. If a 1:1 dilution of a serum sample is made before analyzing the serum chemistries, the results must be multiplied by
     a. One
     b. Two
     c. Ten
     d. One hundred

388. Which of these is least likely to interfere with blood chemistry test results?
     a. Postprandial serum
     b. Icteric serum
     c. Fasting serum
     d. Hemolyzed serum

389. Which of the following statements is true in regard to using hemolyzed serum in a dry chemistry analyzer?
     a. Hemolyzed serum can falsely elevate some results.
     b. Hemolyzed serum can falsely decrease some results.
     c. Hemolyzed serum is corrected by adding saline.
     d. Hemolyzed serum is corrected by adding sterile water.

390. The Ictotest is used to determine
     a. Ketonuria
     b. Bile salts in urine
     c. Bilirubinuria
     d. Proteinuria

391. When preparing cytology samples for microscopic evaluation, what is the best technique to use?
     a. Wet prep
     b. Squash prep
     c. Modified Knott prep
     d. Willis prep

392. Transmission of coccidia occurs by
     a. Ingesting oocysts
     b. Direct bodily contact
     c. Transmammary transmission
     d. Transplacental transmission

393. The period of time when a bitch is receptive to the male is classified as
     a. Metestrus
     b. Proestrus
     c. Anestrus
     d. Estrus

394. Which of the following would be considered an abnormal finding on healthy canine external ear canal cytology?
    a. Cerumen
    b. Epithelial cells
    c. *Malassezia*
    d. Debris

395. The average estrous cycle of the dog lasts ___ days.
    a. 21
    b. 16
    c. 9
    d. 3

396. The main function of the neutrophil is
    a. Phagocytosis
    b. Hypersensitivity reaction
    c. Allergic reaction
    d. Immune response

397. The main function of the eosinophil is
    a. Phagocytosis
    b. Autoimmune reaction
    c. Allergic reaction
    d. Immune reaction

398. What information do the RBC indices yield?
    a. The size, weight, and hemoglobin concentration of an average RBC
    b. The combined size, weight, and hemoglobin concentration of all RBCs
    c. The specific type of anemia present
    d. The packed cell volume

399. Where on the blood smear would you select to start your WBC differential count?
    a. Thickest area
    b. Feathered edge
    c. Monocellular layer
    d. Thinnest area

400. In which of the following species is rouleaux formation common?
    a. Rats
    b. Dogs
    c. Horses
    d. Pigs

401. Döhle bodies are found in what type of blood cell?
    a. Erythrocyte
    b. Neutrophil
    c. Platelet
    d. Nucleated RBC

402. *Anaplasma marginale* is a blood parasite that causes severe anemia in what species?
    a. Reptilian
    b. Avian
    c. Canine
    d. Bovine

403. Given a PCV of 42%, which of the following is the estimated hemoglobin value?
    a. 7 g/dl
    b. 6 g/dl
    c. 14 g/dl
    d. 12 g/dl

404. When counting cells on the hemacytometer, what cells are not counted?
    a. Those on the top and bottom borders
    b. Those on the left and right borders
    c. Those on the left and top borders
    d. Those on the right and bottom borders

405. In addition to birds, which one of the following animals also has white blood cells called *heterophils*?
    a. Llamas
    b. Potbellied pigs
    c. Ferrets
    d. Reptiles

406. Given a WBC count of 10,000/µL and a relative value of 65% neutrophils, calculate the absolute value of neutrophils.
    a. 65/µL
    b. 6500/µL
    c. 650/µL
    d. 65,000/µL

407. In what species are the platelets normally larger than the red blood cells?
    a. Bovine
    b. Canine
    c. Equine
    d. Feline

408. What species has both punctate and aggregate forms of reticulocytes in peripheral blood smears?
    a. Canine
    b. Porcine
    c. Feline
    d. Bovine

409. What would be considered a normal WBC count for a healthy adult horse?
    a. 30×10^3/µl
    b. 8×10^3/µl
    c. 3×10^6/µl
    d. 8×10^6/µl

Correct answers are on pages 293-323.

410. The Unopette system for counting white blood cells uses what diluent?
    a. 0.85% saline
    b. Distilled water
    c. 9% hydrochloric acid
    d. 1% ammonium oxalate

411. The term for red blood cell formation is
    a. Hematopoiesis
    b. Erythropoiesis
    c. Hematopoietin
    d. Leukopoiesis

412. Which list has the cells listed from most immature to most mature?
    a. Rubricyte, reticulocyte, rubriblast, erythrocyte
    b. Rubriblast, reticulocyte, rubricyte, erythrocyte
    c. Rubriblast, rubricyte, reticulocyte, erythrocyte
    d. Reticulocyte, rubriblast, rubricyte, erythrocyte

413. What diagnostic test is used to diagnose autoimmune hemolytic anemia?
    a. Red cell fragility test
    b. Modified Knott
    c. Coombs
    d. Coggins

414. What Vacutainer tube yields plasma via centrifugation?
    a. Red top
    b. Red/black mottled top
    c. Green/gray mottled top
    d. Yellow top

415. In the Gram-stain procedure, which of these is the appropriate staining sequence?
    a. Crystal violet, decolorizer, iodine, safranin
    b. Iodine, crystal violet, decolorizer, safranin
    c. Safranin, iodine, decolorizer, crystal violet
    d. Crystal violet, iodine, decolorizer, safranin

416. Incubation time to grow aerobic bacteria is typically
    a. 6 hours
    b. 12 hours
    c. 24 hours
    d. 48 hours

417. Which of the following is an example of a selective medium?
    a. MacConkey
    b. Mueller-Hinton
    c. Trypticase soy agar with 5% sheep blood
    d. Trypticase soy agar

418. Trypticase soy agar with 5% sheep blood is used
    a. As an enrichment medium
    b. To show hemolytic reactions
    c. To select for *Staphylococcus* spp.
    d. To inhibit growth of *Salmonella* spp.

419. The Fungassay test medium is selective for what organism?
    a. *Trichophyton*
    b. *Trichuris*
    c. *Toxoplasma*
    d. *Tritrichomonas*

420. Chocolate agar is used predominantly to grow
    a. *Proteus vulgaris*
    b. *Escherichia coli*
    c. *Microsporum gypseum*
    d. *Brucella abortus*

421. The causative agent of Lyme disease is
    a. *Bordetella bronchiseptica*
    b. *Borrelia burgdorferi*
    c. *Moraxella bovis*
    d. *Mycoplasma pulmonis*

422. Which of these ectoparasites is zoonotic?
    a. *Demodex*
    b. *Cnemidocoptes*
    c. *Sarcoptes*
    d. *Otodectes*

423. Which of the following mites is commonly found in rabbits and large animals?
    a. *Cnemidocoptes*
    b. *Sarcoptes*
    c. *Psoroptes*
    d. *Otodectes*

424. What endoparasite larva causes creeping eruptions in humans?
    a. Whipworm
    b. Tapeworm
    c. Pinworm
    d. Hookworm

425. What parasite can cause blockage of the cranial mesenteric artery in horses?
    a. *Parascaris equi*
    b. *Oxyuris equi*
    c. *Strongyloides westeri*
    d. *Strongylus vulgaris*

426. Lyme disease is transmitted via
    a. Deer tick
    b. Lone star tick
    c. American dog tick
    d. Brown dog tick

427. Pollakiuria is
   a. Urinating frequently, small volume voided
   b. Complete lack of urine production
   c. Excessive drinking and urinating
   d. Excessive urination at night

428. It is important to keep cytology samples and unstained slides away from ___ so the samples can later be stained properly.
   a. Acetone
   b. Ether
   c. Formalin
   d. Saline

429. A renal cast is
   a. Glycoprotein mold of the renal tubules
   b. Calculi formed in the urinary tract
   c. Crystals stuck together
   d. Calculi formed in the renal medulla

430. The normal pH of an omnivore is generally
   a. Acidic
   b. Alkaline
   c. Neutral
   d. Paradoxical

431. What is the name of the time period between the ingestion of the infective stage of a parasite and the passing of eggs from the adult parasite in the feces?
   a. Pubescent
   b. Prepatent
   c. Paratenic
   d. Vector

432. What protozoan disease causes an ascending paralysis in young dogs and abortion in cattle?
   a. Cryptosporidiosis
   b. EEE
   c. Neosporosis
   d. Brucellosis

433. Cysts of what organism may be seen on a fecal flotation?
   a. *Giardia*
   b. *Mycoplasma (Haemobartonella)*
   c. *Toxoplasmosis*
   d. *Trichomonas*

434. What is a tick-borne organism found in dogs?
   a. *Toxoplasma*
   b. *Isospora*
   c. *Ehrlichia*
   d. *Cryptosporidium*

435. Which of the following terms refers to an infestation with lice?
   a. Myiasis
   b. Acariasis
   c. Paraphimosis
   d. Pediculosis

436. What does the occult heartworm test actually detect?
   a. Microfilariae
   b. L3 larvae
   c. Antibodies
   d. Immature female heartworms

437. What mite is the most damaging to cattle?
   a. *Sarcoptes*
   b. *Chorioptes*
   c. *Psoroptes*
   d. *Demodex*

438. Which of the following is a tapeworm seen in horses?
   a. *Acanthocephala*
   b. *Oxyuris*
   c. *Moniezia*
   d. *Anoplocephala*

439. A skin scraping is used to diagnose what parasite?
   a. *Bovicola*
   b. *Notoedres*
   c. *Otodectes*
   d. *Ctenocephalides*

440. Which of the following is the largest intermediate form of a tapeworm?
   a. Cysticercus
   b. Hydatid cyst
   c. Coenurus
   d. Cysticercoid

441. What protozoan parasite causes a venereal disease in cattle?
   a. *Trypanosoma*
   b. *Giardia*
   c. *Tritrichomonas*
   d. *Babesia*

442. What parasite uses snails as intermediate hosts?
   a. *Toxocara*
   b. *Paragonimus*
   c. *Taenia*
   d. *Dipetalonema*

Correct answers are on pages 293-323.

443. What equine parasite produces microfilariae, which causes patchy alopecia and depigmentation?
    a. *Onchocerca*
    b. *Oxyuris*
    c. *Habronema*
    d. *Psoroptes*

444. What heartworm diagnostic test uses a concentration technique that increases the chance of seeing microfilariae?
    a. Agglutination test
    b. ELISA test
    c. Direct (wet mount)
    d. Filtration test (Difil)

445. What canine parasite causes nodules in the esophagus, which may then become neoplastic?
    a. *Physaloptera*
    b. *Filaroides*
    c. *Spirocirca*
    d. *Neosporum*

446. Which of the following parasites is not zoonotic?
    a. *Toxoplasma*
    b. *Echinococcus*
    c. *Dipylidium*
    d. *Giardia*

447. Observing a "zippy" motility in fresh feces is used to help diagnose the presence of what parasite?
    a. *Toxoplasma*
    b. *Mycoplasma (Haemobartonella)*
    c. *Tritrichomonas*
    d. *Alaria*

448. What fly is responsible for the greatest economic losses in U.S. cattle?
    a. Face fly
    b. Stable fly
    c. Screw worm fly
    d. Horn fly

449. What parasite causes malaria?
    a. *Babesia*
    b. *Trypanosoma*
    c. *Plasmodium*
    d. *Anaplasma*

450. What fecal floatation solution is recommended when looking for *Giardia* cysts?
    a. Saturated sugar
    b. Sodium nitrate
    c. Zinc sulfate
    d. Saturated salt

451. Visceral larval migrans is caused by the larvae of
    a. *Ancylostoma caninum*
    b. *Isospora canis*
    c. *Toxocara canis*
    d. *Taenia canis*

452. Proglottids are produced by what parasite?
    a. Fluke
    b. Tick
    c. Mite
    d. Tapeworm

453. What lungworm is found in cats?
    a. *Dictyocaulus*
    b. *Capillaria plica*
    c. *Filaroides osleri*
    d. *Capillaria aerophila*

454. What is the *least* likely way of transmitting *Toxoplasma* to a human?
    a. Ingesting ova from cat feces
    b. Drinking contaminated water
    c. Skin penetration
    d. Eating undercooked contaminated meat

455. The fecal sedimentation technique is often needed to diagnose the presence of what bovine parasite?
    a. *Dictyocaulus viviparous*
    b. *Fasciola hepatica*
    c. *Moniezia* sp.
    d. *Strongyloides westeri*

456. What small animal parasite ova resemble strongyle ova in horses?
    a. Ascarid
    b. Whipworm
    c. Hookworm
    d. Coccidia

457. Stomach bots are common in horses, but where are bots found in sheep?
    a. Small intestine
    b. Nasal passages
    c. Rumen
    d. Perianal region

458. Occult heartworm infections are those in which
    a. Microfilariae are absent
    b. L3 larvae are absent
    c. Adults are absent
    d. Antibodies are absent

459. What parasite causes blood loss, especially in young animals?
    a. Roundworm
    b. Tapeworm
    c. Heartworm
    d. Hookworm

460. What parasite causes a very pruritic disease in dogs?
    a. *Cheyletiella*
    b. *Sarcoptes*
    c. *Demodex*
    d. *Dermacentor*

461. Myiasis is an infestation of
    a. Flies
    b. Mites
    c. Ticks
    d. Lice

462. What causes the sensitivity of the occult heartworm test to decrease?
    a. No microfilariae present
    b. Female worms only
    c. Male worms only
    d. No clinical signs

463. Which statement is true about *Dirofilaria* infection in the cat?
    a. The life span of heartworms in cats is shorter than in dogs.
    b. Microfilariae are commonly seen in cat infections.
    c. Adult worm burden in cats is similar in numbers to dogs.
    d. *Dirofilaria* causes a severe anemia in cats.

464. An elevated hematocrit can indicate what situation is present?
    a. Hyperglycemia
    b. Anemia
    c. Dehydration
    d. Leukocytosis

465. What is seen in a degenerative left shift?
    a. Leukocytosis
    b. No bands are present.
    c. Lymphocytes outnumber neutrophils.
    d. Bands outnumber mature neutrophils.

466. Which of the following is another term for *icterus*?
    a. Jaundice
    b. Xanthochromia
    c. Ketonemia
    d. Hemoglobinuria

467. What is the function of the megakaryocyte?
    a. Phagocytosis
    b. Produces granulocytes
    c. Produces thrombocytes
    d. Produces plasma cells

468. A normal leukocyte count with an increase in immature PMNs that outnumber the mature PMNs is
    a. Reticulocytosis
    b. Leukopenia
    c. Regenerative left shift
    d. Degenerative left shift

469. What does not occur as you change from the low-power objective to the high-power objective when using a microscope?
    a. The field becomes brighter.
    b. The field of view is smaller.
    c. The image is magnified.
    d. More details are seen.

470. A leukocyte count will be falsely elevated by which of the following in the peripheral blood?
    a. Spherocytosis
    b. Reticulocytes
    c. Metarubricytes
    d. Bands

471. The average canine erythrocyte is often used as a ruler to estimate the sizes of other cells. What is the average diameter of an adult canine red blood cell?
    a. 20 microns
    b. 7 microns
    c. 12 microns
    d. 3 microns

472. What is not associated with a responsive anemia?
    a. Poikilocytosis
    b. Reticulocytosis
    c. Anisocytosis
    d. Polychromasia

473. An antigen epitope is made up of uniquely shaped
    a. Amino acids
    b. Carbohydrates
    c. Cells
    d. Fatty acids

474. The precursor cell to a plasma cell is the
    a. Thymocyte
    b. T cell
    c. Blast cell
    d. B cell

Correct answers are on pages 293-323.

475. The refractometer is used to determine
    a. Hematocrit
    b. Total protein
    c. Hemoglobin
    d. Erythrocyte count

476. What mineral is found in hemoglobin?
    a. Iodine
    b. Calcium
    c. Magnesium
    d. Iron

477. What erythrocyte index gives an indication of the average size of a red blood cell?
    a. MCHC
    b. MCV
    c. M/E ratio
    d. Reticulocyte count

478. What is the most immature cell in the granulocyte series?
    a. Megakaryoblast
    b. Leukoblast
    c. Myeloblast
    d. Progranuloblast

479. A pleomorphic nucleus has
    a. Many colors
    b. Many shapes
    c. Many nucleoli
    d. Undergone many divisions

480. What large cell with multiple separate nuclei is found in bone marrow?
    a. Osteoclast
    b. Megakaryocyte
    c. Osteoblast
    d. Monoblast

481. What marrow finding is consistent with a responsive anemia?
    a. Myeloid hypoplasia
    b. Erythroid hyperplasia
    c. Erythroid hypoplasia
    d. Myeloid metaplasia

482. In a normal marrow sample, what cell should be the most immature?
    a. Prorubricyte
    b. Metamyelocyte
    c. Rubricyte
    d. Myelocyte

483. What test is used to confirm a diagnosis of warfarin (rodenticide) toxicity?
    a. Thrombocyte count
    b. Calcium level
    c. One-step prothrombin time
    d. Partial thromboplastin time

484. What is not seen in a DIC?
    a. Icterus
    b. Hemorrhage
    c. Thrombocytopenia
    d. Prolonged activated clotting time

485. What clotting disorder is stimulated by hypothyroidism?
    a. Hemophilia A
    b. Von Willebrand disease
    c. Disseminated intravascular coagulation
    d. Coumarin toxicity

486. What substance is the final product in the coagulation pathway?
    a. Thrombin
    b. Plasmin
    c. Factor VII
    d. Fibrin

487. Which of the following is a typical specific gravity for dilute porcine urine?
    a. 0.010
    b. 3.055
    c. 1.035
    d. 1.010

488. In what species is ketonuria most commonly found?
    a. Canine
    b. Feline
    c. Equine
    d. Bovine

489. What is the smallest epithelial cell seen on a urine sediment examination?
    a. Leukocyte
    b. Transitional cell
    c. Renal cell
    d. Squamous cell

490. In order for a cast to form, what must be present in the filtrate?
    a. Erythrocyte
    b. Glucose
    c. Protein
    d. Ketones

491. What species has a grossly lobulated kidney?
    a. Bovine
    b. Canine
    c. Equine
    d. Feline

492. In order for glycosuria to occur, which of the following must also be present?
    a. Uremia
    b. Hyperglycemia
    c. Ketonemia
    d. Azoturia

493. Urine specific gravity is actually a measure of which of the following?
    a. Liver function
    b. Renal glomerular function
    c. Renal tubular function
    d. Bladder function

494. What is becoming a common type of urolith in cats?
    a. Oxalate
    b. Silica
    c. Urate
    d. Cystine

495. What test on the urine dipstick is the least useful in animals?
    a. Glucose
    b. Urobilinogen
    c. Protein
    d. Ketones

496. What substance increases in the urine in glomerular disease?
    a. Glucose
    b. Ketones
    c. Bilirubin
    d. Protein

497. What is the most likely constituent of the grit seen in the urethra of male cats?
    a. Oxalate
    b. Uric acid
    c. *Capillaria*
    d. Struvite

498. What breed of dog has the most problems with uric acid stones?
    a. Basenji
    b. German shepherd
    c. Dalmatian
    d. Shetland sheepdog

499. Keeping the urine ___ will keep struvite crystals dissolved in solution.
    a. Acidic
    b. Basic
    c. Isosthenuric
    d. Dilute

500. What is the main constituent of a struvite crystal?
    a. Calcium carbonate
    b. Calcium oxalate
    c. Magnesium phosphate
    d. Silica

501. Basophils share characteristics with what tissue cell?
    a. Macrophage
    b. Mast cell
    c. Phagocyte
    d. Plasma cell

502. Urine often has a sweet odor if which of the following is present?
    a. Ketones
    b. Bacteria
    c. Bilirubin
    d. Protein

503. What type of cast is the most common one found in urine?
    a. Leukocyte
    b. Waxy
    c. Granular
    d. Erythrocyte

504. Fresh urine appears what color when myoglobinuria is present?
    a. Brown
    b. Colorless
    c. Red
    d. White

505. What urinalysis finding is consistent with bacterial cystitis in the dog and cat?
    a. Oliguria
    b. Negative nitrate
    c. Alkaline pH
    d. Glycosuria

506. In what tissue would you normally expect to find the least number of eosinophils?
    a. Skin
    b. Lung
    c. Small intestine
    d. Lymph node

Correct answers are on pages 293-323.

507. What is not considered an electrolyte?
    a. Calcium
    b. Sodium
    c. Potassium
    d. Chloride

508. What is a useful liver test not found on most in-house panels?
    a. Bilirubin
    b. Bile acids
    c. Creatine phosphokinase
    d. Alanine aminotransferase

509. The x-ray film digestion test measures the activity of
    a. Lipase
    b. Fecal amylase
    c. Fecal trypsin
    d. Glucose

510. Hyperkalemia is commonly associated with what endocrine disorder?
    a. Diabetes insipidus
    b. Hyperthyroidism
    c. Hyperparathyroidism
    d. Hypoadrenocorticism

511. What is the most common reason for getting a false positive result on the feline leukemia test that uses test wells?
    a. Reagents added in the wrong order
    b. Low sensitivity of the test
    c. Overwashing
    d. Underwashing

512. What is the term for a substance that stimulates antibody production?
    a. Immunoglobulin
    b. Antigen
    c. T cell
    d. Plasma cell

513. What technology is used in hematology analyzers?
    a. Ion-specific
    b. End-point assay
    c. Impedance
    d. Reflectometry

514. A false positive test result is one in which the
    a. Animal is affected and the test is negative
    b. Animal is not affected and the test is positive
    c. Animal is not affected and the test is negative
    d. Animal is affected and the test is positive

515. What term is used to describe the ability of a test to determine true positives?
    a. Selectivity
    b. Sensitivity
    c. Specificity
    d. Sensibility

516. What should be the course of action for a healthy-appearing cat that tests positive for feline leukemia with an ELISA test?
    a. Euthanasia
    b. Retest in 4 to 8 weeks
    c. Retest in a year
    d. Vaccinate

517. A new in-house test has been developed with 80% sensitivity and 100% specificity. What does this mean?
    a. 20% will be false positive.
    b. 100% of positives will be identified.
    c. 20% will be false negative.
    d. 80% of negatives will be identified.

518. What cell produces immunoglobulins?
    a. Hepatocyte
    b. T lymphocyte
    c. Plasma cell
    d. Myeloblast

519. Which of these immunoglobulins is found on mucous membranes and is stimulated by intranasal vaccines?
    a. IgG
    b. IgM
    c. IgA
    d. IgE

520. The ANA test is the best test to diagnose what disorder?
    a. Immune-mediated hemolytic anemia
    b. Lupus erythematosus
    c. Pemphigus complex diseases
    d. Rheumatoid arthritis

521. What is the best method to diagnose food allergies in dogs?
    a. Measure antibodies.
    b. Try hypoallergenic diets.
    c. Perform ELISA tests.
    d. Perform skin biopsy.

522. What is being measured or tested for when trying to diagnose failure of passive immunity in a foal?
    a. Immunoglobulins
    b. Plasma cells
    c. Lymphocytes
    d. Fibrinogen

523. Combined immunodeficiency is most commonly seen in what animal?
   a. Arabian horses
   b. Jersey cattle
   c. Doberman pinschers
   d. Siamese cats

524. What species has the largest eosinophil granules?
   a. Bovine
   b. Canine
   c. Equine
   d. Feline

525. When analyzing two serum samples (one drawn while the animal is sick, and one drawn later while the animal is convalescent), a positive diagnosis is indicated by
   a. A 50% drop in antibody titers
   b. Two elevated antibody titers
   c. A four fold rise in antibody titer
   d. A rising antigen level

526. In healthy adult horses, the ratio of circulating neutrophils and marginated neutrophils is __.
   a. 80:20
   b. 70:30
   c. 50:50
   d. 25:75

527. What organism is a large, thick-walled yeast, often seen budding, which may infect the skin as well as deeper structures?
   a. *Histoplasma*
   b. *Blastomyces*
   c. *Coccidioides*
   d. *Dermatophilus*

528. Which of the following is most commonly associated with mycotoxicosis?
   a. Grains and forage
   b. Cryptococcosis
   c. Water
   d. Histoplasmosis

529. What systemic fungus is small and often found in the cytoplasm of macrophages?
   a. *Aspergillus*
   b. *Blastomyces*
   c. *Histoplasma*
   d. *Cryptococcus*

530. What is a large, thick-walled yeast surrounded by a wide, nonstaining gelatinous capsule?
   a. *Aspergillus*
   b. *Blastomyces*
   c. *Histoplasma*
   d. *Cryptococcus*

531. Which of the following is a Romanowsky-type stain?
   a. Gram stain
   b. New methylene blue
   c. Diff-Quik
   d. Sedi-Stain

532. What color do fungal organisms stain with Gram stain?
   a. Red
   b. Blue
   c. Green
   d. Black

533. What color do acid-fast organisms stain when stained with an acid-fast stain?
   a. Red
   b. Blue
   c. Green
   d. Black

534. How are diseases caused by prions thought to be transmitted?
   a. By ingestion
   b. By direct contact
   c. By inhalation
   d. By injection

535. What cytologic finding is not associated with neutrophil degeneration?
   a. Pyknosis
   b. Basophilic stippling
   c. Karyolysis
   d. Cytoplasm vacuoles

536. Postprandial lipemia is caused by
   a. Proteins
   b. Chylomicrons
   c. Carbohydrates
   d. Fatty acids

537. Cestodes are
   a. Tapeworms
   b. Flukes
   c. Roundworms
   d. Thorny-headed worms

538. *Macracanthorhynchus hirudinaceus*, the parasite with the longest scientific name among the parasites of domestic animals, is a parasite of
   a. Cattle
   b. Horses
   c. Birds
   d. Pigs

Correct answers are on pages 293-323.

539. What adult parasite would be described as having a slender anterior end with its mouth at the tip and a thickened posterior extremity?
    a. Heartworm
    b. Whipworm
    c. Tapeworm
    d. Hookworm

540. Trematodes are
    a. Tapeworms
    b. Flukes
    c. Roundworms
    d. Thorny-headed worms

541. A gravid proglottid is
    a. An empty tapeworm segment
    b. A tapeworm larvae
    c. A tapeworm segment filled with eggs
    d. The tapeworm segment closest to the head

542. When an *Isospora* oocyst is infective, how many sporozoites does it contain?
    a. 2
    b. 4
    c. 8
    d. 16

543. Which of these is a coccidia organism?
    a. *Giardia*
    b. *Cryptosporidium*
    c. *Bunostomum*
    d. *Taenia*

544. Mesothelial cells are most likely seen in samples from what collection procedure?
    a. Arthrocentesis
    b. Thoracocentesis
    c. Transtracheal aspiration
    d. Cerebrospinal fluid (CSF) tap

545. What cell is most commonly seen in chylothorax?
    a. Neutrophils
    b. Lymphoblasts
    c. Small lymphocytes
    d. Mesothelial cells

546. What cytologic finding on a transtracheal aspiration from a cow is consistent with finding larva of *Dictyocaulus viviparous*?
    a. Eosinophils
    b. Anaplastic epithelial cells
    c. Mesothelial cells
    d. Lymphocytes

547. What color does mucus stain with Diff-Quik stain?
    a. Blue
    b. Red
    c. Brown
    d. Green

548. CSF may be checked for antibodies to help diagnose what disease?
    a. Cryptosporidiosis
    b. Equine protozoal meningitis
    c. Toxoplasmosis
    d. Equine infectious anemia

549. When do most bitches normally ovulate?
    a. Early in estrus
    b. Early in diestrus
    c. Late in estrus
    d. Late in proestrus

550. When does pseudocyesis occur in the bitch's cycle?
    a. Proestrus
    b. Estrus
    c. Diestrus
    d. Anestrus

551. If neutrophils are the predominant cell type seen in an aspirated sample, what else of significance should you look for in the sample?
    a. Extracellular microorganisms
    b. Macrophages
    c. Phagocytized microorganisms
    d. Ruptured RBCs

552. Noncornified epithelial cells and erythrocytes are most commonly seen on a vaginal smear during what phase of the bitchs's cycle?
    a. Anestrus
    b. Diestrus
    c. Estrus
    d. Proestrus

553. What is an example of a cornified vaginal epithelial cell?
    a. Superficial cell
    b. Ciliated columnar epithelial cell
    c. Parabasal cell
    d. Intermediate cell

554. If a milk progesterone test from a cow is positive, it indicates
    a. She is not pregnant.
    b. She is in estrus.
    c. She is in proestrus.
    d. She is not in heat.

555. What sample is normally the least cellular?
 a. Semen
 b. CSF
 c. Synovial fluid
 d. Chylous effusion

556. What is seen in necrospermia on a semen evaluation?
 a. No sperm are present.
 b. No sperm motility
 c. Decreased sperm count
 d. Abnormal sperm cells

557. What animal has a very short estrus with ovulation occurring in metestrus?
 a. Cow
 b. Mare
 c. Queen
 d. Sow

558. What sample normally has the greatest number of cells?
 a. Erythrocyte count
 b. Thrombocyte count
 c. Sperm count
 d. Leukocyte count

559. In what endocrine disorder is polyuria and polydipsia not commonly seen?
 a. Hyperadrenocorticism
 b. Diabetes insipidus
 c. Hyperparathyroidism
 d. Diabetes mellitus

560. Intact erythrocytes in unstained urine sediment may be confused with
 a. Casts
 b. Crystals
 c. Fat cells
 d. Microorganisms

561. Adult heartworms are normally found in the
 a. Left ventricle
 b. Right ventricle
 c. Pulmonary veins
 d. Vena cava

562. How many major canine blood groups have been identified?
 a. 2
 b. 4
 c. 6
 d. 8

563. What has occurred in neonatal isoerythrolysis?
 a. Neonate makes antibodies against its erythrocytes.
 b. Neonate inherits antibodies against its erythrocytes.
 c. Neonate ingests antibodies against its own erythrocytes in the colostrum.
 d. Neonate cannot make T or B cells.

564. What cat blood type is considered the universal donor?
 a. A
 b. O
 c. AB
 d. None exists in the cat.

565. How do transfusion reactions in the cat differ from transfusion reactions in the dog?
 a. More severe in the cat
 b. More acute in the dog
 c. Severe pruritus in the cat
 d. More severe in the dog

566. An acute hemolytic transfusion reaction will occur only in a sensitized ___ dog.
 a. DEA 1.1 positive and DEA 1.2 negative
 b. DEA 1.1 negative and DEA 1.2 positive
 c. DEA 1.1 and DEA 1.2 positive
 d. DEA 1.1 and DEA 1.2 negative

567. A quick check for *Dirofilaria immitis* using a spun hematocrit tube involves microscopically viewing the border between the
 a. Clay plug and plasma
 b. Buffy coat and erythrocytes
 c. Erythrocytes and clay plug
 d. Plasma and buffy coat

568. Decreased total protein can suggest all of the following, except
 a. Dehydration
 b. Renal disease
 c. Overhydration
 d. Gastrointestinal losses

569. When performing a CBC, a stained blood film will not allow you to evaluate the morphology of
 a. Platelets
 b. Small lymphocytes
 c. Large lymphocytes
 d. Macrophages

570. Isosthenuric urine would read ___ on a refractometer.
    a. 1.010
    b. 1.0 g/dl
    c. 7.0 g/dl
    d. 1.101

571. When the spun hematocrit test is done, which of the following can be evaluated?
    a. PCV
    b. Plasma color and PCV
    c. Total protein, buffy coat, plasma color, and PCV
    d. Total protein, buffy coat, plasma color, fibrin, and PCV

572. A monolayer of cells on a blood smear is best described as
    a. A feathered edge
    b. Cells with no overlapping or touching
    c. Cells touching each other very closely with some overlapping
    d. The body of the blood smear

573. A biopsy should be submitted in a solution of formalin at the ratio of
    a. 10 parts formalin to 1 part tissue
    b. 10 parts tissue to 1 part formalin
    c. 5 parts formalin to 1 part tissue
    d. 5 parts tissue to 1 part formalin

574. "Railroad tracks" on a blood smear most often occurs when
    a. The slide is made with inconsistent pressure
    b. The smear is made too fast
    c. The slide is not clean
    d. The blood drop is too big

575. When preparing a large tissue for biopsy, 10% formalin can be
    a. Added to the container to just cover the specimen
    b. Diluted with alcohol for shipping
    c. Injected into the specimen
    d. Diluted with water for shipping

576. What condition could result in myoglobinuria?
    a. Autoimmune hemolytic anemia
    b. Transfusion reaction
    c. Prolonged recumbency
    d. Overeating disease

577. An example of capillary action is
    a. The blood coursing through smaller veins
    b. The perfusion of mucous membranes
    c. The action of blood filling a hematocrit tube
    d. Removing serum from a clot with a pipette

578. Impedance is
    a. Used in analytic instruments to stop a test
    b. Blockage of light or electric current in analytic instruments
    c. Lack of synchronicity between the jugular pulse and the heartbeat
    d. Inability to feel pedal pulses

579. Absolute polycythemia is
    a. Decreased number of circulating leukocytes
    b. Decreased number of circulating erythrocytes
    c. Increased number of circulating leukocytes
    d. Increased number of circulating erythrocytes

580. Which of these is not a random laboratory error?
    a. Variation in glassware
    b. Electronic or optical inconsistency
    c. Anisocytosis
    d. Contamination

581. A standard solution is defined as
    a. A control used to calibrate laboratory instruments
    b. Water used to calibrate laboratory instruments
    c. Alcohol used to calibrate laboratory instruments
    d. Acetone used to calibrate laboratory instruments

582. The best way to decrease light intensity in a microscope, other than to turn the light source down, is to
    a. Open the diaphragm.
    b. Change the ocular.
    c. Move the condenser down.
    d. Move to a lower lens power.

583. A QBC evaluates the blood for
    a. Quantitative buffy coat
    b. Qualitative blood count
    c. Quality blood count
    d. Quantitative buffy cells

584. The scanning objective on a binocular microscope
    a. Is used to focus and orient the viewer when reading a slide
    b. Is the 40× objective
    c. Is the 10× objective
    d. Is used when looking for coccidia

585. When using a liquid reagent–based chemistry analyzer, the higher the concentration of the substance,
    a. The more light that will pass through the solution
    b. The less light that will pass through the solution
    c. The amount of light passing through the solution will remain unchanged.
    d. The more the amount of light passing through the solution will fluctuate

586. A substance that has been lyophilized has been
    a. Dehydrated
    b. Rehydrated
    c. Thawed
    d. Frozen

587. Prolonged exposure of serum to the blood cells before the serum is removed from the clot can result in
    a. Increased serum glucose
    b. Increased serum phosphorus
    c. Increased serum enzyme activity
    d. Increased serum sodium

588. Assuming that there is an average of 100 RBCs per field, what percentage of reticulocytes is on a blood smear if 53 reticulocytes were counted in 10 fields?
    a. 53%
    b. 0.53%
    c. 0.053%
    d. 5.3%

589. What two cell types can be counted using a Unopette and hemocytometer?
    a. Leukocytes and thrombocytes
    b. Epithelial cells and erythrocytes
    c. Thrombocytes and epithelial cells
    d. Monocytes and plasma cells

590. Phagocytes include all of the following, except
    a. Neutrophils
    b. Lymphocytes
    c. Monocytes
    d. Macrophages

591. Eosinophils would most commonly be found in the
    a. Liver
    b. Spleen and greater omentum
    c. Muscle bellies
    d. Lining of the lung

592. Basophils are most commonly found in what tissues?
    a. Eyeball
    b. Near blood vessels
    c. Avascular tissues
    d. Bone marrow

593. Which of the following is correct when describing a large lymphocyte?
    a. It has the same function as a small lymphocyte.
    b. Its primary function is phagocytosis.
    c. It has a small amount of cytoplasm.
    d. Its nucleus stains dark blue with Wright stain.

594. A toxic neutrophil can be identified by all of the following characteristics, except
    a. Cytoplasmic vacuolization
    b. Cytoplasmic basophilia
    c. Hypersegmentation
    d. Döhle bodies

595. A Döhle body is identified with the Diff-Quik stain (modified Wright-Giemsa stain) as
    a. One small dark body on an erythrocyte membrane
    b. A dark blue–staining protuberance on a neutrophil nucleus
    c. Coarse, dark blue dots within an erythrocyte
    d. A small, bluish-gray inclusion in a neutrophil cytoplasm

596. A blast cell is not a characteristic of
    a. An immature cell
    b. An old, degenerating cell
    c. A neoplasm arising in the bone marrow
    d. A lymphocytic reaction to an antigenic stimulus

597. A target cell is also called a
    a. Codocyte
    b. Schistocyte
    c. Spherocyte
    d. Discocyte

598. A crenated cell is also called a/an
    a. Schistocyte
    b. Elliptocyte
    c. Keratocyte
    d. Echinocyte

599. Spherocytes may be seen on a blood smear from a dog suffering from
    a. DIC
    b. IMHA
    c. Ethylene glycol poisoning
    d. Venomous snakebite

Correct answers are on pages 293-323.

600. Acanthocytes are
    a. Crenated cells
    b. Spherocytes
    c. Poikilocytes
    d. Schistocytes

601. A canine RBC is
    a. A biconcave disk-shaped cell
    b. A concave disk-shaped cell
    c. A biconvex disk-shaped cell
    d. A convex disk-shaped cell

602. DIC is commonly represented by schistocytosis. The schistocytes are made when
    a. Normal erythrocytes are phagocytized by leukocytes.
    b. Leukocytes are fragmented.
    c. Fibrin strands cut the erythrocytes apart.
    d. Erythrocytes lose intracellular contents while remaining intact.

603. The destruction of erythrocytes outside of the blood vessels is called
    a. Extravascular hemolysis
    b. Extravascular hemoglobinemia
    c. Intravascular hemolysis
    d. Intravascular hemoglobinemia

604. The third solution of the Diff-Quik (modified Wright-Giemsa) stain is
    a. A counterstain
    b. A fixative
    c. A rinse
    d. Isotonic saline

605. A FeLV snap test is an enzyme-linked immunosorbent assay (ELISA) that tests specially for FeLV group–specific viral
    a. Antigen
    b. Antibody
    c. Antigen and antibody
    d. Antigen or antibody

606. Before beginning other diagnostics of the urine, a ___ examination of urine is recommended.
    a. Darkfield
    b. Gross
    c. Taste
    d. Microscopic

607. Which of these cells is not an epithelial cell type found in urine sediment?
    a. Squamous
    b. Transitional
    c. Renal
    d. Trigeminal

608. The correct medical term for a urinary bladder stone is
    a. Urolith
    b. Cystolith
    c. Renal calculus
    d. Cystic calculus

609. Urine specific gravity readings indicate
    a. Dissolved minerals
    b. Dissolved solids
    c. Number of cells in the urine
    d. Amount of bacteria present

610. *Dirofilaria immitis* adults have not been found in the
    a. Right ventricle
    b. Brain
    c. Anterior chamber of the eye
    d. Subcutaneous tissues

611. Which of these is not a characteristic of *Dirofilaria immitis*?
    a. 310 µ long
    b. Curved tail
    c. Straight tail
    d. Tapered head

612. *Cheyletiella* spp. are
    a. Mites
    b. Nematodes
    c. Lice
    d. Ticks

613. Which of the following is not a fecal flotation medium?
    a. Potassium hydroxide
    b. Zinc sulfate
    c. Sodium nitrate
    d. Sugar solution

614. Which of these is not a stage of a protozoan life cycle?
    a. Trophite
    b. Trophozoite
    c. Cyst
    d. Oocyst

615. What are the tips of *Trichuris vulpis* ova called?
    a. Caps
    b. Opercula
    c. Ends
    d. Morulae

616. *Paragonimus kellicotti* is a
    a. Tapeworm
    b. Tick
    c. Mite
    d. Fluke

617. The ability to obtain the same results, time after time, on the same sample, is
    a. Accuracy
    b. Reliability
    c. Quality control
    d. Precision

618. The extent to which measurements agree with the true value of the quantity measured is
    a. Accuracy
    b. Reliability
    c. Quality control
    d. Precision

619. The ability of a method to be both accurate and precise is
    a. Accuracy
    b. Reliability
    c. Quality control
    d. Precision

620. The process of monitoring instruments, reagents, test procedures, technician performance, and the accuracy of reported results is
    a. Accuracy
    b. Reliability
    c. Quality control
    d. Precision

621. Controls are
    a. Solutions with known constituents analyzed to calibrate instruments
    b. Run on a weekly basis
    c. Solutions with known properties that are analyzed for quality-control purposes
    d. Used if a problem occurs

622. When would you absolutely *not* have to use a control solution?
    a. Two hours after you got acceptable results and no changes have occurred
    b. When you change a lot number of a reagent
    c. When there is a shift change in laboratory personnel
    d. When you perform instrument maintenance

623. The value that occurs most often in a set of observations is
    a. Mean
    b. Mode
    c. Median
    d. Standard deviation

624. The sum of all values divided by the number of values is the
    a. Mean
    b. Mode
    c. Median
    d. Standard deviation

625. The measure of the extent of random variation in a group of observations is
    a. Mean
    b. Mode
    c. Median
    d. Standard deviation

626. The value that represents the center of a set of values is
    a. Mean
    b. Mode
    c. Median
    d. Standard deviation

627. When interpreting quality-control data, a trend is defined as
    a. A change in the analytic system that happens abruptly and continues at a new level
    b. An abrupt change from high to low and then from low to high control levels
    c. A gradual change in control values, either to increase or decrease over a period of 6 consecutive days
    d. An increase or decrease in which control values are distributed on one side of a mean line and maintained at a constant level

628. What nuclear characteristic is associated with the most immature stage of eosinophil maturation?
    a. Segmentation
    b. Hypersegmentation
    c. Chromatin clumping
    d. Nucleoli

629. Which of these is not a function of the lymphatic system?
    a. Transport of waste materials
    b. Leukocyte production
    c. Removal of excess tissue fluid
    d. Protein transport

630. What organ has both lymphatic and hematologic functions?
    a. Spleen
    b. Pancreas
    c. Tonsil
    d. Liver

Correct answers are on pages 293-323.

631. What organ has storage sinuses that hold blood and release it into circulation when the need for oxygen is increased?
    a. Spleen
    b. Pancreas
    c. Parathyroid
    d. Liver

632. What organ releases T cells?
    a. Thyroid
    b. Thymus
    c. Splenic trabeculae
    d. Tonsils

633. What tissue processes B cells before they are sent to peripheral lymphoid tissue?
    a. GLNB
    b. GALB
    c. GALT
    d. GLAN

634. What would not cause shifts or trends in quality-control data?
    a. New lot numbers of reagents
    b. Change in calibration of the instrument
    c. Outdated reagents
    d. Change in laboratory personnel

635. What error is not detectable through use of a quality-control program?
    a. Poor technique
    b. Sample quality
    c. Equipment malfunctions
    d. Reagent contamination or degeneration

636. For proper calibration what solution should be used to calibrate a refractometer?
    a. Tap water
    b. Distilled water
    c. Plasma
    d. Urine

637. To separate serum, whole blood should be spun down in a centrifuge at
    a. 4500 rpm for 30 minutes
    b. 10,000 rpm for 10 minutes
    c. 8500 rpm for 30 minutes
    d. 3500 rpm for 10 minutes

638. When using a centrifuge, it is important to do the following each time you use it, except
    a. Balance the tubes.
    b. Open the lid as the centrifuge is stopping.
    c. Set the timer.
    d. Check tube holders for leaked liquid.

639. As a general rule, enough blood should be collected to run any test at least three times. This compensates for all of the following, except
    a. Instrument error
    b. Technician error
    c. Transcription error
    d. Improper dilution of a sample

640. Ethylenediaminetetraacetic acid (EDTA) is the anticoagulant of choice for hematology because it
    a. Preserves blood cell morphology
    b. Simultaneously stains and preserves blood cells
    c. Destroys red cells while preserving white cells
    d. Destroys white cells while preserving red cells

641. The substance that prevents a blood sample from clotting is
    a. Antihistamine
    b. Chloramphenamine
    c. Heparin
    d. Lithium

642. What is the noncellular portion of coagulated whole blood called after it has been centrifuged?
    a. Serum
    b. Plasma
    c. Anticoagulant
    d. Hemolysin

643. What is the noncellular portion of anticoagulated whole blood called after it has been centrifuged?
    a. Serum
    b. Plasma
    c. Anticoagulant
    d. Hemolysin

644. What is the result of erythrocyte membrane rupture?
    a. Erythroblastosis
    b. Erythrocytosis
    c. Hemoconcentration
    d. Hemolysis

645. When mailing serum samples to a reference laboratory, which of these would you not want to do?
    a. Label all samples.
    b. Include test request papers and case history.
    c. Mail samples out on Saturday.
    d. Pack the sample so that if breakage occurs, the package will not leak.

646. When mailing glass slides, you must not
  a. Send unstained slides.
  b. Send slides with samples preserved in formalin.
  c. Send slides in cardboard mailers.
  d. Send labeled slides.

647. What is the disadvantage of using vacuum blood collection tubes?
  a. Collection tubes can be used sequentially.
  b. Withdrawal pressure is not easily controlled.
  c. Rapid sample collection
  d. Blood enters the tube and mixes rapidly.

648. EDTA, sodium citrate, and sodium oxalate anticoagulants work by
  a. Binding calcium
  b. Chelating potassium
  c. Forming soluble complexes
  d. Removing fibrinogen

649. What anticoagulant inhibits a glycolytic enzyme, thus acting as a preservative for glucose?
  a. Sodium citrate
  b. Lithium heparin
  c. Sodium fluoride
  d. Potassium oxalate

650. What anticoagulant is the first choice for coagulation studies?
  a. Potassium oxalate
  b. Sodium heparin
  c. Calcium oxalate
  d. Sodium citrate

651. Sodium citrate is used for coagulation tests because it chelates calcium, allowing the coagulation process to be easily reversed by addition of
  a. Thrombin
  b. Ionized calcium
  c. Prothrombin
  d. Fibrinogen

652. Serum should be separated from blood cells in a blood sample as soon as possible because
  a. The sample will hemolyze.
  b. It will not clot.
  c. It will become lipemic.
  d. Some chemical constituents will change.

653. What condition will not cause hemolysis?
  a. Removing the needle from the syringe to place blood in a collection tube
  b. Freezing a whole blood sample
  c. Vigorously mixing a sample after collection
  d. Forcing a blood sample through the needle

654. Which of the following is not a consideration when choosing the gauge and length of a needle for blood sample collection?
  a. Amount of blood needed
  b. Condition of phlebotomy sites
  c. Test to be run
  d. Size of the animal

655. If whole blood is allowed to stand at room temperature for an extended time,
  a. Potassium levels may decrease.
  b. Glucose levels may decrease.
  c. There are no chemical changes.
  d. Ammonia levels may increase.

656. If you are unable to perform chemistry tests on a sample for a week, you should
  a. Centrifuge the sample, separate the serum, and freeze it.
  b. Place the sample in the refrigerator.
  c. Place the sample in the freezer.
  d. Centrifuge the sample, separate the serum, and refrigerate it.

657. Diagnostic testing performed in a laboratory setting, outside of the animal's body, is
  a. In vita testing
  b. In viva testing
  c. In vivo testing
  d. In vitro testing

658. Performing a group of blood chemistry tests to evaluate the overall health of an animal is
  a. Biochemical profiling
  b. Quality-control assurance
  c. A complete body count
  d. Prognostic evaluation

659. When plasma is required for blood chemistry analysis, the anticoagulant of choice is
  a. EDTA
  b. Sodium or lithium heparin
  c. Sodium or lithium oxalate
  d. Sodium fluoride

660. The anticoagulant used to preserve blood glucose levels for blood chemistry analysis is
  a. EDTA
  b. Sodium or lithium heparin
  c. Sodium or lithium oxalate
  d. Sodium fluoride

661. The preferred sample for most blood chemistry tests is
  a. Whole blood
  b. Serum
  c. Plasma
  d. Hemolyte

Correct answers are on pages 293-323.

662. As a general rule, sufficient blood should be collected from the animal to yield enough serum, plasma, or whole blood to run each test how many times?
    a. 1
    b. 5
    c. 3
    d. 7

663. In terms of approximate equivalents, one drop of serum is equivalent to
    a. 50 microliters
    b. 100 microliters
    c. 10 microliters
    d. 500 microliters

664. To preserve blood constituents in the event that sample analysis is delayed for 8 hours, serum or plasma should be
    a. Lyophilized and reconstituted before analysis
    b. Refrigerated and warmed to room temperature before analysis
    c. Placed in a 37° C water bath and brought to room temperature before analysis
    d. Left at room temperature until analyzed

665. For most of blood chemistry examinations, serum or plasma samples are stable at room temperature for
    a. 4 to 7 hours
    b. 4 to 7 days
    c. 4 to 7 weeks
    d. 4 to 7 months

666. For most blood chemistry examinations, serum or plasma samples are stable at refrigerated temperatures for
    a. 4 to 7 hours
    b. 4 to 7 days
    c. 4 to 7 weeks
    d. 4 to 7 months

667. For most blood chemistry examinations, serum or plasma samples are stable at frozen temperatures for
    a. 4 to 7 hours
    b. 4 to 7 days
    c. 4 to 7 weeks
    d. 4 to 7 months

668. Centrifuging blood that has been collected in a plain (red-top) vacuum tube and allowed to clot produces
    a. Lipemia
    b. Bilirubinemia
    c. Serum
    d. Plasma

669. False elevations in potassium and inorganic phosphorus levels can be expected in a serum sample that is
    a. Lipemic
    b. Hemolyzed
    c. Icteric
    d. Refrigerated

670. False decreases in serum glucose levels can be caused by
    a. Prolonged contact with red blood cells before separating the serum
    b. Refrigerating the serum sample before analysis
    c. Freezing the serum sample before analysis
    d. A lipemic sample

671. Drawing a blood sample from an animal that has recently eaten may result in a sample that is
    a. Hemolyzed
    b. Lipemic
    c. Icteric
    d. Anemic

672. Centrifuging a blood sample at high speed for a prolonged period may result in
    a. Lipemia
    b. Icterus
    c. Hemolysis
    d. Bacterial contamination

673. Improper handling of a blood sample after it has been collected may result in
    a. Lipemia
    b. Icterus
    c. Hemolysis
    d. Leukocytosis

674. A serum sample that is extremely icteric generally derives its color from an increased level of
    a. Lipids
    b. Total bilirubin
    c. Electrolytes
    d. Glucose

675. Icteric plasma is what color?
    a. Brown
    b. Red
    c. Green
    d. Yellow

676. Which statement is false concerning collection of a plasma sample for blood chemistry analysis?
    a. If a needle and syringe are used, hemolysis can be minimized by removing the needle from the syringe before discharging the blood into a sample tube.
    b. Volume changes caused by evaporation can be minimized by keeping the cap on the blood collection tube as much as possible.
    c. To separate, allow the sample to clot for approximately 30 minutes, gently remove the clot from the sides of the tube, and centrifuge and remove the plasma.
    d. Avoid lipemia by fasting the animal before collecting the sample.

677. What sample condition cannot be minimized by proper animal preparation or proper sample collection and handling?
    a. Hemolysis
    b. Icterus
    c. Lipemia
    d. Evaporation

678. The technology of dry chemistry differs from that of wet chemistry in that the reagents in dry chemistry are supplied
    a. In lyophilized pellets
    b. In liquid solutions
    c. Impregnated on slides, cards, or strips
    d. In powdered capsules

679. In wet chemistry technology, the amount of chemical substance in the blood is determined by measuring the
    a. Light passing through or absorbed by the final sample
    b. Heat generated by the end product
    c. Light reflected from the slide or card
    d. Volume, temperature, and pH of the final sample

680. In dry chemistry technology, the amount of chemical substance in the blood is determined by measuring the
    a. Light passing through or absorbed by the final sample
    b. Heat generated by the end product
    c. Light reflected from the slide, card, or strip
    d. Volume, temperature, and pH of the final sample

681. To verify the accuracy of blood chemistry results in the laboratory, the technician should use
    a. Standard solutions
    b. Quality-control sera
    c. Pooled samples
    d. A reference manual

682. An allergic response that is frequently life threatening is the result of
    a. Agglutination
    b. Hemolysis
    c. DIC
    d. Anaphylaxis

683. Ninety-nine percent of the domestic short-hair cats in the United States have what blood type?
    a. A
    b. B
    c. AB
    d. O

684. Quality-control sera used in most laboratories are supplied in what form?
    a. Liquid
    b. Lyophilized
    c. Pellets
    d. Capsules

685. In blood chemistry assays, reconstituted control serum
    a. Can be used just once a month to assure analyzer reliability
    b. Is used when patient values are abnormal
    c. Can be separated into aliquots, frozen, and thawed for later use
    d. Can be tightly capped and kept in the refrigerator for up to a month

686. In regard to quality control in blood chemistry, what is not a source of a detectable error?
    a. Inconsistent or poor technique
    b. Equipment malfunction
    c. Reagent contamination or degeneration
    d. Random sampling errors

687. Canine blood types are preceded by the letters "DEA." What do these letters stand for?
    a. Detectable Erythrocyte Antibody
    b. Detectable Erythrocyte Antigen
    c. Dog Erythrocyte Antibody
    d. Dog Erythrocyte Antigen

Correct answers are on pages 293-323.

688. Coagulation tests would be useful for diagnosing
    a. Rodenticide poisoning
    b. Thyroid function
    c. Adrenal function
    d. Ethylene glycol poisoning

689. The calibrated device used to deliver a specified volume of patient sample when performing blood chemistry analysis is a
    a. Cuvette
    b. Pipette
    c. Graduated flask
    d. Graduated cylinder

690. The group of values for a particular blood constituent, derived when a laboratory has repeatedly assayed samples from a significant number of clinically normal animals of a given species, is called
    a. The reference range
    b. The biochemical profile
    c. The standard curve
    d. Quality control

691. In blood chemistry testing, the substance on which an enzyme acts is the
    a. Substrate
    b. Sediment
    c. Proenzyme
    d. Product

692. The rate of an enzymatic reaction is measured while it is in progress during what type of reactions?
    a. End point
    b. Kinetic
    c. Thermocouple
    d. Progressive

693. Enzymes with similar activities but different physical and chemical properties, as well as different tissues of origin, are
    a. Isoenzymes
    b. Coenzymes
    c. Cofactors
    d. Activators

694. Which is not detected using ELISA technology?
    a. Heartworms
    b. Feline leukemia virus
    c. T4
    d. Fibrinogen

695. The blood chemistry unit of activity for enzyme concentration is typically expressed as __.
    a. mg/dl
    b. g/dl
    c. IU/L
    d. mEq/L

696. The blood chemistry unit of measurement for the electrolytes—sodium, potassium, bicarbonate and chloride—is
    a. mg/dl
    b. g/dl
    c. IU/L
    d. mEq/L

697. Enzymes are proteins most often found in highest concentration
    a. Inside cells
    b. Outside cells
    c. In the blood
    d. In the urine

698. What condition will not affect the accuracy of a blood chemistry kinetic enzymatic assay?
    a. Temperature of reaction
    b. Time of reaction
    c. Sample volume
    d. Final color change of the sample

699. Laser-flow technology is used in
    a. Hematology analyzers
    b. Chemistry analyzers
    c. Coagulation analyzers
    d. Electrolyte analyzers

700. Reflectometry is used in measuring
    a. White blood cells
    b. Prothrombin time
    c. Blood gases
    d. Blood chemistries

701. A calibration verification on the sensors for PCO_2 and PO_2 is part of the procedure done by an instrument that is measuring
    a. Electrolytes
    b. Hematology parameters
    c. Blood gases
    d. Blood chemistries

702. The Azostix strip is a rapid quantitative test for blood levels of
    a. Aspartate aminotransferase
    b. Alanine transaminase
    c. Glucose
    d. Urea nitrogen

703. Dextrostix and Visidex strips are rapid quantitative tests for blood levels of
a. Aspartate aminotransferase
b. Alanine transaminase
c. Glucose
d. Urea nitrogen

704. An available technology for determination of blood electrolyte levels is
a. Electromagnetic fluctuation
b. Scanning electron microscopy
c. Ion selective electrode
d. Immunoelectrophoresis

705. In dogs and cats the blood chemistry tests most commonly used to evaluate liver function are
a. Alanine transaminase and aspartate aminotransferase
b. Electrolytes and blood urea nitrogen
c. Gamma-glutamyl transferase and sorbitol dehydrogenase
d. Amylase and lipase

706. In horses the blood chemistry tests most commonly used to evaluate liver function are
a. Alanine transaminase and aspartate aminotransferase
b. Electrolytes and blood urea nitrogen
c. Gamma-glutamyl transferase and sorbitol dehydrogenase
d. Amylase and lipase

707. Blood chemistry assays, including dye excretion, ammonia tolerance, and bile acid concentrations, are used to evaluate function of the
a. Pancreas
b. Kidneys
c. Heart
d. Liver

708. Blood levels of cholesterol, triglycerides, and total protein are all used to evaluate function of the
a. Kidneys
b. Liver
c. Pancreas
d. Adrenal glands

709. Blood levels of total bilirubin will not be a significant finding in
a. Hepatocellular damage
b. Bile duct injury or obstruction
c. Hemolytic disorders
d. Acute pancreatitis

710. Blood levels of total bilirubin are used primarily to evaluate function of the
a. Kidneys
b. Liver
c. Pancreas
d. Bile ducts

711. Serum chemistry tests for acute pancreatitis include
a. Amylase and lipase
b. Lipase and trypsin
c. Amylase and trypsin
d. Amylase, lipase, and trypsin

712. A common laboratory test for chronic pancreatitis is a fecal test for
a. Amylase
b. Lipase
c. Trypsin
d. Bilirubin

713. The principal extracellular cation that is commonly measured in a blood chemistry profile is
a. Sodium
b. Potassium
c. Chloride
d. Bicarbonate

714. The principal intracellular cation that is commonly measured in a blood chemistry profile is
a. Sodium
b. Potassium
c. Chloride
d. Bicarbonate

715. Arterial blood is the preferred sample for measurement of blood levels of
a. Bicarbonate
b. Chloride
c. Sodium
d. Magnesium

716. The term *A/G ratio* refers to the blood ratio of
a. Alpha globulins to gamma globulins
b. Albumin to globulin
c. Ammonia to glucose
d. Aspartate aminotransferase to gamma-glutamyl transferase

717. A by-product of muscle metabolism that is commonly used to evaluate glomerular filtration in a blood chemistry profile is
a. Urea nitrogen
b. Creatinine
c. Alanine transaminase
d. Aspartate aminotransferase

Correct answers are on pages 293-323.

718. Serum electrolyte levels should be determined when evaluating function of the
    a. Liver
    b. Pancreas
    c. Kidneys
    d. Heart

719. Kidney disease leads to accumulation of metabolic waste in the blood, a condition known as
    a. Hypernaturia
    b. Hypernatremia
    c. Azotemia
    d. Azoturia

720. In a diabetic animal, blood chemistry analysis is commonly performed to monitor insulin therapy by measuring blood levels of
    a. Sodium
    b. Potassium
    c. Glucose
    d. Insulin

721. In an animal with a history of bone resorption or convulsions, blood chemistry analysis is commonly performed to measure blood levels of
    a. Calcium and phosphorus
    b. Urea nitrogen and creatinine
    c. Aspartate aminotransferase and alanine transaminase
    d. Sodium and potassium

722. What gland is the most active producer of corticosteroids?
    a. Thyroid gland
    b. Pancreas
    c. Pituitary gland
    d. Adrenal glands

723. The gland function that is evaluated by measurement of blood cortisol levels before and after administration of adrenocorticotropic hormone (ACTH) is the
    a. Thyroid gland
    b. Pancreas
    c. Liver
    d. Adrenal glands

724. The gland that is evaluated by measurement of blood levels of T3 and T4 is the
    a. Thyroid gland
    b. Pancreas
    c. Pituitary gland
    d. Thymus

725. Measurement of blood levels of thyroid-stimulating hormone (TSH) and ACTH is used to evaluate function of the
    a. Thyroid gland
    b. Pancreas
    c. Pituitary gland
    d. Adrenal glands

726. Blood chemistry analysis is commonly performed to evaluate function of the ___ in an animal showing lethargy, obesity, mild anemia, infertility, and alopecia.
    a. Thyroid gland
    b. Pancreas
    c. Thymus
    d. Adrenal glands

727. Chemistry evaluation of the kidney includes measurement of metabolic wastes in the blood in the form of
    a. Aspartate aminotransferase and alanine transaminase
    b. Urea nitrogen and creatinine
    c. Ammonia and pyruvic acid
    d. Bilirubin and urobilinogen

728. Ammonia is metabolized by the liver and eliminated by the kidneys. Levels of which metabolic by-product of ammonia are measured to assess kidney function?
    a. Phosphorus
    b. Creatinine
    c. Aspartate aminotransferase
    d. Urea nitrogen

729. Measurement of blood levels of amylase and lipase is used to evaluate function of the
    a. Kidneys
    b. Liver
    c. Pancreas
    d. Adrenal glands

730. *Dioctophyma renale* is often found in the ___ of dogs.
    a. Right kidney
    b. Left kidney
    c. Urinary bladder
    d. Ureters

731. The adult form of the parasite ___ is a fly, and the larval stage is an endoparasite.
    a. *Otobius*
    b. *Capillaria*
    c. *Thelazia*
    d. *Gasterophilus*

732. Bots are
    a. Lice eggs
    b. Fly larvae
    c. Flea feces
    d. Seed ticks

733. Nits are
    a. Lice eggs
    b. Fly larvae
    c. Flea feces
    d. Seed ticks

734. What parasite could cause anemia in horses through blood sucking?
    a. *Strongylus vulgaris*
    b. *Parascaris equorum*
    c. *Anoplocephala perfoliata*
    d. *Dictyocaulus arnfieldi*

735. *Exfoliative cytology* refers to the study of
    a. Cells shed from muscle tissue
    b. Cells shed from body surfaces
    c. Neoplastic cells exclusively
    d. Blood cells exclusively

736. *Pyknosis* is a term used to describe a
    a. Small, condensed, dark, fragmented nucleus
    b. Swollen, lacy, light blue, round nucleus
    c. Cell without a nucleus
    d. Nucleus without a cell

737. Which of the following is not a classification used to describe malignant neoplastic cells?
    a. Bizarre and numerous nucleoli
    b. Increased mitotic index
    c. Uniform size and shape of cells
    d. Rapid growth

738. *Metaplasia* refers to a/an
    a. Increase in cell numbers and mitotic activity in response to a stimulus
    b. Increase in cell size and/or functional activity in response to a stimulus
    c. Increase in cell growth and multiplication that is not dependent on a stimulus
    d. Reversible process in which one mature cell type is replaced by another

739. What is the first step in microscopic evaluation of a cytologic specimen after the smear has been properly stained and dried?
    a. Scan the smear with the 100× objective.
    b. Scan the smear with the 40× objective.
    c. Scan the smear with the 103 objective.
    d. Scan the smear with any objective available.

740. Tissue samples for histopathologic examination should be placed in fluid-tight jars that contain 10% formalin in an amount ___ times the specimen's volume.
    a. 10
    b. 25
    c. 30
    d. 50

741. Which statement concerning cerebrospinal fluid is false?
    a. CSF analysis is useful in diagnosis of some neurologic disorders.
    b. CSF is normally colorless and transparent.
    c. CSF normally has a very low protein concentration.
    d. CSF normally contains large numbers of lymphocytes.

742. Peritoneal fluid of horses
    a. Is normally very thick and viscid
    b. Is normally malodorous
    c. Is frequently examined in cases of colic
    d. Normally contains bacteria

743. Chylothorax is an
    a. Accumulation of milky fluid in the peritoneal cavity
    b. Accumulation of bloody fluid found in the abdomen
    c. Accumulation of bloody fluid found in the pericardial sac
    d. Accumulation of milky fluid found in the pleural cavity

744. The viscosity of synovial fluid is attributable to
    a. Protein
    b. Hyaluronic acid
    c. Bacterial infection
    d. Hyaluronidase

745. Synovial fluid mucin forms a clot when added to
    a. Sodium bicarbonate
    b. Hyaluronic acid
    c. 3% potassium hydroxide
    d. Acetic acid

746. An equine transtracheal wash cannot be performed by passage of a catheter through the
    a. Mouth into an endotracheal tube
    b. Nasal passages
    c. Skin and trachea
    d. Guttural pouch

Correct answers are on pages 293-323.

747. A 10-year-old male Labrador retriever has a soft swelling approximately 10 cm in diameter on its rear leg. You obtain a fine-needle aspirate, make a smear, stain it with new methylene blue, and observe it microscopically. There are cells with numerous dark, basophilic granules in the cytoplasm and a smudged appearance. Your cytology report should indicate the presence of what type of cells?
    a. Macrophages
    b. Mast cells
    c. Lymphocytes
    d. Basophils

748. What stain is used to stain fat?
    a. New methylene blue
    b. Sudan III or IV
    c. Diff-Quik
    d. Giemsa

749. What stain is referred to as a *supravital stain*?
    a. New methylene blue
    b. Camco Quik
    c. Eosin
    d. Sudan III or IV

750. Mrs. T brings her dog to your clinic for routine vaccinations and tells you she thinks her dog has ear problems. A smear from the ear reveals yeast. What is the genus of the most common cause of mycotic (fungal) otitis externa?
    a. *Mucor*
    b. *Malassezia*
    c. *Dermatophilus*
    d. *Phycomycetes*

751. What is considered the minimal percentage of motile sperm in a normal canine ejaculate?
    a. 50%
    b. 25%
    c. 80%
    d. 95%

752. Which statement concerning queens and their reproductive behavior is most accurate?
    a. The average interval between estrous periods is 45 days.
    b. Queens are seasonally polyestrous, and coitus is necessary for ovulation.
    c. Vaginal smears do not accurately predict estrus in the queen.
    d. The gestation period of the queen is 45 days.

753. The correct classification of vaginal epithelial cells from the deepest layer near the basement membrane, progressing superficially to the layer near the vaginal lumen, is
    a. Parabasal, basal, intermediate, superficial
    b. Superficial, intermediate, parabasal, basal
    c. Basal, parabasal, intermediate, superficial
    d. Intermediate, superficial, parabasal, basal

754. The largest cell seen in vaginal smears is
    a. Intermediate
    b. Basal
    c. Parabasal
    d. Superficial

755. Name the stage of estrus that exhibits the following changes on the vaginal smear: epithelial cell type changes quickly to the noncornified cell, red blood cells disappear completely, and white blood cells appear in great numbers.
    a. Proestrus
    b. Estrus
    c. Diestrus
    d. Anestrus

756. What cells predominate during anestrus?
    a. Parabasal and intermediate
    b. Neutrophils and superficial
    c. Intermediate and superficial
    d. Neutrophils and intermediate

757. In conjunctival and corneal scrapings, what cell combination suggests an allergic reaction?
    a. Lymphocytes and monocytes
    b. Neutrophils and monocytes
    c. Plasma cells and neutrophils
    d. Eosinophils and mast cells

758. What cells are predominant in conjunctival smears from animals with conjunctivitis?
    a. Monocytes
    b. Neutrophils
    c. Mast cells
    d. Lymphocytes

759. Which of the following is not a characteristic of a normal cell population?
    a. Equal distribution of cells
    b. Clearly differentiated cells
    c. Absence of foamy cytoplasm and nucleoli
    d. Pyknotic nuclei

760. Which statement concerning vaginal cytology is false?
    a. Vaginal epithelial cells on smears made during proestrus may appear very similar to smears made in diestrus (metestrus).
    b. During proestrus, red blood cells may be abundant.
    c. Parabasal cells are larger than superficial cells.
    d. Vaginal smears from animals with pyometra or metritis usually contain large numbers of degenerated neutrophils.

761. What stain should you use on a conjunctival scraping if you are interested in classifying bacteria?
    a. Diff-Quik
    b. New methylene blue
    c. Gram
    d. Eosin

762. After proper staining of a normal bone marrow sample, what should you see on the smear?
    a. A uniform population of cells
    b. Mature red blood cells and immature white blood cells
    c. Both immature and mature blood cells
    d. Immature red blood cells and mature white blood cells

763. When performing a major crossmatch in anticipation of a canine blood transfusion,
    a. Red cells from the recipient are mixed with red cells from the donor.
    b. Red cells from the recipient are mixed with serum from the donor.
    c. Red cells from the donor are mixed with serum from the recipient.
    d. Red cells from the donor and mixed with whole blood from the recipient.

764. What sample collection technique will result in the poorest quality sample?
    a. Swabbing
    b. Scraping
    c. Aspirating
    d. Debriding

765. Before making an impression smear from a specimen collected during surgery or necropsy,
    a. The specimen should be blotted with clean absorbent material.
    b. The specimen should be cleaned with alcohol.
    c. The specimen should be soaked in formalin.
    d. The specimen should be seared with a hot spatula.

766. What needle would you give the veterinarian to use for a fine-needle aspirate?
    a. 14 gauge
    b. 16 gauge
    c. 20 gauge
    d. 22 gauge

767. Eosinophilia is commonly seen with a
    a. Bacterial infection
    b. Parasitic infection
    c. Viral infection
    d. Hormonal disorder

768. What is the underlying cause of icterus?
    a. Anemia
    b. Hyperbilirubinemia
    c. Ketonuria
    d. Hyperhemoglobinemia

769. Basophilic stippling is often associated with
    a. Lead poisoning
    b. Autoimmune disease
    c. Anemia
    d. Neoplasia

770. A common finding on a stained blood smear from an animal with autoimmune hemolytic anemia is
    a. Lymphocytosis
    b. Basophilic stippling
    c. Spherocytosis
    d. Leukemia

771. Denatured hemoglobin found in erythrocytes is
    a. A Heinz body
    b. A Howell-Jolly body
    c. An *Anaplasma* body
    d. A spherocyte

772. Fresh frozen plasma can be stored up to ___ and still contain clotting factors.
    a. 1 month
    b. 12 months
    c. 36 months
    d. 60 months

773. What cell produces antibodies?
    a. Hepatocyte
    b. Plasma cell
    c. Thymocyte
    d. T cell

Correct answers are on pages 293-323.

774. What appears as a blue spheric nuclear remnant seen in some Wright-stained erythrocytes?
    a. Reticulocyte
    b. Howell-Jolly body
    c. Heinz body
    d. Leptocyte

775. Frozen fresh plasma (FFP) must be separated and frozen within __ hours to maintain all coagulation factors in normal concentrations.
    a. 2
    b. 8
    c. 12
    d. 6

776. Which of the following stimulates antibody production?
    a. Immunoglobulin
    b. Antigen
    c. T cell
    d. Plasma cell

777. Physiologic leukocytosis can be caused by
    a. Bacterial infection
    b. Parasite infection
    c. Toxemia
    d. Excitement

778. A normal leukocyte count with an increase in immature neutrophils that outnumber mature neutrophils is
    a. Leukocytosis
    b. Leukopenia
    c. A regenerative left shift
    d. A degenerative left shift

779. A total leukocyte count can be falsely elevated by which of the following in the peripheral blood?
    a. Spherocytes
    b. Reticulocytes
    c. Metarubricytes
    d. Bands

780. What is the half life of neutrophils in the peripheral blood of dogs?
    a. 6 hours
    b. 24 hours
    c. 7 days
    d. 120 days

781. Where is the storage pool of granulocytes found?
    a. Pancreas
    b. Bone marrow
    c. Liver
    d. Capillaries

782. A variation in erythrocyte size is known as
    a. Polycytosis
    b. Anisocytosis
    c. Poikilocytosis
    d. Erythrocytosis

783. What is a nonnucleated, immature erythrocyte found in small numbers in the peripheral blood of dogs called?
    a. Reticulocyte
    b. Metarubricyte
    c. Rubriblast
    d. Rubricyte

784. What sample is recommended for hemoglobin testing?
    a. Serum
    b. Plasma
    c. Whole blood
    d. Blood smear

785. What part of the CBC is the most accurate procedure?
    a. Erythrocyte count
    b. Hemoglobin determination
    c. Leukocyte count
    d. Hematocrit

786. What part of the CBC cannot be done manually with adequate accuracy?
    a. Erythrocyte count
    b. Leukocyte count
    c. Packed cell volume
    d. WBC differential

787. A neutrophil in which the cytoplasm is more basophilic than normal and contains vacuoles is also known as a
    a. Band cell
    b. Toxic neutrophil
    c. Metamyelocyte
    d. Hypersegmented neutrophil

788. Which of the following is not part of a stress leukogram?
    a. Leukocytosis
    b. Neutrophilia
    c. Monocytosis
    d. Eosinophilia

789. Four purple-top tubes with blood samples from four different animals are left standing in the laboratory. In what sample will the RBCs settle the fastest?
    a. Goat sample
    b. Cat sample
    c. Cow sample
    d. Horse sample

790. What would you expect to see on a Diff-Quik stained blood smear from an animal with regenerative anemia?
   a. Schistocytosis
   b. Reticulocytosis
   c. Eosinophilia
   d. Polychromasia

791. What cell is described as a central rounded area of hemoglobin surrounded by a clear zone, with a dense ring of hemoglobin around the periphery?
   a. Plasma cell
   b. Target cell
   c. Spherocyte
   d. Reticulocyte

792. Which of the following is the least common granulocyte seen in the peripheral blood of a healthy adult cow?
   a. Monocyte
   b. Basophil
   c. Eosinophil
   d. Metarubricyte

793. *Babesia equi* and *Babesia caballi* are intracellular parasites found within the ___ of horses.
   a. Erythrocytes
   b. Neutrophils
   c. Reactive lymphocytes
   d. Tissue macrophages

794. What equine parasite produces microfilaria?
   a. *Setaria equina*
   b. *Strongylus vulgaris*
   c. *Oxyuris equi*
   d. *Strongyloides westeri*

795. What parasite is the equine pinworm?
   a. *Setaria equina*
   b. *Strongylus vulgaris*
   c. *Oxyuris equi*
   d. *Strongyloides westeri*

796. Where in an adult cow would you expect to find adult *Haemonchus* sp. parasites?
   a. Trachea
   b. Bronchioles
   c. Abomasum
   d. Perianal region

797. What causes plasma to appear red?
   a. Lipemia
   b. Chyle
   c. Icterus
   d. Hemolysis

798. What is the minimum amount of whole blood needed from a healthy adult sheep to yield 1 ml of serum?
   a. 2 ml
   b. 3 ml
   c. 10 ml
   d. 20 ml

799. Reticulocytes are never found in the peripheral blood of
   a. Horses
   b. Cattle
   c. Dogs
   d. Cats

800. What cell becomes a macrophage once it enters the tissues?
   a. Plasma cell
   b. Lymphocyte
   c. Neutrophil
   d. Monocyte

801. Which leukocyte count is in the normal reference range for a dog, cat, cow, or horse?
   a. 35,000/dl
   b. 5,750,000/dl
   c. 7,500/dl
   d. 275,000/dl

802. What cell is produced by megakaryocytes?
   a. Erythrocyte
   b. Lymphocyte
   c. Neutrophil
   d. Thrombocyte

803. In which of these would you expect to find a predominance of lymphocytes on the differential WBC count?
   a. Garfield
   b. Billy Goat Gruff
   c. Tweety Bird
   d. Lassie

804. What cell is produced at a site other than bone marrow?
   a. Erythrocytes
   b. Neutrophils
   c. Lymphocytes
   d. Monocytes

805. Lymphocytic leukemia is indicated by finding what cells in a peripheral blood smear?
   a. Large lymphocytes
   b. Lymphoblasts
   c. Small lymphocytes
   d. Plasma cells

Correct answers are on pages 293-323.

806. What species normally has the smallest erythrocytes?
    a. Horses
    b. Cats
    c. Cattle
    d. Goats

807. What is an intracellular parasite of erythrocytes?
    a. *Babesia*
    b. *Ehrlichia*
    c. *Trypanosoma*
    d. *Toxoplasma*

808. Where is the buffy coat found on the refractometer?
    a. Beneath the packed red cells
    b. Above the packed red cells
    c. Above the plasma
    d. Buffy coats are not seen on refractometers.

809. What is the major difference between serum and plasma?
    a. Plasma has higher protein levels.
    b. Serum has higher electrolyte levels.
    c. Plasma has a darker color.
    d. Serum will clot.

810. What is the term used to describe plasma that appears white or milky?
    a. Leukemia
    b. Lipemia
    c. Chylemia
    d. Lactemia

811. What is the term used to describe the situation in which many of the erythrocytes stain varying shades of lavender?
    a. Anemia
    b. Anisocytosis
    c. Polychromasia
    d. Poikilocytosis

812. Reticulocytes are reported as
    a. g/dl
    b. % $\times 10^3$
    c. #/1000 cells
    d. %

813. Which of the following is a breakdown product of hemoglobin?
    a. Bilirubin
    b. Erythropoietin
    c. Urea
    d. Carotene

814. Which of the following is associated with clotting problems?
    a. Anemia
    b. Leukopenia
    c. Thrombocytopenia
    d. Reticulocytosis

815. How long must the typical microhematocrit tube be centrifuged for packed cell volume determination?
    a. 1 minute
    b. 5 minutes
    c. 10 minutes
    d. 15 minutes

816. What measure determines the average size of an erythrocyte?
    a. Mean corpuscular volume
    b. Packed cell volume
    c. Mean corpuscular hemoglobin concentration
    d. Mean corpuscular hemoglobin

817. What is normally the most numerous leukocyte seen in bovine blood?
    a. Monocyte
    b. Neutrophil
    c. Lymphocyte
    d. Eosinophil

818. What is normally the most numerous leukocyte seen in canine blood?
    a. Monocyte
    b. Neutrophil
    c. Lymphocyte
    d. Eosinophil

819. What blood cell resembles the mast cell found in tissues?
    a. Eosinophil
    b. Reticulocyte
    c. Neutrophil
    d. Basophil

820. What parasite resembles Howell-Jolly bodies?
    a. *Babesia cati*
    b. *Mycoplasma haemofelis (Haemobartonella sp.)*
    c. *Trypanosoma cruzi*
    d. *Ehrlichia canis*

821. Basophilic stippling is seen in
    a. Mature neutrophils
    b. Toxic neutrophils
    c. Erythrocyte cytoplasm
    d. Activated lymphocytes

822. What term indicates an abnormally high lymphocyte count?
    a. Lymphocytosis
    b. Leukosis
    c. Lymphocytopenia
    d. Lymphosarcoma

823. What type of anemia is associated with icterus?
    a. Responsive
    b. Nonresponsive
    c. Hemolytic
    d. Megaloblastic

824. What is the most immature erythrocyte that can be identified in bone marrow?
    a. Prorubricyte
    b. Rubriblast
    c. Erythrocytoblast
    d. Multipotent stem cell

825. The abbreviation "seg" refers to what blood cell?
    a. Lymphocyte
    b. Monocyte
    c. Band neutrophil
    d. Neutrophil

826. Which blood cell can have vacuoles in its cytoplasm when seen in peripheral blood from a healthy animal?
    a. Monocyte
    b. Lymphocyte
    c. Neutrophil
    d. Thrombocyte

827. The dark-staining material in the nuclei of lymphocytes and neutrophils is called __.
    a. Leukopoietin
    b. Chromatin
    c. Mitochondria
    d. Endoplasmic reticulum

828. What species normally has eosinophils with small, round, red-staining cytoplasmic granules?
    a. Feline
    b. Canine
    c. Bovine
    d. Equine

829. At what stage in granulopoiesis do the specific or definitive granules first appear?
    a. Metamyelocyte
    b. Progranulocyte
    c. Myeloblast
    d. Myelocyte

830. How does a band cell differ in appearance from a mature neutrophil?
    a. The mature neutrophil is larger.
    b. The band nucleus has smooth, parallel sides.
    c. The band cytoplasm does not contain granules.
    d. The mature neutrophil has bluer cytoplasm.

831. A canine erythrocyte that is smaller than normal, with no pale area in the center, is a
    a. Rubricyte
    b. Metarubricyte
    c. Spherocyte
    d. Rubriblast

832. Rouleaux formation is most commonly seen on blood smears from
    a. Horses
    b. Goats
    c. Dogs
    d. Cats

833. An MCV value below the normal reference range suggests
    a. Hyperchromasia
    b. Hypochromasia
    c. Macrocytosis
    d. Microcytosis

834. If you count 40 reticulocytes per 1000 erythrocytes, what is the observed reticulocyte count?
    a. 2%
    b. 4%
    c. 20%
    d. 40%

835. What bovine erythrocyte parasite resembles *Haemobartonella felis* in cats?
    a. *Anaplasma*
    b. *Babesia*
    c. *Dirofilaria*
    d. *Ehrlichia*

836. What is indicated by a neutrophil with a nucleus with six lobes?
    a. Toxemia
    b. Female animal
    c. Old cell
    d. Normal cell

837. What animal has oval erythrocytes?
    a. Normal horse
    b. Normal llama
    c. Anemic cat
    d. Toxemic dog

Correct answers are on pages 293-323.

838. What causes dark granules called *Döhle bodies* in the cytoplasm of canine neutrophils?
    a. Leukemia
    b. Parasitic infection
    c. Immaturity
    d. Toxemia

839. What is normally the largest mature blood cell in peripheral blood of domestic species?
    a. Monocyte
    b. Neutrophil
    c. Eosinophil
    d. Lymphocyte

840. Mature erythrocytes are normally nucleated in
    a. Miniature horses
    b. Ferrets
    c. Camels
    d. Birds

841. Which leukocyte has a kidney-bean–shaped nucleus?
    a. Promyelocyte
    b. Myelocyte
    c. Metamyelocyte
    d. Band neutrophil

842. Which of these is an artifact?
    a. Agglutination
    b. Crenation
    c. Rouleaux
    d. Schistocyte

843. When preparing a direct smear from feces, what liquid should be mixed with the feces?
    a. Tap water
    b. Distilled water
    c. Hydrogen peroxide
    d. Saline

844. With the exception of cats, most animals have a total blood volume equivalent to ___ of their body weight.
    a. 7%
    b. 15%
    c. 25%
    d. 40%

845. What is tested in a minor crossmatch?
    a. T-cell production
    b. Recipient serum against donor erythrocytes
    c. Recipient erythrocytes against donor serum
    d. Recipient urine against donor erythrocytes

846. What anticoagulant is used most commonly in animal-blood collection for CBCs?
    a. Sodium heparin
    b. Potassium oxalate
    c. Potassium ethylenediaminetetraacetic acid
    d. Sodium citrate

847. What anticoagulant is used to determine activated partial thromboplastin time and one-stage prothrombin time?
    a. Heparin
    b. Citrate
    c. Fluoride
    d. EDTA

848. What structure is normally found in the nuclei of immature blood cells?
    a. Nucleolus
    b. Golgi apparatus
    c. Heinz body
    d. Döhle body

849. A cat has a total leukocyte count of 15,000/dl. On the differential count, 65% of the cells are neutrophils. What is the absolute neutrophil count?
    a. 975/dl
    b. 6500/dl
    c. 9750/dl
    d. 5250/dl

850. Certain oxidant drugs can denature hemoglobin and cause production of round structures in erythrocytes called
    a. Howell-Jolly bodies
    b. Russell bodies
    c. Döhle bodies
    d. Heinz bodies

851. What is the most common cause of hypochromia in erythrocytes?
    a. Hypertonic drugs
    b. Decreased hemoglobin
    c. Iron toxicity
    d. Increased erythrocyte production

852. What is the primary function of fibrinogen?
    a. Antibody production
    b. Phagocytosis
    c. Hemostasis
    d. Complement fixation

853. What nucleated erythrocyte is the first one you'll see in peripheral blood if an animal has used all of its reserves of mature erythrocytes in the bone marrow?
    a. Reticulocyte
    b. Metarubricyte
    c. Rubricyte
    d. Prorubricyte

854. *Haemobartonella felis* is seen most commonly in the erythrocytes of
    a. Cats
    b. Cattle
    c. Dogs
    d. Horses

855. An increased number of bands in the peripheral blood indicate
    a. Leukemia
    b. Autoimmune hemolytic anemia
    c. Left shift
    d. Neutropenia

856. When using the 100× oil-immersion lens with the standard 10× ocular, what is the magnification of cells observed through the microscope?
    a. 90×
    b. 100×
    c. 110×
    d. 1000×

857. The first line of defense that the body has against foreign invaders is the
    a. Hair
    b. Neutrophils
    c. Primary lymphoid tissue
    d. Skin

858. Which of these white blood cells migrate through tissue as macrophages and function to remove and destroy bacteria, damaged cells, and neoplastic cells?
    a. Lymphocytes
    b. Neutrophils
    c. Monocytes
    d. Eosinophils

859. Which immunoglobulin is the first antibody produced in a primary immune response?
    a. IgG
    b. IgA
    c. IgM
    d. IgD

860. Which immunoglobulin is most abundant in the serum and plays the major role in humoral immunity?
    a. IgG
    b. IgM
    c. IgA
    d. IgD

861. Immunity that is generated by an animal's immune system following exposure to a foreign antigen is referred to as
    a. Passive immunity
    b. Active immunity
    c. Responsive immunity
    d. Colostral immunity

862. Which immunoglobulin is the only one that can cross the placenta?
    a. IgG
    b. IgM
    c. IgA
    d. IgD

863. Which of the following is not a major function of macrophages or a result of macrophage activity?
    a. Phagocytosis
    b. Fever
    c. Inflammation
    d. Peroxidase production

864. Which of the following correctly lists the progressive stages of phagocytosis?
    a. Adherence, chemotaxis, ingestion, digestion
    b. Ingestion, adherence, chemotaxis, digestion
    c. Chemotaxis, adherence, ingestion, digestion
    d. Ingestion, digestion, chemotaxis, adherence

865. An attenuated vaccine is one in which
    a. Microorganisms have been killed.
    b. Microorganisms are weakened but still alive.
    c. Microorganisms are 100% virulent.
    d. No microorganisms are found.

866. Which statement concerning passive immunity is least accurate?
    a. It involves antibodies that have been produced in a donor animal.
    b. It provides immediate but short-lived immunity.
    c. It may be natural or artificial.
    d. It develops after exposure to a pathogen.

Correct answers are on pages 293-323.

867. Cytokines are
    a. Chemicals that elicit a hormonal response after glandular stimulation
    b. Chemicals that attract white blood cells to an area and activate macrophages
    c. Chemicals secreted by monocytes after they ingest a foreign substance
    d. Chemicals found in eosinophil granules that cause them to stain red

868. Anaphylactic shock is
    a. A mild reaction that causes destruction of erythrocytes
    b. A moderate reaction that causes hives
    c. A severe life-threatening reaction that occurs seconds after an antigen enters the circulation
    d. A severe reaction caused by rapid loss of large volumes of blood or other body fluid

869. Combined immunodeficiency is a condition in which the animal fails to produce functioning __ .
    a. Plasma cells
    b. B cells
    c. T cells
    d. B and T cells

870. Which of the following is not a malfunction of the immune system?
    a. Allergy
    b. Immunodeficiency
    c. Autoimmune disease
    d. Immunity by vaccination

871. What cells are chiefly concerned with production and secretion of antibodies?
    a. B lymphocytes
    b. T lymphocytes
    c. Neutrophils
    d. Monocytes

872. What cells respond more quickly to a second antigen exposure than to the initial exposure?
    a. Thymocytes
    b. Monocytes
    c. Memory B cells
    d. Neutrophils

873. Serology is the branch of science involved with detection of
    a. Bacteria or fungi
    b. Viruses or prions
    c. Antibodies or antigens
    d. Endoparasites and ectoparasites

874. ELISA is an acronym for
    a. Electro-linked immunosorbent assay
    b. Enzyme-linked immunosorbent assay
    c. Enzyme-linked immunoassay
    d. Electrolytic isoantibody assay

875. Which statement concerning ELISA testing is true?
    a. The test specificity is very low.
    b. Washing is a critical step in the methodology.
    c. It may be used to detect only antibodies in the serum.
    d. It is not available in kit form.

876. What serologic test is used for diagnosis of autoimmune hemolytic anemia?
    a. Coombs test
    b. Coggins test
    c. Intradermal testing
    d. Latex agglutination test

877. Which of these parasites sucks blood from its host?
    a. *Macracanthorhynchus hirudinaceus*
    b. *Onchocerca* cervicalis
    c. *Metastrongylus apri*
    d. *Ctenocephalides felis*

878. Which of these pig parasites can be diagnosed by muscle biopsy?
    a. *Trichinella spiralis*
    b. *Oesophagostomum dentatum*
    c. *Eimeria suis*
    d. *Fasciola hepatica*

879. Vaccines may be given by any of the following routes, except
    a. Subcutaneously
    b. Intramuscularly
    c. Intranasally
    d. Intraperitoneally

880. Which statement concerning antigen-antibody complexes is true?
    a. They rapidly result in death.
    b. They resemble a lock and key in principle.
    c. They cannot be detected with serologic tests.
    d. They form only when an antigen meets any antibody.

881. Which of the following is least likely to cause vaccine failure?
    a. Improper storage
    b. Administration during anesthesia
    c. Interference by maternal antibodies
    d. Improper route of administration

882. Which of these parasites is a tapeworm?
    a. *Strongyloides westeri*
    b. *Paranoplocephala mamillana*
    c. *Parascaris equorum*
    d. *Oxyuris equi*

883. Which of these parasites is classified as coccidia?
    a. *Cryptosporidium parvum*
    b. *Bunostomum phlebotomum*
    c. *Moniezia expansa*
    d. *Haemonchus contortus*

884. Pemphigus is a group of autoimmune disorders that affect the
    a. Blood and lymph systems
    b. Skin and oral mucosa
    c. Eyes
    d. Hooves and claws

885. Signs of immune-mediated thrombocytopenia include all of these conditions, except
    a. Petechiae
    b. Ecchymoses
    c. Thrombocytosis
    d. Anemia

886. Where does red blood cell production take place in a healthy adult goat?
    a. Yellow bone marrow
    b. Red bone marrow
    c. Red pulp of the spleen
    d. Liver

887. Where does neutrophil production take place in a healthy adult sheep?
    a. Red bone marrow
    b. Red pulp of the spleen
    c. White pulp of the spleen
    d. Liver

888. Which of these cells is the most immature?
    a. Rubricyte
    b. Metarubricyte
    c. Prorubricyte
    d. Reticulocyte

889. Which of these cells should not be found in the peripheral blood of a healthy adult pig?
    a. Metarubricyte
    b. Small lymphocyte
    c. Monocyte
    d. Eosinophil

890. What is one possible site of extramedullary hematopoiesis in times of increased blood cell production?
    a. Spleen
    b. Kidney
    c. Umbilicus
    d. Bone cortex

891. The definitive host for *Baylisascaris procyonis* is
    a. Rabbits
    b. Raccoons
    c. Foxes
    d. Ferrets

892. *Baylisascaris procyonis* larvae have been shown to cause ___ in humans.
    a. Pneumonia
    b. Hemolytic anemia
    c. Brain damage
    d. Bloody diarrhea

893. Hemagglutination is
    a. Clumping of erythrocytes
    b. Lysing of erythrocytes
    c. Crenation of erythrocytes
    d. Swelling of erythrocytes

894. What test is routinely used to diagnose equine infectious anemia?
    a. Indirect fluorescent antibody test
    b. Coggins test
    c. Coombs test
    d. Electrophoresis

895. If an erythrocyte loses part of its membrane but still remains intact, it will appear as a ___ on a stained peripheral blood smear.
    a. Reticulocyte
    b. Acanthocyte
    c. Target cell
    d. Spherocyte

896. An erythrocyte that does not contain its full amount of hemoglobin will appear as ___ on a stained peripheral blood smear.
    a. Polychromasia
    b. Hypochromasia
    c. Basophilia
    d. Hyperchromasia

897. A neutrophil with a four-segmented nucleus would be classified as a
    a. Hypersegmented neutrophil
    b. Immature neutrophil
    c. Normal neutrophil
    d. Aged neutrophil

Correct answers are on pages 293-323.

898. *Polymorphonuclear* is another name commonly used for what cell?
  a. Macrophage
  b. Monocyte
  c. Eosinophil
  d. Neutrophil

899. Diagnostic seroconversion results from a ___ between the time the acute blood sample is drawn and the convalescent blood sample is drawn.
  a. Doubling of the antibody titer
  b. Fourfold increase in the antibody titer
  c. Fourfold decrease in the antibody titer
  d. Cutting of the antibody titer in half

900. After infection is eliminated, the immune response is reduced by
  a. B lymphocytes
  b. B-memory lymphocytes
  c. Monocytes
  d. T-suppressor cells

901. During an allergic response, what do sensitized cells produce in abnormal quantities when an allergen reappears after an initial exposure?
  a. Antihistamines
  b. Histamine
  c. Toxins
  d. Lysins

902. Gram-positive microorganisms stain ___ using a Gram stain.
  a. Purple
  b. Red
  c. Orange
  d. Lavender

903. Acid-fast stains are used to identify
  a. Coccidia
  b. Yeast
  c. Fungi
  d. Mycobacteria

904. What cells are sensitized by IgE to produce large quantities of histamines?
  a. Mast cells and basophils
  b. Eosinophils and basophils
  c. Monocytes and lymphocytes
  d. Neutrophils and eosinophils

905. T killer cells function to
  a. Release histamine.
  b. Recognize cancer cells as abnormal cells and eliminate them.
  c. Coat cancer cells with antibody.
  d. Release endorphin.

906. Spherocytes are ___ when viewed on a peripheral blood smear.
  a. Microcytic erythrocytes
  b. Macrocytic erythrocytes
  c. Polychromatophilic erythrocytes
  d. Hypochromic erythrocytes

907. Cats exposed to feline leukemia virus typically respond in any of the following ways, except
  a. Not becoming infected at all
  b. Becoming temporarily infected, developing immunity, and overcoming the infection
  c. Becoming infected and continuing to shed the virus indefinitely without becoming ill
  d. Becoming infected, becoming ill within 3 days, and dying within a week

908. Acid-fast positive organisms stain ___ when using an acid-fast stain.
  a. Yellow
  b. Blue
  c. Pink
  d. Brown

909. What is the predominant method of transmission of feline immunodeficiency virus in cats?
  a. Grooming
  b. Bite wounds
  c. Urine
  d. Feces

910. In assessing titers, how long after the first serum sample is collected should the second sample be collected?
  a. 7 days
  b. 3 days
  c. 2 to 6 weeks
  d. 14 weeks

911. Large numbers of bacteria growing in a broth media will cause the broth to become
  a. Red
  b. Gel
  c. Colorless
  d. Turbid

912. What microorganisms are not free living?
  a. Algae
  b. Fungi
  c. Bacteria
  d. Viruses

913. What is the correct way to write the genus and species of bacteria?
  a. *Streptococcus Pyogenes*
  b. *streptococcus pyogenes*
  c. **Streptococcus pyogenes**
  d. *Streptococcus pyogenes*

914. The acid-fast stain is used to identify the organism that causes
  a. Anaplasmosis
  b. Colibacillosis
  c. Ringworm
  d. Tuberculosis

915. What type of microbiologic media is used when a specific pathogen is sought from an area where there is normally extensive normal flora?
  a. Selective
  b. Indicator
  c. Nutrient
  d. Reducing

916. *Escherichia coli* 0157 infections are most likely obtained from eating infected
  a. Steak
  b. Hamburger
  c. Frozen chicken
  d. Cold cuts

917. Gram-negative organisms appear as what color when stained with Gram stain?
  a. Blue
  b. Red
  c. Green
  d. Clear

918. Which of the following is not a collection device for microbiologic samples?
  a. Sterile swab
  b. New toothbrush
  c. Syringe with fine-gauge needle
  d. Needle with EDTA tube

919. Which of the following best describes what happens when a bacterial cell is placed in a solution that contains 5% NaCl?
  a. No change is evident; the solution is isotonic.
  b. The cell undergoes osmotic lysis.
  c. Water moves out of the cell.
  d. Water moves into the cell.

920. Which of the following does not kill endospores?
  a. Autoclaving
  b. Incineration
  c. Hot-air sterilization
  d. Pasteurization

921. What method is best used to sterilize heat-sensitive medical equipment?
  a. Dry heat
  b. Autoclaving
  c. Gas sterilization
  d. Pasteurization

922. Viruses are best described as
  a. Free-living organisms
  b. Obligatory interstitial parasites
  c. Obligatory intracellular parasites
  d. Eukaryotic cells

923. The test that uses an enzyme that causes the conversion of hydrogen peroxide to hydrogen and oxygen when a bacterial colony is placed in the hydrogen peroxide is
  a. Coggins
  b. Coagulase
  c. Catalase
  d. Coombs

924. A positive catalase test will be indicated by the presence of
  a. A color change
  b. Gel formation
  c. Bubbles
  d. Fibrin

925. The test that will differentiate *Staphylococcus aureus* from other, less pathogenic staphylococci is the ___ test.
  a. Deaminase
  b. Urease
  c. Oxidase
  d. Coagulase

926. A nosocomial infection is
  a. Always present but not apparent at the time of hospitalization
  b. Always acquired during the course of hospitalization
  c. Always caused by medical personnel
  d. Always acquired during surgery

927. Proliferation of an organism such as *Bacillus anthracis* in the blood of cattle would be classified as a
  a. Blood dyscrasia
  b. Focal infection
  c. Local infection
  d. Septicemia

928. When normal flora prevent overgrowth of pathogens, it is called
  a. Microbial commensalism
  b. Microbial symbiosis
  c. Microbial antagonism
  d. Microbial parasitism

Correct answers are on pages 293-323.

929. "Gram-positive cocci that are arranged in grape like clusters" describes what genus of bacteria?
    a. *Escherichia*
    b. *Staphylococcus*
    c. *Streptococcus*
    d. *Actinomyces*

930. A collection of viral particles in a cell is known as a/an
    a. Viral accumulation
    b. Inclusion body
    c. Precipitate
    d. Granule

931. "Facultatively anaerobic gram-negative rods that live in the intestinal tracts of healthy and sick animals" describes what genus of bacteria?
    a. *Clostridium*
    b. *Bacillus*
    c. *Escherichia*
    d. *Corynebacterium*

932. Generally, endotoxins are products of
    a. Viruses
    b. Gram-negative bacteria
    c. Gram-positive bacteria
    d. Fungi

933. The microscopic morphology of *Streptococcus* is described as a
    a. Coccus in chains
    b. Coccus in grape like clusters
    c. Bacillus in chains
    d. Bacillus in a random arrangement

934. What organism will most likely grow on mannitol salt agar?
    a. *Streptococcus pyogenes*
    b. *Bacillus subtilis*
    c. *Clostridium perfringens*
    d. *Staphylococcus aureus*

935. What organism ferments mannitol?
    a. *Streptococcus pyogenes*
    b. *Staphylococcus epidermidis*
    c. *Staphylococcus aureus*
    d. *Streptococcus mutans*

936. *Streptococcus pyogenes* is classified as Lancefield
    a. Group A
    b. Group B
    c. Group C
    d. Group D

937. The organism that grows in and is considered a pathogen mainly of the mammary gland is
    a. *Streptococcus pyogenes*
    b. *Staphylococcus aureus*
    c. *Streptococcus agalactiae*
    d. *Escherichia coli*

938. The CAMP test is specific for
    a. *Streptococcus pyogenes*
    b. *Staphylococcus aureus*
    c. *Streptococcus agalactiae*
    d. *Staphylococcus epidermidis*

939. Warts are caused by what virus?
    a. Papilloma
    b. Variola
    c. Herpes
    d. Pox

940. Dermatophytosis pertains to a
    a. Venereal yeast infection
    b. Cutaneous mycosis
    c. Cutaneous bacterial infection
    d. Pyoderma

941. What organism exhibits fluorescence under ultraviolet light?
    a. *Microsporum gypseum*
    b. *Trichophyton mentagrophytes*
    c. *Microsporum canis*
    d. *Epidermophyton floccosum*

942. Pinkeye or contagious conjunctivitis in cattle is caused by
    a. *Hemophilus aegypti*
    b. *Moraxella bovis*
    c. *Streptococcus pyogenes*
    d. *Staphylococcus aureus*

943. Dermatitis characterized by a blue-green purulent discharge is most likely caused by
    a. *Streptococcus pyogenes*
    b. *Staphylococcus aureus*
    c. *Corynebacterium pyogenes*
    d. *Pseudomonas aeruginosa*

944. What organism often causes encephalitis in feedlot animals and encephalitis in people?
    a. *Listeria monocytogenes*
    b. *Clostridium botulinum*
    c. *Proteus vulgaris*
    d. *Pseudomonas aeruginosa*

945. What species has the highest concentration of the tetanus organism in its feces?
    a. Dogs
    b. Cats
    c. People
    d. Horses

946. What sign is most likely to be caused by botulism toxicity in water fowl?
    a. Diarrhea
    b. Vomiting
    c. Tetanic spasms
    d. Limberneck

947. What organism causes tularemia?
    a. *Yersinia pestis*
    b. *Francisella tularensis*
    c. *Escherichia coli*
    d. *Fusobacterium necrophorum*

948. The major source of tularemia exposure in people is
    a. Beavers
    b. Rats
    c. Rabbits
    d. Deer

949. Bang method is a serum test used to detect
    a. *Proteus vulgaris*
    b. *Pseudomonas aeruginosa*
    c. *Streptococcus pyogenes*
    d. *Brucella abortus*

950. In most areas of the world, rats are the reservoir host of the plague organism. However, in the Western United States, the most common species harboring this organism is
    a. Dogs
    b. Cats
    c. Beavers
    d. Prairie dogs

951. What bacterium is pleomorphic?
    a. *Streptococcus*
    b. *Mycobacterium*
    c. *Pasteurella*
    d. *Corynebacterium*

952. The kennel cough syndrome in dogs is often caused by a combination of boarding at a kennel, a viral infection, and infection with
    a. *Pasteurella multocida*
    b. *Staphylococcus aureus*
    c. *Corynebacterium diphtheriae*
    d. *Bordetella bronchiseptica*

953. The tuberculin test uses what reagent?
    a. A freeze-dried tuberculin antigen
    b. A small dose of a live bacterin
    c. A purified protein derivative of *Mycobacterium tuberculosis*
    d. An organism closely related to *Mycobacterium tuberculosis*

954. What organism often causes bacterial pneumonia in newborn foals?
    a. *Streptococcus pneumoniae*
    b. *Klebsiella pneumoniae*
    c. *Mycoplasma pneumoniae*
    d. *Diplococcus pneumoniae*

955. Potomac horse fever is caused by *Ehrlichia risticii*, which is a/an
    a. Gram-negative bacillus
    b. Gram-positive bacillus
    c. Obligate extracellular parasite
    d. Obligate intracellular parasite

956. What virus is most difficult to destroy on an inanimate surface?
    a. Coronavirus
    b. Rotavirus
    c. Hepatitis virus
    d. Parvovirus

957. Cystitis is most often caused by
    a. Gram-negative cocci
    b. Gram-negative bacilli
    c. Gram-positive cocci
    d. Gram-positive bacilli

958. What organism is a spirochete?
    a. *Corynebacterium pyogenes*
    b. *Streptococcus pyogenes*
    c. *Mycobacterium tuberculosis*
    d. *Leptospira grippotyphosa*

959. What organism causes strangles in horses?
    a. *Staphylococcus aureus*
    b. *Streptococcus equi*
    c. *Corynebacterium equi*
    d. *Strongylus vulgaris*

960. What characteristic is unique to *Mycobacterium*?
    a. It is a spore former.
    b. It is anaerobic.
    c. It is easily killed by antibiotics.
    d. It survives phagocytosis.

Correct answers are on pages 293-323.

961. What resistant stage of a protozoan is usually passed in the feces?
    a. Trophozoite
    b. Cyst
    c. Egg
    d. Larva

962. What organism has a cell membrane instead of a cell wall?
    a. Fungus
    b. Protozoan
    c. Yeast
    d. Alga

963. Which of the following is not a simple stain?
    a. Methylene blue
    b. Crystal violet
    c. Safranin
    d. Gram stain

964. Ergot is a toxin produced by
    a. Bacteria
    b. Viruses
    c. Protozoa
    d. Fungi

965. Acquired active immunity results from
    a. Vaccination
    b. Antitoxin administration
    c. Ingestion of colostrum
    d. Administration of gamma globulin

966. In culturing a bacterial sample, use of aseptic technique ensures that
    a. All of the bacteria in the sample are destroyed.
    b. Only the bacteria in the sample are transferred to the culture medium.
    c. Nothing will grow on the culture medium.
    d. Multiple bacterial species will grow on the culture medium.

967. *Escherichia coli* is normally found
    a. On the skin
    b. In the intestinal tract
    c. In the respiratory tract
    d. In the stomach

968. An organism that requires oxygen to grow and survive is defined as a/an
    a. Obligate anaerobe
    b. Aerobe
    c. Obligate aerobe
    d. Facultative anaerobe

969. The main disadvantage of quaternary ammonium compounds is that
    a. They weaken with evaporation.
    b. They easily stain skin.
    c. Organic compounds interfere with their activity.
    d. They lose the oxygen radical and become water.

970. On a blood agar plate, an area of complete hemolysis is classified as
    a. Alpha
    b. Beta
    c. Gamma
    d. Delta

971. The enzyme catalase is used by bacteria to break down
    a. Proteins
    b. Superoxides
    c. Hydrogen peroxide
    d. Starches

972. Trophozoites and cyst forms are associated with
    a. Protozoans
    b. Cestodes
    c. Trematodes
    d. Nematodes

973. *Dipylidium caninum* is a
    a. Trematode
    b. Nematode
    c. Arthropod
    d. Cestode

974. *Fasciola hepatica* is a
    a. Nematode
    b. Cestode
    c. Trematode
    d. Protozoan

975. All of the following are blood-borne parasites, but which one does not belong in the same classification group as the other three?
    a. *Dirofilaria* species
    b. *Haemobartonella* species
    c. *Toxoplasma* species
    d. *Anaplasma* species

976. Flotation solutions usually have a specific gravity between
    a. 1.350 and 1.400
    b. 1.250 and 1.300
    c. 1.100 and 1.150
    d. 1.200 and 1.250

977. What method does not concentrate ova?
   a. Centrifugal flotation
   b. Direct smear
   c. Simple flotation
   d. Sedimentation

978. What method favors detection of fluke ova?
   a. Sedimentation
   b. Centrifugal flotation
   c. Simple flotation
   d. Direct smear

979. What is unique about fluke ova that requires a special detection procedure?
   a. They are found in fewer numbers than most other ova.
   b. They have a lower specific gravity than most other ova.
   c. The cysts are the detectable form in feces.
   d. They have a higher specific gravity than most other ova.

980. Cellophane tape is traditionally used to detect the ova of ___ in horses.
   a. Roundworms
   b. Pinworms
   c. Whipworms
   d. Flukes

981. Which of the following is not a fecal flotation solution?
   a. Sodium sulfate
   b. Sugar
   c. Sodium chloride
   d. Sodium nitrate

982. To examine for trophozoites, it is best to use a mixture of fresh feces and ___.
   a. Sodium chloride
   b. Sodium nitrate
   c. Zinc sulfate
   d. Physiologic saline

983. A puppy infected with *Dirofilaria immitis* the day it is born will not test positive for heartworm microfilariae until it is ___ old.
   a. 12 months
   b. 6 to 7 months
   c. 3 to 4 months
   d. 1 month

984. The ELISA heartworm test kit detects the antigens of
   a. Heartworm microfilariae
   b. Female adult heartworms
   c. Adult heartworms and microfilariae
   d. Toxins produced by adult heartworms

985. *Dirofilaria immitis* is a
   a. Cestode
   b. Arthropod
   c. Nematode
   d. Trematode

986. *Otodectes cynotis* is a
   a. Cestode
   b. Arthropod
   c. Nematode
   d. Trematode

987. Transmission of lice is mostly via
   a. Blood-sucking arthropods
   b. Direct contact
   c. Ingestion
   d. Fecal contamination

988. A dog becomes infected with *Dipylidium caninum* by ingestion of
   a. Saliva from an infected dog
   b. Feces from an infected dog
   c. Tissues of an infected rabbit
   d. Infected fleas

989. A spurious parasite infection would occur if
   a. *Dipylidium caninum* ova were found in feline feces.
   b. *Moniezia expansa* ova were seen in canine feces.
   c. *Strongyloides stercoralis* larvae were found in canine feces.
   d. *Isospora felis* oocysts were found in feline feces.

990. In puppies, transplacental transmission is the primary route of infection for
   a. *Dipylidium*
   b. *Toxocara*
   c. *Ancylostoma*
   d. *Trichuris*

991. The most common intermediate host of *Taenia pisiformis* is a
   a. Ruminant
   b. Flea
   c. Fly
   d. Rabbit

992. The parasite whose adult resembles a whip and whose eggs have bipolar plugs is
   a. *Strongyloides stercoralis*
   b. *Trichuris vulpis*
   c. *Toxocara canis*
   d. *Toxascaris leonina*

Correct answers are on pages 293-323.

993. *Taenia* eggs closely resemble the eggs of
   a. *Echinococcus*
   b. *Isospora*
   c. *Toxocara*
   d. *Capillaria*

994. The genus of tapeworm that releases its eggs in packets is
   a. *Taenia* species
   b. *Echinococcus* species
   c. *Dipylidium* species
   d. *Moniezia* species

995. *Trichophyton mentagrophytes* causes ___ in cats.
   a. Tick fever
   b. Pediculosis
   c. Mange
   d. Ringworm

996. Pediculosis is an infestation of
   a. Ticks
   b. Flies
   c. Lice
   d. Mites

997. In people, *Toxocara canis* is the causative agent of
   a. Creeping eruption
   b. Scabies
   c. Hydatidosis
   d. Visceral larva migrans

998. A large ciliate protozoa that may be found in swine feces is
   a. *Balantidium* species
   b. *Trichomonas* species
   c. *Giardia* species
   d. *Histomonas* species

999. Smegma may be examined for the presence of
   a. *Tritrichomonas* species
   b. *Thelazia* species
   c. *Dictyocaulus* species
   d. *Stephanurus* species

1000. The parasite diagnosed by vaginal washing is
   a. *Tritrichomonas* species
   b. *Dictyocaulus* species
   c. *Dioctophyma* species
   d. *Anaplasma* species

1001. The parasite diagnosed by tracheal wash is
   a. *Tritrichomonas* species
   b. *Dictyocaulus* species
   c. *Dioctophyma* species
   d. *Anaplasma* species

1002. The parasite diagnosed by examining urine is
   a. *Tritrichomonas* species
   b. *Dictyocaulus* species
   c. *Dioctophyma* species
   d. *Anaplasma* species

1003. The parasite diagnosed by examining blood is
   a. *Tritrichomonas* species
   b. *Dictyocaulus* species
   c. *Dioctophyma* species
   d. *Anaplasma* species

1004. The parasite also known as a *brown dog tick* is
   a. *Rhipicephalus sanguineus*
   b. *Ixodes dammini*
   c. *Dermacentor variabilis*
   d. *Dermacentor albipictus*

1005. The parasite also known as *a winter tick*
   a. *Rhipicephalus sanguineus*
   b. *Ixodes dammini*
   c. *Dermacentor variabilis*
   d. *Dermacentor albipictus*

1006. The parasite also known as the *American dog tick* is
   a. *Rhipicephalus sanguineus*
   b. *Ixodes dammini*
   c. *Dermacentor variabilis*
   d. *Dermacentor albipictus*

1007. The parasite also known as *a dear tick*
   a. *Rhipicephalus sanguineus*
   b. *Ixodes dammini*
   c. *Dermacentor variabilis*
   d. *Dermacentor albipictus*

1008. The parasite that lives in ears is
   a. *Sarcoptes* species
   b. *Demodex* species
   c. *Chorioptes* species
   d. *Otodectes* species

1009. The parasite that lives on the skin's surface is
   a. *Sarcoptes* species
   b. *Demodex* species
   c. *Chorioptes* species
   d. *Otodectes* species

1010. The parasite that burrows into the skin is
   a. *Sarcoptes* species
   b. *Demodex* species
   c. *Chorioptes* species
   d. *Otodectes* species

1011. The parasite that lives in hair follicles is
    a. *Sarcoptes* species
    b. *Demodex* species
    c. *Chorioptes* species
    d. *Otodectes* species

1012. What equine parasite genus has three species?
    a. *Parascaris* species
    b. *Strongylus* species
    c. *Oxyuris* species
    d. *Strongyloides* species

1013. Which stage of the tick life cycle has six legs?
    a. Nymphal
    b. Larval
    c. Adult female
    d. Adult male

1014. A flea is the intermediate host for
    a. *Trichuris vulpis*
    b. *Taenia pisiformis*
    c. *Dipylidium caninum*
    d. *Strongyloides stercoralis*

1015. A rabbit is the intermediate host for
    a. *Trichuris vulpis*
    b. *Taenia pisiformis*
    c. *Dipylidium caninum*
    d. *Strongyloides stercoralis*

1016. *Cheyletiella* mites use ___ as their hosts.
    a. Dogs, cats, and rabbits
    b. Dogs, rabbits, and birds
    c. Cats, birds, and rodents
    d. Cats, dogs, and rodents

1017. Infection of this parasite is via skin penetration.
    a. *Trichuris vulpis*
    b. *Taenia pisiformis*
    c. *Dipylidium caninum*
    d. *Strongyloides stercoralis*

1018. People may serve as the intermediate host of
    a. *Echinococcus granulosus*
    b. *Anoplocephala magna*
    c. *Taenia pisiformis*
    d. *Moniezia benedeni*

1019. What parasite ova have a single operculum?
    a. *Trichuris* species
    b. *Taenia* species
    c. *Alaria* species
    d. *Moniezia* species

1020. What parasite ova have three pairs of hooklets?
    a. *Trichuris* species
    b. *Taenia* species
    c. *Alaria* species
    d. *Moniezia* species

1021. What parasite ova have bipolar plugs?
    a. *Trichuris* species
    b. *Taenia* species
    c. *Alaria* species
    d. *Moniezia* species

1022. What parasite ova have radial striations?
    a. *Trichuris* species
    b. *Taenia* species
    c. *Alaria* species
    d. *Moniezia* species

1023. Fish are intermediate hosts of what parasite?
    a. *Diphyllobothrium* species
    b. *Hymenolepis* species
    c. *Paragonimus* species
    d. *Fasciola* species

1024. What parasite has ova found in sputum?
    a. *Diphyllobothrium* species
    b. *Hymenolepis* species
    c. *Paragonimus* species
    d. *Fasciola* species

1025. The double-pore tapeworm is
    a. *Paragonimus kellicotti*
    b. *Moniezia expansa*
    c. *Dipylidium caninum*
    d. *Echinococcus granulosus*

1026. The parasite that infects the liver of its host is
    a. *Diphyllobothrium* species
    b. *Hymenolepis* species
    c. *Paragonimus* species
    d. *Fasciola* species

1027. The parasite whose larvae encyst in the subcutaneous tissue of rabbits is
    a. *Gasterophilus* species
    b. *Hypoderma* species
    c. *Oestrus* species
    d. *Cuterebra* species

1028. The parasite whose eggs are cemented to the hair of horses is
    a. *Gasterophilus* species
    b. *Hypoderma* species
    c. *Oestrus* species
    d. *Cuterebra* species

Correct answers are on pages 293-323.

1029. The parasite whose larvae form warbles in subcutaneous tissue along the back of cattle is
    a. *Gasterophilus* species
    b. *Hypoderma* species
    c. *Oestrus* species
    d. *Cuterebra* species

1030. The parasite whose larvae enter the nasal cavity of sheep is
    a. *Gasterophilus* species
    b. *Hypoderma* species
    c. *Oestrus* species
    d. *Cuterebra* species

1031. What parasite completes its life cycle on or in its host?
    a. *Ctenocephalides* species
    b. *Otodectes* species
    c. *Hypoderma* species
    d. *Dermacentor* species

1032. What species causes a disease known as *walking dandruff*?
    a. *Trombicula* species
    b. *Sarcoptes* species
    c. *Demodex* species
    d. *Cheyletiella* species

1033. Scabies is caused by
    a. *Trombicula* species
    b. *Otodectes* species
    c. *Melophagus* species
    d. *Sarcoptes* species

1034. The parasite also known as the *hookworm* is
    a. *Bunostomum* species
    b. *Ostertagia* species
    c. *Trichostrongylus* species
    d. *Haemonchus* species

1035. The parasite also known as the *stomach hair worm* is
    a. *Bunostomum* species
    b. *Ostertagia* species
    c. *Trichostrongylus* species
    d. *Haemonchus* species

1036. The parasite also known as the *brown stomach worm* is
    a. *Bunostomum* species
    b. *Ostertagia* species
    c. *Trichostrongylus* species
    d. *Haemonchus* species

1037. The parasite also known as the *barber's pole worm* is
    a. *Bunostomum* species
    b. *Ostertagia* species
    c. *Trichostrongylus* species
    d. *Haemonchus* species

1038. Choose the correct size sequence, from largest ova to smallest ova.
    a. *Trichostrongylus, Nematodirus, Strongyloides, Eimeria*
    b. *Nematodirus, Trichostrongylus, Strongyloides, Eimeria*
    c. *Eimeria, Nematodirus, Trichostrongylus, Strongyloides*
    d. *Nematodirus, Strongyloides, Trichostrongylus, Eimeria*

1039. The parasite found in the abomasal gastric glands of ruminants is
    a. *Oesophagostomum* species
    b. *Ostertagia* species
    c. *Haemonchus* species
    d. *Dictyocaulus* species

1040. The parasite that sucks blood in the abomasum of ruminants is
    a. *Oesophagostomum* species
    b. *Ostertagia* species
    c. *Haemonchus* species
    d. *Dictyocaulus* species

1041. The parasite that matures in the lungs is
    a. *Oesophagostomum* species
    b. *Ostertagia* species
    c. *Haemonchus* species
    d. *Dictyocaulus* species

1042. The parasite that forms nodules in the intestinal mucosa is
    a. *Oesophagostomum* species
    b. *Ostertagia* species
    c. *Haemonchus* species
    d. *Dictyocaulus* species

1043. The most common parasite found in pigs is
    a. *Ascaris* species
    b. *Metastrongylus* species
    c. *Oesophagostomum* species
    d. *Trichuris* species

1044. Skin penetration is a means of entry into a host by
    a. *Toxocara* species
    b. *Taenia* species
    c. *Anaplasma* species
    d. *Ancylostoma* species

1045. A client has found a large number of roundworms in her puppy's feces at home. A logical explanation may be that
   a. The dog has been treated recently for roundworms.
   b. The puppy ate something that looks like worms that were passed in the feces.
   c. It is a period in the life cycle of roundworms that results in the passage of large numbers of worms.
   d. The roundworms pass out in large numbers when the dog has diarrhea.

1046. Coughing and increased numbers of eosinophils in peripheral blood suggest
   a. *Trichuris* infection
   b. *Toxocara* infection
   c. *Dipylidium* infection
   d. *Giardia* infection

1047. Choose the correct size sequence, from smallest ova to largest ova.
   a. *Isospora, Uncinaria, Ancylostoma, Toxocara*
   b. *Isospora, Ancylostoma, Toxocara, Uncinaria*
   c. *Isospora, Ancylostoma, Uncinaria, Toxocara*
   d. *Ancylostoma, Isospora, Uncinaria, Toxocara*

1048. Anemia in puppies is most likely associated with infection with
   a. *Isospora* species
   b. *Paragonimus* species
   c. *Strongyloides* species
   d. *Ancylostoma* species

1049. A common sign of giardiasis is
   a. Chronic diarrhea
   b. Hemolytic anemia
   c. Acute coughing
   d. Bloody vomit

1050. The parasite also known as a *liver fluke* is
   a. *Dioctophyma* species
   b. *Fasciola* species
   c. *Paragonimus* species
   d. *Capillaria* species

1051. The parasite also known as a *lung fluke* is
   a. *Dioctophyma* species
   b. *Fasciola* species
   c. *Paragonimus* species
   d. *Capillaria* species

1052. The parasite also known as the *kidney worm* is
   a. *Dioctophyma* species
   b. *Fasciola* species
   c. *Paragonimus* species
   d. *Capillaria* species

1053. The parasite also known as a *lungworm* is
   a. *Dioctophyma* species
   b. *Fasciola* species
   c. *Dipylidium* species
   d. *Capillaria* species

1054. *Trichuris* ova most resemble the ova of
   a. *Isospora* species
   b. *Taenia* species
   c. *Ancylostoma* species
   d. *Capillaria* species

1055. A chewing louse of dogs is
   a. *Trichodectes* species
   b. *Haematopinus* species
   c. *Felicola* species
   d. *Damalinia* species

1056. A chewing louse of cats is
   a. *Trichodectes* species
   b. *Haematopinus* species
   c. *Felicola* species
   d. *Damalinia* species

1057. A sucking louse of cattle is
   a. *Trichodectes* species
   b. *Haematopinus* species
   c. *Felicola* species
   d. *Damalinia* species

1058. A chewing louse of cattle is
   a. *Trichodectes* species
   b. *Haematopinus* species
   c. *Felicola* species
   d. *Damalinia* species

1059. The genus name for the spinose ear tick is
   a. *Otodectes*
   b. *Otobius*
   c. *Oestrus*
   d. *Oxyuris*

1060. What species is not parasitized by pinworms?
   a. Horses
   b. Dogs
   c. Rodents
   d. Humans

1061. An intestinal fluke is
   a. *Alaria* species
   b. *Fascioloides* species
   c. *Stephanurus* species
   d. *Metastrongylus* species

Correct answers are on pages 293-323.

1062. The parasite also known as a *lungworm* is
   a. *Alaria* species
   b. *Fascioloides* species
   c. *Stephanurus* species
   d. *Metastrongylus* species

1063. The parasite also known as a *kidney worm* is
   a. *Alaria* species
   b. *Fascioloides* species
   c. *Stephanurus* species
   d. *Metastrongylus* species

1064. The parasite also known as the *large American liver fluke* is
   a. *Alaria* species
   b. *Fascioloides* species
   c. *Stephanurus* species
   d. *Metastrongylus* species

1065. Which statement concerning fleas is true?
   a. "Flea dirt" is flea feces.
   b. Fleas are host specific.
   c. Adults cannot survive long periods without feeding.
   d. Flea eggs are not sticky and fall off into the environment.

1066. The parasite that causes generalized pruritus is
   a. *Ancylostoma* species
   b. *Melophagus* species
   c. *Notoedres* species
   d. *Echinococcus* species

1067. The parasite that causes creeping eruption in people is
   a. *Ancylostoma* species
   b. *Melophagus* species
   c. *Notoedres* species
   d. *Echinococcus* species

1068. A gravid proglottid would be found in a
   a. Mite
   b. Tick
   c. Arthropod
   d. Tapeworm

1069. The parasite that causes feline scabies is
   a. *Ancylostoma* species
   b. *Melophagus* species
   c. *Notoedres* species
   d. *Echinococcus* species

1070. The parasite that is a protozoan is
   a. *Psoroptes* species
   b. *Mallophaga* species
   c. *Cryptosporidium* species
   d. *Anoplura* species

1071. Johnes disease in sheep is caused by
   a. *Campylobacter jejuni*
   b. *Mycobacterium paratuberculosis*
   c. *Corynebacterium diphtheriae*
   d. *Mycoplasma gallisepticum*

1072. A sucking louse is a/an
   a. Protozoan
   b. Trematode
   c. Cestode
   d. Arthropod

1073. Which of these parasites is a mite?
   a. *Psoroptes* species
   b. *Mallophaga* species
   c. *Cryptosporidium* species
   d. *Anoplura* species

1074. The urine of an animal with hematuria is most likely to be
   a. Cloudy and red
   b. Clear and brown
   c. Red and clear
   d. Brown and cloudy

1075. The specific gravity of a patient's urine is so high you cannot measure it. You dilute the sample 1:2 with distilled water. Now the specific gravity is 1.032. What is the sample's true specific gravity?
   a. 2.032
   b. 1.016
   c. 2.064
   d. 1.064

1076. The specific gravity of urine is a measure of
   a. The weight of urine compared with the weight of water
   b. The weight of urine compared with the weight of physiologic saline
   c. The weight of urine
   d. The weight of urine minus the weight of water

1077. Calcium carbonate crystals are often seen in ___ urine.
   a. Dog
   b. Horse
   c. Cat
   d. Cattle

1078. In a urine sample, a red blood cell may be easily confused with a/an
   a. Fat droplet
   b. Degenerate white blood cell
   c. Renal epithelial cell
   d. Amorphous crystal

1079. All of the following are assessed in a routine urinalysis, except
    a. pH
    b. Occult blood
    c. Urobilinogen
    d. Blood urea nitrogen

1080. The Ictotest is used to detect ___ in urine.
    a. Blood
    b. Fat
    c. Urobilinogen
    d. Bilirubin

1081. What can you do if the specific gravity of a urine sample is greater than 1.065?
    a. Multiply the results by 2
    b. Dilute it 2:1 with distilled water
    c. Dilute it 1:2 with distilled water
    d. Read it using the total protein scale

1082. Dipsticks for urine chemical analysis should always be
    a. Shaken before used
    b. Stored in the refrigerator
    c. Stored with desiccant
    d. Reconstituted with physiologic saline

1083. A control should be run on the urine dipstick
    a. After the dipstick has been reconstituted
    b. Before each urinalysis is begun
    c. After each urinalysis is completed
    d. When there is a shift change in personnel

1084. What crystal is commonly described as having a coffin-lid appearance?
    a. Bilirubin crystal
    b. Calcium oxalate crystal
    c. Cystine crystal
    d. Triple phosphate crystal

1085. An ammonium biurate crystal is sometimes described as
    a. Shaped like an envelope
    b. Shaped like a pyramid
    c. Looking like a thorny apple
    d. Looking like a bicycle wheel

1086. The best urine sample from a housebroken dog is collected in
    a. Late evening
    b. Afternoon
    c. Midmorning
    d. Early morning

1087. Urine samples collected in the morning from housebroken dogs tend to be
    a. Unacceptable for sediment analysis
    b. The most concentrated samples
    c. Bright orange
    d. The least concentrated samples

1088. What are the two preferred methods of collecting a urine sample for culture?
    a. Catheterization and voiding
    b. Expressing the bladder and cytocentesis
    c. Cytocentesis and catheterization
    d. Cytocentesis and voiding

1089. Polyuria is
    a. Lack of urine production
    b. Production of excessive amounts of urine
    c. Lack of water intake
    d. Excessive protein in the urine

1090. Oliguria is
    a. Excessive eating
    b. Green urine
    c. Excessive bilirubin in the urine
    d. Decreased urine output

1091. Anuria is
    a. Decreased urine output
    b. Decreased drinking
    c. Complete lack of urine production
    d. Excessive drinking

1092. Isosthenuria is urine that would most likely have a specific gravity
    a. Of 1.010
    b. Below 1.006
    c. Of 1.000
    d. Above 1.065

1093. How would you expect the specific gravity of dilute, colorless urine to compare with that of dark yellow urine?
    a. Slightly higher
    b. Moderately higher
    c. Much higher
    d. Lower

1094. An alkaline urine pH can be the result of
    a. Urinary tract obstruction
    b. Uncontrolled diabetes
    c. Prolonged diarrhea
    d. Starvation

Correct answers are on pages 293-323.

1095. What part of the urinalysis is measured by a refractometer?
    a. Protein
    b. Glucose
    c. Ketones
    d. pH

1096. A urine specimen collected by free catch at 8 A.M. and left at room temperature until the afternoon could be expected to have
    a. Decreased numbers of bacteria
    b. Increased numbers of bacteria
    c. Decreased numbers of epithelial cells
    d. Increased numbers of epithelial cells

1097. Blood in the urine is reported as
    a. Dysuria
    b. Hematuria
    c. Pyuria
    d. Proteinuria

1098. Pus in the urine is reported as
    a. Dysuria
    b. Hematuria
    c. Pyuria
    d. Proteinuria

1099. Painful urination is recorded as
    a. Dysuria
    b. Hematuria
    c. Pyuria
    d. Proteinuria

1100. Corticosteroid treatment results in a hemogram characterized by
    a. Increased lymphocytes and increased neutrophils
    b. Increased lymphocytes and decreased neutrophils
    c. Decreased lymphocytes and decreased neutrophils
    d. Decreased lymphocytes and increased neutrophils

1101. In dogs the normal neutrophil-to-lymphocyte ratio is
    a. 1:1
    b. 3.5:1
    c. 1:5
    d. 7.5:1

1102. In horses the normal neutrophil-to-lymphocyte ratio is
    a. 4:1
    b. 1:5
    c. 3:1
    d. 1:1

1103. Dark yellow, cloudy urine generally would be expected to have a
    a. pH of 5.0 or below
    b. Low specific gravity
    c. High specific gravity
    d. pH of 8.0 or above

1104. In pigs how long can a stress neutrophilia last?
    a. 30 minutes
    b. 60 minutes
    c. 2 hours
    d. 8 hours

1105. Pancytopenia is characterized by
    a. Decreased numbers of white blood cells
    b. Decreased numbers of all blood cells
    c. Decreased numbers of red blood cells
    d. Decreased numbers of granulocytes and monocytes

1106. Toxic change is evaluated in
    a. Eosinophils
    b. Erythrocytes
    c. Neutrophils
    d. Monocytes

1107. A urine sample that shows 3+ occult blood on a dipstick and is grossly red and clear would most likely contain
    a. Mucus
    b. Red blood cells
    c. Hemoglobin
    d. Crystals

1108. Chronic infections are often associated with
    a. Monocytosis
    b. Erythrocytosis
    c. Basopenia
    d. Eosinopenia

1109. It is easier to observe the elements in urine sediment by
    a. Lowering the condenser to increase the light
    b. Raising the condenser to increase the light
    c. Lowering the condenser to reduce the light
    d. Raising the condenser to lower the light

1110. Carnivores generally have
    a. Very high protein levels in urine
    b. Acidic urine
    c. Alkaline urine
    d. High glucose levels in urine

1111. Vegetable diets generally yield
    a. Acidic urine
    b. High levels of ketones in urine
    c. Low levels of ketones in urine
    d. Alkaline urine

1112. The sulfosalicylic acid test of urine is used to detect
    a. Bilirubin
    b. Protein
    c. Glucose
    d. Hemoglobin

1113. Urine samples should be centrifuged at a
    a. Low speed (1000 to 3000 rpm) for 20 minutes
    b. High speed (6000 to 10,000 rpm) for 20 minutes
    c. Low speed (1000 to 3000 rpm) for 5 minutes
    d. High speed (6000 to 10,000 rpm) for 5 minutes

1114. Erythropoietin is produced in the
    a. Bone marrow
    b. Kidney
    c. Liver
    d. Pituitary gland

1115. You could observe a right shift on a stained blood smear of blood
    a. Drawn from an artery
    b. Frozen before a smear was made
    c. Stored at room temperature for a week
    d. Collected in the wrong anticoagulant

ANSWERS

1. **a** Vibrios are gram negative, curved rods.

2. **a**

3. **a** Bacterial endospores are "survival capsules" that allow the organisms to survive harsh environments, but they are not a form of reproduction.

4. **d**

5. **b** Iodine fixes crystal violet in gram-positive bacteria.

6. **a**

7. **a** Antisepsis is destruction or inhibition of microbes on skin or living tissue; disinfection is the same but on inanimate objects. Sterilization is the complete destruction of living organisms.

8. **c**

9. **b**

10. **a** *Borrelia* is the genus.

11. **b**

12. **b** B cells produce antibodies used for humoral immunity.

13. **b** Lentiviruses cause slowly developing diseases.

14. **c**

15. **b**

16. **b**

17. **c**

18. **c**

19. **d**

20. **c** The WBC response to infections and inflammation will vary depending on the severity and longevity of the condition. Not all WBCs are phagocytic all of the time.

21. **b**

22. **b**

23. **a** The rest are all gram-negative organisms.

24. **b** The rest are gram-positive or non-Gram staining.

25. **d** Because viruses multiply in living host cells only, selective toxicity is difficult to achieve.

26. **b** Despite its name, most cases occur far from the Rocky Mountains.

27. **a**

28. **c**

29. **d** Following decolorization, safranin stains gram-negative bacteria pink.

30. **d** Most bacteria prefer a neutral pH.

31. **b**

32. **a**

33. **c** Viruses multiply in living cells only.

34. **d**

35. **c**

36. **a**

37. **b**

38. **a**

39. **c** The *Brucella* bacteria can cause a fluctuating, or undulant, fever in humans that is a symptom of human brucellosis.

40. **c**

41. **d** There is a great deal of redundancy built into the kidneys.

42. **d** Blood urea nitrogen (BUN) is a breakdown product of protein that healthy, functioning kidneys remove. SGTP is a liver function test, creatinine is a breakdown product of muscle creatine that the kidneys also normally remove. Increased glucose levels may indicate diabetes.

43. **a**

44. **b** Urea is produced by the metabolism of protein.

45. **a** Albumin is produced by the liver.

46. **b**

47. **a**

48. **a**

49. **c**

50. **a**

51. **b** All contain anticoagulants; purple = EDTA, blue = citrate, gray = sodium fluoride.

52. **b**

53. **a** Urea is excreted by the kidneys, and up to 40% is reabsorbed by the tubules for reexcretion. Rate of reabsorption is inversely proportional to the amount of urine output; therefore, urea evaluates both filtration and function.

54. **a** With loss of fluid, both the urine and the plasma will become more concentrated.

55. **c** The patient is already stressed because of a preexisting condition, and the body may have already begun to produce ADH; therefore, it is not a good scientific baseline.

56. **a** Excess glucose is flushed from the body into the urine.

57. **a**

58. **b** Cells continue to utilize glucose at a rate of 7% to 10% per hour.

59. **c**

60. **a**

61. **d**

62. **b**

63. **a** Test method should be specific to the species being tested, or the horse specimen should be diluted before beginning the testing.

64. **c** Lipase is a test for pancreatitis.

65. **d**

66. **d**

67. **a** A popular electrolyte analyzer, the IDEXX VetLyte, uses ion-specific electrodes to measure sodium, potassium, and chloride.

68. **d**

69. **b**

70. **d** T4, thyroxine, is typically elevated in hyperthyroidism, which may be seen in older cats. Luteinizing hormone (LH) is measured for reproductive studies, cortisol for Cushing disease, and bile acids for liver abnormalities.

71. **c**

72. **b** This is necessary to concentrate any cells present; they are then removed from the supernatant.

73. **d**

74. **c**

75. **a**

76. **b**

77. **b** 10× objective

78. **a** 40× objective

79. **d** Also highly refractile

80. **a**

81. **d**

82. **b**

83. **d** These are retained primary granules.

84. **b**

85. **c**

86. **c**

87. **a** They can be hard to distinguish from macrophages once they have been activated.

88. **b**

89. **a**

90. **c**

91. **b**

92. **a** The entire blood supply is replenished approximately every 3 months.

93. **c**

94. **a**

95. **c** Individuals produce antibodies to a specific antigen.

96. **d**

97. **b**

98. **c**

99. **c** Leukocytes secrete various interleukins. These small, soluble proteins stimulate cellular activities, such as cell proliferation, cell activation, and release or inhibition of more cytokines, all of which help regulate the immune response.

100. **b**

101. **a**

102. **c** IgA is found in body secretions such as tears, mucus, and colostrum.

103. **d**

104. **d** IgE is found on the surfaces of mast cells and attracts eosinophils to the site of inflammation.

105. **a**

106. **b**

107. **d**

108. **a**

109. **b**

110. **c**

111. **b**

112. **c**

113. **a** An example of epitasis is the case of a black cat with tabby stripes; the stripes cannot be seen because of the black color.

114. **a**

115. **d**

116. **a**

117. **c**

118. **c** Anomalies would include things such as malocclusions, hip dysplasia, and collie eye.

119. **d** One female homozygous polled, one male homozygous polled, one female heterozygous polled, and one male heterozygous polled

120. **d**

121. **c**

122. **a**

123. **b** Selective media contain inhibitors to growth of other types of bacteria, for example, CNA.

124. **b**

125. **d**

126. **c**

127. c

128. d

129. c

130. a

131. a

132. a

133. a

134. b

135. b

136. d

137. a

138. d

139. b

140. c A Howell-Jolly body is the last remaining remnant of the nucleus before it is totally gone from the immature RBC. Hypochromasia may very well be present with RBC regeneration but is not a sign: crenation is an artifact, and Döhle bodies are a sign of toxic change in neutrophils.

141. a Anemic blood is thinner in consistency, and using the normal angle creates too long a smear. Increasing the angle shortens the smear.

142. c MCV, mean cell volume; MCH, mean cell hemoglobin; MCHC, mean cell hemoglobin concentration; MPV, mean platelet volume

143. b Total WBC counts done either manually or by instrument will result in increased WBCs, because the nuclei of the immature RBCs do not lyse and are counted as nucleated WBCs.

144. d Nucleated platelets and free nuclei from lysed avian RBCs cannot be distinguished from WBCs. An indirect method of determining the avian WBC count that avoids this problem is done by using the eosinophil Unopette and special calculations.

145. c Cat platelets have a tendency to clump, so it is important to examine the blood smear for clumping if a machine count gives a low reading. The other species' platelets do not clump as easily.

146. c Acanthocytes have a few projections and may be of uneven length. Crenated cells have shorter projections that are evenly spaced around the cell. Schistocytes are pieces of RBCs, and anisocytes are RBCs that show varying sizes (anisocytosis).

147. a Polychromasia is a slight bluish tinge caused by RNA that is not completely gone from the RBC. A hypochromic RBC is a cell that has insufficient hemoglobin and has more central pallor than normal. Hyperchromasia is a condition that does not really exist, but spherocytes look hyperchromic; they appear darker than normal. Crenated RBCs have evenly spaced, short projections all around the cells, which are artifacts.

148. c Absolute numbers are based on the total WBC count; percentages are based on 100 cells counted on the differential. Relative numbers and decimal numbers do not pertain.

149. d Fibrinogen rises in inflammatory processes, and its detection is useful, especially in ruminants.

150. b If the WBCs and/or platelets are elevated, you can see the larger, white layer on top of the RBC column in a spun-down hematocrit tube.

151. c Neutrophils and macrophages (called *monocytes* in the blood) are the phagocytes. Granulocytes include basophils and eosinophils and have other primary functions.

152. c Monocyte nuclei are not segmented and are usually lobed, although occasionally they may be round or band shaped. Then you must identify on the basis of other characteristics.

153. c The same number of cells are counted, no matter what objective is used. Poor positioning of the condenser obscures the WBCs. Too much time on the hemocytometer dries the diluted blood and could affect the count. Mini clots trap WBCs and would affect the count.

154. c Spherocytes are seen with immune-mediated hemolytic anemia and will cause RBC regeneration. All other responses are signs of regeneration.

155. a *Left shift* typically refers to increased numbers of immature neutrophils that may include any stage, from bands to more immature forms.

156. **b** New methylene blue is used to detect reticulocytes. Lactophenol cotton blue is used for identification of fungal elements, Gram stain is for bacteria, and acridine orange is a special stain used in a hematology analyzer.

157. **b** Choice **d** is would also be correct, except it is missing the metamyelocyte stage that follows the myelocyte.

158. **c** Any cell name ending in *blast* is the most immature cell that can be visually identified on a bone marrow or blood smear.

159. **c** Kittens are most likely to become infected with roundworms by nursing on an infected queen.

160. **d** The infective L$_3$ larvae can penetrate the skin and migrate eventually to the intestine.

161. **a** There are many ova that look alike; to correctly identify them, you must know the origin of the feces.

162. **b** Proglottids or tapeworm segments may be found around the anus before dropping to the ground. Dogs are not hosts to pinworms.

163. **c** Several species of mosquitoes serve as intermediate hosts for heartworms.

164. **d** The prepatent period is 6 to 7 months, and the detection antibody in the serology kit is directed at the adult heartworms. Therefore, it is not possible to immediately detect heartworm infection.

165. **d** After killing the adult worms, the animal is treated to kill the circulating microfilariae.

166. **d** They are all protozoans, but *Giardia* belongs to a different phylum.

167. **a** *Giardia* cysts are the infective form and are passed in formed feces; the trophozoite form is more apt to be seen in watery feces.

168. **a** Oocyst size for *Isospora canis* is 32 to 53 by 26 to 43 microns, compared to *Toxocara canis* ova, which is 90 by 75 microns.

169. **d** *Strongylus* sp. is a large strongyle, *Oxyuris* is the pinworm, and *Anoplocephala* is a tapeworm.

170. **d** *Strongylus spp.* cannot be identified by the appearance of their ova.

171. **b** These parasites and canine hookworms all belong to the order Strongylidae, and all have typical "strongyle" (or "strongylid") eggs.

172. **a** *Tritrichomonas* causes reproductive problems; the other three can cause diarrhea.

173. **a** The kidneys would preserve water but still remove the wastes, resulting in more concentrated urine.

174. **d** The presence of WBCs indicates inflammation somewhere in the urogenital tract, and the presence of RBCs indicates bleeding in the urogenital tract.

175. **c** A third name for these crystals is *ammonium-magnesium-phosphates.*

176. **b** Often crystal formation is temperature dependent. If allowed to cool, dissolved substances come out of solution. Sometimes there is a correlation between crystalluria and the presence of uroliths.

177. **d** Blood urea nitrogen (BUN) is a chemical analyte in the blood whose increase is associated with kidney disease.

178. **a** The size ranges for the two cell types overlap.

179. **d** Fat droplets and RBCs may be similar in appearance, but fat droplets are more variable in size. Adding acetic acid further identifies the structures in question.

180. **c** Amorphous crystals are granular in appearance and may be confused with cocci; however, many bacteria found in urine are rods that do not look like these crystals.

181. **c** Casts are cylinders composed of protein that is secreted by the renal tubules and may contain cells of various stages of disintegration, if they were present in the tubule regions.

182. **c** In kidney disease, excessive amounts of protein enter the glomerular filtrate and are not reabsorbed, resulting in protein in the urine.

183. **d** When carbohydrates are not metabolized in the normal way, or there is a lack of sufficient carbohydrates, the animal's body uses fat as its energy source. Breakdown of fat results in ketones in the urine.

184. **b** Mucus threads may be seen occasionally in other species. They are easily overlooked because of their faint appearance in the background.

185. **d** Choice **a**, cystine crystals; **b**, tyrosine crystals; **c**, ammonium biurate crystals

186. **c** Microbial contamination is more likely to occur with the other three collection methods.

187. **b** Feline renal epithelial cells have a high fat content, and fat droplets are released when these cells disintegrate.

188. **d** The crystal violet stain washes out of the gram-negative bacteria, and they pick up the pink counterstain, safranin.

189. **b** The other three media are differential media used to help identify isolated bacteria, especially gram-negative bacteria.

190. **a** BAP supports growth of both gram-positive and gram-negative bacteria; mannitol salt agar selects for staphylococci, and Mueller-Hinton is used for antimicrobial sensitivity testing.

191. **b** These tests help differentiate the gram-positive cocci and small gram-positive bacilli bacteria.

192. **c** This is a characteristic of *Proteus mirabilis* and *Proteus vulgaris* that helps in their identification but can also hinder isolation of other bacteria growing on the same plate.

193. **d** This is a yeast that is thought to have at least a secondary role in some cases of otitis externa.

194. **a** *Microsporum canis* accounts for a large percentage of canine and feline ringworm cases; two species of *Trichophyton* also cause the infection in dogs and cats.

195. **c** *Bacillus* spp. are among the most common laboratory contaminants, but *Bacillus anthracis* is a pathogen of many mammals.

196. **d** This organism can wall itself off from treatment but can still produce toxins that may kill the host.

197. **a** *Streptococcus* spp. are normally present in the environment, intestine, and oral cavities but are important pathogens.

198. **b** A strain of this organism, *Escherichia coli* O157:H7, is a cause of food-borne illness associated with eating undercooked, contaminated ground beef.

199. **c** The normal habitat of these small, gram-negative rods are the intestinal tracts of animals and humans and the soil.

200. **d** A few drops of a 10% solution of potassium hydroxide (KOH) is added to the specimen and is allowed to sit for several hours to clear the sample of debris.

201. **c** A temperature of 37° C is close to body temperature of many animals and supports the growth of most pathogens.

202. **b** Sabouraud's is for fungi, MacConkey selects for gram-negative bacteria, and Kligler iron is for differential for enterobacteriaceae.

203. **d** Glucose is released for increased energy needs.

204. **c** Uric acid is increased in the blood of both avians and Dalmatians with kidney disease.

205. **b** Measuring cholesterol is useful, because the thyroid hormone controls synthesis and destruction of cholesterol.

206. **b** A diabetic animal does not have sufficient insulin to metabolize the glucose load given at the beginning of the test.

207. **c** In dehydration, fluid leaves the blood to enter the dehydrated tissues, leaving the blood concentrated.

208. **a** In addition, the kidney maintains homeostasis by regulating water and electrolyte levels and producing the hormone important in RBC production.

209. **b** In addition, the pancreas secretes insulin and glucagon to regulate glucose metabolism.

210. **c** Bile acids are synthesized by the liver from cholesterol and released into the intestine.

211. **c** Acute inflammation or tissue damage can elevate fibrinogen.

212. **c** The three major proteins comprising total protein are fibrinogen, albumin, and globulin. By using serum, the fibrinogen is gone, leaving only the albumin and globulin fractions.

213. **d** Bicarbonate is the second most common plasma anion and can be measured indirectly from the blood gas CO_2 measurement.

214. **c** Electrolyte measurements help assess the severity of the fluid loss.

215. **d** Albumin levels may be decreased in liver disease.

216. **a** In dogs, this is one of the most common causes of hypercalcemia.

217. **c** EDTA combines with calcium to prevent clot formation, resulting in a falsely decreased blood calcium concentration.

218. **b** A sensitivity of 95% implies that the assay will identify positive samples 95 out of 100 times when the patient has the disease. Specificity refers to the ability of a test to identify negative samples when the disease is absent.

219. **c** Establishing normal ranges must be done in a statistically correct manner and is usually something an individual clinic will not do.

220. **c** Abnormal test results (outside of the normal reference range) imply disease conditions; but sometimes a test result is outside of the reference range, but the animal really does not have the disease. This is called a *false positive*.

221. **a** Some action must be taken, and even simply repeating the test and getting a good value shows that the out-of-range value was probably a simple outlier, especially when you know the control usually falls within its normal range.

222. **c** The analyzers used in today's veterinary clinics are programmed to do many self-checks, and any necessary calibration for the instrument is done or is supplied by the manufacturer.

223. **b** Normal values and reference ranges are synonymous, referring to the range of values that is established when running a test on many healthy animals of the same species.

224. **c** Only separated serum from this list can be frozen; freezing the other specimens would alter test results.

225. **d** *Rimming* or *ringing* the clot means loosening the clotted blood from the tube, which may help release serum trapped in the clot.

226. **a** Physiologic saline is most like serum in composition.

227. **d** Many of the kits today can even use a drop of whole EDTA blood. There is a built-in mechanism for separating the plasma from the whole blood in the test card.

228. **d** Although negligible, even tiny clots may alter test results. Therefore, good laboratory procedure is to never use clotted blood of any degree.

229. **a** Newborns rely on the antibodies they receive from the colostrum the first few days of life for protection against infectious disease. These antibodies are gamma globulins.

230. **b** Kinetic reaction refers to the way in which enzymes are measured.

231. **c** The humoral immune response involves the B-lymphocyte production of antibodies.

232. **b** Monoclonal antibodies are very specific antibodies that are commercially produced for use against specific antigenic portions of a disease organism.

233. **d** Dogs and cats cannot be hyposensitized to foods, so eliminating the foods the animal is allergic to is the best form of treatment.

234. **c** The other three responses are typical signs of allergies.

235. **d** Cornified and superficial are the same, but *cornified* conjures the image of a cell with "corners," which makes it easy to identify the cell.

236. **d** The presence of many superficial cells is the predominant feature on a vaginal smear of a dog in heat.

237. **d** A hematocrit is a blood test; an example of a transudate is the fluid of ascites from congestive heart failure; an example of an exudate is the fluid collected from septic peritonitis.

238. **c** This is one way to prepare a smear from aspirated material from a solid mass, particularly samples of high cellularity.

239. **b** Diseased tissue removed during a surgical procedure is cut, and the exposed portion is pressed to a microscope slide and stained for cytologic analysis.

240. **c** Single laboratory tests are more conveniently done in-house. Samples sent out to commercial laboratories are not as fresh, and results are delayed when compared to those done in an in-house laboratory. Commercial veterinary laboratories have rigorous quality control standards.

241. **d** Toenail clips yield only very small blood samples and are painful, so they are not commonly used for blood sample collection.

242. **c** Excess anticoagulant will dilute the blood sample, affecting both morphology and cell counts.

243. **c**

244. **b** The anticoagulant of choice for blood gas analysis is heparin.

245. **b**

246. **c** The jugular and cutaneous ulnar vein (wing vein), along with the medial metatarsal vein, are the most common blood collection sites in this species.

247. **b** Venous blood is generally used for all of the listed laboratory tests, except for blood gases.

248. **c** The magnification of the ocular lens multiplied by the magnification of the objective used equals the total magnification.

249. **c** All of the tubes contain anticoagulant except for the red-top tube. When blood is collected into a tube containing anticoagulant, the tube must be gently inverted several times to adequately mix the sample.

250. **d** Sheep is the only species listed whose erythrocytes are anucleate.

251. **b** Granulocytes are those leukocytes that contain granules, including neutrophils, eosinophils, and basophils. Lymphocytes and monocytes are agranulocytes.

252. **d** Basophils are a rare finding in peripheral blood.

253. **a** Macrocytosis is usually an indication that there is ongoing regeneration of erythrocytes, because immature cells are larger in size than fully mature erythrocytes.

254. **b** The major sites for production for lymphocytes are the lymphoid organs and peripheral lymphoid tissue (thymus, lymph nodes, spleen, tonsils); they are produced only secondarily in the bone marrow.

255. **c** Horse erythrocytes are round and anucleated. Bird and reptile erythrocytes are usually oval in shape and nucleated. Only red blood cells of llamas are ovoid and devoid of a nucleus.

256. **c**

257. **d**

258. **b** All of the species listed have round to globoid granules in their eosinophils. Only the cat has rod-shaped granules.

259. **d**

260. **c** Spherocytosis is a considered a classic finding in patients with autoimmune hemolytic anemia (AIHA).

261. **b** The MCHC is considered the most accurate of all the indices.

262. **c** A large buffy coat would be expected in a patient with an infection, because the buffy coat is composed of leukocytes, and an elevated white cell count is to be expected in response to infection.

263. **c** The most common cause of an elevated hematocrit is dehydration. This is a relative increase, resulting from a decreased blood fluid component.

264. **c**

265. **b** Normal erythrocyte cell counts are in the millions.

266. **d**

267. **d** Platelets are the smallest elements found in a peripheral blood smear, and thus a higher magnification is necessary to view them adequately.

268. **b**

269. **a** Howell-Jolly bodies are remnants of nuclear material found in erythrocytes, not leukocytes.

270. **c** Buccal mucosal bleeding time is the only test listed that evaluates primary hemostasis. The others evaluate secondary hemostasis.

271. **b**

272. **b**

273. **a** Vascular spasm and platelet plug formation occur during primary hemostasis. Clot lysis occurs after the traumatized tissue has healed.

274. **d** As an erythrocyte develops, it becomes smaller and pinker, its nucleus becomes smaller, and the nuclear chromatin becomes denser.

275. **d** Trauma during venipuncture interferes with the results of a coagulation profile by increasing the blood's coagulability. Samples are collected in blue citrate–containing Vacutainer. It is not necessary to immediately test the sample.

276. **b** Because von Willebrand disease is a disorder of primary hemostasis—that is, the coagulation cascade is normal—buccal mucosal bleeding time (BMBT) is the best screening test of those listed.

277. **b** The sciatic nerve is located in the gluteal region, in close proximity to the proximal femur.

278. **c**

279. **b**

280. **d** Petechiae, epistaxis, and hematuria are all symptoms of a bleeding disorder.

281. **d**

282. **d** All of these ectoparasites are macroscopic except for mites, which normally require microscopic examination for visualization.

283. **c** Members of the family *Psoroptidae* reside on the surface of the skin or within the external ear canal. All other mites listed live under the surface of the skin.

284. **c** Of the choices, only the sarcoptic mange mite is highly contagious to other animals and humans.

285. **d** *Demodex* is not contagious.

286. **a** *Cheyletiella*, also known as *walking dandruff*, is commonly known as the *fur mite* because of where it is normally found.

287. **b**

288. **d**

289. **d** *Oxyuris*, or pinworm, ova are most often collected with cellophane tape from the perianal region of horses.

290. **b**

291. **d**

292. **a**

293. **d**

294. **b** Only the PCV uses a sample collected in a microhematocrit tube and centrifuged. This procedure is necessary for examination of the buffy coat as well.

295. **b** The Difil is a filter test that detects the presence of microfilariae only, whereas the ELISA test may detect presence of the antigen of adult parasites in an occult infection.

296. **a** Because the eggs of *Fasciola hepatica* are heavy, they sink rather than float.

297. **a**

298. **c**

299. **c**

300. **c** Fecal sedimentation is a concentrating method that tests a large sample. A direct smear is quick to perform, yet tests only a very small sample. Both these methods contain much fecal debris, making examination difficult.

301. **b**

302. **c** Eosinophils are often found in greater numbers in the blood of animals that are allergic or who have parasitic infections.

303. **d** Common tapeworm eggs of dogs and cats are not usually seen on flotation tests or direct smears, because they usually leave the host in tapeworm segments.

304. **a** All of the techniques are concentrating methods, except for the direct examination of a whole blood sample.

305. **d** *Trichuris* and *Capillaria* are barrel-shaped, with bipolar plugs. *Dipetalonema* and *Dirofilaria* are both filaroid. *Toxocara canis* and *Toxocara cati* are both round, ascarid-type ova. The pairs differ primarily in size. On the other hand, *Ancylostoma* and *Toxascaris* are easily differentiated by their distinctive shapes, and so comparative measurement of ova size is not necessary in this instance.

306. **d**

307. **b**

308. **b** Fecal samples that do not stand for a long enough time may not reveal the presence of ova. Standing for an excessive amount of time may distort the ova present, complicating their identification.

309. **c**

310. **a** All of the tests listed are tests specific for heartworm. Only the differential cell count, for which a blood smear is examined, may accidentally or incidentally reveal the presence of microfilariae.

311. **c**

312. **b** The more concentrated a flotation solution, the more likely it is to distort ova.

313. **d**

314. **d** Only the ova of the hookworm fit the description.

315. **b**

316. **b**

317. **a** EDTA will best preserve any cells present in the sample.

318. **c** Penetration of a joint or body cavity demands the same aseptic preparation as for a surgical procedure.

319. **d** *Cheyletiella*, or *walking dandruff* mites, are best collected from the surface of the animal's fur with cellophane tape.

320. **c**

321. **b** Bone marrow smears are much thicker than blood smears, and so a longer period of staining time is necessary to adequately identify the various cells present.

322. **b**

323. **c**

324. **a**

325. **a**

326. **a** If the urethra is not patent, it will not be possible to pass a urinary catheter. If there is a partial obstruction, it is still possible to manually express the bladder or collect a sample by free catch. Cystocentesis involves direct puncture of the bladder, entirely bypassing the urethra.

327. **c** Casts generally dissolve in basic urine, that is, urine that has been standing for some time before being examined. The rest of the statements are true.

328. **b** Urine becomes more basic over time, raising the pH rather than lowering it.

329. **d** A state of dehydration causes the kidneys to conserve body water, thereby decreasing the amount of urine produced and increasing the concentration of urine excreted.

330. **b**

331. **a** Small amounts of bilirubin are considered a normal finding in dogs.

332. **b** Animals in the final stages of chronic renal failure are isosthenuric, that is, they have urine specific gravities of between 1.008 to 1.012.

333. **c** The tests for leukocytes, specific gravity, and nitrites on biochemical strips are generally considered inaccurate in veterinary patients.

334. **c** Only the free-catch method involves no iatrogenic traumatization of the patient's urinary tract.

335. **d**

336. **d** A horse is an herbivore. Herbivores are more likely to have a basic urine pH, whereas carnivores have an acidic urine pH.

337. **a** An overhydrated patient's body would need to excrete the excessive fluids, thereby increasing the amount of urine produced, diluting it, and thus lowering its specific gravity.

338. **d** Ketones are produced as a result of the breakdown of fatty acids. Because diabetic patients cannot normally utilize glucose, they get their energy from the breakdown of fatty acids.

339. **c** Cystocentesis is the method of choice for collecting a sterile urine sample. All other methods listed yield a sample that is potentially contaminated.

340. **d** UTIs with nitrate-reducing bacteria cause nitrite formation. However, this test does not seem to be as sensitive in dogs and cats as it is in people, therefore it is important to look for bacteria in the sediment.

341. **d** Bilirubin tends to break down on exposure to ultraviolet light.

342. **a** The first urine sample of the morning tends to be most concentrated, thereby indicating the ability of the patient's kidney to concentrate urine.

343. **b** Hematuria is the presence of intact red blood cells in the urine. During centrifugation, only intact red blood cells settle out, changing the color of the supernatant from red to clear.

344. **b**

345. **d** Patients, especially females, need to be sedated before urinary catheterization.

346. **d** Crystal presence does not change the pH of urine, rather certain types of crystals are more likely to form if the urine is acidic or basic.

347. **d** Squamous epithelial cells are derived from the lower urinary passageways. Cystocentesis bypasses these tissues, and so there is virtually no possibility of retrieving these cells when performing a cystocentesis.

348. **c** Hemolysis and lipemia are the most common factors that affect clinical chemistry analysis.

349. **c**

350. **c** Creatinine is the most reliable indicator of renal function.

351. **d** Only the cortisol/creatinine ratio is a test of urine. All other tests listed use blood.

352. **c**

353. **a** BUN and creatinine are biochemical tests of the renal profile.

354. **b** Globulin is not measured directly, rather it is calculated by subtracting serum albumin from the total protein value. In this case, 7.3 – 3.5, or 3.8 g/dl. The A/G ratio would be 3.5 divided by 3.8, which is 0.92.

355. **c** Steatorrhea is the presence of fecal fat. Fat will appear as red-orange droplets in the feces when stained with Sudan III or Sudan IV.

356. **d**

357. **b**

358. **b** All tests listed evaluate liver function, but bile acids, preprandial and postprandial, are considered the function test of choice.

359. **d**

360. **c** 8° C is approximately 46° F, which is refrigerator temperature (F = 9/5 C + 32).

361. **a**

362. **b**

363. **d**

364. **a** When using the Neubauer hemocytometer, leukocytes are counted in the nine large primary squares.

365. **b** When using the Neubauer hemocytometer, platelets are counted in the 25 secondary squares within the central primary square.

366. **c** Birds have heterophils instead of neutrophils.

367. **a**

368. **a** Azotemia means there is presence of urea or other nitrogenous elements in the blood.

369. **c** Prerenal azotemia is due to a pathologic condition that occurs prerenally, resulting from decreased blood flow, shock, and heart disease.

370. **c** Nonspecific or nonadaptive immunity includes physical and chemical barriers in the body to ward off antigen attacks.

371. **c** The PMN, or polymorphonuclear cell, refers to the neutrophil.

372. **b** They have turbid urine because of calcium carbonate crystals.

373. **d** A refractometer is the most reliable; it estimates density based on the refractive index of fluid. A urinometer uses a glass cylinder with a float and is less reliable, and the reagent test strips are the least reliable.

374. **d**

375. **c** Cats have two forms of reticulocytes, punctate and aggregate; only the aggregate form is counted.

376. **b** Pathologic conditions occurring after the kidney, in the bladder and urethra, result in anuria or oliguria.

377. **d** Healthy animals have sufficient insulin to drop the increased glucose load to normal levels in approximately 2 hours. Animals with diabetes mellitus typically still show hyperglycemia and glucosuria in this same time period.

378. **d** The neutrophil is the white cell that responds most quickly to the presence of microorganisms. It leaves the circulation, enters tissue, and becomes phagocytic.

379. **a** The total white cell count of milk is reflected by the degree of precipitation or gel formation.

380. **a**

381. **b** Lithium heparin causes the least amount of morphologic changes in avian and reptile cells.

382. **b** Blood should be allowed to thoroughly form the fibrin clot matrix by resting at room temperature 20 to 30 minutes before centrifugation.

383. **d** Red-top tubes should never be placed on a rocker, because it can cause hemolysis of the cells.

384. **c**

385. **d** Refrigeration (0° C to 4° C) is the best method of preservation for whole blood. Allow the sample to warm up to room temperature before analysis.

386. **a**

387. **b** One part sample, one part diluent

388. **c** Lipemic, icteric, and hemolyzed sera may interfere with chemistry testing.

389. **a** Hemolysis and lipemia may elevate the enzyme concentration.

390. **c** The Ictotest is used to determine bilirubinuria.

391. **b** The squash preparation yields excellent cytologic smears.

392. **a**

393. **d** It is the only stage in which the bitch will not only attract the male but also will be receptive to him.

394. **c** *Malassezia pachydermatis* is a common cause of otitis externa.

395. **c**

396. **a**

397. **c**

398. **a**

399. **c** The monolayer is selected because the cells are barely touching one another but not so far apart that you would not be able to count 100 WBCs.

400. **c** Horses may have pronounced rouleaux formation of the red cells normally.

401. **b**

402. **d** *Anaplasma marginale* affects cattle predominantly.

403. **c** The PCV value is divided by 3 to determine the estimated hemoglobin value.

404. **c** This is done to avoid double counting cells on shared borders of the squares.

405. **d** Birds, rabbits, hamsters, reptiles, amphibians, some fish, and guinea pigs all have heterophils. Heterophils may be confused with eosinophils.

406. **b** The white blood cell count is multiplied by the relative value (%) to determine the absolute value of each type of cell present.

407. **d** Cat platelets are large compared with their relatively small red blood cells. This can lead to inaccurate electronic blood cell counts when the cells are not differentiated by size.

408. **c** Felines have both punctate and aggregate reticulocytes, although only the aggregate is counted.

409. **b**

410. **d** A 1% ammonium oxalate is the diluent for the WBC Unopette, because it lyses the RBCs.

411. **b**

412. **c**

413. **c**

414. **c**

415. **d**

416. **c**

417. **a** Selective agar "selects for" a particular type of growth, like gram-negative organisms. Most gram-positive organisms will not grow on MacConkey's. The other three will grow both gram-negative and gram-positive organisms.

418. **b** *Alpha hemolysis* refers to partial hemolysis of the RBCs and shows as a greenish color; *beta hemolysis* refers to total hemolysis of the RBCs surrounding the colonies and results in a clear zone.

419. **a** Ringworm organisms use the dextrose in Fungassay agars.

420. **d** Chocolate agars are used to grow organisms that cause sexually transmitted diseases (STDs); *Brucella* is considered an STD.

421. **b** *Borrelia burgdorferi* is the causative agent of Lyme disease transmitted via the deer tick.

422. **c** *Sarcoptes* mites are transmittable to humans, a condition referred to as *scabies*.

423. **c**

424. **d** Hookworms are a zoonotic parasite that causes a disease in humans known as *cutaneous larval migrans*.

425. **d**

426. **a** The deer tick *Ixodes scapularis*

427. **a** Pollakiuria is commonly seen in blocked cats, who squat frequently to urinate but void small amounts only.

428. **c** Formalin fumes can affect the staining quality of cytology samples.

429. **a** Casts are cylindrical molds of the renal tubules in which they are formed and are made up of glycoprotein.

430. **a**

431. **b**

432. **c**

433. **a** In addition, the trophozoite form may be seen in diarrheic feces, but cysts are the infective stage.

434. **c** Ehrlichiosis is a tick-borne disease seen in dogs. Toxoplasmosis, coccidiosis, and cryptosporidiosis are not spread by ticks.

435. **d** Pediculosis refers to an infestation with lice. Myiasis is fly larvae penetration of living tissue (maggots). Acariasis is a mite or tick infestation.

436. **c**

437. **c** *Psoroptes* is very contagious and psoroptic mange is a reportable disease.

438. **d**

439. **b** The skin scraping is used to diagnose the mite *Notoedres*, which infests cats. *Bovicola* is a louse, and *Otodectes* is an ear mite. *Ctenocephalides* is a flea.

440. **b** The hydatid cyst is the largest intermediate form of a tapeworm. Cysticercus, coenurus, and cysticercoid are all smaller intermediate forms of tapeworms.

441. **c**

442. **b** *Paragonimus*, the lung fluke of dogs and cats, uses snails as intermediate hosts.

443. **a**

444. **d** The Difil test uses a membrane to filter the blood and capture microfilariae. Although microfilariae may be seen on the direct wet mount; they are not concentrated on a filter, and only a drop of blood is screened, versus 1 ml of blood in the Difil procedure.

445. **c** *Spirocirca* is a canine parasite that causes nodules in the esophagus, which may then become neoplastic. *Physaloptera* is the canine stomach worm. *Filaroides* is the canine lungworm. *Neosporum* is a protozoan that causes neurologic disease in pups.

446. **c**

447. **c** *Tritrichomonas* in fresh feces have a very "zippy" movement. *Giardia* trophozoites, on the other hand, have what is called a "falling leaf" movement.

448. **d** The horn fly, *Haematobia irritans*, is responsible for the greatest economic losses in U.S. cattle because of reduced weight gain and reduced milk production.

449. **c** Various species of *Plasmodium* cause malaria in humans and birds.

450. **c**

451. **c** Visceral larval migrans is due to the migration of the larva of *Toxocara canis*, the canine roundworm. Larvae of *Ancylostoma caninum*, the canine hookworm, cause cutaneous larval migrans.

452. **d** Proglottids are tapeworm segments, often appearing like rice grains around the anus or in the feces.

453. **d** *Capillaria aerophila* is a lungworm found in cats. The ova resemble those of *Trichuris vulpis*, the whipworm. *Capillaria plica* is the bladder worm and similar ova are seen in the urine. *Dictyocaulus* is the ruminant lungworm. *Filaroides osleri* is the canine lungworm.

454. **c** *Toxoplasma* does not enter through the skin; choices **a** and **d** are the most common sources of *Toxoplasma* ova.

455. **b** The sedimentation technique is often needed to diagnose the presence of *Fasciola hepatica*, which is a fluke with heavy ova that may not float.

456. **c** Hookworm ova are similar to strongyle ova often seen in horses. Ascarids are roundworms. The whipworm has an operculated egg. Coccidia oocysts are smaller than strongyle ova.

457. **b** *Oestrus ovis*, sheep nose bot fly, deposits larvae in the nostrils.

458. **a** Occult heartworm infections are those in which microfilariae are absent; this is very common.

459. **d** Hookworm larvae can be transmitted to puppies transplacentally. After the puppies are born the hookworms mature and attach to the intestinal lining and begin sucking blood.

460. **b**

461. **a** Myiasis is caused by flies laying eggs in living tissue, which then hatch, and the larvae eat the tissue.

462. **c** The sensitivity of the occult heartworm test is zero when only male worms are present.

463. **a** Heartworms in cats usually live 2 to 3 years, compared to 5 to 7 years in dogs. They also have fewer and smaller adult worms, and microfilaremia is uncommon. Cats overall are more resistant hosts of heartworms than are dogs.

464. **c** An elevated hematocrit usually indicates dehydration is present. A low hematocrit indicates anemia is present.

465. **d** Leukocytosis is seen in a regenerative left shift. The leukocyte count is normal or depressed, and the immature neutrophils outnumber the mature neutrophils in a degenerative left shift.

466. **a**

467. **c** The megakaryocyte is a large cell found in the bone marrow that produces thrombocytes (platelets).

468. **d** A normal leukocyte count with an increase in immature cells that outnumber the mature cells is called a *degenerative left shift*. A *regenerative left shift* is when the leukocyte count is elevated, and the segments outnumber the bands.

469. **a** As you change from the low-power objective to the high-power objective when using a microscope, the image is magnified, the field of view is smaller, more details are seen, and the field becomes darker, not lighter, so you need to increase the light.

470. **c** A leukocyte count will be falsely elevated because of metarubricytes, nucleated erythrocytes, in the peripheral blood, because the counting procedures count all nucleated cells.

471. **b** The average canine erythrocyte is 7 microns in diameter and can be used as a ruler to estimate the sizes of other cells.

472. **a** Poikilocytosis, which is a variation in the red cell shape, is not associated with a responsive anemia. Anisocytosis, reticulocytosis, and polychromasia are all seen in responsive anemias.

473. **a**

474. **d**

475. **b**

476. **d** Iron is an essential mineral found in hemoglobin.

477. **b** The mean corpuscular volume (MCV) gives an indication of the average size of a red blood cell. The mean corpuscular hemoglobin concentration (MCHC) gives an indication of the average amount of hemoglobin in a red blood cell.

478. **c** The myeloblast, an immature granulocyte, is the most immature cell in the granulocyte series. The megakaryoblast is the most immature cell in the thrombocyte series.

479. **b**

480. **a** The osteoclast is a normal large cell in the marrow with separate multiple nuclei. The megakaryocyte is similar, except that the nuclei are all attached and not separate. The osteoblast and monoblast are also large cells, but they have a single nucleus.

481. **b** Erythroid hyperplasia, increased red cell production in the marrow, is consistent with a responsive anemia.

482. **a**

483. **c** The one-step prothrombin time, which measures the extrinsic coagulation pathway, is used to confirm a diagnosis of warfarin (rodenticide) toxicity.

484. **a** Icterus is not seen in disseminated intravascular coagulation (DIC). Because this is an abnormal activation of all of the coagulation pathways, hemorrhage, thrombocytopenia, and a prolonged activated clotting time (ACT) are all seen.

485. **b** Von Willebrand disease is stimulated by hypothyroidism, resulting in the appearance of clinical signs.

486. **d**

487. **d** A typical specific gravity for dilute porcine urine is 1.010. The values 0.010 and 3.055 are invalid numbers; 1.035 is a high specific gravity that suggests that the urine is concentrated.

488. **d** Ketonuria, ketones in the urine, is most commonly found in the bovine because of the way that they metabolize carbohydrates.

489. **c** The renal cell is the smallest epithelial cell seen on a urine sediment examination. A leukocyte is smaller, but it is not an epithelial cell.

490. **c**

491. **a**

492. **b**

493. **c**

494. **a** Oxalate is becoming a common type of urolith, a stone in the urinary tract, in cats.

495. **b** The urobilinogen test on the urine dipstick is the least useful in animals, because it is designed to detect a blocked bile duct, which rarely occurs in animals.

496. **d** Protein often increases in the urine in glomerular disease because of leakage of the large protein molecules through the glomerular filter.

497. **d** Struvite, composed of ammonium, magnesium, and phosphate, is the most likely constituent of the grit seen in the urethra of male cats.

498. **c** Dalmatians have the most problems with uric acid stones, because they lack the enzyme uricase to break down the uric acid.

499. a

500. c

501. b

502. a

503. c

504. a

505. c

506. d

507. a Calcium, a mineral, is not considered an electrolyte.

508. b

509. c The x-ray film digestion test actually measures fecal trypsin, which is lacking in pancreatic atrophy.

510. d Hyperkalemia is commonly associated with hypoadrenocorticism, also known as *Addison disease.*

511. d

512. b

513. c Ion-specific technology is used in electrolyte analyzers; end-point analysis is a type of technology used in liquid chemistry analyzers; reflectometry is used in dry chemistry analyzers.

514. b A false positive test is one in which the animal is not affected and the test is positive. A false negative is when the animal is affected and the test is negative.

515. b Sensitivity is the ability of a test to determine true positives. Specificity is the ability of a test to determine true negatives.

516. b The course of action for a normal-appearing cat that tests positive with an ELISA test for feline leukemia should be to retest in 4 to 8 weeks, or run an IFA test.

517. c An 80% sensitivity and 100% specificity for a test procedure means that 20% of the tests will result in false negative results. The 100% specificity indicates that all the negative patients will be determined.

518. c Plasma cells produce immunoglobulins, also known as *antibodies.*

519. c

520. b

521. b The best method to diagnose food allergies in dogs is to place them on hypoallergenic diets for 10 weeks with no other foods.

522. a

523. a Combined immunodeficiency is a genetic disease commonly seen in Arabian horses or Arabian crosses.

524. c

525. c

526. c The circulating pool of neutrophils and the marginal pool of neutrophils are the same size.

527. b

528. a Grains and forage are most commonly associated with mycotoxicosis, which is due to a toxin produced by certain types of fungi growing on the feedstuffs.

529. c

530. d

531. c

532. b Fungal organisms stain blue (gram-positive) with Gram stain.

533. a

534. a Diseases caused by prions, such as the spongiform encephalopathies, are thought to be transmitted by ingestion.

535. b Basophilic stippling is seen in erythrocytes.

536. b

537. a

538. d

539. b

540. b

541. c

542. c Each oocyst contains eight infective sporozoites.

543. b *Giardia* is a protozoa, but not a coccidian. *Bunostomum* is a hookworm. *Taenia* is a tapeworm.

544. b Mesothelial cells, from the body wall, are most likely seen from thoracocentesis.

545. c Small lymphocytes are most commonly seen in chylothorax, which is usually due to a ruptured thoracic duct.

546. a

547. b

548. b In equine protozoal meningitis (EPM), the diagnostic test requires CSF to measure antibodies.

549. a

550. c Pseudocyesis, or false pregnancy, is a normal event in the bitch and occurs during diestrus.

551. c This would help differentiate an inflammatory response (no microorganisms) from an infectious response (neutrophils are phagocytizing microorganisms). Extracellular microorganisms could be the result of contamination.

552. d

553. a The superficial cell, which often resembles a potato chip, is an example of a cornified vaginal epithelial cell.

554. d

555. b The CSF is normally the least cellular with only 5 to 25 cells/mm^3.

556. b In necrospermia all of the sperm are dead, and there is no motility or movement. This may also occur if the sample is cold. The term for "no sperm are present" is *azoospermia*.

557. a In the cow, estrus is 12 hours only, and ovulation occurs in metestrus.

558. c Sperm counts are usually in excess of 100,000,000 cells/mm^3. Erythrocyte counts are in the 6 to 10 million cells/mm^3 range, thrombocytes are in the 250,000 to 500,000 cells/mm^3 range, and leukocyte counts are in the 5000 to 20,000 cells/mm^3 range.

559. c Polydipsia/polyuria (PU/PD) is not commonly seen in hyperparathyroidism. In hyperadrenocorticism, diabetes insipidus, and diabetes mellitus, PU/PD is a common clinical sign.

560. c

561. b Also in the pulmonary arteries

562. d

563. c In neonatal isoerythrolysis, the neonate gets antibodies against its own erythrocytes in the colostrum. This occurs naturally in thoroughbred and standard-bred horses and can also be seen in bitches that have had transfusions. The young animal develops a hemolytic anemia.

564. d There is no universal cat blood donor, because cats have isoantibodies against other blood types. The good news is that most cats in the United States have the same blood type, A.

565. a Although rare, transfusion reactions in the cat are much more severe than those in the dog and may occur with the first transfusion, which does not occur in the dog.

566. d

567. d Microfilariae circulate in the bloodstream, and when spun down in a hematocrit tube, they become trapped in the upper layers of the buffy coat. They look like clear spaghetti at the buffy coat plasma separation in the tube under a microscope at 10×.

568. a An increased total protein is most indicative of dehydration.

569. d Macrophages are tissue cells.

570. a Isosthenuria generally indicates dilute urine, commonly seen with diabetic animals and end stage renal disease.

571. c The spun hematocrit gives you the packed red cell volume, plasma color, and appearance; an estimate of white blood cells and platelets in the buffy coat; and a refractometer reading of total protein from the separated plasma.

572. b A monolayer (mono means "one") is a layer of cells one cell thick only; therefore, there is no overlapping of blood cells, and they are not bunched together, distorting shape.

573. **a** To ensure adequate fixation, tissue submitted for biopsy should be less than 1 cm in any given plane and should be placed in 10 times the specimen's volume of 10% formalin.

574. **a** Railroad tracks do not allow a nice monolayer for viewing and occur during the push/pull phase of a blood smearing, when too much pressure or inconsistent pressure is maintained on the push/pull slide.

575. **c** Ideally a biopsy specimen should have formalin contact within a centimeter of tissue. Large masses that cannot be sliced for smaller specimens should be injected with formalin for better preservation.

576. **c** Myopathy from prolonged recumbency could result in excess myoglobin being released.

577. **c** Capillary action, or capillarity, occurs when a liquid pushes against a solid and is caused to rise, such as blood entering a capillary tube.

578. **b** Impedance is commonly used to test blood samples in an instrument that passes a current of light or electricity through the sample. The change in current is measured as impedance.

579. **d**

580. **c** Anisocytosis is the only selection that would be an abnormality of the substance being evaluated. All of the other answers are mechanical properties of the instrumentation, and any inconsistencies with these will cause laboratory error.

581. **a** A standard solution is commonly distilled water; it is a solution that acts as a control to equilibrate laboratory instruments.

582. **c** Doing any of the other selections will actually increase the light source availability that is refracted into the lens.

583. **a** QBC stands for quantitative buffy coat, in which a machine quantitates the numbers of various white blood cells that are concentrated in the buffy coat of a spun, specialized hematocrit tube.

584. **a** The scanning objective on a binocular microscope is the lowest magnification power (usually 4×) and should be the first objective used to bring the sample into view and focus.

585. **b** This is the principle of Beer's law.

586. **a**

587. **b** Glucose will decrease, enzyme activity may be decreased, and potassium, not sodium, will increase.

588. **d** $53/1000 \times 100 = 5.3\%$

589. **a** RBC Unopettes are inaccurate. WBCs and platelets can still be counted using a Unopette for dilution and a hemacytometer for the count. It is not possible to accurately differentiate WBC types on the hemocytometer. Epithelial cells are not counted; they are a skin contaminant from the blood draw.

590. **b** Lymphocytes act in the body's immune system. All of the other cells can phagocytize.

591. **d** Eosinophils are usually localized to surface tissues.

592. **b** Basophils are localized around the blood vessels.

593. **a** The function of the lymphocyte does not change, regardless of size.

594. **c** Hypersegmentation is a normal change in an aging neutrophil that has been in circulation for a long time.

595. **d** Small dark dot on an RBC is most likely a nuclear remnant; Döhle bodies are retained RNA in neutrophils, not erythrocytes.

596. **b** A blast cell, by definition, is a reactive and/or young cell.

597. **a** *Codocyte* is an archaic term still seen in some texts. *Target cell* is a more descriptive term (an RBC looks like a target).

598. **d** Echinocytes are crenated RBCs with 10 to 30 spicules; they resemble a sea urchin (echinoderm).

599. **b** Immune-mediated hemolytic anemia may be characterized by spherocytes; you may see RBC fragments (schistocytes) in DIC and echinocytes in snake-bite. Look for the monohydrate form of calcium oxalate crystals in urine sediment in antifreeze poisoning.

600. **c** Acanthocytes are a descriptive morphologic change in the shape of red blood cells.

601. a *Discocyte* is an archaic term for the biconcave disk shape of an RBC.

602. c DIC causes the body's clotting abilities to malfunction, and fibrin strands slice through RBCs, destroying their ability to function as well.

603. a Key words are "outside the blood vessels." *Extra,* outside; *vascular,* vessels; *hemo,* blood cell; *lysis,* breakdown.

604. a The blood smear slide is dipped first in the fixative, followed by the red eosinophilic stain, and then the blue basophilic counterstain.

605. a

606. b Gross examination, looking at the sample in its presenting form, is required for all samples, including urine, blood, and feces, before beginning diagnostics.

607. d There is no such thing as a trigeminal cell.

608. a *Uro* means "urinary bladder"; *lith* means "stone."

609. b Urine specific gravity tests for the dissolved solids in urine.

610. d *Dirofilaria* can be found in all other fluid-bathed sites but is most common in the blood circulation.

611. b *Dirofilaria immitis* has a straight tail.

612. a *Cheyletiella* spp. are mites commonly found on rabbits, dogs, and cats and are commonly called the *walking dandruff* mite.

613. a Potassium hydroxide is used to clear hair during fungal examinations.

614. a The trophozoite is the motile stage of a flagellate protozoon and is the vegetative multiplying form. The cyst is the encysted form that has lost the flagellum. Schistocytes are the infective stage of coccidia.

615. b The opercula are the clear dots or caps on the ends of the *Trichuris vulpis* ova.

616. d The lung fluke of the dog and cat

617. d

618. a

619. b

620. c

621. c Controls are run for quality-control purposes only. They are not used to calibrate instruments.

622. a

623. b

624. a

625. d

626. c

627. c

628. d

629. b Leukocyte production takes place in bone marrow.

630. a

631. a

632. b The thymus processes thymocytes and releases them as T cells.

633. c Gut-associated lymph tissue (GALT) is often compared to the bursa of Fabricius in birds, where B lymphocytes are processed before being sent to peripheral lymphoid tissue.

634. d Quality-control data should not change when the people who conduct the tests are well trained and conscientious.

635. b It is not possible to tell, through the use of quality-control measures, whether the samples are of acceptable quality. Example: A red-top tube may have not been handled properly before separating, but the instrument may still produce a value; however, it may not be accurate.

636. b Refractometers should be checked daily with distilled water to ensure that they zero to a specific gravity of 1.000.

637. d Centrifuging a sample at too high a speed or for an extended period may cause hemolysis.

638. b The lid should be kept closed until the centrifuge comes to a complete stop.

639. **c** Transcription errors are clerical errors and do not require extra use of a sample.

640. **a**

641. **c**

642. **a**

643. **b**

644. **d**

645. **c** Samples should not be mailed over the weekend because of the delayed delivery and because laboratory personnel are typically not present to process samples.

646. **b** Slides should not be sent in the same package as formalin samples, because the fumes can affect the slides.

647. **b** Withdrawal pressure can be controlled with a syringe but not with a vacuum-tube system.

648. **a** Most anticoagulants work by forming insoluble complexes with calcium.

649. **c**

650. **d** Sodium citrate, because the anticoagulation is easily reversed by addition of ionized calcium

651. **b**

652. **d**

653. **a**

654. **c**

655. **b**

656. **a**

657. **d**

658. **a**

659. **b** Heparin interferes the least with chemical assays.

660. **d**

661. **b** Serum is usually preferred over plasma, because some anticoagulants interfere with tests results. Fibrin clots in some plasma samples may also interfere but can be removed by further centrifugation. Whole blood is usually unacceptable because of the presence of blood cells and the potential for hemolysis.

662. **c** Technician, reagent, or equipment error may result in the need to repeat a test. Some results may require dilution of the sample and retesting. It is good practice to initially collect enough blood in case repeat testing is necessary.

663. **a**

664. **b** Refrigeration is an acceptable means of preserving chemical constituents; the period or preservation varies for each constituent. Freezing prolongs the preservation of chemicals but may affect some test results. Samples stored at room temperature are not as stable; however, refrigerated or frozen samples should be allowed to warm to room temperature before analysis.

665. **a** General recommendation; chemicals in serum or plasma are least stable at room temperature.

666. **b** General recommendation; chemicals in serum or plasma are more stable when refrigerated than at room temperature.

667. **d** General recommendation; chemicals in serum or plasma are stable the longest when frozen, although freezing may affect some tests.

668. **c** Blood collected in this manner (without an anticoagulant), centrifuged, and separated after clotting will yield serum. Plasma is obtained when blood is collected in a tube that contains anticoagulant, is centrifuged, and then separated.

669. **b** Hemolysis (rupture of erythrocytes) releases intracellular components into the surrounding fluid (serum or plasma). Among these intracellular components, potassium is the principal cation; levels of potassium in the serum or plasma, therefore, increase in hemolysis. Most of the phosphorus found in whole blood is organic phosphorus inside erythrocytes; inorganic phosphorus is found in the serum or plasma. Organic phosphorus released in hemolysis may interfere with the phosphorus assay performed on serum or plasma.

670. **a** Erythrocytes use glucose for energy; serum and plasma must be separated from cells as soon as possible after blood collection.

671. **b** Postprandial lipemia is common in a nonfasted animal.

672. **c**

673. **c**

674. **b** Icterus is caused by an increase in the total bilirubin in the blood; total bilirubin is a combination of conjugated and unconjugated bilirubin. Icteric (or yellow) serum or plasma is frequently seen in animals with liver disease or hemolytic anemia.

675. **d**

676. **c** A blood sample drawn for obtaining plasma should be collected using an anticoagulant; it should not clot.

677. **b** Icterus is a condition that cannot be corrected or prevented by proper sample collection or handling. It is frequently seen in animals with liver disease or hemolytic anemia. Hemolysis is most commonly attributed to technician error, although hemolysis may occur in some anemias. Lipemia can usually be prevented or minimized by fasting the animal before collection.

678. **c**

679. **a** Light passing through the sample is measured as the percent of transmittance (T), and light not passing through is measured as absorbance.

680. **c** Technology of reflective photometric principles are used in dry chemistry analyzers.

681. **b** Quality-control serum is freeze-dried (lyophilized) and must be rehydrated before use. It contains specific quantities of chemical constituents; the range of acceptable values for each chemical constituent is provided by the manufacturer. It is analyzed as if it were patient serum, and the results are compared with the known values provided. Control serum is used for technician, reagent, and instrument assessment. Results within the acceptable ranges provided by the manufacturer help ensure the accuracy of test results.

682. **d**

683. **b** Purebred cats more often have type A blood.

684. **b** Quality-control sera are generally lyophilized (freeze-dried) and must be reconstituted before use.

685. **c** Reconstituted control serum is not stable for more than a few days when refrigerated, and an entire bottle is rarely used before it expires. After reconstituting one bottle, several aliquots are placed in small tubes and frozen. These aliquots can be thawed one at a time, thereby extending the use of the serum and cutting supply costs.

686. **d** Choices **a**, **b**, and **c** are each detectable through use of quality-control sera; random sampling errors are not.

687. **d**

688. **a** Rodenticides act by prolonging coagulation times.

689. **b** A pipette is usually automatic and delivers microliter volumes of patient sample.

690. **a**

691. **a** Each enzyme has a specific substrate; enzymes are often named for the substrate on which they act.

692. **b** Kinetic methods measure the rate of an enzymatic reaction while it is in progress and usually involve serial measurements of the product per unit of time. In end-point reactions, the product formed from enzyme activity is measured after the reaction has stopped.

693. **a** Some enzymes found in different tissues occur as isoenzymes. The serum concentration of an enzyme that occurs as isoenzymes is the total of the concentrations of all of the isoenzymes present. The source of a particular isoenzyme can be identified by determining which isoenzyme is present in a patient's sample.

694. **d** Fibrinogen can be estimated by using a heat precipitation test.

695. **c** IU/L = international units per liter, sometimes expressed as U/L = units per liter

696. **d**

697. **a**

698. **d** Kinetic reactions are measured while the reaction is in progress, not at the end. Temperature, time, and sample volume are all factors in a kinetic enzymatic assay.

699. **a** Laser-flow technology is used to determine blood cell concentrations, white blood cell differential, and other hematology parameters.

700. **d** Chemistry analyzers using reflectometry measure the amount of light reflected off the reagent slide.

701. **c** Dissolved carbon dioxide and oxygen are blood gases.

702. **d** These test strips estimate the amount of BUN.

703. **c** These test strips estimate the amount of blood glucose.

704. **c** Ion selective electrode and flame photometry are two methods of measuring electrolytes. Some electrolytes can also be measured using photometric or dry chemistry methods.

705. **a** These enzymes are found in hepatocytes and are used in small animals to evaluate liver function; GGT and SDH are primarily measured to evaluate liver function in horses.

706. **c** See answer 705.

707. **d**

708. **b**

709. **d**

710. **b** The liver conjugates bilirubin; it is a test of liver function.

711. **a** Although amylase, lipase, and trypsin are produced and secreted by the pancreas, only amylase and lipase are measured in the serum. Trypsin can be qualitatively measured in the feces as an assessment of chronic pancreatitis.

712. **c** See answer 711.

713. **a**

714. **b**

715. **a** Bicarbonate levels are often assayed in blood gas analysis to detect alterations in acid–base balance. The preferred sample is heparinized arterial whole blood.

716. **b** The A/G ratio is commonly determined as part of a liver profile.

717. **b**

718. **c** The kidneys play a role in electrolyte regulation.

719. **c** Elevated levels of nitrogenous waste products accumulate in the blood, especially urea nitrogen. Hypernatremia is an increase in sodium levels in the blood; hypernaturia is an increase in sodium levels in the urine.

720. **c** Insulin's effect on blood glucose levels is monitored in a diabetic animal.

721. **a** Calcium plays a role in bone development, transmission of nerve impulses, and muscle contraction. Calcium concentrations are usually inversely related to phosphorus concentrations.

722. **d** The adrenal cortex produces numerous steroids; cortisol is the major steroidal hormone released in domestic animals.

723. **d** ACTH stimulates the adrenal cortex to secrete cortisol. In the ACTH response test, cortisol levels are measured before and after administration of ACTH.

724. **a** The thyroid gland secretes thyroid hormone (thyroxine), which is a combination of T3 and T4; T4 is also converted to T3 in the tissues.

725. **c** TSH and ACTH are both secreted by the anterior pituitary (adenohypophysis) gland, which is under the control of the hypothalamus. Blood levels of these hormones may be used to evaluate pituitary gland function.

726. **a** These are all signs of hypothyroidism.

727. **b** Urea nitrogen and creatinine are metabolic wastes measured to evaluate renal function.

728. **d** Ammonia is converted to urea by the liver; BUN is often decreased in hepatic disease and elevated in renal disease.

729. **c** The pancreas secretes these digestive enzymes; levels are elevated in acute pancreatitis.

730. **a** *Dioctophyma renale* is the largest parasitic nematode.

731. **d** The larvae of *Gasterophilus* are known as bots and are equine parasites. The fly deposits eggs on the host's hair. The eggs hatch and the emerging larvae enter the mouth and migrate to the stomach where they attach to the inner lining.

732. **b**

733. **a**

734. **a** This is one of the large strongyles of horses; **b** is an ascarid, **c** is a tapeworm, and **d** is the lungworm.

735. **b**

736. **a** Pyknosis is a thickening and degeneration of a cell in which the nucleus shrinks and the chromatin condenses into a solid, structureless mass.

737. **c** Bizarre and numerous nucleoli, increased mitotic index and rapid growth are used to classify malignancy.

738. **c** Metaplasia is the change of a mature cell into a form that is abnormal for that tissue.

739. **c**

740. **a**

741. **d**

742. **c**

743. **d**

744. **b** Hyaluronic acid is a mucopolysaccharide and is the cement substance of tissues; it forms a gel in intercellular spaces.

745. **d**

746. **d**

747. **b** Mast cells are sometimes referred to as *dirty cells* because of the dark basophilic granules found in their cytoplasm. Basophils are blood cells found in circulating blood.

748. **b**

749. **a** New methylene blue is a supravital dye that precipitates basophilic material (RNA) and stains it blue.

750. **b**

751. **c**

752. **b**

753. **c**

754. **d**

755. **c**

756. **a**

757. **d**

758. **b** Neutrophils are essential for phagocytosis and proteolysis of bacteria, cellular debris, and solid particles, all of which may be present in association with conjunctivitis.

759. **d**

760. **c** The parabasal cells are smaller than the intermediate or superficial (anuclear) cells. The nucleus is also more prominent, and the cytoplasm stains darker.

761. **c** The Gram stain is the classic bacteriologic stain used to separate bacteria according to their gram reaction, classified as gram-positive (blue) or gram-negative (red).

762. **c** Bone marrow also contains fat that appears as large unstained vacuoles.

763. **c**

764. **d**

765. **a** Specimens that are to be used to make impression smears should be blotted with clean, absorbent material to remove fresh blood, thus giving a more representative view of the cells making up the lesion.

766. **d**

767. **b**

768. **b**

769. **a**

770. **c**

771. **a**

772. **b** After 1 year it has to be relabeled as frozen plasma (FP).

773. **b** Lymphocytes transform to plasma cells, which produce antibodies.

774. **b**

775. **b**

776. **b**

777. **d**

778. **d** A degenerative left shift is seen when the leukocyte count is normal or low and when bands outnumber mature neutrophils.

779. **c** Metarubricytes (nucleated erythrocytes) in the peripheral blood falsely elevate the leukocyte count.

780. **a**

781. **b**

782. **b**

783. **a**

784. **c**

785. **d**

786. **a** The erythrocyte Unopette is no longer available, and the cell counts done manually were not sufficiently accurate. Packed cell volume (hematocrit) remains a manual procedure that gives an indication of the red blood cell population.

787. **b**

788. **d** Absolute eosinopenia is seen in a stress leukogram.

789. **d** Because of rouleaux, the RBCs will be heavier and settle faster.

790. **d** Reticulocytes are seen with a new methylene blue stain.

791. **b**

792. **b**

793. **a**

794. **a**

795. **c**

796. **c** *Haemonchus* is one of the trichostrongyles of ruminants that are found in the abomasum and intestines.

797. **d**

798. **b**

799. **a** The horse does not release immature erythrocytes into the peripheral blood.

800. **d**

801. **c** Although the upper limit of normal leukocyte counts varies from species to species, 7500/dl is well within the normal range for all of these species.

802. **d**

803. **b** Goats are ruminants, and ruminants tend to have more lymphocytes than any other WBC in peripheral blood.

804. **c** Lymphoid tissue, not bone marrow, is the major site of lymphocyte production.

805. **b** Lymphoblasts may be seen in the peripheral blood in lymphocytic leukemia.

806. **d**

807. **a** *Babesia* is an intracellular parasite of erythrocytes in dogs, cattle, and horses.

808. **d** The buffy coat layer is found between the packed red cells and plasma in a spun microhematocrit tube.

809. **a** Plasma has not been allowed to clot, therefore it still contains the plasma protein fibrinogen.

810. **b**

811. **c** Polychromasia occurs when the erythrocyte cytoplasm contains hemoglobin (stains red) and cytoplasmic RNA (stains blue). This is seen with immature RBCs.

812. **d**

813. **a** Hemoglobin breaks down to bilirubin, iron, and globin.

814. **c**

815. **b** The standard microhematocrit centrifuge takes 5 minutes to run the PCV.

816. **a** Mean corpuscular volume is the average size of an erythrocyte.

817. **c**

818. **b**

819. **d** Basophils that contain blue granules resemble mast cells.

820. **b**

821. **c**

822. **a**

823. **c** Hemolytic anemia, especially if acute and massive, produces icterus from released hemoglobin breakdown products.

824. **b**

825. **d** A *seg* is another name for the segmented neutrophil.

826. **a**

827. **b**

828. **c**

829. **d**

830. **b** The band nucleus has smooth, parallel sides compared with the irregular, twisted, or segmented nucleus of the mature neutrophil.

831. **c** A spherocyte is a densely stained erythrocyte that is smaller than the others.

832. **a**

833. **d**

834. **b** Forty is 4% of 1000.

835. **a**

836. **c** Hypersegmented neutrophils that contain more than five nuclear lobes occur as the cells age.

837. **b** Members of the camel family, which include the llama, normally have oval erythrocytes.

838. **d**

839. **a**

840. **d** Birds, reptiles, and fish normally have mature nucleated erythrocytes.

841. **c** The nucleus is not round as in choices **a** and **b** and is less than 50% indented.

842. **b**

843. **d**

844. **a**

845. **c** In a minor crossmatch, donor serum is mixed with red cells from the recipient.

846. **c** Potassium and sodium EDTA are the most common anticoagulants used in blood collection.

847. **b**

848. **a**

849. **c** 65% of 15,000 is 9750.

850. **d**

851. **b**

852. **c** Fibrinogen functions in the last step in the hemostatic process.

853. **b** Metarubricytes are the most common immature erythrocytes seen in the peripheral blood of dogs and cats.

854. **a** *Haemobartonella felis* is a common feline blood parasite.

855. **c**

856. **d** Multiply the 10× by 100× to get 1000× magnification with the oil-immersion lens.

857. **d**

858. **c** Monocytes are derived from promonocytes, which are bone marrow stem cells. Once monocytes enter the bloodstream, they remain there for only a few days before entering tissues and developing into macrophages.

859. **c** IgM is the first antibody produced in the primary immune response and represents about 20% of the serum antibodies.

860. **a** IgG is the most abundant of the five classes of immunoglobulins, representing about 80% of serum immunoglobulin protein.

861. **b**

862. **a** IgG is the major component of passive maternal antibody transfer.

863. **d** Peroxidase is an enzyme found in granulocytes, not in monocytes.

864. **c**

865. **b** Attenuation is a process that reduces the virulence of an organism until, although still alive, it is no longer capable of producing disease. The organism still retains its ability to produce an immune response.

866. **d**

867. **b** Cytokines are soluble biologic messenger proteins that control macrophages and lymphocytes taking part in the cell-mediated immune reaction.

868. **c**

869. **d** Combined immunodeficiency occurs in approximately 2% to 3% of Arabian foals. The foals fail to produce functional T or B cells. They may receive maternal immunoglobulins as they suckle successfully, but when the maternal immunoglobulins have been used, the foal cannot produce its own antibodies. All foals stricken usually die within 4 to 6 months as a result of infection.

870. **d**

871. **a**

872. **c** Plasma cells are B cells that produce antibodies to the antigen, but the most correct answer is *memory* B cells. Memory B cells are produced during the initial exposure and remain to produce antibodies more quickly in case there is a second exposure to the antigen.

873. **c**

874. **b**

875. **b** Complete washing of test wells used in ELISA is the critical step to ensure accurate results. Follow the manufacturer's instructions explicitly regarding washing procedures.

876. **a** Coombs tests are used to detect certain antigen–antibody reactions, one of which is used for diagnosis of autoimmune hemolytic anemia.

877. **d** Fleas suck blood.

878. **a**

879. **d**

880. **b**

881. **b**

882. **b**

883. **a**

884. **b**

885. **c**

886. **b**

887. **a**

888. **c** The sequence of maturation for RBCs is rubriblast, prorubricyte, rubricyte, metarubricyte, reticulocyte, and mature RBC.

889. **a**

890. **a**

891. **b**

892. **c**

893. **a**

894. **b** The Coggins test is an agar-gel, double-diffusion, immunodiffusion test used to detect antibodies against equine infectious anemia.

895. **d**

896. **b**

897. **c**

898. **d**

899. **b** In order for the antibody response to be considered significant and diagnostic of the suspected antigen stimulus (the cause of a specific disease), the antibody titer must increase fourfold between the two samples.

900. **d** T-suppressor cells are a type of lymphocyte that suppresses B-lymphocyte activity.

901. **b** Histamine is released in allergic and inflammatory reactions and causes dilatation of capillaries, decreased blood pressure, increased release of gastric juices, and constriction of the smooth muscles of the bronchi and uterus.

902. **a**

903. **d**

904. **a** Mast cells and basophils normally produce a small quantity of histamine, but when they are sensitized by IgE, they react abnormally, producing large quantities of histamines and other chemicals. These chemicals cause allergic attacks (such as runny noses, and swollen tissues).

905. **b**

906. **a**

907. **d**

908. **c**

909. **b** Because FIV is found in saliva, bite wounds serve as a means of transmission.

910. **c** Titer is a measure of antibody units per unit volume of serum. Titer testing is performed immediately after infection (acute phase) and 2 to 6 weeks after collection of the first serum sample (convalescent phase).

911. **d**

912. **d** Viruses are not free living, because they are obligatory intracellular parasites. They use host cell structures for reproduction.

913. **d** Genus and species names are both italicized, and the genus name is capitalized.

914. **d** *Mycobacterium* causes tuberculosis.

915. **a** Selective media will eliminate the unwanted organisms (normal flora) with chemicals or antimicrobials.

916. **b** *Escherichia coli* 0157 may contaminate meat during slaughter. Grinding the meat increases the chances of infection by introducing the organism into the center of the meat.

917. **b**

918. **d**

919. **c** 0.9% NaCl is isotonic; 5% NaCl is hypertonic. Water moves toward the higher solute concentration, which, in this case, is outside of the cell.

920. **d** The standard technique for pasteurization heats a liquid to 63° C for 30 minutes. To kill endospores, the temperature must reach 121° C and be maintained for 15 minutes.

921. **c** Ethylene oxide can be used.

922. **c**

923. **c**

924. **c**

925. **d**

926. **b**

927. **d** Septicemia is the presence of pathogenic bacteria in the blood.

928. **c**

929. **b**

930. **b**

931. **c** All of the others are gram-positive rods.

932. **b**

933. **a**

934. **d**

935. **c** *Staphylococcus aureus* ferments the mannitol, resulting in a color change of yellow in the medium.

936. **a**

937. c

938. c

939. a

940. b

941. c

942. b

943. d

944. a

945. d

946. d *Clostridium botulinum* causes flaccid paralysis.

947. b

948. c

949. d

950. d

951. d

952. d

953. c

954. b

955. d

956. d Parvoviruses are resistant to most common disinfectants, except sodium hypochlorite.

957. b Many cases of cystitis are caused by retrograde infections by gram-negative enteric organisms.

958. d

959. b

960. d

961. b

962. b

963. d Gram-stain is a differential stain.

964. d

965. a All of the other answer choices are examples of acquired passive immunity.

966. b

967. b *Escherichia coli* organisms are among the normal flora of the intestines.

968. c

969. c

970. b Alpha is incomplete hemolysis, beta is complete hemolysis, and gamma is no hemolysis.

971. c Catalase causes the release of O_2 from hydrogen peroxide (H_2O_2).

972. a

973. d *Cestodes* refer to the subclass Cestoda, the tapeworms.

974. c *Trematodes* refer to the class Trematoda, the flukes.

975. a *Dirofilaria immitis* is a nematode; the others are protozoans.

976. d

977. b Direct smears use only a small amount of feces. The other techniques increase the chances of seeing ova by concentrating the ova from a large amount of feces in a small sample, such as under the cover slip or in the top or bottom layer of flotation solution.

978. a Some fluke ova have a higher specific gravity than many other ova and therefore do not float in flotation solutions.

979. d

980. b Pinworm eggs are deposited on the skin around the anus and are not normally seen in the feces. The cellophane tape is pressed against the skin around the anus, pulled off, and stuck to a microscope slide. The eggs will adhere to the tape and be visible under the microscope.

981. a

982. d Trophozoites may collapse in nonisotonic flotation solutions and may be difficult to recognize.

983. **b** It takes 6 to 7 months for the heartworm to mature and produce microfilariae.

984. **b**

985. **c**

986. **b** *Otodectes cynotis* is an ear mite.

987. **b**

988. **d** The infective stage of *Dipylidium caninum* is found in the flea. Rabbits are hosts for *Taenia pisiformis,* another tapeworm of dogs and cats.

989. **b** A spurious infection is not a true parasite infection. The ova are present because the dog has ingested ruminant feces that contain *Moniezia.*

990. **b**

991. **d**

992. **b**

993. **a** *Taenia* and *Echinococcus* ova are so similar that definitive diagnosis can be made only by examination of the adult worms.

994. **c**

995. **d**

996. **c**

997. **d** These are all zoonotic diseases. Visceral larva migrans is caused by ingestion of *Toxocara* eggs that hatch and develop into larvae that migrate through the abdominal viscera; creeping eruption is caused by skin penetration by *Ancylostoma* larvae; scabies is caused by the sarcoptic mange mite; hydatidosis is infection with the hydatid cyst of *Echinococcus.*

998. **a** All are protozoans. *Giardia* and *Trichomonas* are flagellates.

999. **a** Smegma is a secretion found within the prepuce, where the protozoa live. *Thelazia* species are eyeworms whose larvae may be found in tears. Embryonated ova or hatched larvae from the lungworm *Dictyocaulus* may be found in feces. *Stephanurus* passes eggs that are found in urine.

1000. **a** *Tritrichomonas foetus* is a protozoan parasite of cattle.

1001. **b** *Dictyocaulus* species are lungworms found in the trachea and bronchi of cattle and sheep.

1002. **c** *Dioctophyma renale* is the giant kidney worm of wild carnivores and other species. Its eggs are found in urine sediment.

1003. **d** *Anaplasma* is an intracellular parasite of bovine red blood cells.

1004. **a**

1005. **d**

1006. **c**

1007. **b**

1008. **d**

1009. **c**

1010. **a**

1011. **b**

1012. **b** There are three species of large strongyles and more than 40 species of small strongyles of horses.

1013. **b** All of the other stages have eight legs.

1014. **c**

1015. **b**

1016. **a**

1017. **d**

1018. **a** *Echinococcus granulosus* produces larvae that form hydatid cysts in the intermediate hosts, such as people.

1019. **c**

1020. **d**

1021. **a**

1022. **b**

1023. **a** The second intermediate host of *Diphyllobothrium latum* is a fish.

1024. **c** Ova of *Paragonimus kellicotti,* the lung fluke, are found in the sputum or feces of dogs and cats.

1025. c

1026. d

1027. d

1028. a

1029. b

1030. c

1031. **b** Mites may live off of their host for a short time, but they propagate only while on their host.

1032. d

1033. d

1034. a

1035. c

1036. b

1037. d

1038. b

1039. b

1040. c

1041. d

1042. a

1043. a

1044. d

1045. a

1046. **b** Larvae migrate to the liver and then to the lungs.

1047. c

1048. **d** Hookworms feed on blood from the intestinal wall and can produce profound anemia.

1049. **a** *Giardia* is a flagellate protozoan that invades the small intestine and causes chronic diarrhea.

1050. b

1051. c

1052. a

1053. d

1054. **d** Both *Trichuris vulpis* and *Capillaria aerophila* ova have bipolar plugs, but the *Capillaria* ovum is smaller and tends to be more asymmetric than the *Trichuris* ovum.

1055. a

1056. c

1057. b

1058. d

1059. b

1060. b

1061. a

1062. d

1063. c

1064. b

1065. **d** Flea eggs are not sticky and drop off into the environment.

1066. **b** *Melophagus ovinus* bites cause pruritus over much of the sheep's body.

1067. **a** *Ancylostoma* larvae penetrate the skin of people but can develop no further.

1068. d

1069. **c** *Notoedres cati* is the cause of feline scabies, also known as *notoedric mange*.

1070. **c** *Cryptosporidium* is a small protozoan that is associated with chronic diarrhea.

1071. b

1072. d

1073. **a** *Psoroptes ovis* causes common mange in cattle and sheep.

1074. **a** It is cloudy because of the presence of intact red blood cell membranes.

1075. **d** Multiply only the last two digits of the specific gravity by the dilution factor. Specific gravity is always in the range of 1.0×.

1076. **a**

1077. **b**

1078. **a** Red blood cells and fat droplets are often the same size. However, fat droplets come in various sizes.

1079. **d** BUN is not part of a routine urinalysis.

1080. **d**

1081. **c** Dilute the urine 1:2 with distilled water and multiply the last two digits of the specific gravity by 2.

1082. **b**

1083. **d** Controls need to be run only once during a shift unless a problem occurs.

1084. **d**

1085. **c**

1086. **d** The urine from an early morning sample is concentrated, which allows for detection of substances that may not be present in a more dilute sample.

1087. **b**

1088. **c** Cystocentesis and catheterization provide good samples for urinalysis that are free of contamination from the distal genital tract and external areas.

1089. **b**

1090. **d**

1091. **c**

1092. **a**

1093. **d**

1094. **a** The other conditions would be associated with acidic urine.

1095. **a**

1096. **b** Bacterial numbers continue to increase if the sample is left at room temperature.

1097. **b**

1098. **c**

1099. **a**

1100. **d**

1101. **b**

1102. **d**

1103. **c** Dark yellow urine is generally more concentrated; therefore, the specific gravity is higher.

1104. **d**

1105. **b**

1106. **c**

1107. **c** Urine that contains blood typically has a high protein content.

1108. **a**

1109. **c** If the light is too bright, it is hard to see some of the elements in the urine.

1110. **b**

1111. **d** Vegetable diets may cause the urine to be alkaline.

1112. **b** Sulfosalicylic acid is used to detect protein in the urine.

1113. **c** Urine samples should be centrifuged at low speed for 5 minutes.

1114. **b**

1115. **c** A right shift is characterized by hypersegmented neutrophils (>5 nuclear lobes). This would most likely be seen on a smear of old, nonpreserved blood, because the neutrophils will continue to mature in the blood sample until they die of old age. This is why it is important to make the blood smear from the freshest blood, preferably before it goes into anticoagulant.

Animal Nursing

Animal Care

Sarah Wagner

QUESTIONS

1. In general, how many days should be allowed for diet changes in dogs and cats?
   a. 5 to 7 days
   b. 1 to 3 days
   c. 48 to 72 hours
   d. 28 days

2. As a dog or cat transitions from immature to mature, the recommended diet change is for
   a. Increase in calories
   b. Decrease in fat, increase in fiber
   c. Addition of table scraps
   d. Decrease in fiber

3. Which of the following is/are antioxidants?
   a. Lipoic acids, vitamin E, vitamin C
   b. L-Carnitine
   c. Vitamin K
   d. Krebs cycles

4. Which of the following has the least influence on the acceptability of food to dogs and cats?
   a. Salt content
   b. Size
   c. Shape
   d. Color

5. On the average, an adult horse consumes approximately how many gallons of water per day?
   a. 10 to 15
   b. 5 to 7
   c. 25
   d. 1

6. Horses and rabbits are
   a. Ruminants
   b. Omnivores
   c. Cecum fermenters
   d. Carnivores

7. Puppies, kittens, and nursing mothers require
   a. Similar levels of protein in their diet
   b. Vitamin supplementation
   c. High levels of fiber for energy
   d. Few calories

8. What ratio is compromised by feeding a diet high in bran to horses?
   a. Na/Cl
   b. Ca/P
   c. Vitamins A/D
   d. Mg/CO_2

9. Oversupplementation of vegetable oils can result in
   a. Increase in serum nitrogen
   b. Decrease in absorption of vitamins A, D, E, and K
   c. Greasy coat
   d. Predisposition to autoimmune disease

10. Birds are attracted to
    a. Pelleted foods
    b. Human foods
    c. Brightly colored feed
    d. Foods high in salt

Correct answers are on pages 349-359.

11. Psyllium is a source of
    a. Fat
    b. Protein
    c. Fiber
    d. Carbohydrates

12. A factor included in body condition score
    of dogs and cats is
    a. Age
    b. Visible waist
    c. Weight
    d. Palpation of ribs

13. Which of the following is/are examples of
    preservatives?
    a. Omega-3 oils
    b. Sucrose, dextrose
    c. Lactated Ringer
    d. Potassium sorbate

14. Thyroid medication, corticosteroids, and
    anabolic steroids
    a. Decrease appetite
    b. Stimulate tear production
    c. Increase appetite
    d. Decrease energy

15. Chondroitin sulfates are an example of
    a. Flavor enhancement
    b. A nutraceutical
    c. FDA-approved treatment
    d. Parenteral medication

16. Failure to decrease the grain intake for a horse
    that transitions from training/work to an idle
    status may cause
    a. Polydipsia
    b. Azoturia
    c. Anorexia
    d. Pyrexia

17. Which of the following vitamins is/are water
    soluble?
    a. Vitamins A and D
    b. Vitamin E
    c. Vitamin B_{12}
    d. Vitamin K

18. Hypoallergenic diets oftentimes contain
    a. Soybean
    b. Corn
    c. Rice
    d. Ethoxyquin

19. Patients with pancreatitis or hyperlipidemia
    should avoid foods high in
    a. Fiber
    b. Dextrose
    c. Fats
    d. Water

20. Taurine and L-carnitine have been found to aid
    a. Inappetence
    b. Dysphagia
    c. Cardiac muscle function
    d. Temperament

21. Which of the following is most often associated
    with cancer patients?
    a. Cachexia
    b. Obesity
    c. Polyphagia
    d. Increased appetite

22. Potassium is critical for
    a. Muscle function
    b. Weight gain
    c. Palatability
    d. Digestion

23. Metabolizable energy differs from gross calorie
    content by
    a. Pertaining to canned foods only
    b. Measuring the usable energy in a food
    c. Measuring only the nutrients in a food
    d. Pertaining to dry foods only

24. When feeding horses, it is recommended to
    measure feed
    a. By volume, not weight
    b. As a per-day ration
    c. By weight, not volume
    d. According to supplementation

25. Nutrient content as *dry matter* means
    a. Analysis after water has been added
    b. Analysis of nutrient after moisture has been
       removed
    c. Nutrient content of canned foods only
    d. Nutrient analysis of dry foods only

26. Diet recommendation for diabetic patients is
    a. Foods that are high in fat for weight gain
    b. Foods that are high in sugar for energy
    c. Foods that are high in fiber for slow release of
       nutrients
    d. Foods that are high in moisture for
       compensatory hydration

27. Horses are generally fed grain to meet what need?
    a. Appetite
    b. Energy
    c. Digestion
    d. Vitamin

28. Oversupplementation of which of the following can be detrimental?
    a. Vitamin C
    b. Vitamin K
    c. Selenium
    d. Biotin

29. Appetite may be stimulated by all of the following, except
    a. Certain medications
    b. Warming the food
    c. Sense of smell
    d. Refrigerating the food

30. Deficiency of which of the following major nutrients is likely to have the most rapid negative effect on an animal?
    a. Water
    b. Protein
    c. Fat
    d. Carbohydrates

31. Flaxseed is an especially good source of
    a. B vitamins
    b. Vitamin C
    c. Omega-3 and six vitamins
    d. Vitamin D

32. Enteral feeding is
    a. Intravenous supplementation
    b. Feeding at timed intervals
    c. Feeding orphans
    d. Feeding via the gastrointestinal tract

33. If the percent dry matter on the label reads protein 45.7% and fat 30.5%, what patient should not eat this food?
    a. A dog with pancreatitis
    b. A malnourished 8-week-old kitten
    c. A malnourished 8-week-old puppy
    d. A postsurgical patient

34. Pet food labels list ingredients
    a. In descending order by weight
    b. In ascending order by volume
    c. By animal-derived ingredients first
    d. By nonanimal ingredients first

35. The amino acid found in animal tissue that is required by cats but not dogs is
    a. Methionine
    b. Taurine
    c. Lysine
    d. Arginine

36. Which of the following is a normal urine pH for a cat?
    a. 6.2
    b. 6.0
    c. 7.0
    d. 7.5

37. AAFCO
    a. Oversees pet food advertising
    b. Substantiates nutrition claims by implementing procedures for animal feeding tests
    c. Differentiates between soy- and meat-based diets
    d. Sets parameters for pet food prices

38. When a product is labeled as *flavored*, it must contain at least what percent of said ingredient?
    a. 10%
    b. 28%
    c. 3%
    d. 12%

39. Alfalfa is a palatable source of protein for herbivores. In what macromineral is alfalfa also abundant?
    a. Cobalt
    b. Calcium
    c. Zinc
    d. Iron

40. Protein that is not used by the body is converted to energy, and the waste
    a. Is stored as fat for energy
    b. Is excreted by the kidneys
    c. Is filtered by the liver
    d. Is reabsorbed as amino acids

41. Which of the following animals can easily become hyperthermic if chased?
    a. Hogs and sheep
    b. Goats and sheep
    c. Goats and hogs
    d. Cattle and goats

42. What is the best method to encourage a goat to stand still?
    a. Lift up the head and chin
    b. Cover an eye
    c. Hold up a front leg
    d. Tie to a fence

Correct answers are on pages 349-359.

43. What breed is usually worked in stanchions or headlocks?
    a. Holstein cow
    b. Simmental bull
    c. Angus heifer
    d. Jersey bull

44. Which is a dairy breed?
    a. Simmental
    b. Charolais
    c. Hereford
    d. Guernsey

45. A deficiency in the essential amino acid taurine in a feline diet can result in
    a. Anemia
    b. Dilated cardiomyopathy
    c. Calcium oxalate uroliths
    d. Fatty liver

46. What type of energy-producing nutrient is a dog or cat able to manufacture, if it is not available in the animal's body?
    a. Soluble carbohydrates
    b. Insoluble carbohydrates
    c. Essential amino acids
    d. Nonessential amino acids

47. What species has the highest protein requirement?
    a. Cats
    b. Dogs
    c. Rabbits
    d. Sheep

48. What is an example of a soluble carbohydrate?
    a. Lignin
    b. Glucose
    c. Cellulose
    d. Pectin

49. Fats are required for absorption, transportation, and storage of what vitamins?
    a. A, D, E, and K
    b. A, B complex, C, and D
    c. B complex, D, E, and K
    d. B complex and C

50. A dishwasher and a good quality detergent can be used for disinfecting nondisposable food and water bowls. The recommended temperature to kill most organisms is
    a. 100° F
    b. 180° F
    c. 212° F
    d. 220° F

51. What nutrient is sometimes referred to as *ash*?
    a. Vitamins
    b. Carbohydrates
    c. Proteins
    d. Minerals

52. What mineral is considered to be a trace mineral?
    a. Calcium
    b. Potassium
    c. Iodine
    d. Sodium

53. A deficiency of what nutrient can cause anemia?
    a. Iron
    b. Zinc
    c. Iodine
    d. Manganese

54. Orphaned kittens no longer need stimulation for urination and defecation at what age?
    a. Kittens do not need external stimulation for urination and defecation
    b. 4 to 7 days
    c. 10 to 14 days
    d. 16 to 21 days

55. At what age is a kitten fully able to control its body temperature?
    a. 61 days
    b. 45 days
    c. 28 days
    d. 12 days

56. Cow's milk should not be given to puppies or kittens as a milk replacer because of its
    a. Low protein and fat levels
    b. High fat and protein levels
    c. Low fat and higher protein levels
    d. High fat and lower protein levels

57. What is the normal body temperature of a kitten during the first 2 weeks of its life?
    a. 102° F
    b. 100° F
    c. 95° F
    d. 104° F

58. At what core temperature does a newborn kitten's digestive tract become less functional?
    a. 90° F
    b. 95° F
    c. 100° F
    d. 103° F

59. Which of these species is an omnivore?
    a. Chinchilla
    b. Hamster
    c. Rabbit
    d. Gerbil

60. Calcium in the diet must be carefully regulated for what species?
    a. Chinchilla
    b. Hamster
    c. Rabbit
    d. Guinea pig

61. Rabbits should have an unlimited amount of
    a. Alfalfa hay
    b. Alfalfa pellets
    c. Grass hay
    d. Fresh fruits and vegetables

62. Which is not true about rabbit cecal pellets?
    a. Also known as "day droppings"
    b. Are eaten by the rabbit
    c. Are soft, are dark in color, have a strong odor, and are coated in mucus
    d. Are formed in the cecum and are rich in vitamins and nutrients

63. Vitamin C supplements must be added to prevent scurvy in what species?
    a. Chinchilla
    b. Hamster
    c. Rabbit
    d. Guinea pig

64. The vitamin C levels in guinea pig food decline after how many months of storage?
    a. 3 months
    b. 6 months
    c. 9 months
    d. 12 months

65. What species is not nocturnal?
    a. Hamster
    b. Gerbil
    c. Hedgehog
    d. Sugar glider

66. Which statement about housing rabbits is accurate?
    a. Rabbits should be housed in a warm and humid environment.
    b. Two female rabbits housed together will fight.
    c. Two male rabbits housed together will fight.
    d. Solid-walled cages with wire mesh flooring are best.

67. What species is not a social animal and should be housed alone?
    a. Chinchilla
    b. Hamster
    c. Gerbil
    d. Guinea pig

68. Parvovirus causes what disease in cats?
    a. Panleukopenia
    b. Rhinotracheitis
    c. Infectious peritonitis
    d. Infectious anemia

69. Feline distemper is caused by the same type of organism as what canine disease?
    a. Canine distemper
    b. Canine parvovirus
    c. Parainfluenza
    d. Adenovirus type 2

70. What disease is not characterized by diarrhea, vomiting, and dehydration?
    a. Feline infectious enteritis
    b. Feline infectious peritonitis
    c. Feline panleukopenia
    d. Feline distemper

71. What type of floor is the most difficult to disinfect?
    a. Tile
    b. Cement
    c. Wood
    d. Dirt

72. A dog has a history of not eating for 2 days and has lost 10% of its body weight. This weight loss is most likely due to a loss of
    a. Lean body mass
    b. Fat
    c. Glycogen
    d. Water

73. The most important factor in assuring weight loss in an obese cat is
    a. Proper diet
    b. A healthy cat
    c. Diet pills
    d. Owner compliance

74. Scent glands in the male goat are located
    a. Around the tail base
    b. Around the horn base
    c. In the groin area
    d. In the axial area

Correct answers are on pages 349-359.

75. The reason that adult dogs and cats will often have diarrhea after consuming a large quantity of milk is because
    a. They are allergic to lactose.
    b. They have an inability to absorb lactose.
    c. The protein in milk causes a toxic reaction to the microvilli of the small intestine, thus decreasing the amount of nutrient that can be absorbed.
    d. Milk coats the intestine, preventing the reabsorption of water, thus leading to diarrhea.

76. Why should you not feed dog food to a cat?
    a. Cats have a lower requirement for essential fatty acids than dogs.
    b. Cats have a lower requirement for arginine than dogs.
    c. Cats have a higher requirement for essential carbohydrates than dogs.
    d. Cats have a higher requirement for taurine than dogs.

77. Cholesterol would be found in the highest concentration in
    a. Corn oil
    b. Peanut butter
    c. Turkey breast without the skin
    d. Celery

78. An all-meat diet will cause a deficiency in
    a. Iron
    b. Calcium
    c. Zinc
    d. Magnesium

79. Lack of what nutrient is associated with prolonged clotting times?
    a. Vitamin B_{12}
    b. Vitamin A
    c. Vitamin C
    d. Vitamin K

80. A cat fed only fish would be most at risk for which of the following problems?
    a. Pansteatitis
    b. Encephalomalacia
    c. Anemia
    d. Mulberry heart disease

81. Feeding an animal raw egg whites would put the animal at risk of a(n)
    a. Iron deficiency
    b. Vitamin E deficiency
    c. Biotin deficiency
    d. Protein deficiency

82. Cats should not be fed dog food because
    a. It is unpalatable.
    b. It will give them diarrhea.
    c. The fat content is too low.
    d. The amino acid content is too low.

83. Great care must be taken when dehorning a goat with a hot electric dehorner because.
    a. The hair may catch fire.
    b. The smell of burning skin scares goats.
    c. It is difficult to control dehorning pain in goats.
    d. The heat may damage their brains.

84. A cat being fed a homemade vegetarian diet could be expected to be deficient in all of the following, except
    a. Vitamin A
    b. Niacin
    c. Vitamin B_{12}
    d. Protein

85. Which of these signs is not seen in fearful animals?
    a. Constricted pupils
    b. Standing or lying tensely at the rear of the cage
    c. Facing the back corner of the cage, glancing over the shoulder to keep people in sight
    d. Ears pulled back

86. The reason why lamb was used in the past as the protein source in many hypoallergenic veterinary diets was because
    a. Lamb is more digestible than beef and poultry products.
    b. Lamb causes less pancreatic stimulation.
    c. There was a time when most dogs and cats had not eaten lamb before.
    d. Lamb has a higher biologic value than other typical meat products.

87. If there were no contraindications for the following feeding routes, the best route would be via
    a. The cephalic vein
    b. The jugular vein
    c. A gastric tube
    d. Femoral artery

88. An advantage of a nasoesophageal (NE) tube over a gastrostomy tube is
    a. It does not require general anesthesia to put the tube in.
    b. You can use regular dog or cat canned food with the NE tube.
    c. The NE tube can be left in place longer than a gastrostomy tube.
    d. There is less chance of aspiration pneumonia with an NE tube.

89. After more than 1 day of not eating, animals are deriving most of their energy from
    a. Fat stores
    b. Glycogen stores
    c. Protein stores
    d. Fiber pockets

90. After more than 1 day of not eating, animals are deriving most of their glucose from
    a. Fat stores
    b. Glycogen stores
    c. Lean body mass
    d. Fiber pockets

91. The following would all be good methods of inducing a cat to eat except
    a. Heating the food
    b. Covering the cage door with a towel
    c. Sprinkling the food with onion powder to increase the olfactory properties of the food
    d. Placing the food in a wide bowl

92. What condition is not exacerbated by obesity?
    a. Joint problems
    b. Diabetes
    c. Hyperthyroidism
    d. Anesthetic complications

93. What is not commonly associated with food allergies?
    a. Bilateral otitis externa
    b. Diarrhea
    c. A sudden change in diet
    d. A nonseasonal pruritus

94. When using an elimination diet to test whether a dog has a food allergy, improvement should be seen within
    a. 24 hours
    b. 2 days
    c. 1 week
    d. 1 month

95. What has been demonstrated to prevent periodontal disease?
    a. Tartar-control diets
    b. Chew toys
    c. Instrumental dental cleaning
    d. Dry food

96. For large-breed dogs, in addition to a genetic predisposition, research has also incriminated ___ in obesity.
    a. A high percent of the calories in the diet from protein
    b. A high percent of the calories in the diet from carbohydrates
    c. A high percent of the calories in the diet from fat
    d. An energy-dense food provided *ad libitum* to puppies

97. Which of the following would be most detrimental to feed a growing puppy?
    a. An over-the-counter multivitamin
    b. Multivitamin tablet
    c. Vitamin C tablet
    d. Calcium supplement

98. Greasy, foul-smelling feces usually indicates
    a. Too high protein content in the diet
    b. Too high fat content in the diet
    c. Too high carbohydrate content in the diet
    d. A problem with fat absorption

99. The best measure of whether an animal is eating the right amount of food is
    a. If the proximate analysis of the food is correct for the life stage of the animal
    b. If the CHO/fat/protein ratio is adjusted correctly for the animal
    c. If the animal has a 3 out of 5 body condition score
    d. If the animal eats all of the food it is given

100. A dog's ideal weight is 20 kg and its actual weight is 30 kg. If each day you fed the dog 200 kcal less than what it would take for the dog to maintain its ideal weight, how long would it take for the animal to reach its ideal weight?
    a. 3 weeks
    b. 3 months
    c. 6 months
    d. 1 year

101. Which of the following is not an advantage to feeding a dog with lymphosarcoma a diet high in fat?
    a. High-fat diets are usually very palatable.
    b. Fat would increase the energy density of the diet.
    c. Lymphosarcoma cells cannot use fat for energy.
    d. Fats are beneficial to digestion.

Correct answers are on pages 349-359.

102. A common complaint that clients make after their overweight dog has been switched to a high-fiber diet is
    a. Anemia
    b. Lethargy
    c. Vomiting
    d. Flatulence

103. The guaranteed analysis statement on the label of a bag of food will not give any information on the
    a. Minimum amount of fat in the diet
    b. Minimum amount of protein in the diet
    c. Maximum amount of fiber in the diet
    d. Digestibility of the protein in the diet

104. A problem with giving guinea pigs a diet appropriate for rabbits is
    a. Guinea pigs have a higher requirement for protein than rabbits.
    b. Rabbits have a higher requirement for copper, which is toxic to guinea pigs.
    c. Guinea pigs have a higher requirement for vitamin C than rabbits.
    d. Rabbits do not need vitamin B_{12}.

105. Advantages of giving an animal in respiratory distress a high-fat diet would not include which of the following?
    a. Less CO_2 is produced from the metabolism of fat.
    b. Fat is more energy dense.
    c. Diets are more palatable.
    d. Fat in the diet will cause an animal to breathe slower.

106. Which of the following would be the most accurate estimate of the energy a foodstuff would contribute to an animal?
    a. Gross energy
    b. Net energy
    c. Digestible energy
    d. Metabolizable energy

107. Which of the following terms would most likely predict forage with a high ADF value?
    a. Stemmy
    b. Prebloom
    c. Leafy
    d. Green

108. By determining the nitrogen content of a food sample, one can estimate the amount of ___ in the diet.
    a. Fat
    b. Fiber
    c. Carbohydrate
    d. Protein

109. A client of your practice calls you up with a question about the diet that was prescribed for her cat. This client noticed on the label that the cat food contains several kinds of animal protein. The client says that because all animal protein contains cholesterol, she wondered whether the food contained good cholesterol or bad cholesterol. Which of the following statements would not be included in your answer?
    a. Plant products and animal products contain cholesterol.
    b. Cholesterol is an essential nutrient in the body used for estrogen, testosterone, bile, and so forth.
    c. What is referred to as "good cholesterol" is actually a lipoprotein (HDL) that carries cholesterol from peripheral tissues to the liver.
    d. Bad cholesterol is actually a lipoprotein (LDL) that carries cholesterol to the peripheral tissues.

110. A client asks you about a new nutraceutical that you have never heard about. The least important question, as far as your ability to judge the efficacy of the product, would be
    a. Has any research been done by an independent organization?
    b. Have any results been reported in a refereed journal?
    c. Have any toxicity studies been done?
    d. How expensive is the product?

111. Which of the following would be least likely to induce diarrhea in a cat?
    a. Increased fiber in the diet
    b. Panleukopenia
    c. Food allergy
    d. Increased salt content in the diet

112. Which of the following would be an unlikely treatment for chronic diarrhea?
    a. Increasing fiber in the diet
    b. Decreasing fiber in the diet
    c. Increasing digestibility of the food
    d. Increasing the amount of vitamin C in the diet

113. Goiter can be caused by
    a. Deficiency of iodine
    b. Deficiency of iron
    c. Deficiency of vitamin C
    d. Deficiency of essential fatty acids

114. Which of the following does not result in glucose in the blood?
    a. Diet
    b. Conversion of protein to glucose via gluconeogenesis in the liver
    c. Breakdown of glycogen
    d. Conversion of fatty acids to glucose via gluconeogenesis in the liver

115. Food allergies are usually due to which constituent of the diet?
    a. Fat
    b. Antioxidants
    c. Preservatives
    d. Protein

116. Typical sources of fiber in dog food would include all of the following, except
    a. Peanut hulls
    b. Beet pulp
    c. Cellulose
    d. Cornstarch

117. The primary difference in a diet to decrease hairballs in cats as compared with other cat diets is
    a. Amount of protein
    b. Amount of fat
    c. Amount of fiber
    d. Amount of salt

118. Of the following, the least dangerous if consumed in excessive amounts over requirements would be
    a. Vitamin A
    b. Vitamin B_{12}
    c. Copper
    d. Calcium

119. The most common nutritionally caused problems in dogs and cats is/are
    a. Joint problems
    b. Cardiac problems
    c. Reproductive problems
    d. Obesity

120. The best plan to get an overweight pet to lose weight is to
    a. Increase the amount of fiber in the diet.
    b. Decrease the amount of fat in the diet.
    c. Give the pet diet pills.
    d. Feed the pet less and exercise it more.

121. Acidifying diets will help prevent what type of bladder stones?
    a. Struvite
    b. Oxalate
    c. Biurate
    d. Ammonium

122. If a cat is eating grass, then you know that the
    a. Cat wants to vomit
    b. Cat has worms
    c. Cat has a nutritional deficiency
    d. Cause is unknown

123. Which of the following housing conditions is most likely to aggravate chronic obstructive pulmonary disease (heaves) in horses?
    a. Low temperature in the stable
    b. Feeding dusty hay
    c. Screen partitions between stalls
    d. Fresh wood shavings for bedding

124. What species is least likely to require frequent cage cleaning?
    a. Rats
    b. Mice
    c. Gerbils
    d. Hamsters

125. The most useful preventive measures against kennel cough in a shelter would be
    a. Frequently cleaning exercise areas of feces
    b. Frequently cleaning kennels of urine
    c. Aggressively cleaning and disinfecting food and water dishes
    d. Ensuring that air circulation is good

126. Low environmental humidity puts neonatal puppies and kittens at risk for
    a. Chilling
    b. Dehydration
    c. Diarrhea
    d. Retardation

127. The minimum relative humidity in a neonatal puppy housing unit should be
    a. 30%
    b. 50%
    c. 70%
    d. 90%

Correct answers are on pages 349-359.

128. During the first week of life, orphaned puppies and kittens should be reared in an environmental temperature of
    a. 32.2° C (90° F)
    b. 26.7° C (80° F)
    c. 21.1° C (70° F)
    d. 15.6° C (60° F)

129. To keep animals germ free inside a barrier unit, the air pressure inside compared with that outside must be
    a. Higher
    b. Lower
    c. Equal
    d. Much lower

130. In an isolation unit where sick animals are housed, the air pressure in the unit compared with that in the quarters housing healthy animals must be
    a. Higher
    b. Lower
    c. Equal
    d. Much higher

131. Very low humidity in a colony of rats may precipitate a problem known as
    a. Stud tail
    b. Wet tail
    c. Fan tail
    d. Ring tail

132. A roll-bar in a farrowing crate keeps the sow from contacting the pen wall as she lies down; the function of the roll-bar is to prevent
    a. Injuring the teats
    b. Upsetting the food
    c. Crushing the young
    d. Breaking the pen wall

133. The squeeze-back is a desirable feature in cage housing for
    a. Cats
    b. Rats
    c. Dogs
    d. Monkeys

134. Adult males of what species should not be group-housed?
    a. Rats
    b. Mice
    c. Guinea pigs
    d. Gerbils

135. For good sanitation, outdoor runs should have floors constructed of
    a. Dirt
    b. Grass
    c. Concrete
    d. Wood

136. "Red tears" (chromodacryorrhea) in rats is caused by
    a. Stress
    b. Infection
    c. Toxins
    d. Impaired blood clotting

137. Ducks and geese that eat moldy feed frequently succumb to
    a. Dermatophytosis
    b. Aspergillosis
    c. Pediculosis
    d. Actinobacillosis

138. Filter caps on rodent shoebox cages reduce the
    a. Ammonia levels
    b. Horizontal transmission of pathogens
    c. Cage temperatures
    d. Litter sizes of pregnant females

139. The most common health problem encountered in cattle that have been recently shipped is
    a. Pneumonia
    b. Diarrhea
    c. Lameness
    d. Pinkeye

140. Which of the following is not required of a well-built doghouse?
    a. Windproof against drafts
    b. Raised off the ground
    c. Insulated against cold
    d. Spacious and roomy inside

141. Which of these is not a common strategy for managing heat stress in dairy cattle?
    a. Feeding early in the day
    b. Placing fans over housing areas
    c. Sprinkling or misting cows with water
    d. Cooling the holding pen near the milking parlor

142. The best type of feeding bowl for dogs is one made of
    a. Plastic
    b. Steel
    c. Enamel
    d. Ceramic

143. Although there is good serologic evidence that animals in shelters are exposed to many of the same pathogens, not all shelters experience a disease problem. The difference can best be explained by variance in the
    a. Degrees of pathogenic virulence
    b. Standards of management practice
    c. Prevailing weather conditions
    d. Genetic makeup of the animals

144. An inappropriate use of a puppy crate is for
    a. Housebreaking
    b. Traveling
    c. Punishing
    d. Sleeping

145. When young livestock are exposed to poor ventilation or cold stress, what outbreaks often occur?
    a. Pinkeye
    b. Dermatophilosis
    c. Pneumonia
    d. Polioencephalomalacia

146. If you are visiting all of the housing areas on a farm, in what order should you view or examine the animals?
    a. Cows, weaned heifers or steers, calves
    b. Weaned heifers or steers, calves, cows
    c. Calves, cows, weaned heifers or steers
    d. Calves, weaned heifers or steers, cows

147. An especially important period of puppy development that is critical to normal behavior as an adult is
    a. The nursing period
    b. Whelping
    c. Weaning
    d. The socialization period

148. Puncture wounds in horses and other species pose a particular risk for the development of
    a. Rabies
    b. Colibacillosis
    c. Tetanus
    d. Strangles

149. The height of a nipple watering device must be adjusted according to the size of the pigs in the pen. It should be set at a level that is
    a. Even with the elbow of the pigs
    b. Just above the shoulder of the pigs
    c. Halfway between the shoulder and the elbow of the pigs
    d. Comfortably reachable when the pigs are lying down

150. The number of nipple watering devices in group pens varies according to the size and number of animals involved. A pen of 20 pigs should have a minimum of
    a. 1 nipple per pen
    b. 2 nipples per pen
    c. 3 nipples per pen
    d. 4 nipples per pen

151. What is a newborn piglet's lower critical temperature?
    a. 70° to 75° F
    b. 65° to 70° F
    c. 110° to 115° F
    d. 90° to 95° F

152. What does it mean when piglets lie in a pile, with some on top of others?
    a. They are well fed.
    b. They are well socialized.
    c. They are hungry.
    d. They are cold.

153. The environmental temperature should be monitored routinely in a farrowing unit. Where should thermometers be placed?
    a. At the herdsman's eye level
    b. At the herdsman's waist
    c. Near the entrance to the room
    d. Near the floor at the pigs' level

154. What can a producer do to provide an acceptable environment for a lactating sow and her offspring?
    a. Keep the sow comfortable, and let the piglets huddle against her for warmth.
    b. Heat the entire farrowing area to a comfortable level for the piglets, and let the sow cool herself through perspiration.
    c. Keep the overall area comfortable for the sow, and provide zones of supplemental heat for the piglets.
    d. Set the room temperature at a level halfway between the two extremes.

155. Fences and dividers between groups of pigs should be constructed so that
    a. The slats are positioned horizontally.
    b. The slats are positioned vertically.
    c. The top of the fence is no higher than the largest pig's back.
    d. The bottom of the fence is at least 8 inches above the floor of the pen.

Correct answers are on pages 349-359.

156. As you walk through the nursery section of a swine production unit, you notice that many of the pigs have rectal prolapses. What does this observation tell you about their behavior?
    a. The pigs are not active enough.
    b. The pigs are piling up.
    c. The pigs are eating too much.
    d. The pigs are well socialized.

157. Frequently, the most challenging aspect of housing goats is
    a. Building materials
    b. Fencing
    c. Heating
    d. Size considerations

158. Where is the dunging area most likely to be located in a pen that has adequate space for hogs?
    a. Near the front
    b. All over
    c. In the center
    d. At the rear

159. What common vice might become apparent if pigs are crowded into a pen with insufficient space for the number of animals?
    a. Tail biting
    b. Hyperactivity
    c. Self-mutilation
    d. Bar biting

160. Excessive carbon monoxide levels in a swine barn are usually associated with
    a. Too many animals in a building or room
    b. Overheating of the animals in a building or room
    c. Incomplete combustion of fuel in a heater
    d. Excessive waste buildup in the pits

161. Chutes used for moving swine should be constructed so that the sides
    a. Have no openings
    b. Have vertical bars
    c. Have horizontal bars
    d. Are wider at the bottom than at the top

162. Feeders in finishing hog pens should have
    a. One feeder space per pig
    b. Wide openings so that two pigs can eat per hole
    c. One feeder space per 6 to 10 pigs
    d. Shallow feeder spaces

163. In finishing buildings with pits, exhaust fans should pull air out of the building from the
    a. Pit area
    b. Ceiling
    c. Sides of the building
    d. Ends of the building

164. What nutrient is not an energy-producing nutrient?
    a. Sugars
    b. Amino acids
    c. Minerals
    d. Fatty acids

165. Fiber serves as a major energy source for
    a. Monogastric mammals
    b. Herbivorous animals
    c. Carnivorous animals
    d. Snakes

166. Adenosine triphosphate (ATP) is a high-energy storage molecule used directly or indirectly to drive other cellular processes that require energy. What process is not driven by ATP?
    a. Transport of molecules and ions across cell membranes against concentration gradients that maintain the internal environment of the cell
    b. Synthesis of chemical compounds
    c. Contraction of muscle fibers and other fibers producing motion of the cells
    d. Synthesis of other low-energy compounds

167. Of the following, which takes priority in the use of amino acids in an animal?
    a. Growth and lactation
    b. Maintenance
    c. Exertional work
    d. Exercise

168. The most important ingested nutrient is
    a. Minerals
    b. Fats
    c. Vitamins
    d. Water

169. Which of the following is an example of a dietary macromineral?
    a. Iron
    b. Calcium
    c. Zinc
    d. Copper

170. The definition of *nutrients* is
    a. Materials used to manufacture a finished feed
    b. Quantitative distribution of the individual nutrients within the finished formula
    c. A nourishing substance, food, or component of food, including minerals, vitamins, fats, protein, carbohydrates, and water
    d. Portions and select ingredients

171. A normal growth rate for puppies (per kilogram of anticipated adult weight) is
    a. 2 to 4 g/day
    b. 4 to 5 g/day
    c. 1 to 2 g/day
    d. 3 to 6 g/day

172. What vitamin is not fat soluble?
    a. A
    b. D
    c. E
    d. C

173. What condition does not cause obesity in companion animals?
    a. Overfeeding
    b. Genetic predisposition
    c. Insufficient exercise
    d. Surgical neutering of males and females

174. What would provide the best information on the mineral status of a horse?
    a. Feed analysis
    b. Muscle analysis
    c. Blood and urine analyses
    d. Hair analysis

175. Sudden ration changes would not cause
    a. Cachexia
    b. Laminitis
    c. Diarrhea
    d. Colic

176. Enteral feeding is indicated in a horse with
    a. Rabies
    b. Dementia
    c. Ileus
    d. Dysphagia

177. Prolonged undernutrition in adult horses adversely affects all of the following except
    a. Wound healing
    b. Immune system
    c. Skeletal structures
    d. Gastrointestinal tract

178. A horse with cardiac disease may not require a major dietary change. The only change may be to restrict intake of
    a. Hay
    b. Grain
    c. Salt
    d. Water

179. Horses with active laminitis should be fed
    a. Grain only
    b. Alfalfa hay and grain
    c. Alfalfa hay only
    d. Average-quality hay and no grain

180. Horses prone to esophageal obstruction should not be fed
    a. Pellets
    b. Grain
    c. Hay
    d. Salt

181. What nutrient is not required for normal horn and hoof formation?
    a. Lipids
    b. Vitamin K
    c. Amino acids
    d. Protein

182. A first line of attack to improving voluntary feed intake in a hospitalized patient is to
    a. Initiate vitamin supplementation.
    b. Improve palatability of feeds.
    c. Feed stimulants.
    d. Treat the primary condition.

183. During pregnancy, goats require extra dietary energy during the last
    a. 4 months
    b. 3 months
    c. 2 months
    d. 1 week

184. Urea toxicity in small ruminants typically occurs within 1 hour after ingestion. What is not a sign of urea toxicity?
    a. Low packed cell volume (PCV)
    b. Frequent urination and defecation
    c. Incoordination
    d. Muscle and chin tremors

Correct answers are on pages 349-359.

185. In goats, night blindness, poor appetite, weight loss, unthrifty appearance with a poor hair coat, and a thick nasal discharge have resulted from a lack of vitamin
    a. B
    b. K
    c. D
    d. A

186. Lack of what vitamin in goats can cause nutritional muscular dystrophy (white muscle disease)?
    a. E
    b. B
    c. D
    d. A

187. Lack of what nutrients can cause retarded growth and rickets in goat kids?
    a. Vitamin B and magnesium
    b. Vitamins E and C
    c. Vitamin C and calcium
    d. Vitamins A and B

188. Most scent glands in male goats can be destroyed at the time of
    a. Birth
    b. Weaning
    c. Foot trimming
    d. Dehorning

189. Goats are most at risk for developing the metabolic condition termed *ketosis* during
    a. Middle of gestation
    b. Late lactation
    c. Early gestation
    d. Late gestation

190. Ruminants that consume excessive concentrates may be predisposed to
    a. Ketosis
    b. Rumen acidosis
    c. Rumen alkalosis
    d. Parturient paresis

191. Consumption of unaccustomed quantities of grain, or of lush pasture when first turned out in the spring, by goats or sheep can lead to incomplete digestion, overgrowth of clostridia in the small intestine, and production of epsilon toxin. This syndrome is called
    a. Parturient paresis
    b. Urolithiasis
    c. Posthitis
    d. Enterotoxemia

192. A llama's stomach is functionally similar to, but anatomically different from, a true ruminant stomach. How many compartments does a llama's stomach have?
    a. 2
    b. 3
    c. 4
    d. 5

193. Llamas, like true ruminants, can break down what feed constituent into short-chained fatty acids with the assistance of bacteria and protozoa?
    a. Cellulose
    b. Water
    c. Calcium
    d. Phosphorus

194. Which statement concerning feeding of llamas is most accurate?
    a. They must be fed once daily.
    b. They must be fed twice daily.
    c. They must be fed free choice.
    d. They should be fed on a regular schedule.

195. A predominant deficiency of what nutrient causes angular limb deformities, given current North American feeding practices of llamas?
    a. Phosphorus
    b. Calcium
    c. Vitamin A
    d. Vitamin D

196. What nutrient represents the greatest fraction of dairy cattle diets after weaning and is essential to optimizing milk production?
    a. Minerals
    b. Vitamins
    c. Carbohydrates
    d. Protein

197. Overfeeding of the nutrient class ___ to ruminants or horses predisposes them to laminitis, or *founder*.
    a. Vitamins
    b. Minerals
    c. Energy
    d. Protein

198. Cattle add large quantities of saliva to their feed during chewing and also regurgitate during rumination. The most important effect of this is to
    a. Add more moisture to forage materials
    b. Buffer the acids produced in the rumen
    c. Aid chewing and swallowing
    d. Keep the tongue moist

199. Which of the following comprises the major gaseous energy loss as a result of fermentation in the rumen?
    a. Oxygen
    b. Ethane
    c. Carbon dioxide
    d. Methane

200. Neonates unable to tolerate gastrointestinal feeding are often administered TPN. What do the letters *TPN* stand for?
    a. Thiamin/protein/nitrogen mix
    b. Total parenteral nutrition
    c. Typical program for neonates
    d. Triglyceride potassium nutrients

201. To supply nearly adequate nutrition via the intravenous route, solutions used must be
    a. Hypertonic
    b. Hypotonic
    c. Isotonic
    d. Catatonic

202. What foal type has the greatest nutritional requirement?
    a. Healthy, active foal
    b. Foal with an umbilical infection
    c. Newborn foal
    d. Premature foal with septicemia

203. Hyperlipidemia is usually caused by intolerance of lipids and is characterized by cloudy serum and
    a. Hypoglycemia
    b. Hyperactivity
    c. Increased serum triglycerides
    d. Acidosis

204. Which of the following is not recommended for a weak foal?
    a. Bucket feeding
    b. Bottle feeding
    c. Nasogastric intubation
    d. Intravenous nutrition

205. What condition is not associated with weight loss?
    a. Anorexia
    b. Increased nutrient demands
    c. Protein calorie malnutrition
    d. Hyperadrenocorticism

206. To avoid abomasal bloat in calves, milk replacer must
    a. Be low in protein
    b. Be fed at body temperature
    c. Be well mixed
    d. Contain antibiotics

207. Successful strategies for preventing diarrhea in unweaned dairy calves include all of the following, except
    a. Vaccination of the dam
    b. Dry, draft-free housing
    c. Colostrum feeding
    d. Limiting the amount of milk fed

208. When a calf suckles and ingests warm milk, the reticular groove is stimulated to close so that milk and saliva pass directly into the
    a. Abomasum
    b. Rumen
    c. Reticulum
    d. Duodenum

209. When the newborn lamb receives no nutrition at all in cold environmental conditions, fat reserves last about
    a. 4 hours only
    b. 1 to 2 days only
    c. 5 days only
    d. 1 week only

210. The neonatal calf is a preruminant. What factor most influences rumen development?
    a. The sex of the calf
    b. The season
    c. The breed of the calf
    d. The calf's diet

211. What is a freemartin?
    a. A beef breed calf
    b. A heifer calf born twinned to a bull
    c. A calf with extra teats
    d. A premature calf with birth defects

212. Lack of what vitamin can cause deafness, tissue malfunction, and large coarse skin lesions in dogs?
    a. A
    b. K
    c. B_1
    d. B_{12}

213. The vitamin that is synthesized in the intestinal tract of dogs and other animals under normal conditions is
    a. Vitamin E
    b. Vitamin K
    c. Vitamin B_1
    d. Vitamin B_{12}

Correct answers are on pages 349-359.

214. The vitamin needed by dogs in heavy training to facilitate development of erythrocytes to carry oxygen from the lungs to the muscles is
  a. Vitamin E
  b. Vitamin K
  c. Vitamin B_1
  d. Vitamin B_{12}

215. The vitamin that is very important in reproduction, is a biologic antioxidant, and is considered necessary for several bodily functions is
  a. Vitamin E
  b. Vitamin K
  c. Vitamin B_1
  d. Vitamin B_{12}

216. What vitamin is also known as *thiamine*?
  a. Vitamin E
  b. Vitamin K
  c. Vitamin B_1
  d. Vitamin B_{12}

217. The major consideration in evaluating a dog's diet is
  a. Maintenance requirements
  b. Reproduction and lactation
  c. Carbohydrate content
  d. Digestibility

218. What term refers to the quantities of nutrients necessary to maintain a constant body weight in mature dogs at rest?
  a. Maintenance requirements
  b. Reproduction and lactation
  c. Palatability
  d. Digestibility

219. What condition is most likely to increase a dog's nutritional requirements?
  a. Sedentary lifestyle
  b. Pregnancy and lactation
  c. Old age
  d. Obesity

220. Lack of the dietary nutrient ___ will cause problems in the shortest amount of time.
  a. Water
  b. Protein
  c. Carbohydrates
  d. Vitamins

221. What nutrient makes up the greatest part of most dog rations and supplies energy?
  a. Protein
  b. Fat
  c. Carbohydrates
  d. Vitamins and minerals

222. During lactation, the feed intake of queens typically
  a. Stays the same
  b. Increases about 1.5 times
  c. Increases about 2 to 3 times
  d. Increases about 50%

223. In home-cooked diets for dogs and cats, what are the most common nutritional deficits?
  a. Protein and fat
  b. Water and magnesium
  c. Vitamin A and copper
  d. Salt and protein

224. Because of their high fiber content and bulky nature, dry dog food should not be fed to dogs with
  a. Diarrhea
  b. Ascites
  c. Anemia
  d. Pancreatitis

225. What clinical condition is often mistaken for obesity and may conceal malnutrition?
  a. Diarrhea
  b. Ascites
  c. Anemia
  d. Pancreatitis

226. What clinical condition is associated with acute overconsumption of a high-fat meal in dogs but is rarely seen in horses and pigs?
  a. Diarrhea
  b. Ascites
  c. Anemia
  d. Pancreatitis

227. In what condition should dietary ash be reduced and 5 g of NaCl per pound of food be added to stimulate water intake and thus achieve moderate diuresis?
  a. Diarrhea
  b. Ascites
  c. Pancreatitis
  d. Crystalluria

228. Newborn piglets raised in confinement must be supplemented with
  a. Zinc
  b. Iron
  c. Copper
  d. Manganese

229. Why do piglets need an iron supplement?
    a. The calcium obtained from nursing binds the mineral and makes it useless.
    b. They are born without any and must have it to survive.
    c. They are born with low levels in their tissue and do not have an adequate dietary source while nursing.
    d. It is depleted during digestion.

230. Swine must have access to drinking water at all times. If deprived of water for an extended period, they may
    a. Develop sodium chloride toxicity
    b. Become hyperactive
    c. Begin to bite the tail of other pigs in the same pen
    d. Develop potassium deficiency

231. Goose-stepping in swine (excessive lifting of the rear legs during walking) is most likely to be caused by a deficiency of
    a. Copper
    b. Vitamin D
    c. Zinc
    d. Pantothenic acid

232. Soybean meal is often a basic component of swine diets. What does this ingredient provide?
    a. Fat
    b. Protein
    c. Minerals
    d. Vitamins

233. A nursery pig is presented for necropsy. The history states that it was healthy yesterday afternoon and was found dead this morning. Necropsy reveals "mulberry heart disease." What dietary deficiency is the most likely cause of this pig's sudden demise?
    a. Vitamin E
    b. Vitamin C
    c. Vitamin K
    d. Vitamin B_2

234. What nutrient will provide the most calories per gram?
    a. Carbohydrates
    b. Fats
    c. Vitamins
    d. Proteins

235. A diet high in vegetable protein will cause the animal to produce ___ urine.
    a. Cloudy
    b. Clear
    c. Alkaline
    d. Acidic

236. Sows often develop constipation during late gestation and early lactation. What should the producer do to minimize this problem and keep them in optimal health?
    a. Increase the daily ration.
    b. Add fiber to the ration.
    c. Confine the animals to prevent exercise.
    d. Decrease the daily ration.

237. Finely ground hog feed (particle size 600 to 800 microns) can increase the incidence of
    a. Gastric ulcers
    b. Reproductive problems
    c. Respiratory infections
    d. Lameness

238. Antibacterial drugs are routinely added to hog feed to increase performance and feed efficiency. What group of animals benefits the most from this practice?
    a. Breeding boars
    b. Breeding sows
    c. Finishing hogs
    d. Nursery and grower pigs

239. What ingredient can be added to the diet of hogs to provide increased energy and reduce dust in the feed?
    a. Fat
    b. Water
    c. Soybean meal
    d. Silage

240. Which statement regarding disinfecting kennels is false?
    a. Mixing different disinfectants together can be dangerous.
    b. The disinfectant must be allowed to stay in contact with all of the surfaces for 30 seconds, or it will not kill the disease organism.
    c. The area should be rinsed thoroughly after the appropriate contact time.
    d. The area should be dried before the animal is returned to the cage.

241. Bleach diluted ___ has consistently been found to be a good disinfectant for both routine use and for use during a disease outbreak.
    a. 1:12 with alcohol
    b. 1:50 with alcohol
    c. 1:2 with water
    d. 1:32 with water

242. What is a trichobezoar?
    a. Hairball
    b. Laceration
    c. Abscess on the body surface
    d. Any ingested metal foreign body

Correct answers are on pages 349-359.

243. If used improperly, what restraint instrument is most likely to cause broken bones, strangulation, and death?
    a. Cat bag
    b. Nose lead
    c. Restraint gloves
    d. Capture pole

244. Because of their bellows-like breathing, what species should be held loosely if grasped around the thorax?
    a. Birds
    b. Ferrets
    c. Cats
    d. Hamsters

245. If a bird is presented to you in a cage that contains toys, perches, and water and food dishes, what is the best procedure for capturing the bird?
    a. Throw a towel over the bird and grasp it.
    b. Turn the lights down and reach in behind the bird.
    c. Talk gently and coax the bird to stand on your finger.
    d. Remove all of the paraphernalia from the cage and then reach in behind the bird.

246. To collect blood from the cephalic vein of a dog or cat, you should place the animal in
    a. A sitting or sternal position and lift the head to expose the ventral aspect of the neck
    b. Lateral recumbency and steady the uppermost back leg
    c. A sitting or sternal position and steady a front leg
    d. Lateral recumbency and lift the uppermost rear leg out of the way to expose the medial surface of the other rear leg

247. For oral administration of liquid medication to a dog or cat, you should
    a. Tilt the head up slightly and roll the lips over the canine teeth to open the mouth.
    b. Leave the head in a horizontal position and administer the liquid between the lips and cheek.
    c. Tilt the head straight up and open the mouth, using the index finger of your other hand.
    d. Tilt the head straight up, administer the liquid between the lips, and stroke the throat.

248. Of the following steps to place a cat in a cat bag, which should be first?
    a. Close the zipper
    b. Place the bag on the table
    c. Hook the bag around the cat's neck
    d. Place the cat in the center of the bag

249. In prolonged attempts to capture a sheep or pig in a paddock or pen, it is extremely easy to cause
    a. An abortion
    b. Hyperthermia
    c. A limb fracture
    d. Death from shock

250. When applying a chain twitch to a horse, you should
    a. Place it on the upper lip and tighten with intermittent pressure.
    b. Place it on the upper lip and tighten as much as possible.
    c. Place it on the ear and tighten with intermittent pressure.
    d. Place it on the lower lip and tighten as much as possible.

251. What piece of restraint equipment is most commonly used on horses?
    a. Twitch
    b. Hobbles
    c. Cradle
    d. Halter

252. When disturbed by attempts at physical restraint, a horse's initial response is usually to
    a. Kick
    b. Bite
    c. Run
    d. Rear

253. When restraining a foal for treatment or diagnostic procedures, you should
    a. Lead the mare out of sight of the foal
    b. Keep the mare nearby, within sight of the foal
    c. Leave the mare with the foal but heavily sedate the mare
    d. Pick the foal up off the ground so it cannot run away

254. What piece of restraint equipment usually remains permanently attached to bulls used for breeding?
    a. Halter
    b. Nose lead
    c. Bull staff
    d. Nose ring

255. What animals have the strongest instinct to remain in a group when threatened?
    a. Sheep
    b. Goats
    c. Pigs
    d. Chickens

256. The knot or hitch used to tie together two ropes of different sizes is a
    a. Bowline
    b. Sheet bend
    c. Halter tie
    d. Clove hitch

257. The knot or hitch that can be used for breeding hobbles is a
    a. Bowline on a bight
    b. Clove hitch
    c. Halter tie
    d. Reefer

258. The knot or hitch used to secure a lead rope to a stationary object is a
    a. Square
    b. Clove hitch
    c. Bowline
    d. Halter tie

259. The knot or hitch used to secure a rope to a vertical bar without slippage is the
    a. Clove hitch
    b. Halter tie
    c. Half hitch
    d. Bowline

260. A nonslip knot or hitch that is safe to place around an animal's neck is the
    a. Bowline
    b. Halter tie
    c. Clove hitch
    d. Sheet bend

261. When "tail jacking" a cow, grasp the tail
    a. By the end and pull it to one side as far as possible
    b. At the base and elevate it dorsally and to the right
    c. By the end and elevate it dorsally and to the left
    d. At the base and elevate it dorsally and directly in the midline

262. When carrying a rabbit, it is important to support its hindquarters, so the animal does not
    a. Scratch you with its hind feet
    b. Struggle and possibly fracture its spine
    c. Injure its ear
    d. Defecate and urinate

263. After securing a mouse by its tail, the head and body can be restrained by
    a. Twirling the mouse until it is dizzy and then quickly grasping the scruff of its neck
    b. Placing the mouse on a smooth surface, pulling caudally on its tail, and then quickly grasping the scruff of its neck
    c. Grasping the loose skin along its back
    d. Placing the mouse on a grate, pulling back on its tail, and then quickly grasping the scruff of its neck

264. The apparatus usually used to restrain beef cattle is the
    a. Halter
    b. Stock
    c. Squeeze chute
    d. Nose ring

265. The apparatus used to restrain horses is the
    a. Stock
    b. Squeeze chute
    c. Stanchion
    d. Tilt table

266. The apparatus used to restrain adult pigs is the
    a. Snare
    b. Squeeze chute
    c. V-trough
    d. Hobbles

267. The apparatus ideal for restraining a bull to facilitate hoof trimming is the
    a. Stock
    b. Squeeze chute
    c. Tilt table
    d. Alley way

268. What procedure is not a distraction technique?
    a. Taping the legs together
    b. Firm petting
    c. Twitching
    d. Blowing on the face

269. What is the best time of day to restrain sheep in the summer?
    a. Midafternoon
    b. Afternoon
    c. Early morning
    d. Midmorning

Correct answers are on pages 349-359.

270. To judge whether a dog is being aggressive, observe its body language. An aggressive dog
    a. Looks from side to side
    b. Holds its head low between the shoulders
    c. Wags its tail
    d. Has eyes that dart from one thing to another

271. To judge whether a dog is nervous, observe its body language. A nervous dog usually
    a. Holds its head low between the shoulders
    b. Stares straight at you
    c. Remains in a "sit" position
    d. Has eyes that dart from one thing to another

272. To protect yourself when attacked by a dog, you should
    a. Run.
    b. Kick or hit at it.
    c. Roll yourself into a ball and protect your neck and face with your arms.
    d. Stand still and call for help.

273. When confronted by a dog inside a kennel that is snarling, growling, and lunging at the bars, what restraint instrument is safest for you and the dog?
    a. Restraint gloves
    b. Capture pole
    c. Blanket
    d. Rope leash

274. A cat that was quiet and manageable before going into a cage has turned into a snarling mass of fangs and claws. What is the most likely cause of this behavior change?
    a. Someone hit it or beat it.
    b. It has been frightened.
    c. It is defending its territory.
    d. It is lonely.

275. The cardinal rule when working with cats is to
    a. Make sure doors, windows, and hiding places are firmly closed.
    b. Always wear restraint gloves.
    c. Put them in a cat bag for easier handling.
    d. Always cover their head with a blanket or towel.

276. Normal behavior for a healthy, well-socialized cat in a new place is to
    a. Cower in a corner
    b. Lose bladder and bowel control
    c. Sit in one spot
    d. Look around and investigate

277. Which of these is not a warning sign of an angry cat?
    a. Hissing and spitting
    b. Rubbing up against the cage bars
    c. Ears lowered
    d. Crouching low with tail lashing

278. When restraining a rooster, be most careful of the
    a. Beak
    b. Spurs
    c. Wings
    d. Feet

279. When restraining a large parrot, be most careful of its
    a. Beak
    b. Wings
    c. Talons
    d. Spurs

280. Of domestic fowl, which poses the least threat to a handler?
    a. Ducks
    b. Geese
    c. Turkeys
    d. Chickens

281. Of the caged birds listed, which one has the least tolerance for handling?
    a. Cockatiels
    b. Canaries
    c. Parrots
    d. Conures

282. The most common cause of fear-based aggression in adult dogs is
    a. Abuse
    b. Neglect
    c. Hunger
    d. Poor socialization

283. What restraint equipment is most useful when moving pigs from one place to another?
    a. A bucket
    b. Small fences
    c. A portable barrier
    d. A dog

284. It is acceptable and humane to lift a newborn pig by the
    a. Tail
    b. Ear
    c. Front leg
    d. Back leg

285. Of the cattle listed, which is most likely to be docile?
  a. Dairy bull
  b. Beef bull
  c. Dairy cow
  d. Beef cow

286. When handling cattle with horns, stand
  a. Directly in front of the animal
  b. To the left of the animal
  c. To the left and in front of the animal
  d. To one side, directly behind the horns

287. If you need to tie a cow's tail out of the way, it is best to tie it to
  a. The cow's own body
  b. A fence rail no higher than its hock
  c. A nail directly overhead
  d. The front of the chute or stanchion

288. To lift a full-grown rabbit out of its cage, you should grasp it by the
  a. Ears
  b. Lumbar vertebrae
  c. Shoulders
  d. Scruff of the neck

289. Rats can be safely and humanely picked up by
  a. The scruff of the neck
  b. Grasping them over the shoulders
  c. Grasping the tail
  d. Grasping a back leg

290. What species can have a seizure if handled too harshly?
  a. Gerbils
  b. Guinea pigs
  c. Mice
  d. Rats

291. To restrain a snake, you should
  a. Grasp it behind the head and let the rest of the body hang down.
  b. Grasp it behind the head and support the rest of the body with your other hand.
  c. Grasp it with one hand at midupper body and the other at midlower body.
  d. Grasp it by the tail and let the rest of the body hang down.

292. A horse standing with its ears erect and moving and its head erect is most likely
  a. Depressed
  b. Nervous
  c. Alert
  d. Angry

293. The safest place to stand next to a horse is
  a. Directly in front
  b. On the left side
  c. On the right side
  d. On the left and to the front

294. Unlike other large animals, horses usually
  a. Respond to voice commands
  b. Back away when approached
  c. Chase you if you make them angry
  d. Scatter if you try to round up an entire herd

295. When tying a horse to a fence rail, keep the rope
  a. Knee high with about 3 feet of slack
  b. Knee high with about 8 feet of slack
  c. Wither high with about 8 feet of slack
  d. Wither high with about 3 feet of slack

296. Horses respond to a handler's body language more than other large animals. If you are nervous about handling horses, you should
  a. Talk loudly.
  b. Move quietly but confidently and say nothing.
  c. Whistle.
  d. Move quickly and talk constantly.

297. A chain shank is used with the halter as an added restraint device. Where should it be placed?
  a. Over the ears
  b. Under the throat
  c. Between the jaws
  d. Over the nose, dorsal to the nostrils

298. When restraining a sheep, what body part should not be grabbed?
  a. Front leg
  b. Head
  c. Back leg
  d. Wool

299. The "shepherd's crook" is used around the
  a. Front leg
  b. Chest
  c. Back leg
  d. Neck

300. To capture a herd of goats, it is best to
  a. Chase them with a dog.
  b. Capture the lead goat and the rest will follow.
  c. Use small panels to block off escape.
  d. Stand in front of the barn and call.

Correct answers are on pages 349-359.

301. To restrain a kid for dehorning, you should
    a. Fold the legs into your lap and grasp the scruff of the neck.
    b. Fold the legs into your lap and place each hand alongside the cheeks, holding the ears out of the way with your thumbs.
    c. Grasp both legs on one side with one hand, and the other legs with the other hand, and flip the animal onto your chest.
    d. Grasp all four legs in one hand, and hold the neck stretched out with the other.

302. How high can goats commonly jump?
    a. 6 feet
    b. 5 feet
    c. 4 feet
    d. 3 feet

303. A hog snare is used to catch and restrain pigs. For the snare to be effective, it should be placed over the
    a. Base of the animal's ear
    b. Entire mouth and nose
    c. Snout and as far back in the mouth as possible
    d. Hind leg above the hock

304. For a sow to exit a farrowing crate, she must back up. What device works best to force her to back out of the crate?
    a. A herding panel
    b. A bucket
    c. A hog snare
    d. A broom

305. Pigs can be challenging animals to handle. When working with swine, understand that
    a. There is no cause for concern about personal safety.
    b. Pigs are not normally vicious, but caution is advised when working with them.
    c. Lactating sows are calm and do not mind if their piglets are handled.
    d. All pigs are extremely dangerous and will attack humans without provocation.

306. You and the veterinarian are called to a local farm, where several litters of pigs are suffering from diarrhea. The piglets are 7 to 10 days old and are housed with their dams in conventional farrowing crates. The veterinarian prescribes immediate antibiotic injections, followed by oral medication for 3 days. The sows are extremely agitated by the presence of strangers and seem to be protective of their offspring. To minimize a sow's reaction to handling her piglets, you should remove them from her presence. Generally, the piglets will not squeal if you lift them by grasping the
    a. Tail
    b. Hind leg
    c. Foreleg
    d. Chest

307. What restraint device would you choose to safely and easily collect blood samples from crated sows?
    a. Hog snare
    b. Sling
    c. V trough
    d. Rope snare

308. It is July, and the weather is hot and humid. For what time of day should an appointment be made to blood test a group of replacement gilts?
    a. Early morning
    b. Late afternoon
    c. Midmorning
    d. It does not matter

309. A local swine producer calls your clinic to schedule an appointment for blood testing a group of replacement gilts. The gilts are currently penned in a large pasture but are fed daily on a fenced concrete pad. It is July, and the weather is hot and humid. What instructions would you give to the producer about penning the gilts before you and the veterinarian arrive?
    a. Fence them in their current mud wallow.
    b. Pen the animals in the corner of the pasture the night before and withhold water.
    c. No special instructions are necessary.
    d. Entice the animals into the feeding area and confine them on the concrete pad just before the scheduled appointment time.

310. A group of gilts is very nervous, because they have been caught with a snare several times in the past. What would you use to facilitate snaring them?
    a. A cane or herding stick
    b. A lariat
    c. A pair of hog tongs
    d. A bucket placed over the pig's head

311. While blood is being collected from a gilt during hot weather, she begins to show signs of porcine stress syndrome. What should you do?
    a. Let go and refrain from stressing her further.
    b. Cover her with a blanket to preserve body heat.
    c. Continue restraining her to avoid exciting the other gilts.
    d. Continue with the blood collection and ignore the reaction.

312. When choosing a muzzle for a Boston terrier, you should
    a. Use a muzzle made from roll gauze.
    b. Use a leather strap muzzle.
    c. Use a basket-style muzzle.
    d. Use an open-ended style muzzle.

313. Pigs exhibit territorial behavior. When several unfamiliar animals are mixed in a group pen, fighting may occur. If the animals are of similar size, the aggressive behavior
    a. Will begin shortly after the animals are introduced and will be short term
    b. Will not begin until several days after the pigs are introduced to the pen
    c. Will continue as long as the pigs are in the same pen
    d. Will not occur

314. Cattle have a visual blind spot located
    a. Off their shoulder points
    b. Behind their rear
    c. Directly in front of their nose
    d. Back from the level of their ears

315. A herd of cattle must be moved from the holding pen in a well-lit barn into a trailer sitting outside at night. The cattle are reluctant to leave the pen and move into the trailer. How can you most easily move the cattle?
    a. Find the lead cow and force her into the trailer.
    b. Wait until dawn.
    c. Turn on a light in the trailer that does not shine in the cattle's faces.
    d. Turn off the lights in the barn.

316. Grazing animals have the best depth perception when
    a. An object is at their side
    b. An object is toward their rear
    c. Their heads are up
    d. Their heads are down

317. A herding panel is useful when handling
    a. Cattle
    b. Swine
    c. Cats
    d. Goats

318. An animal-care facility is having a problem with coccidioidomycosis. Treatment of runs and pens for this problem will be most successful using a
    a. Steam-cleaner with bleach
    b. Stain-remover with aldehydes
    c. Detergent
    d. Disinfectant

319. Use of a detergent cage-washer is an example of
    a. Disinfection
    b. Sanitation
    c. Sterilization
    d. Chelation

320. All of the following disinfectants can be used on surgical instruments except
    a. Quaternary ammonium compounds
    b. Phenolics
    c. Alcohols
    d. Halogens

321. Which of the following is useful for dissolving urine scale from rabbit pans?
    a. Alkalies
    b. Anionics
    c. Acids
    d. Chelators

322. Rubber and plastic articles should be disinfected with
    a. Alcohols
    b. Halogens
    c. Detergents
    d. Aldehydes

323. Effective cage washing necessitates a temperature at some point in the cycle of at least
    a. 50.4° C (123° F)
    b. 71.5° C (161° F)
    c. 82.2° C (180° F)
    d. 100.3° C (213° F)

Correct answers are on pages 349-359.

324. What disinfectant should not be used around cats or other felines?
   a. Quaternary ammonium compounds
   b. Phenolics
   c. Halogens
   d. Alcohols

325. Disinfection is most difficult following contamination of premises with
   a. Canine distemper virus
   b. Feline leukemia virus
   c. Canine parvovirus
   d. Feline calicivirus

326. Solutions of bleach mixed with water are useful for disinfection for up to
   a. 24 hours
   b. 2 to 3 days
   c. A week
   d. 2 to 3 weeks

327. A product that destroys 100% of bacteria is classified as a
   a. Sterilant
   b. Disinfectant
   c. Sanitizer
   d. Germicide

328. Chelating agents in cleaners remove
   a. Oil and grease
   b. Hard water minerals
   c. Urine scale
   d. Blood and serum

329. For a disinfectant cleaner to be registered by EPA as hospital strength, it must be effective at its recommended dilution in killing ___ of the targeted pathogens.
   a. 75%
   b. 90%
   c. 100%
   d. 95%

330. Hazardous components of a cleaner or disinfectant are stated in the manufacturer's
   a. SOPS
   b. GLPS
   c. VFAS
   d. MSDS

331. Alcohol's optimum disinfecting ability occurs at a dilution factor of
   a. 50%
   b. 70%
   c. 90%
   d. 95%

332. When hypochlorite solution comes in contact with formaldehyde, the gas produced is a very
   a. Effective disinfectant
   b. Dangerous carcinogen
   c. Pleasant deodorant
   d. Weak antiseptic

333. When disinfecting using two products, the rule is to
   a. Use one disinfectant at a time.
   b. Mix the disinfectants together.
   c. Dilute each disinfectant by half.
   d. Select one bactericidal and one bacteriostatic disinfectant.

334. Selection of a disinfectant ideally depends on the
   a. Result required
   b. Purchase price
   c. Ease of application
   d. Product stability

335. Ultrasonic cleaners are used to
   a. Sanitize instruments
   b. Disinfect instruments
   c. Sterilize instruments
   d. Lubricate instruments

336. Ultrasonic cleaners work through creating
   a. Steam under pressure
   b. High-frequency sound waves
   c. Mechanical scrubbing
   d. Radiation

337. In hand-cleaning equipment after surgery, the degree of cleanliness is most influenced by the
   a. Contact time with the cleaner
   b. Degree of mechanical friction
   c. Thoroughness of subsequent rinsing
   d. Temperature of the wash water

338. Floors are cleaned best using a
   a. Wet vacuum
   b. Dry vacuum
   c. Wet mop
   d. Dry mop

339. During busy days in surgery, the area in the suite most likely to need decontamination is the
   a. Doorway to the operating room
   b. Cabinets holding surgical packs
   c. Scrub sink floor and walls
   d. Air conditioning and heating duct grills

340. When washing hands, it is important to remember that the highest density of bacteria occurs
a. Under the nails
b. Over the knuckles
c. Between the digits
d. On the palm

341. Nursing mares and foals should not be put into pastures that were grazed the previous year by
a. Stallions
b. Mares
c. Foals
d. Yearlings

342. Pastures should be free of
a. Rocks
b. Ponds
c. Trees
d. Fences

343. If stabling horses on clay floors, you should ___ once a year.
a. Apply a sealant to the clay floor.
b. Soak the floor with disinfectant.
c. Replace the clay surface.
d. Culture the clay for microbes.

344. For effective sanitation, lights in the surgical suite should be
a. Recessed into the ceiling
b. Close to the air inlet
c. Fitted with fluorescent bulbs
d. Activated by entry of personnel

345. Soap for hand washing is most likely to harbor microbes if it is in
a. A pressurized dispensing pump
b. Solid bar form
c. An aerosol canister
d. A sponge-brush combination

346. Before it is taken into the surgery room, portable equipment should be
a. Wiped with a dry sterile cloth
b. Fumigated with formaldehyde gas
c. Damp dusted with a disinfectant
d. Scrubbed with a sanitizer

347. Chlorine bleach must never be combined with ammonia because of the potential production of
a. An iodophor
b. Chlorhexidine
c. Chlorine gases
d. Alcohol

348. A healthy, adult horse can drink up to ___ of water a day.
a. 5 gallons
b. 12 gallons
c. 25 quarts
d. 10 quarts

349. What animal would you expect to have the highest water intake?
a. Heifer
b. Bull
c. Lactating cow
d. Dry cow

350. The ___ hay, if processed correctly, has the highest nutritional value when compared to other hays.
a. Alfalfa
b. Bluegrass
c. Oat
d. Timothy

ANSWERS

1. **a** Limits digestive upset by allowing for a slow change and adjustment

2. **b** Fewer calories are required once growth is complete, and fiber is beneficial for GI function.

3. **a**

4. **d** Has some effect on birds but not so much on small animals

5. **a**

6. **c** The fermentation process in the cecum constitutes the bulk of the digestion process.

7. **a** High-protein diets are necessary for lactation and growth.

8. **b** Bran is high in phosphorous.

9. **b** Fat-soluble vitamins

10. **c** Vision stimulation

11. **c** Husks are a fermentable, gel-forming source and a common ingredient in fiber supplements.

12. **b** Should show an hourglass profile when viewed from above

13. **d** Potassium sorbate is fungistatic.

14. **c** Thyroid hormone, corticoid steroids, and anabolic steroids increase appetite due to altered metabolism.

15. **b** A coined phrase from *nutrition* and *pharmaceutical*

16. **b** Buildup of waste products leading to a diseased state of renal function

17. **c** B vitamins are water-soluble.

18. **c** Protein source with low allergic potential

19. **c** Require increased digestibility

20. **c** Significant amino acids and proteins for muscle function

21. **a** Cancer patients often lose weight even if their intake of food does not diminish.

22. **a** Intracellular cation essential for smooth, skeletal, and cardiac muscle contraction

23. **b** Energy derived from the end products of digestion

24. **c** The horse stomach can hold approximately 5 lb at a time.

25. **b** Used to make direct comparison with products of variable moisture content

26. **c** Aids in maintaining consistent glucose levels

27. **b** Generally inadequate with forage diet only

28. **c** Signs of selenium toxicity include nervousness, anorexia, and ataxia.

29. **d** Decreases palatability and odor

30. **a** Signs of dehydration can develop quickly if an animal's intake of water is deficient.

31. **c**

32. **d**

33. **a** High fat and protein diets are contraindicated.

34. **a** Ingredients are listed in descending order by weight in accordance with AAFCO guidelines.

35. **b** Deficiencies can result in cardiomyopathy and retinal atrophy.

36. **a** The normal urine pH range for cats is 6.2 to 6.6.

37. **b** AAFCO is the Association of American Feed Control Officials.

38. **c** Per AAFCO guidelines

39. **b** The others are microminerals.

40. **b** Feeding excess protein is expensive, and it goes to waste.

41. **a** The hog's insulating layer of fat and the sheep's thick wool will contribute to overheating if these animals are chased or handled for long periods.

42. **c** Most goats, large or small, will calmly stand in one place if a front leg is lifted.

43. **a** Dairy cows are worked in stanchions or headlocks.

44. **d**

45. **b** Anemia can be caused by a deficiency of iron, calcium oxalate uroliths may be caused by reduced dietary magnesium, and fatty liver can be caused by a deficiency of riboflavin.

46. **d** Soluble and insoluble carbohydrates and essential amino acids must be fed or supplemented. Nonessential amino acids are not essential in the diet.

47. **a** Cats are carnivores and therefore require more protein than herbivores and omnivores.

48. **b** Lignin, cellulose, and pectin are all dietary fiber or insoluble carbohydrates.

49. **a** Vitamin B complex and vitamin C are both water soluble.

50. **b**

51. **d**

52. **c** Calcium, potassium, and sodium are all macrominerals.

53. **a** Deficiencies in zinc can cause skin lesions and poor coat condition, iodine can cause hypothyroidism, and manganese deficiency can cause defective growth and reproduction.

54. **d**

55. **c** At 28 days, kittens are no longer dependent on the ambient temperature and are able to control their body temperature. At this time they begin to explore their surroundings and become more independent.

56. **a** Puppies and kittens require a significantly higher level of fat and protein in their milk formulas than cow milk provides.

57. **c** Kittens lack the shiver response and are able to raise their body temperature only 12° F higher than the ambient temperature.

58. **a** The digestive tract becomes nonfunctional, and the kitten should not be fed until the core temperature is greater than 90° F.

59. **b** Hamsters, like rats and mice, are omnivores. Chinchillas, rabbits, and gerbils are herbivores.

60. **c** Rabbits have an unusual metabolism of calcium. Excessive amounts can lead to uroliths; deficiencies can cause osteodystrophy.

61. **c** Alfalfa hay is high in calcium; too much can lead to uroliths. Alfalfa pellets can cause obesity, heart, liver, and kidney disease if given excessive amounts. Too many fresh fruits and vegetables can cause digestive upset.

62. **a** Cecal pellets are also known as *night droppings*.

63. **d** Like humans and other primates, guinea pigs are prone to scurvy with an inadequate amount of vitamin C.

64. **a**

65. **b** The gerbil and the mouse are diurnal.

66. **c** Rabbits need a cool but dry environment. The cage should have good circulation with a solid floor area for resting and to prevent sore hocks.

67. **b** Hamsters are solitary in nature.

68. **a** Coronavirus causes feline infectious peritonitis, and a rickettsial parasite causes feline infectious anemia.

69. **b** Feline distemper (feline panleukopenia) is caused by a parvovirus similar to the canine parvovirus.

70. **b** Feline infectious peritonitis is characterized by abdominal distention resulting from ascites.

71. **d**

72. **d** Acute weight loss is typically due to water loss.

73. **d** Getting the owner (and the rest of the family) to feed only the prescribed amount of food is the primary problem in getting pets to lose weight.

74. **b** Scent glands in male goats are located around the horn base and may be destroyed at dehorning.

75. **b** This is an example of a food intolerance, not a food allergy. These animals lack the necessary enzyme, lactase, needed to break lactose into simple sugars for absorption.

76. **d** Cats have higher requirements for essential fatty acids and arginine than dogs, and there are no essential carbohydrates for cats or dogs.

77. **c** Cholesterol is found in animal tissues only.

78. **b** Meat without bones has very little Ca^{++}. The high phosphorus content of meat will cause a mobilization of Ca^{++} from bones, eventually to the point that they will become so fragile they will fracture just from the weight of the animal.

79. **d** Vitamin K is essential for normal blood clotting.

80. **a** A high amount of unsaturated fatty acids without supplemented vitamin E puts a cat at risk of yellow fat disease or pansteatitis.

81. **c** Avidin in egg whites will bind to biotin, making it unavailable.

82. **d** Cats require more arginine and taurine than dogs.

83. **d** Goats have thinner skulls than calves and may suffer brain damage if too much heat is applied to their heads with a dehorner.

84. **d** A diet meeting all of a cat's essential nutrient requirements cannot be entirely derived from plant products.

85. **a** Fearful animals have dilated pupils.

86. **c**

87. **c** If the gut works, use it.

88. **a**

89. **a** Glycogen stores are exhausted in about 24 hours. Fat is burned to make volatile fatty acids for energy.

90. **c** Muscle is burned for glucose; fat is burned for volatile fatty acids.

91. **c** Onions can cause Heinz body anemia in cats.

92. **c**

93. **c** On the average, animals have been on a diet for 2 years before developing a food allergy to that food.

94. **d** Clients need to be informed that it may take a month before any improvement is seen and that it is essential that no other food be given to the animal.

95. **c** Diets and toys have been shown to decrease calculus and tartar, but they have not been shown to prevent periodontal disease.

96. **d**

97. **d** Remodeling of bones is a necessary component of growth in a puppy. Excess calcium will prevent the necessary breakdown of bones and lead to bone deformities.

98. **d** Also called *steatorrhea*

99. **c** The best measure is if the animal is maintaining its ideal weight.

100. **d** An animal will derive approximately 7700 kcal from 1 kg of adipose tissue.

(10 kg × 7700 kcal/kg = 77,000 kcal needed to lose 77,000 kcal/200 kcal lost a day = 385 days)

101. **d** Animals with cancer typically do not have much of an appetite, therefore a highly palatable, energy-dense diet is preferred. It has been demonstrated for lymphosarcoma cells, and is probably true for other types of cancer, that they are restricted to anaerobic metabolism, that is, glucose.

102. **d** Owners need to be forewarned that often when animals are switched to a high-fiber diet, especially during the first week, there likely will be an increase in flatulence.

103. **d** Guaranteed analysis statements address quantities of contents only, not the quality of contents.

104. **c**

105. **d**

106. **b** The *net energy* of any feed is the amount of energy left after deducting from the metabolizable energy the energy lost in the so-called "work of digestion."

107. **a** Acid detergent fiber (ADF) and neutral detergent fiber (NDF) are tests to analyze the fiber content of a forage. In general, the higher the ADF or NDF, the less digestible the forage.

108. **d** Protein is a nitrogenous compound.

109. **a**

110. **d**

111. **d**

112. **d** Fiber can be used to decrease the passage rate of food through the gut, thus allowing for more water to be reabsorbed, leading to a firmer stool. Nevertheless, if the cause of the diarrhea is a food allergy, fiber will prolong the contact of the antigen with the gut wall, so decreasing the amount of fiber in a diet for chronic diarrhea is also frequently tried.

113. **a**

114. **d** Fatty acids cannot be converted to glucose.

115. **d**

116. **d** Cornstarch is a source of energy.

117. **c** It has been proposed that fiber aids in the passage of hairballs through the digestive tract.

118. **b** Excess water-soluble vitamins are eliminated via the urine.

119. **d** It has been estimated that more than 50% of pet dogs and cats in the United States are overweight and 25% are obese.

120. **d**

121. **a** Acidifying diets may decrease the formation of struvite (triple phosphate) stones and contribute to the formation of oxalate stones.

122. **d** It is unknown why cats and dogs eat grass.

123. **b** The cause of heaves is not entirely environmental, but, in predisposed animals, the feeding of dusty hay can aggravate the condition.

124. **c**

125. **d**

126. **b** Dry air is dehydrating.

127. **b**

128. **a** Neonatal puppies and kittens usually stay right next to their dams, in an environment nearing body temperature. Orphaned neonates require a similar environment.

129. **a** Higher pressure inside will prevent entry of outside contaminants when the door is opened.

130. **b** This will prevent air from travelling from sick-animal areas to well-animal areas.

131. **d** Low humidity and overabsorbent bedding may predispose rats to "ringtail," or tail necrosis.

132. **c** This kind of housing is typical for preventing injuries to piglets.

133. **d** Primates may be difficult to handle, so it is important to have a way to restrain them without requiring direct contact between the handler and the animal.

134. **b** Male mice housed together will frequently display aggressive behavior.

135. **c** Most outdoor kennels have floors made of concrete or some other impervious material.

136. **a** Stress can cause rats to secrete red porphyrin pigments in their tears.

137. **b**

138. **b** Filters on the only opening in shoebox-type housing will filter out small particles, such as pathogens.

139. **a** Cattle that undergo transport stress are at increased risk for pneumonia, also called *shipping fever*.

140. **d** A doghouse need only be big enough for the dog to stand and turn around, but the other items are required.

141. **a** Typically, all farms feed early all of the time, plus it is imperative that cows have feed in front of them at all times.

142. **b** Steel bowls are nonporous for thorough cleaning and not susceptible to breaking.

143. **b** Proper husbandry helps animals maintain good immune function for resistance to disease.

144. **c** A puppy or dog must regard its crate as a "den," where it feels safe and comfortable.

145. **c** Cold stress and poor ventilation decrease immune resistance to the pathogens that cause pneumonia.

146. **d** The risk of spreading disease is reduced by visiting the stock in order, from youngest to oldest.

147. **d**

148. **c** The anaerobic environment of a puncture wound is favorable for the growth of *Clostridium tetani*, the pathogen that causes tetanus.

149. **b** The pig should have to reach up slightly to drink from a nipple watering device to minimize waste. In addition, the pigs are less likely to come into contact with the nipple, which could cause damage to themselves or to the device.

150. **b** Providing two nipples in a pen of 20 pigs allows all of the animals access to water. Generally, swine producers are encouraged to install a minimum of two watering devices per pen.

151. **d** Newborn piglets do not have the ability to regulate their body temperature, and supplemental heat must be provided to near adult body temperature.

152. **d** Piling of piglets is a sign of cold stress.

153. **d** The environmental temperature can fluctuate in the room. Thermometers should be placed at the pigs' level to ensure that the pigs are comfortable.

154. **c** If a sow is too warm, milk production decreases, resulting in smaller pigs. In addition, an uncomfortable sow changes position often and could crush her pigs. Keeping her comfortable is, therefore, to the advantage of the piglets. They should be provided with a source of heat well away from the sow.

155. **b** Vertical slats prevent the pigs from climbing the fence.

156. **b** Piling up increases the risk of rectal prolapse in piglets.

157. **b** Goat housing does not need to be sophisticated, and goats can handle hot and cold with proper shelter. However, they are good climbers, and fencing must be secure and 4 to 6 feet high.

158. **d** Pigs tend to defecate in a far corner of the pen, because they are in a vulnerable position at this time.

159. **a** Tail biting is commonly seen when pigs are overcrowded. Producers often remove the tails from newborn piglets to alleviate this vice as the animals grow older.

160. **c**

161. **a** If pigs see obstructions or movement in front of them, they stop moving.

162. **c** One feeder space per 6 to 10 pigs allows the animals ample access to the food supply and is economical for the producer to provide.

163. **a** Animal wastes that collect in the pits produce noxious gases that should not be pulled back into the building. Exhaust fans must be set up so that they move the air from the pit area out of the building.

164. **c** Minerals are necessary in the diet, but they do not provide energy.

165. **b** Grazing animals; mammals lack fiber-degrading enzyme systems, so fiber is not digested in a monogastric carnivore, whereas herbivores are able to ferment fiber to produce energy.

166. **d** Should be "synthesis of other *high*-energy components."

167. **a**

168. **d** Dehydration is a common clinical problem in sick patients unwilling or unable to eat and drink.

169. **b** Iron, zinc, and copper are examples of microminerals.

170. **c**

171. **a** 2 to 4 g/day/kg of anticipated adult weight; Puppies should be weighed when there is concern about lactation.

172. **d** Vitamin C is water soluble.

173. **c** Neutering can be associated with obesity, but it does not cause it.

174. **a**

175. **a** Cachexia is a profound and marked state of malnutrition.

176. **d** Dysphagia; Difficulty in swallowing is an indication for enteral feeding.

177. **c** Skeletal structures are maintained in the face of malnutrition in horses.

178. **c** Salt restriction is a common dietary adjustment in many species with heart failure; it may help reduce blood pressure and the work of the heart.

179. **d** Grain and alfalfa hay are high in energy; high-energy feeds may exacerbate laminitis.

180. **a** Pellets are more likely to form an obstruction than other forms of feed.

181. **b**

182. **d**

183. **c** Fetal growth is greatest during the last 2 months of gestation.

184. **a** An elevated PCV is seen with small ruminants with urea toxicity due to dehydration.

185. **d**

186. **a**

187. **c**

188. **d** Most scent glands are located around the base of the horn buds and can be destroyed during electric dehorning.

189. **d** The disease is also termed *pregnancy toxemia* and occurs when energy demands in the doe exceed intake.

190. **b** Fermentation of carbohydrates acidifies the contents of the rumen.

191. **d** Enterotoxemia due to clostridial overgrowth is also called *overeating disease*. Sheep and goats are commonly vaccinated against the disease.

192. **b** A llama's stomach has three compartments, whereas ruminants, like sheep, goats, and cattle, have four.

193. **a** Ruminants convert cellulose into energy through a process of fermentation.

194. **d** Owners may have a lifestyle whereby they feed twice a day or free choice. The most important point is that they should feed regularly.

195. **a**

196. **c**

197. **c** Overfeeding to hoofed stock increases their risk of developing laminitis.

198. **b** Saliva in cattle is basic and helps buffer the acidic products of ruminal fermentation.

199. **d** Methane is a product of rumen fermentation.

200. **b**

201. **a**

202. **d** Infection increases nutrient needs; septicemia is a more infectious process than umbilical infection.

203. **c** Triglycerides are lipids.

204. **b** Bottle feeding may cause aspiration pneumonia in a weak foal.

205. **d** Hyperadrenocorticism is not usually associated with weight loss.

206. **c** Poorly mixed milk replacer contributes to bloat in preweaned calves.

207. **d** Vaccination of the cow and calf, proper housing, and proper colostrum management will help prevent diarrhea. Limiting the amount of milk fed will not prevent diarrhea.

208. **a**

209. **b**

210. **d** Development of rumen papillae and function is stimulated by consumption of high-energy feed such as calf starter.

211. **b** Heifers born with bull twins are called *freemartins*, and they are almost always infertile.

212. **a**

213. **b**

214. **d**

215. **a**

216. **c**

217. **d**

218. **a** Maintenance includes basic nutrient requirements only.

219. **b**

220. **a**

221. **c** Carbohydrates supply most of the energy in the diet.

222. **c**

223. **c**

224. **a**

225. **b** Ascites create the appearance of a pendulous abdomen, which may be confused with obesity.

226. **d**

227. **d** Increased urine production may help prevent crystalluria from developing into urolithiasis.

228. **b** Piglets raised outdoors obtain iron from the dirt lots, whereas piglets raised in confinement are generally given iron injections.

229. **c** Piglets are born with very low iron reserves and do not obtain much iron while nursing the sow.

230. **a** With water deprivation, sodium accumulation can lead to convulsions and death. Affected pigs should be rehydrated slowly over a period of several hours.

231. **d** A deficiency of pantothenic acid in the diet leads to deterioration of the sciatic nerve. Affected pigs exhibit an abnormal gait.

232. **b** Soybean meal provides a readily available source of protein (44% to 48.5%) and satisfies the amino acid requirements of pigs.

233. **a** Mulberry heart disease is a classic finding in pigs that suffer from vitamin E deficiency; it is characterized by degeneration of cardiac muscle.

234. **b** One gram of fat provides 2.25 times more calories than a gram of protein or carbohydrate. Vitamins are not a source of calories.

235. **c**

236. **b** Sows are limit-fed to prevent obesity. More fiber adds bulk to the diet without increasing calories.

237. **a** Studies show that the production of digestive acids increases when the pig ingests finely ground particles of feed.

238. **d** Young pigs grow rapidly, and addition of antibacterial drugs to the diet increases feed efficiency and the rate of gain during this period of the pig's life.

239. **a** Fats or oils provide a readily available source of energy to the diet, with the added benefit of reducing the level of dustiness of the feed.

240. **b** Disinfectants must remain on the surfaces for varying lengths of time. The manufacturer's instructions must be followed.

241. **d** If the bleach is not properly diluted, it can be irritating to mucous membranes. There should be no bleach odor detectable with the proper dilution.

242. **a**

243. **c** Restraint gloves decrease your tactile perception to the extent that you could cause strangulation, broken bones, and, ultimately, death.

244. **a** The lungs of birds cannot inflate if the thorax is grasped tightly.

245. **d** Removing all paraphernalia reduces the chance that the bird will injure itself in attempts to escape.

246. **c** The cephalic vein is on the cranial surface of the front leg.

247. **b** The head should remain horizontal and the mouth closed. Stroking the throat induces swallowing.

248. **b** Place the open bag on the table.

249. **b** The insulation of a sheep's heavy wool coat and a pig's layer of body fat can lead to overheating if the animal is chased excessively.

250. **a** The twitch is placed on the upper lip, with pressure applied intermittently to keep the horse's attention on the twitch and at the same time preserve circulation to the lip.

251. **d** The halter is the main tool of restraint for horses.

252. **c** Running is a horse's first instinct when threatened. If it cannot run away, it will fight.

253. **b** The foal and mare should remain within eyesight of each other. If not, both will fret and struggle to be reunited.

254. **d** Nose rings are permanently inserted through the nasal septum of bulls.

255. **a**

256. **b**

257. **a** When this knot is tied in the middle of a long rope, it forms a nonslip noose that can go around the animal's neck. The long ends can be wrapped around the rear legs and secured so the mare cannot kick.

258. **d** This quick-release knot should be the only knot used to tie a lead rope to a stationary object.

259. **a** A clove hitch will not slip, even when one end is pulled.

260. **a**

261. **d** The tail should be grasped at the base and elevated straight up. Moving the tail toward one side or holding the tail by the end can damage the tail.

262. **b** Rabbits carried without support of the rear legs can struggle to the extent that they fracture their spine.

263. **d** A mouse will instinctively grasp a grate with its forefeet. You can then quickly grasp it by the scruff of the neck.

264. **c** A squeeze chute is usually used to restrain beef cattle. Dairy cattle are usually restrained in stanchions.

265. **a** Stocks are used to protect the veterinarian or technician while working on a horse.

266. **a** Adult pigs are routinely restrained using a snare around the snout.

267. **c** A tilt table is ideal for trimming cattle hooves.

268. **a** Taping the legs is considered a restraint technique.

269. **c** Early morning is the coolest time and allows the owner to observe the flock for signs of distress throughout the rest of the day.

270. **b** Head held low between the shoulders is a classic stance of an aggressive dog.

271. **d**

272. **c** This position will protect you and prevent further stimulation of the dog.

273. **b** The capture pole allows you to remain a safe distance from the dog, and the noose will not cause the animal to choke if used properly.

274. **c** Cats are territorial and establish territory quickly.

275. **a** Cats can squeeze through very small spaces. To prevent escape from a cage, examination room, or hospital, all doors should remain securely latched.

276. **d** The cat's natural instinct is to investigate a new territory.

277. **b**

278. **b** The spurs on a rooster's feet are sharp and can cause injury.

279. **a** Parrots may bite.

280. **a** A duck's bill is blunt and can pinch but will not break the skin. Also, ducks are small; consequently, their wings do not cause painful bruises.

281. **b** The canary is typically the most affected by handling, although the other birds can also have an adverse reaction to rough treatment.

282. **d** Poor socialization is a more common cause of fear aggression than outright abuse or neglect.

283. **c** A hurdle or barrier made of a solid piece of plastic or fiberglass placed in the path of a pig will turn it in the desired direction.

284. **d** Lifting by any of the other body parts may cause injuries.

285. **c** Dairy cows are usually accustomed to handling and do not react as the other three may.

286. **c** This the safest area, as long as you stand well beyond the reach of the animal's head.

287. **a** Never tie a tail to anything but the animal's body. If you forget to untie the tail and the cow bolts, the tail may be pulled off.

288. **d** Anywhere else, the rabbit or handler may be injured.

289. **b** Anywhere else, the rat may be injured.

290. **a**

291. **b** A snake's head must be controlled, and the body must be supported in the middle so that the vertebrae are not damaged.

292. **c** When the ears are erect and still, the horse may be becoming nervous.

293. **b** One should stand on the left side near the shoulder.

294. **a** Most horses are trained to respond to "whoa" or "hold still" and a few other commands.

295. **d** Anything lower or longer, and the animal can get tangled in the rope.

296. **b** Horses are very adept at reading body language and may detect signs of nervousness.

297. **d** Placing it anywhere else will cause extreme discomfort to the horse.

298. **d** Pulling on the wool of sheep can damage subcutaneous tissues and the fleece, and it may cause hemorrhages.

299. **c** Using a crook anywhere else can harm the animal.

300. **b** Save steps and aggravation by learning which goat is the lead goat. A dog will cause them to only scatter more.

301. **b**

302. **a** All fences and paddocks must be at least 6 feet high, because a goat can easily jump anything lower.

303. **c** The snare must control the pig's head. When the pig feels the pressure of the snare, it will pull backward.

304. **d** The sow's vision will be effectively blocked, causing her to back up. The other items mentioned might work, but the handler's hand and arms would be at risk from the bars of the crate.

305. **b**

306. **b** A 7- to 10-day-old pig weighs too much for the animal to be lifted from the ground by the tail alone.

307. **d** The rope snare can be placed around the sow's snout, and the end can be secured to the bars of the crate. A large sow can swing a regular hog snare against the bars of the crate and severely injure the handler's arms and hands.

308. **a** Pigs cannot dissipate heat, because they do not have functional sweat glands. It is always wise to schedule such activities early in the day to avoid overheating the animals.

309. **d** It is always easier to catch pigs when they are confined in a small area. Bringing them into the area just before the arrival of the veterinarian can avoid problems associated with water deprivation.

310. **c** Hog tongs facilitate snaring. One handler applies the tongs to the back of the neck, which causes the animal to squeal. As soon as a second person places the snare, the tongs are released. This procedure is usually less stressful than chasing the gilt around the pen.

311. **a** If the restraint is continued, the reaction may progress, and the gilt will die.

312. **c** A basket-style muzzle will not interfere with the dog's breathing.

313. **a** Pigs are territorial and establish a dominance order when new animals are introduced. It is important to pen together pigs of similar size to minimize fighting. The aggression is normally short-lived, because the pigs determine the dominance order.

314. **b** Cattle have wide-angle vision and can see behind themselves without turning their heads, except for an area directly behind their rear.

315. **c** Cattle will move to a light source, as long as it is not shining brightly in their eyes.

316. **d** Grazing animals have poor depth perception when they are moving with their heads up. It does not matter where the object is placed, their heads have to be down in order to have the best depth perception.

317. **b** The handler should easily be able to manipulate the herding panel, which is used to block the pig's vision. A pig will not attempt to walk through a solid panel.

318. **a**

319. **b**

320. **d** Halogens easily penetrate the protective coating on stainless steel and cause corrosion of the metal.

321. **c** Urine scale is high in calcium, which can be dissolved using acids.

322. **d** Aldehydes will disinfect rubber and plastic without causing damage.

323. **c** Temperature must be achieved for at least 3 minutes to accomplish disinfection.

324. **b** Cats, birds, and some reptiles are more sensitive to phenol toxicity than other species.

325. **c** Parvovirus can survive in the environment for months.

326. **a** Bleach solutions become ineffective 24 hours after mixing.

327. **b** Disinfectants are products that destroy pathogens, such as bacteria.

328. **b** Chelating agents bind minerals.

329. **c**

330. **d** Material Safety Data Sheets (MSDSs) outline the hazards of chemical products.

331. **b**

332. **b**

333. **a** Using disinfectants in sequence will maximize efficacy and minimize the risk of producing toxic mixes of compounds.

334. **a**

335. **a**

336. **b**

337. **b** Instruments must be wiped or scrubbed for optimal cleaning.

338. **a**

339. **c**

340. **a**

341. **c** Avoiding putting foals in the same pasture year after year will help reduce parasite levels in the foals.

342. **b** Ponds may serve as reservoirs of pathogens.

343. **c** Clay surfaces may become uneven with wear and soaked with urine and should be replaced periodically.

344. **a** These are not the surgery lights but the lights used to illuminate the room.

345. **b** Handling bar soap may contaminate it.

346. **c** Items taken into the surgery should be clean and dust-free, but scrubbing is not necessary.

347. **c** Chlorine gases are poisonous.

348. **b**

349. **c** A lactating cow has to replace the body fluids used to produce milk.

350. **a**

Emergency Care

Thomas Colville

QUESTIONS

1. A dog that experiences shock may have fluid replacement provided by all of the following. The least desirable is
   a. Crystalloids
   b. Hypertonic saline
   c. Dextrose
   d. Colloids

2. The first drug of choice for a cat that experiences status epilepticus is
   a. Pentobarbital
   b. Diazepam
   c. Potassium bromide
   d. Propofol

3. Tension pneumothorax occurs when
   a. Pressure in the thoracic cavity is less than atmospheric pressure.
   b. Pressure in the thoracic cavity is equal to atmospheric pressure.
   c. Pressure in the thoracic cavity is greater than atmospheric pressure.
   d. Pressure in the thoracic cavity is constant as animal breathes in and out.

4. Vomiting should not be induced in patients that have ingested
   a. Organophosphates
   b. Salicylates
   c. Kerosene
   d. Ethylene glycol

5. The mucous membranes of a dog in septic shock are
   a. Icteric
   b. Pale
   c. Cyanotic
   d. Brick red

6. The least desirable anesthetic protocol for an emergency cesarean section is
   a. Epidural block
   b. Barbiturate anesthetic
   c. Neuromuscular blocker
   d. Propofol and isoflurane

7. The underlying disease for most cases of feline aortic thromboembolism is
   a. Renal failure
   b. Myocardial disease
   c. Hepatic disease
   d. Diabetes mellitus

8. To reduce intracranial pressure that results from trauma, ___ may be administered every 4 to 8 hours.
   a. Mannitol
   b. Atropine
   c. Diazepam
   d. Solu-Delta

9. Which of the following groupings of conditions has been triaged in the correct order?
   a. Unconsciousness, dyspnea, abscesses
   b. Dystocia, severe hemorrhage, aural hematoma
   c. Hematuria, insect sting, gaping wound
   d. Fracture, prolapsed eye, minor burn

10. Avulsed incised wounds may be closed by first-intention healing
    a. 4 hours after injury
    b. 8 hours after injury
    c. 12 hours after injury
    d. At any point after injury

11. A patient is experiencing cardiopulmonary arrest. The least effective route of drug administration is
    a. Intratracheal
    b. Intracardiac
    c. Cephalic
    d. Intraosseous

12. Fluid administration of 24 hours or more is recommended to be administered via a(n)
    a. Winged-tip catheter
    b. Over-the-needle catheter
    c. Hypodermic needle
    d. Through-the-needle catheter

13. A dog that has been hit by a car and has no palpable pulse or detectable heartbeat may need rhythmical compressions to stimulate the heart. These compressions should be performed at the
    a. First to second ribs
    b. Second to third ribs
    c. Third to sixth ribs
    d. Eight to tenth ribs

14. To minimize hemorrhage to the head of a canine trauma patient, pressure should be applied
    a. At the thoracic inlet in both jugular grooves
    b. At the thoracic inlet of the left jugular groove
    c. To the area adjacent and ventral to the mandible
    d. To the lateral points of the temporomandibular joint

15. A trauma patient has had a primary survey performed. During the secondary survey, it is noted that in lateral recumbency the patient demonstrates a jugular vein with normal distention time but protracted relaxation time. This may indicate all of the following except
    a. Hypovolemia
    b. Chronic right heart failure
    c. Chronic liver disease
    d. Acute heart failure

16. A cat has significant arterial bleeding from a distal extremity. It is best to
    a. Use a blood pressure cuff inflated to 30 mm Hg above systolic pressure distal to the bleeding.
    b. Use a blood pressure cuff inflated to 30 mm Hg above systolic pressure proximal to the bleeding.
    c. Use a tourniquet to apply pressure distal to the bleeding.
    d. Use a tourniquet to apply pressure proximal to the bleeding.

17. In emergency care cases in which it is not possible to administer large volumes of desired fluids, it may be beneficial to properly administer
    a. Isotonic saline
    b. Hypertonic saline
    c. Hypotonic saline
    d. D_5W

18. During emergency intubation, the cranial nerve ___ may be stimulated, resulting in ___.
    a. I; bradycardia
    b. X; tachycardia
    c. X; bradycardia
    d. XII; tachycardia

19. A man phones the clinic where you work to say that he has just hit a dog with his car, and it is now lying on the side of the road. It appears to be breathing with minimal distress, there is blood coming from both nostrils, there is a small river of dark blood coming from a laceration on the lateral side of its hind leg, and it can raise its head and is attempting to stand. In advising the man, your recommendation is to do all of the following except
    a. Be aware for any signs of aggression.
    b. Tie the mouth securely closed with your shoelace.
    c. Transport the dog on a board lying on its side.
    d. Apply direct pressure to the wound.

20. A normal CVP range is
    a. 20 to 30 cm H_2O
    b. 0 to 10 cm H_2O
    c. 10 to 20 cm H_2O
    d. 50 to 100 cm H_2O

21. Facilitation of the placement of a jugular catheter in an obese animal may be achieved by
    a. Placing the animal in dorsal recumbency
    b. Placing the animal in lateral recumbency
    c. Placing the animal in sternal recumbency
    d. Placing the animal in a sitting position

22. When monitoring patients on fluids and/or patients that undergo diuresis, urine output is an important consideration. The normal urine production for a healthy dog or cat is approximately
    a. 5 to 10 ml/kg/hr
    b. 1 to 2 ml/kg/hr
    c. 15 to 20 ml/kg/hr
    d. 25 to 30 ml/kg/hr

23. Multiple parameters are measured to determine a category of shock that an animal may be experiencing. The central venous pressure is high in which of the following types of shock?
    a. Traumatic
    b. Septic
    c. Hypovolemic
    d. Cardiogenic

24. Hypoglycemia is *most* common in patients that experience
    a. Neurogenic shock
    b. Cardiogenic shock
    c. Septic shock
    d. Anaphylactic shock

Correct answers are on pages 372-377.

25. In treating a shock patient it was necessary to bandage both hind limbs and the caudal abdomen. The correct way to remove the bandages is to
   a. Remove bandages as quickly as possible from hind limbs, but leave the abdomen bandaged for another 24 hours.
   b. Remove bandages slowly from the abdomen, but leave hind-limb bandages on for another 24 hours.
   c. Remove all bandages as quickly as possible, so the animal can resume circulation to the area.
   d. Slowly remove all bandages while monitoring the patient's heart rate and blood pressure.

26. Although the use of corticosteroids for the treatment of hypovolemic shock is controversial, it is generally agreed that their administration is most beneficial
   a. Once the animal has been stabilized
   b. In the early stages after initial fluid administration
   c. 24 hours after the event, to treat pain
   d. As a continuous, slow infusion over the entire treatment period

27. The Schiff-Scherrington motor posture is characterized by
   a. Bilateral extensor rigidity of forelimbs and bilaterally flaccid or paralyzed hind limbs or both
   b. Bilateral extensor rigidity of forelimbs and bilaterally flexed hind limbs
   c. Bilateral extensor rigidity of fore and hind limbs
   d. Bilateral flexing of fore and hind limbs

28. The Schiff-Scherrington motor posture is indicative of
   a. Injury to C1 to T6
   b. Injury to T2 to L4
   c. Injury to cerebellum
   d. Injury to brainstem

29. The PCV of the abdominal fluid of an animal with urologic injury is
   a. The same as the peripheral PCV
   b. Higher than the peripheral PCV
   c. Lower than the peripheral PCV
   d. Noncontributory to a diagnosis

30. NSAIDs are also referred to as
   a. Proprostaglandins
   b. Prostaglandoids
   c. Antiprostaglandins
   d. Neoprostaglandins

31. Which of the following is a colloid solution?
   a. Blood
   b. Lactated Ringer
   c. Normosol-R
   d. Plasmalyte 148

32. Defibrillation is the passing of an electrical current through the heart to
   a. Cause the already depolarized cardiac cells to repolarize in a uniform manner
   b. Cause the cardiac cells to depolarize and then repolarize in a uniform manner
   c. Prevent the cardiac cells from depolarizing, thus maintaining rhythm
   d. Prevent any contractile activity of the cardiac cells temporarily

33. Which of the following is not a sign of shock?
   a. Elevated body temperature
   b. Increased respiratory rate and effort
   c. Tachycardia
   d. Pale mucous membranes

34. Gastric dilatation/volvulus (GDV) is a life-threatening emergency. Its main damaging effect is the obstruction of the
   a. Renal vein
   b. Portal vein
   c. Femoral vein
   d. Splenic vein

35. The unit of measurement for insulin is
   a. Milliliters
   b. Microliters
   c. Milligrams
   d. International units

36. The placement of a urinary catheter in a male cat with a urethral obstruction usually serves all of the following purposes, except
   a. Ability to document rate of urine formation
   b. Prevent reobstruction within 24 hours
   c. Decompress bladder
   d. Administration of in situ antibiotics

37. Dystocia in the dog or cat may be defined as active straining without delivery of a fetus for
   a. More than 20 minutes
   b. More than 30 minutes
   c. More than 40 minutes
   d. More than 60 minutes

38. When approaching an animal that requires emergency treatment, the recommended way is to approach
   a. Caudally
   b. Laterally
   c. Rostrally
   d. Let the animal try to come to you.

39. Ocular exposure to a toxin has occurred in a dog. On examination, it is discovered that there is possible damage to the corneal epithelium. Which of the following procedures is contraindicated?
    a. Continuous flushing with physiologic saline
    b. Provision of mild sedative or analgesic or both
    c. Corticosteroid administration to prevent inflammation
    d. Use of antibiotic cream after flushing

40. A client calls the clinic where you are working to say that 6 hours ago, her cat drank some ethylene glycol. Everyone else is at lunch, and you immediately page the veterinarian; however, the client wants to make her cat vomit to rid it of the toxin. You advise her
    a. To use 3% hydrogen peroxide at 1 tbs/20 lb
    b. To use salt on the back of the tongue
    c. To use dry mustard powder only
    d. Not to induce vomiting and to immediately bring in the cat

41. Eclampsia produces elevated body temperatures, resulting from
    a. Increased level of endotoxins present
    b. Large fetal mass present
    c. Heat produced through muscle movement
    d. Eclampsia does not result in elevated body temperature.

42. A frantic client calls to say that her horse is acting strangely; the horse does not appear to be able to eat or drink and is moving with a stiff gait, there is a pink membrane present in the medial aspect of the eye, and it seems to be very agitated by loud noises. Considering this description, the horse is apparently suffering from
    a. Night blindness
    b. Potomac horse fever
    c. Tetanus
    d. Equine herpes virus 4

43. You have paged the veterinarian to go to the farm of the client in question 42; until the veterinarian arrives, you advise the client to
    a. Bathe the horse with cold water to cool it.
    b. Encourage the horse to drink lots of water.
    c. Keep the horse walking slowly.
    d. Put the horse in a quiet, dark, well-bedded stall.

44. To place a nasal oxygenation catheter in a dog, you would
    a. Measure a standard 1.5 inch of catheter length.
    b. Measure to the beginning of the ear.
    c. Measure to the medial canthus of the eye.
    d. Measure to the pharynx.

45. A client calls to say she has come home to find her cat lying with the lamp cord in its mouth. You advise her to
    a. Immediately place the cat in a carrier, and bring it to clinic.
    b. Explain how to perform CPR.
    c. Immediately disconnect the plug of the lamp cord from the wall socket.
    d. Take note of the amperage of the lamp.

46. The most common artery to use when assessing the pulse of a dog or cat is the
    a. Jugular
    b. Femoral
    c. Carpal
    d. Tarsal

47. In small breeds of dogs examined in the veterinary clinic, the pulse rate can often exceed
    a. 400 beats/min
    b. 600 beats/min
    c. 200 beats/min
    d. 500 beats/min

48. A pulse deficit is when the pulse is
    a. In complete alignment with the heartbeat
    b. Lagging behind the heartbeat
    c. Covering up the heartbeat, making it difficult to hear
    d. Totally absent, including the heartbeat

49. A sinus arrhythmia occurs when the pulse
    a. Varies in a regular manner with every breath
    b. Varies in an irregular manner with every breath
    c. Does not vary with breathing
    d. Does not vary with the ventricles and is out of alignment with the atria

50. *Hyperpnea* means
    a. Excessively high temperatures
    b. Excessively high heart rate
    c. Excessively high respiratory rate
    d. Excessive amount of muscular contractions

51. When doing physical therapy, which routine has the greatest capacity to reduce pain and muscle spasm?
    a. Wet heat produced by applying warm wet compresses to the area
    b. Dry heat
    c. Cold applied every 20 minutes
    d. Cold applied every 10 minutes

Correct answers are on pages 372-377.

52. A part of physical therapy of the respiratory tract is to
    a. Pinch the trachea to stimulate coughing.
    b. Apply hot compresses to the neck area.
    c. Avoid turning a recumbent patient often.
    d. Place hands over the patient's nose to slow down rapid respiration.

53. What size needles are the most suitable for subcutaneous injections of fluids in dogs and cats?
    a. 21 to 25 gauge
    b. 18 to 20 gauge
    c. 25 to 27 gauge
    d. 14 to 18 gauge

54. The proper site for intraperitoneal injection is
    a. On the lateral abdominal wall just caudal to the rib cage
    b. 2 to 3 inches caudal to the umbilicus on the midline
    c. At the level of the umbilicus to the right or left of the midline
    d. 2 to 3 inches anterior to the umbilicus on the midline

55. When administering liquids via the oral route to a dog,
    a. Flush a large bolus of fluid directly into the mouth.
    b. Flush a very small bolus of fluid directly into pharyngeal area.
    c. Place fluid between the teeth and the cheek, and allow the patient to swallow on its own accord.
    d. Place the fluid between the teeth and the cheek in large enough amounts so that the patient will be forced to swallow.

56. When assessing skin turgor in a canine patient, which area of the body is best to avoid?
    a. The neck
    b. The thoracolumbar junction
    c. The lumbar area
    d. The chest area

57. Where is the popliteal lymph node located?
    a. At the angle of the mandible and the neck
    b. In the inguinal area under the hind leg
    c. Proximal to the stifle at the caudal aspect of the leg
    d. Ventral aspect of the foreleg where it meets the body

58. Knuckling is
    a. A normal phenomenon in some breeds of dogs and cats
    b. A neurologic abnormality
    c. An abnormality of the respiratory system
    d. A swelling usually observed on the carpus or tarsus

59. The rapid intravenous administration of large amounts of potassium can result in
    a. Weight gain
    b. Cardiac arrest
    c. Increased urination
    d. A need to double the required fluid for rehydration

60. Potassium solutions can be administered to dogs and cats without causing severe pain by what routes?
    a. Intravenous only
    b. Subcutaneous only
    c. Intramuscular only
    d. Intravenous and subcutaneous

61. If a dog that receives parenteral fluids is pyrexic, how much additional fluid should be added to the maintenance fluid dose?
    a. 20%
    b. 15%
    c. 25%
    d. 10%

62. Which of the following is not a contraindication for fluid therapy?
    a. Pulmonary edema
    b. Cerebral edema
    c. Pitting of the soft tissues
    d. Swollen soft tissue from bruising caused by trauma

63. Which of the following is used to monitor fluid therapy?
    a. Appetite
    b. Bowel movements
    c. Temperature
    d. Urine output

64. What part of the eye can be used to indicate fluid overload?
    a. Conjunctiva
    b. Lens
    c. Pupil
    d. Nictitating membrane

65. Rapid fluid replacement is contraindicated in conditions of
    a. Severe dehydration
    b. Shock
    c. Cerebral edema
    d. Renal failure

66. A common colloid preparation administered intravenously is
    a. Lactated Ringer solution
    b. Normosol-R solution
    c. Sodium chloride 9%
    d. Pentastarch

67. Fluid-therapy solutions administered subcutaneously are
    a. Isotonic
    b. Hypertonic
    c. Hypotonic
    d. Colloids

68. The best route for rapid fluid administration of large amounts of fluids to patients with poor venous access is
    a. Subcutaneous
    b. Oral
    c. Intraosseus
    d. Intraperitoneal

69. In trauma cases, fluid therapy should be used with caution in which of the following scenarios?
    a. Severe shock
    b. Mild shock
    c. Pulmonary contusions
    d. Severe skin damage

70. What is the primary objective of first aid for a critically injured animal?
    a. Keep the animal alive.
    b. Make the animal comfortable.
    c. Make the owner comfortable.
    d. Relieve pain.

71. Which of the following is the safest and most effective first aid for frostbite?
    a. Apply warm towels and massage the area.
    b. Immerse the effected area in hot water.
    c. Immerse the effected area in lukewarm water.
    d. Rub the effected area with snow.

72. Which of the following methods of controlling hemorrhage from a traumatic wound is least likely to cause further damage to the animal?
    a. Clamping the wound with a hemostat
    b. Direct pressure
    c. Tourniquet
    d. Applying silver nitrate

73. Which would be considered the least important physical measure evaluated during triage of a patient?
    a. Heart rate
    b. Respiratory rate
    c. Capillary refill time
    d. Weight

74. Patients in shock have
    a. An initial decrease in heart rate that then increases as the patient nears death
    b. A decreased heart rate
    c. An initial increase in heart rate that then decreases as the patient nears death
    d. An increased heart rate

75. The mucous membranes of patients in hemorrhagic shock are
    a. Cyanotic
    b. Pale or white
    c. Brick red
    d. Unusually warm

76. The mucous membranes of patients with severe anemia and respiratory distress are
    a. White
    b. Purple or blue
    c. Brick red
    d. Pink

77. Normal urine output in cats and dogs is
    a. 1 to 2 ml/kg/hr
    b. 3 to 4 ml/kg/hr
    c. 0.5 ml/kg/hr
    d. 10 ml/kg/hr

78. According to the principles of triage, which patient should first be seen by the veterinarian?
    a. Cat with a closed fracture
    b. Dog in respiratory distress
    c. Dog with otitis externa
    d. Cat with a small laceration on a paw pad

79. Petechial hemorrhages on the mucous membranes can indicate
    a. Trauma
    b. Methemoglobinemia
    c. Anemia
    d. Thrombocytopenia

80. Which of these is not a characteristic of traumatic shock?
    a. White mucous membranes
    b. Cool extremities
    c. Capillary refill time under 1 second
    d. Weak femoral pulses

Correct answers are on pages 372-377.

81. According to the principles of triage, which patient should be seen first by a veterinarian?
    a. Dog with a small laceration on a pinna
    b. Dog with acute gastric dilatation/volvulus
    c. Cat with dystocia, not in shock, no kitten in birth canal
    d. Cat with possible linear foreign body in the bowel

82. Which of these signs is not an indication of dystocia?
    a. Green or black vulvar discharge
    b. Profuse vulvar hemorrhage
    c. Pup or kitten in the birth canal for 5 minutes
    d. More than 1 hour of vigorous contractions with no pup or kitten produced

83. What is not usually a sign of acute gastric dilatation/volvulus?
    a. Unproductive attempts to vomit
    b. Hypersalivation
    c. Abdominal distention
    d. Profuse diarrhea

84. Crackles on thoracic auscultation indicate
    a. Asthma
    b. Upper-airway obstruction
    c. Fluid in the lungs
    d. Pleural space disease

85. A client describes his male cat as lethargic and constipated; he has observed the cat straining in the litter box. You suspect that the cat is actually suffering from
    a. Peritonitis
    b. Urethral obstruction
    c. Intestinal obstruction
    d. An upper respiratory viral infection

86. If the hindquarters are elevated in a dog with a severe diaphragmatic hernia, what effect does this have on respiration?
    a. There is no change in respiratory rate or depth.
    b. Respiratory rate decreases and respiration becomes less labored.
    c. Respiration becomes more labored.
    d. A cough is induced.

87. You are assessing a cat with a spinal injury. When you pinch its toe, a positive response to deep pain is indicated by
    a. No response
    b. Withdrawal of the foot without vocalizing
    c. Vomiting
    d. Withdrawal of the foot and vocalizing

88. Signs of impending cardiopulmonary arrest include all of the following except
    a. Alertness
    b. Dilated pupils
    c. Agonal breathing
    d. No femoral pulse

89. A patient with multiple pelvic fractures has not urinated in over 24 hours. You suspect the patient may also have
    a. A ruptured urinary bladder
    b. A diaphragmatic hernia
    c. Renal failure
    d. Urethral calculi

90. A free-roaming dog is brought to your clinic for listlessness and dyspnea. When performing venipuncture, you notice that the animal seems to have a prolonged clotting time. You suspect that the patient may have ingested
    a. Anticoagulant rodent poison
    b. Ethylene glycol
    c. Strychnine
    d. Organophosphate insecticide

91. Which statement concerning status epilepticus is most accurate?
    a. It occurs in geriatric animals only.
    b. It is a life-threatening medical emergency.
    c. It is treated by administering acepromazine.
    d. It will resolve spontaneously.

92. Signs of organophosphate toxicity include all of the following except
    a. Salivation
    b. Lacrimation
    c. Dyspnea
    d. Dilated pupils

93. Normal capillary refill time in dogs is
    a. Under 1 second
    b. 1 to 2 seconds
    c. 2 to 4 seconds
    d. 4 to 6 seconds

94. A client calls your clinic and tells you that his cat has just been hit by a car. You should recommend that he
    a. Immediately bring the cat in to be examined by a veterinarian.
    b. Observe the cat at home for an hour, and call back if problems occur.
    c. Bring the cat for examination by a veterinarian the following day.
    d. Bring the cat to you for initial examination, so you can determine whether the animal needs to be seen by a veterinarian.

95. A dog has been hit by a car, and the client calls your clinic. The client says the dog has a dangling leg. You recommend to the client that he
    a. Immediately start cardiopulmonary resuscitation, then bring the pet to the clinic.
    b. Observe the pet at home for an hour, and bring it to the clinic if there is no improvement.
    c. Observe the pet at home for 24 hours, and bring it to the clinic if there is no improvement.
    d. Splint the leg, if possible, and immediately bring the pet to the clinic.

96. A client calls your clinic and tells you that his puppy has just eaten rat poison that contains an anticoagulant. What should you recommend?
    a. Do not induce emesis, and immediately bring the pet to the clinic for examination and treatment.
    b. Induce emesis then immediately bring the pet to the clinic for examination and treatment.
    c. Induce emesis; no further treatment is required.
    d. Induce emesis then bring the pet to the clinic only if it shows signs of toxicity.

97. A client calls your clinic and tells you that his cat has just ingested antifreeze (ethylene glycol). What should you recommend?
    a. Do not induce emesis and immediately bring the pet to the clinic for examination and treatment.
    b. Induce emesis then immediately bring the pet to the clinic for examination and treatment.
    c. Induce emesis; no further treatment is required.
    d. Induce emesis then bring the pet to the clinic only if it shows signs of toxicity.

98. A client of a diabetic cat calls your clinic and says that her cat has just had a seizure and collapsed. She gave the cat its usual dose of insulin that morning, but the animal has not eaten anything during the day. You should recommend that she give
    a. Another dose of insulin, then bring the cat to the clinic for medical attention
    b. Some corn syrup or sugar solution on the gums, then observe the cat at home
    c. Some corn syrup or sugar solution on the gums, then bring the cat to the clinic for medical attention
    d. Another dose of insulin, then observe the cat at home

99. A client has just treated his 5-week-old kitten with a flea dip that contains lindane. The cat is acting slightly lethargic, and the client then notices that the label on the dip reads "for dogs only." The client calls your clinic. You should advise him to
    a. Observe the kitten at home.
    b. Wash the kitten with mild dish soap, rinse well, and then bring the animal to the clinic for examination.
    c. Wash the kitten with mild dish soap, rinse well, and then administer acetaminophen for discomfort.
    d. Induce emesis and observe the kitten at home.

100. A client calls your clinic because he has noticed that his cat has a string protruding from under the tongue. You should advise him to
    a. Attempt to gently pull out the string.
    b. Induce emesis.
    c. Cut the string and administer laxatives at home.
    d. Bring the cat to the clinic for examination.

101. A client calls your clinic because she has noticed a barbed fishhook embedded in her dog's lower lip. You should advise her to
    a. Attempt to gently pull out the fishhook.
    b. Observe the dog at home; most fishhooks fall out spontaneously within 24 hours.
    c. Attempt to gently push the fishhook through the skin, then cut and remove it. If this is not possible or successful, bring the animal to see the veterinarian as soon as possible.
    d. Administer aspirin for discomfort, and see the veterinarian within 48 hours for treatment.

102. The first measure to control active external bleeding should be
    a. Direct digital pressure
    b. A tourniquet
    c. A pressure bandage
    d. Electrocautery

103. A dog has a lacerated paw pad. The client has placed a small bandage over the wound, but blood is soaking through. The appropriate treatment is to
    a. Remove the bandage and apply digital pressure to the wound.
    b. Apply a pressure bandage over the client's original bandage.
    c. Remove the bandage and apply a tourniquet to the limb.
    d. Do nothing; no further treatment is required if the bleeding is not excessive.

Correct answers are on pages 372-377.

104. A client calls the clinic and tells you that her small poodle has stopped breathing, and she cannot feel a heartbeat. What should you recommend?
    a. Attempt no treatment; immediately transport the pet to the hospital.
    b. Attempt mouth-to-mouth resuscitation and chest compressions; immediately transport the pet to the hospital.
    c. Close the dog's mouth and attempt mouth-to-nose resuscitation and chest compressions; immediately transport the pet to the hospital.
    d. Attempt resuscitation; transport the pet to the hospital if attempts at resuscitation are unsuccessful.

105. A patient with a head or neck injury should be transported to the hospital in what position?
    a. Head elevated, neck neutral
    b. Head elevated, neck flexed
    c. Head lowered, neck neutral
    d. Head lowered, neck flexed

106. A patient with a possible herniated intervertebral disk should be
    a. Allowed to move freely; if no improvement is evident in 24 hours, see the veterinarian
    b. Allowed to move freely; immediately see the veterinarian
    c. Kept strictly quiet and confined; if no improvement is evident in 24 hours, see the veterinarian
    d. Kept strictly quiet and confined; see the veterinarian immediately

107. Which of these items would be least useful on a crash cart used for emergency situations?
    a. Laryngoscope
    b. Intravenous catheter
    c. Otoscope
    d. Ambu bag

108. A patient who is apneic and cyanotic comes to your clinic. A quick oral examination reveals a hard ball lodged in the glottal opening. You should
    a. Place the patient in an oxygen cage.
    b. Attempt to pass a nasal oxygen catheter.
    c. Attempt to pass an endotracheal tube.
    d. Perform the Heimlich maneuver; if unsuccessful, prepare the patient for tracheotomy.

109. A 16-year-old, 3-kg poodle, cyanotic with agonal respirations and frothy fluid coming from the nose and mouth, comes to your clinic. You should
    a. Administer intravenous fluids at 90 ml/kg/hr.
    b. Administer furosemide intramuscularly, then place the patient in an oxygen cage.
    c. Swing the patient to remove as much fluid as possible from the airway, then initiate cardiopulmonary resuscitation.
    d. Prepare the patient for immediate tracheostomy.

110. The veterinarian for whom you work has authorized you to start infusing intravenous fluids in a 0.25-kg Yorkshire terrier puppy that is critically ill. You are unable to insert a catheter into a jugular or cephalic vein. An alternate site that can be used to administer large volumes of fluids is the
    a. Medullary cavity of the femur
    b. Carotid artery
    c. Lingual vein
    d. Ear vein

111. The veterinarian for whom you work has directed you to give a whole blood transfusion to a 0.3-kg kitten with severe anemia from flea infestation. You are unable to insert a catheter into a vein. Which of the following would be the most effective alternate route to effectively administer the blood?
    a. Subcutaneous injection
    b. Intramuscular injection
    c. Intraperitoneal injection
    d. Per os

112. You are instructing a client to apply an emergency muzzle to his injured dog. Which of these is the least appropriate material for the muzzle?
    a. Rope
    b. Metal chain dog leash
    c. Pantyhose
    d. Necktie

113. Which of the following is least likely to be available for at-home induction of emesis?
    a. Apomorphine
    b. Syrup of ipecac
    c. Hydrogen peroxide
    d. Salt

114. All of the following should be included in the first-aid procedure for acute gastric dilatation/volvulus except
    a. Induce emesis.
    b. Treat for shock.
    c. Attempt to pass a stomach tube.
    d. Trocarize the stomach.

115. All of the following should be included in the first-aid procedure for epistaxis except
    a. Elevate the nose.
    b. Apply warm compresses to the nose.
    c. Apply an ice pack to the nose.
    d. Keep the patient quiet.

116. Which statement concerning administration of activated charcoal via stomach tube is least accurate?
    a. Check tube placement by administering a small amount of water; listen for coughing or gagging.
    b. Measure the tube from the tip of the nose to the area of the 9th through 13th ribs.
    c. Measure the tube from the tip of the nose to the area of the thoracic inlet.
    d. Use a roll of tape as a speculum to keep the mouth open and prevent the animal from biting the tube.

117. Oxygen can be administered to a patient via any of the following routes except
    a. Endotracheal tube
    b. Tracheotomy tube
    c. Chest tube
    d. Nasal oxygen catheter

118. The initial first-aid procedure for a patient with heat stroke is
    a. Intravenous fluid administration
    b. Cool-water enema
    c. Oxygen administration
    d. Cool-water bath

119. First aid for a dog with paraphimosis includes all of the following, except
    a. Lubricate the penis.
    b. Apply ice packs to the penis.
    c. Apply hypertonic solutions to the penis.
    d. Apply a warm compress to the penis.

120. Initial first-aid treatment for a dog with an open fracture includes all of the following except
    a. Copiously clean and flush the wound.
    b. Cover the wound.
    c. Apply a temporary splint to the limb.
    d. Take radiographs of the fracture.

121. Which statement concerning first aid for a seizure is most accurate?
    a. Grasp the animal's tongue and pull it forward to prevent airway obstruction.
    b. Administer oral anticonvulsants.
    c. Keep the animal quiet, and prevent it from injuring itself.
    d. Immediately start infusion of intravenous fluids.

122. A client calls your hospital and says that his Pekingese has suffered an eye proptosis. Your advice to the client should include all of the following except
    a. Apply pressure to the globe to replace it in the socket.
    b. Protect the globe from further trauma.
    c. Keep the globe moist.
    d. Immediately bring the dog to the veterinarian.

123. A client calls and says that his Rottweiler has been shot in the abdomen but appears perfectly fine. What should you recommend?
    a. Observe the animal at home for vomiting or abdominal pain.
    b. See the veterinarian immediately.
    c. See the veterinarian at your earliest convenience.
    d. Observe the animal for hemorrhage.

124. Initial treatment for a cat with an open pneumothorax may include all of the following except
    a. Thoracocentesis
    b. Oxygen administration
    c. Covering the wound
    d. Radiographic examination

125. Which statement concerning emergency treatment of cats with urethral obstruction is least accurate?
    a. Cats must always be sedated to have a urinary catheter passed.
    b. Sometimes the obstruction can be relieved by massaging the tip of the penis.
    c. Cats with a slow, irregular heart rate probably have a high serum potassium level.
    d. If the obstruction is not relieved, the cat will die.

126. What procedure is not routinely performed to resuscitate neonates following cesarean section?
    a. Clean the nose and mouth of secretions.
    b. Rub them with a towel to stimulate breathing.
    c. Administer a drop of oxytocin under the tongue.
    d. Ligate the umbilical cord.

Correct answers are on pages 372-377.

127. Inducing emesis after ingestion of a solid toxin is probably no longer of value after how much time has elapsed since ingestion?
    a. 10 minutes
    b. 30 minutes
    c. 1 to 4 hours
    d. 24 hours

128. Which is not an immediate consideration in cardiopulmonary resuscitation?
    a. Airway
    b. Circulation
    c. Analgesia
    d. Breathing

129. During cardiopulmonary arrest, what route is the least effective for drug administration?
    a. Intraosseous
    b. Intratracheal
    c. Intramuscular
    d. Intravenous

130. At what rate should cardiac compressions be administered to a small dog in cardiopulmonary arrest?
    a. 80 to 120/min
    b. 60 to 80/min
    c. 110 to 140/min
    d. 25 to 30/min

131. What is the most common vessel used to assess the pulse in a dog?
    a. Dorsal pedal artery
    b. Aorta
    c. Sublingual vein
    d. Femoral artery

132. All of the following are signs of shock, except
    a. Weak and thready pulse
    b. Vasodilation
    c. Prolonged capillary refill time
    d. Tachycardia

133. Central venous pressure is used in monitoring
    a. Pulse quality
    b. Temperature
    c. Hydration status
    d. Heart rate

134. All of the following can be used to check mucous membrane color except the
    a. Sclera
    b. Gingiva
    c. Lining of vulva
    d. Lining of prepuce

135. Dehydration is assessed by all of the following, except
    a. Moistness of mucous membranes
    b. Skin turgor
    c. Packed cell volume and total plasma protein
    d. Nasal discharge

136. A 20-kg Springer spaniel is brought to the clinic because of anorexia and lethargy. Dehydration is estimated at 8%. The maintenance requirement of fluids is 66 ml/kg/day. To correct this dog's dehydration, how much fluid should it receive over the first 24 hours?
    a. 2920 ml
    b. 1600 ml
    c. 1320 ml
    d. 1336 ml

137. A 20-kg Springer spaniel is brought to the clinic because of anorexia and lethargy. Dehydration is estimated at 8%. The maintenance requirement of fluids is 66 ml/kg/day. What is the hourly rate of fluid infusion to provide two times the daily maintenance requirements?
    a. 55 ml
    b. 110 ml
    c. 235 ml
    d. 1320 ml

138. Placement of a jugular catheter is contraindicated in which of these situations?
    a. Vomiting
    b. Pancreatitis
    c. Thrombocytopenia
    d. Renal failure

139. What is the first consideration in cardiac arrest?
    a. Ventilate the animal.
    b. Apply cardiac compressions.
    c. Be sure the airway is patent.
    d. Intravenous catheter placement

140. Tissue perfusion can be assessed by all of the following except
    a. Capillary refill time
    b. Blood pressure
    c. Mucous membrane color
    d. Rectal temperature

141. During triage, which patient should be attended to first?
    a. Dog with a penetrating wound of the abdomen
    b. Cat in respiratory arrest
    c. Cat with an intestinal foreign body
    d. Dog with gastric dilatation/volvulus

142. Signs seen during cardiopulmonary arrest include all of the following except
    a. Absence of pulse
    b. No breathing
    c. Loss of consciousness
    d. Tachycardia

143. Hyperthermic patients should be treated immediately with
    a. A cool-water bath
    b. Ice packs
    c. Corticosteroid injection
    d. An alcohol bath

144. What is the recommended dosage for intratracheal drug administration during cardiac arrest?
    a. 1.5 times the intravenous dosage
    b. Same as the intravenous dosage
    c. Double the intravenous dosage
    d. Half the intravenous dosage

145. A client calls you on the telephone and is worried about her Irish wolfhound. The dog ran loose in the neighborhood, and it is now retching without bringing anything up and pacing the floor. The abdomen looks a little distended. What should you do?
    a. Record the client's phone number and tell her the doctor will call her back.
    b. Tell the client to immediately bring the dog in for examination.
    c. Advise the client to give 3% hydrogen peroxide to induce vomiting.
    d. Tell the client that the dog may have eaten garbage and to call the hospital in the morning if the animal is not feeling better.

146. A 6-year-old mongrel is brought to your hospital with anisocoria, loss of consciousness, and involuntary urination. What is the most likely cause of these signs?
    a. Urethral obstruction
    b. Warfarin poisoning
    c. Epileptic seizure
    d. Organophosphate poisoning

147. A 3-year-old female cat is brought to your hospital with petechiae on her abdomen, bleeding gums, and lethargy. What is the most likely cause of these signs?
    a. Head trauma
    b. Heatstroke
    c. Seizure
    d. Rat poison exposure

148. When advising a client to move an injured animal, all of the following are appropriate except
    a. If a back injury is suspected, place the animal on a board to move it.
    b. Muzzle the injured animal, because it may bite when being moved.
    c. Call the veterinary hospital to notify it of your expected arrival time.
    d. Give a baby aspirin to reduce pain before moving the animal.

149. Intraosseous infusion can be used in all of the following cases except
    a. Young and debilitated animals
    b. Epinephrine and atropine administration in an arrest
    c. Animals with septicemia
    d. Rapid access to the circulatory system in hypovolemic animals

150. What is the preferred route of fluid administration in a critically ill animal?
    a. Intravenous
    b. Subcutaneous
    c. Oral
    d. Intramuscular

151. Which of the following is a colloid?
    a. Hypertonic saline
    b. Lactated Ringer solution
    c. Hetastarch
    d. Dextrose

152. Whole blood is indicated over packed red blood cells in what case?
    a. Acute blood loss during surgery
    b. Disseminated intravascular coagulation
    c. Autoimmune hemolytic anemia
    d. Acute blood loss caused by trauma

153. Nutritional support can be given in several ways. What is the preferred method?
    a. Per os
    b. Partial parenteral nutrition
    c. Total parenteral nutrition
    d. Per rectum

154. A small breed dog is considered tachycardic if the heart rate is
    a. Greater than 180
    b. Lower than 180
    c. Greater than 100
    d. Lower than 100

Correct answers are on pages 372-377.

155. Which of the following is not a sign of a blood transfusion reaction?
   a. Fever
   b. Vomiting
   c. Tachycardia
   d. Seizure

156. The normal blood pH for a dog is
   a. 6.4
   b. 7.0
   c. 7.4
   d. 8.0

157. What electrolyte imbalance is most likely to be found in a cat with total urethral obstruction?
   a. Hyperkalemia
   b. Hypokalemia
   c. Hyponatremia
   d. Hypercalcemia

158. All of the following are ways to monitor the heart rate in an unanesthetized animal except
   a. Stethoscope
   b. Electrocardiographic monitor
   c. Pulse rate
   d. Esophageal stethoscope

159. All of the following are noninvasive ways of monitoring a critically ill patient except
   a. Blood pressure measurement using a Doppler unit
   b. Temperature measurement using a tympanic thermometer
   c. Blood pressure measurement using an arterial catheter hooked to a transducer
   d. Blood pressure estimation based on pulse strength

160. Which of these has the lowest priority when preparing to treat a critical patient?
   a. Oxygen source
   b. Endotracheal tubes
   c. Heating pad
   d. Intravenous catheters

ANSWERS

1. **c** Dextrose is least desirable, because one of its major disadvantages is that the water will not stay in the intravascular space to provide the much-needed expansion. Instead, it moves to the intracellular space.

2. **b** Status epilepticus is a prolonged seizure that the animal is unable to come out of. Diazepam is the recommended first-choice drug to stop seizures; if successful, then it is continued as a constant-rate infusion. If the animal is not responsive to diazepam, then pentobarbital may be administered.

3. **c** Pneumothorax is air in the pleural space. Tension pneumothorax occurs when the pressure becomes greater than atmospheric pressure; air is allowed to enter the pleural cavity but cannot escape.

4. **c** Kerosene is a corrosive material. Do not induce vomiting, because it is caustic and can cause damage on its way back up.

5. **d** Septic shock is a "distribution" problem. There is a flow maldistribution; therefore mucous membranes are congested.

6. **b** Barbiturates readily cross the placenta and therefore stand the risk of reaching and depressing the fetuses.

7. **b** The thrombi develop in the heart (left atrium). From there they enter the systemic arteries and eventually lodge in distal aorta.

8. **a** Mannitol has the effect of increasing the intravascular volume and reducing the blood viscosity. As a result, there is an increase in cerebral blood flow. In addition, there is some effect of osmotic dehydration of the brain.

9. **a** They are in the correct order from the most to the least potentially serious conditions.

10. **a** The only possible answer is choice **a**. Once 8 hours or more have elapsed after injury, wounds are left to heal by second intention, because edges are less viable and there is an increased chance of infection and so forth.

11. **c** It is best to place a jugular intravenous catheter. The more peripheral the vein, the longer it takes to get into the central circulation in the correct concentration.

12. **d** Through-the-needle catheters are usually placed in the jugular, which is the route of choice for extended administration of fluids.

13. **c** Best location to compress the heart

14. **c** This area has the most effect on blood flow to the head without restricting air flow.

15. **a** In a case of hypovolemia, there is not a normal distention time.

16. **b** Tourniquets are not recommended, because they have the most potential to cause vascular and neurologic damage. Pressure should be proximal to stop arterial blood flow.

17. **b** Hypertonic solution (7% NaCl) causes a fluid shift from the intracellular space to the extracellular space. This improves venous return and cardiac output.

18. **c** Cranial nerve X is the vagus nerve, and compressing it results in bradycardia.

19. **b** The blood from the nostrils may be an indication of airway trauma. The animal may need to breathe from its mouth; therefore do not tie its mouth closed with a muzzle.

20. **b**

21. **d** This position allows maximum exposure to the vessel and allows skin and subcutaneous fat to be held taut for withdrawal.

22. **b**

23. **d**

24. **c**

25. **d**

26. **b** Corticosteroids have the effects of improving oxygen transport to peripheral tissue, stabilizing cell and organelle membranes, and enhancing cellular metabolism.

27. **a**

28. **b**

29. **c** Lower because of the hemodilution with urine

30. **c** NSAIDs inhibit cyclooxygenase (COX 1 and COX 2), which in turn synthesize prostaglandins.

The COX 2 group of prostaglandins mediate the inflammatory response.

31. **a** Colloids contain large insoluble molecules such as gelatin or proteins. Blood, which contains large protein molecules, is a colloid. The other choices are all crystalloids.

32. **b** A fibrillating heart has a chaotic, asynchronous electrical activity. If you depolarize and then repolarize with defibrillation, a resumption of normal coordinated electrical activity can be generated.

33. **a** Shock patients have a low body temperature, because the body is shutting down.

34. **b** The distention and/or rotation of the stomach partially or completely blocks the portal vein.

35. **d**

36. **d** Immediately on presentation and catheterization, there is no need for in situ antibiotics; if there were, a more appropriate route would be selected.

37. **d**

38. **c** Allows for observation of the animal's behavior and state of mind

39. **c** Corticosteroids delay corneal healing and possibly exacerbate infection.

40. **d** Six hours have elapsed; would only advise inducing vomiting if less than 3 hours.

41. **c** Heat is generated by muscle tremors.

42. **c** Tetanus causes the signs described.

43. **d**

44. **c** If too shallow, air hisses out; if too far—that is, nasopharyngeal—cough is provoked.

45. **c** First stop the flow of electricity.

46. **b** The femoral artery is easily accessed on the medial side of the hind leg. It is easy to find and causes the least amount of stress to the patient during physical examination.

47. **c** Small dog breeds are often excited when visiting the veterinarian, and heart rates can be in the high normal ranges (normal range is 60 to 200 beats/min).

48. **b** Pulse deficit occurs when the pulse lags behind the auscultated heartbeat.

49. **a** Sinus arrhythmia occurs when the heartbeat varies in a regular manner, with each breath resulting from changes in pressure occurring in the chest.

50. **c** *Hyperpnea* means a higher than normal respiration rate.

51. **b** Dry heat has the greatest effect on reducing pain and muscle spasm.

52. **a** Pinching the trachea will stimulate coughing to allow expansion of the lungs and prevent atelectasis.

53. **b** Eighteen- to 20-gauge needles allow subcutaneous fluids to be administered in a reasonable period of time without causing undue pain to the patients. Smaller sizes should be used in pediatric or very small patients.

54. **c** At the level of the umbilicus, to the right or left of the midline, is the site that will result in the smallest chance of causing damage to abdominal contents.

55. **c** The patient should be allowed to swallow on its own accord so that aspiration pneumonia can be prevented. Administration of the fluid between the cheeks and the teeth will also reduce the risks of aspiration.

56. **a** The neck in the dog often has extra skin, making the skin tent test inaccurate in this area.

57. **c** The popliteal lymph node is easily assessable at the caudal aspect of the hind leg inside the muscle group dorsal to the stifle.

58. **b** Knuckling is a symptom of malfunction of the nervous system. The patient walks on the dorsal surface of the paws.

59. **b** Rapid intravenous administration of potassium can lead to cardiac arrest.

60. **d** Potassium can be administered both intravenously and at no more than 30 mEq/L subcutaneous without causing pain to the patient.

61. **d** Fever (pyrexia) increases a patient's metabolic rate and, therefore, its fluid need. Ten percent additional fluid is added to the maintenance requirement for pyrexic patients.

62. **d** Car accidents and other forms of trauma to soft tissue are usually indications for fluid shock therapy.

63. **d** Urine output gives us an indication of the amount of water the body is eliminating through the kidneys and thus can be used to monitor fluid input.

64. **a** Chemosis of the eye (conjunctival edema) can result from fluid overload.

65. **c** Rapid fluid replacement adds to the intracranial pressure, making cases of cerebral edema worse.

66. **d** Pentastarch is a colloid. All of the other solutions listed are crystalloids.

67. **a** Only isotonic solutions can be safely administered subcutaneously.

68. **c** Intraosseous administration of fluids (injection into the marrow cavity of a large bone) is the only method listed that allows rapid administration of large fluid volumes.

69. **c** Pulmonary contusion may lead to pulmonary edema, which is a contraindication to rapid fluid therapy.

70. **a** Keeping a critically injured animal alive is more important than the other three choices.

71. **c** The other choices could cause more tissue damage.

72. **b** The other choices have greater potential to cause damage.

73. **d** The patient's weight does not reveal the seriousness of its condition.

74. **c** Compensatory mechanisms initially cause an increase in heart rate; as the patient nears death, these mechanisms fail, and the heart rate drops.

75. **b** Blood loss causes pale mucous membranes as a result of diminished peripheral vascular perfusion.

76. **a** Patients must have adequate amounts of hemoglobin before cyanosis is demonstrated.

77. **a**

78. **b** Of the listed conditions, respiratory distress is the most critical.

79. **d** Abnormally low platelet counts interfere with blood clotting. One sign of thrombocytopenia may be petechial hemorrhages on mucous membranes.

80. **c** Traumatic shock is characterized by capillary refill times over 2 seconds.

81. **b** Of the conditions listed, acute gastric dilatation/volvulus is the most critical.

82. **c** Pups and kittens normally take longer than 5 minutes to traverse the birth canal.

83. **d** Diarrhea is not associated with gastric dilatation/volvulus.

84. **c** Crackles are produced as air is forced through fluid-filled airways.

85. **b** One should suspect urethral obstruction in male cats that are straining in the litter box until that problem is ruled out.

86. **c** Entry of abdominal organs into the chest cavity causes labored breathing.

87. **d** The patient must indicate somehow, such as with vocalization, that it feels deep pain. Withdrawal alone with no indication of feeling pain is a spinal reflex.

88. **a** The patient's mental status is not a reliable indicator of impending arrest.

89. **a** Trauma sufficient to cause multiple pelvic fractures may also cause a ruptured urinary bladder.

90. **a** Ingestion of sufficient anticoagulant rodenticides can cause prolonged clotting times.

91. **b** Status epilepticus (prolonged grand mal seizures that do not stop) is a life-threatening medical emergency. Without prompt treatment, brain damage or death may result.

92. **d** Organophosphate toxicity causes miosis (constricted pupils).

93. **b**

94. **a** Because of the potential for serious injury, all animals hit by a car should be immediately examined by a veterinarian.

95. **d** All animals hit by a car should be evaluated immediately. The fractured leg should be splinted, if possible, to prevent further injury during transport.

96. **b** Emesis should be induced, because this is a noncorrosive toxin. The pet should be brought for antidotal treatment before signs of toxicity occur.

97. **b** Emesis should be induced, because this is a noncorrosive toxin. The pet should be brought in for antidotal treatment before signs of toxicity occur.

98. **c** Because the cat had a morning dose of insulin but did not eat, hypoglycemia most likely caused the seizure. Applying corn syrup or sugar solution to the gums can help raise the blood glucose level.

99. **b** All cutaneous toxins should be removed via thorough washing as soon as possible.

100. **d** All of the other choices are potentially harmful to the cat.

101. **c** Barbed fishhooks must be pushed through the skin for removal.

102. **a** Direct pressure has little potential for damage and can be used while other means of hemostasis are being secured.

103. **b** Removing the bandage would remove any clot that had started to form. For most lacerated extremities, a pressure bandage is applied; tourniquets are used only when bandages cannot effect hemostasis.

104. **c** Mouth-to-nose resuscitation is more successful in most small patients and should be initiated during transport to the hospital.

105. **a** Elevating the head reduces intracranial pressure; a neutral neck minimizes spinal cord compression or possible vertebral fracture displacement.

106. **d** A patient with a possible herniated disk should be strictly confined to minimize further spinal cord damage. It should be immediately examined by a veterinarian to assess the extent of injury and start appropriate therapy.

107. **c** All other equipment is used for cardiopulmonary resuscitation and life support.

108. **d** The Heimlich maneuver is used to relieve upper airway obstruction; if unsuccessful, a tracheotomy will be necessary.

109. **c** This patient is in cardiopulmonary arrest. The airway should be cleared of secretions before instituting other resuscitation measures.

110. **a** The medullary cavity of the femur can accept large volumes of fluid.

111. **c** Although this route is not ideal, intact red blood cells will be absorbed from the peritoneal cavity.

112. **b** A metal chain may injure the animal and is difficult to apply.

113. **a** Apomorphine is a controlled drug unlikely to be found in a home.

114. **a** Inducing emesis is contraindicated in gastric dilatation/volvulus. Vomitus cannot be passed if the stomach is twisted.

115. **b** Warm compresses may increase circulation and worsen the epistaxis (nosebleed).

116. **c** If reaching the area of the thoracic inlet only, the tube will not reach the stomach. It will be in the esophagus.

117. **c** Administration of oxygen via a chest tube would result in pneumothorax.

118. **d** This initial first aid can be performed by the client at home.

119. **d** A warm compress may increase circulation and worsen the paraphimosis (prolonged erection).

120. **d** Radiographs are not a first-aid measure and should be taken only when wounds are cleaned and when the patient's condition is stable.

121. **c** The other measures may be contraindicated or unnecessary.

122. **a** Pressure may cause further injury to the globe.

123. **b** Because of the high risk of peritonitis, most emergency clinicians recommend exploratory surgery as soon as possible after penetrating abdominal injuries.

124. **d** A radiographic examination should not be performed until the patient's condition is stabilized.

125. **a** Cats with prolonged urethral obstruction may be comatose and often require no sedation for urinary catheterization.

126. **c** Doxapram is usually administered under the tongue; oxytocin is not given to neonates.

127. **c** After this length of time, the toxin has been absorbed into the system.

128. **c** The others are all principles of cardiopulmonary resuscitation.

129. **c** Drugs administered by the intramuscular route in patients with cardiac arrest are not absorbed quickly because of decreased perfusion of muscles.

130. **a**

131. **d** The femoral artery is the largest superficial blood vessel used to palpate the pulse, and it is usually easy to feel.

132. **b** Vasoconstriction occurs in shock.

133. **c**

134. **a** The conjunctiva of the eye, not the sclera, is used.

135. **d**

136. **a** $0.08 \times 20 \times 1000 = 1600$ ml; $20 \times 66 = 1320$ ml; (1600 ml + 1320 ml = 2920 ml)

137. **b** $20 \times 132 = 2640/24 = 110$ ml/hr

138. **c** Low platelet count causes higher risk of bleeding. The jugular vein should not be used for fear of causing a large hematoma near the trachea.

139. **c**

140. **d**

141. **b** Respiratory function is an immediate concern.

142. **d** Bradycardia or asystole are seen during cardiopulmonary arrest.

143. **a** Ice packs may shock the system; alcohol may cause toxicity.

144. **c**

145. **b** The signs fit gastric dilatation/volvulus. Time is critical, because this is a life-threatening condition.

146. **c** *Anisocoria* means unequal pupil size.

147. **d** Petechiae are small pinpoint areas of hemorrhage. They indicate a blood clotting disorder.

148. **d** Medication should not be given without the doctor's consent.

149. **c** Intraosseous infusion may cause osteomyelitis in animals with septicemia.

150. **a** The intravenous route provides direct access to the intravascular space.

151. **c** The others are crystalloids.

152. **b** Platelets are needed in disseminated intravascular coagulation; platelets are not present in packed red blood cells.

153. **a** *Per os* means orally.

154. **a**

155. **d**

156. **c**

157. **a** Hyperkalemia is too high a level of potassium in the blood. Because the potassium cannot be properly eliminated from the body, the cat becomes hyperkalemic.

158. **d** An animal must be anesthetized to insert an esophageal stethoscope.

159. **c** An arterial catheter is invasive.

160. **c** Ensuring adequate respiratory and cardiovascular functions is the first priority in critical patients. Body temperature is important, but it is secondary in importance in this case.

Pocket Pets/Laboratory Animals

Marianne Tear

QUESTIONS

1. The genus and species name for the rabbit is
   a. *Oryctolagus cuniculus*
   b. *Mesocricetus auratus*
   c. *Meriones unguiculatus*
   d. *Cavia porcellus*

2. The genus and species name for the hamster is
   a. *Oryctolagus cuniculus*
   b. *Mesocricetus auratus*
   c. *Meriones unguiculatus*
   d. *Cavia porcellus*

3. The genus and species name for the gerbil is
   a. *Oryctolagus cuniculus*
   b. *Mesocricetus auratus*
   c. *Meriones unguiculatus*
   d. *Cavia porcellus*

4. The genus and species name for the guinea pig is
   a. *Oryctolagus cuniculus*
   b. *Mesocricetus auratus*
   c. *Meriones unguiculatus*
   d. *Cavia porcellus*

5. The sex of juvenile guinea pigs is determined by
   a. Palpation of the pelvic region
   b. Behavioral traits
   c. Secondary sex characteristics
   d. Anogenital distance

6. The term for *parturition* in the guinea pig is
   a. Kindling
   b. Queening
   c. Farrowing
   d. Littering

7. The term for *parturition* in the rabbit is
   a. Kindling
   b. Queening
   c. Farrowing
   d. Littering

8. The laboratory animal species most likely to experience dystocia is a
   a. Rat
   b. Gerbil
   c. Hamster
   d. Guinea pig

9. The sex of juvenile mice is determined by
   a. Palpation of the pelvic region
   b. Behavior traits
   c. Secondary sex characteristics
   d. Anogenital distance

10. The cage type frequently used for housing nonhuman primates is
    a. Rack
    b. Squeeze
    c. Cabinet
    d. Metabolism

11. The scientific name of the mouse pinworm is
    a. *Eimeria*
    b. *Aspiculuris*
    c. *Hymenolepis*
    d. *Oxyuris*

12. Which of the following is the most commonly used species in research?
    a. Rabbit
    b. Guinea pig
    c. Rat
    d. Mouse

13. The species with the shortest gestation period is the
    a. Hamster
    b. Gerbil
    c. Mouse
    d. Rabbit

14. What is the correct term for a female guinea pig?
    a. Doe
    b. Queen
    c. Bitch
    d. Sow

15. All of the following are rodents, except the
    a. Guinea pig
    b. Rabbit
    c. Hamster
    d. Gerbil

16. A common problem that results from incorrect restraint of a gerbil is
    a. Prolapsed rectum
    b. Fractured back
    c. Proptosed eyes
    d. Tail slip

17. A common disease of juvenile hamsters is
    a. Wet tail
    b. Seizures
    c. Snuffles
    d. Leukemia

18. Seizures are a common problem in the
    a. Rabbit
    b. Hamster
    c. Mouse
    d. Gerbil

19. A male rabbit is called a
    a. Boar
    b. Bull
    c. Buck
    d. Barrow

20. The Animal Welfare Act is administered and enforced by the
    a. United States Department of Agriculture
    b. American Humane Society
    c. National Institutes of Health
    d. American Association for Laboratory Animal Science

21. The disease of rats and mice caused by low humidity is
    a. Sore hocks
    b. Wet tail
    c. Sore nose
    d. Ring tail

22. Ferrets are very susceptible to
    a. Canine distemper
    b. Feline panleukopenia
    c. Canine hepatitis
    d. Feline rhinotracheitis

23. A type of inbred albino mouse is
    a. DBA
    b. Swiss
    c. C57/BL
    d. BALB/C

24. Sacculus rotundus, appendix, and cecum are parts of what laboratory animal's gastrointestinal tract?
    a. Mouse
    b. Rabbit
    c. Hamster
    d. Guinea pig

25. What type of guinea pig has long, silky hair?
    a. Abyssinian
    b. English
    c. Peruvian
    d. Duncan-Hartley

26. What laboratory animal species has a gestation period similar to that of cats?
    a. Gerbil
    b. Mouse
    c. Rabbit
    d. Guinea pig

27. Normal body temperature is highest in the
    a. Pigeon
    b. Hamster
    c. Rat
    d. Rabbit

28. Dutch and New Zealand are types of
    a. Guinea pigs
    b. Rabbits
    c. Hamsters
    d. Rats

29. The major causative agent of chronic respiratory disease in rats is
    a. *Pseudomonas*
    b. *Mycobacterium*
    c. *Pasteurella*
    d. *Mycoplasma*

30. Caudal paralysis, as a consequence of injury to the spinal cord from a fractured back, occurs commonly in the
    a. Gerbil
    b. Rabbit
    c. Hamster
    d. Guinea pig

31. What organization's major focus is voluntary accreditation of laboratory animal facilities?
    a. American Association for Accreditation of Laboratory Animal Care
    b. American Society of Laboratory Animal Practitioners
    c. American Association for Laboratory Animal Science
    d. American College of Laboratory Animal Medicine

32. What laboratory animal species has cheek pouches and callous pads on its buttocks?
    a. Hamster
    b. Guinea pig
    c. Rabbit
    d. Rhesus monkey

Correct answers are on pages 393-400.

33. A rabbit with a purulent nasal discharge and conjunctivitis would most likely be affected by
    a. Kennel cough
    b. Venereal disease
    c. Ringworm
    d. Snuffles

34. A diet rich in vitamin C must be provided to what species because they cannot synthesize their own?
    a. Guinea pigs and nonhuman primates
    b. Hamsters and rabbits
    c. Rabbits and guinea pigs
    d. Nonhuman primates and gerbils

35. What species normally has two types of feces, day feces and night feces?
    a. Hamster
    b. Gerbil
    c. Guinea pig
    d. Rabbit

36. What laboratory animal species has ventral sebaceous glands?
    a. Gerbil
    b. Mouse
    c. Hamster
    d. Rat

37. All of the following are Old World monkeys, except the
    a. Rhesus
    b. Squirrel
    c. Cynomolgus
    d. Stump tail

38. Offspring of what laboratory animal species are born fully furred and with open eyes?
    a. Guinea pig
    b. Mice
    c. Hamster
    d. Rabbit

39. What caging material with high-impact strength is transparent and can withstand high temperatures?
    a. Polystyrene
    b. Polypropylene
    c. Polydextran
    d. Polycarbonate

40. What group reviews animal research protocols to be sure that the methods of care and use are appropriate and in compliance with federal and institutional guidelines?
    a. American Association for Laboratory Animal Science
    b. Institutional Animal Care and Use Committee
    c. American Humane Society
    d. American Veterinary Medical Association

41. For a strain to be considered inbred, a minimum of how many generations of brother to sister or parent to offspring must occur?
    a. 20
    b. 16
    c. 10
    d. 8

42. The laboratory animal species with hip glands is the
    a. Gerbil
    b. Rat
    c. Hamster
    d. Mouse

43. A greasy hair coat of a gerbil indicates that the ambient
    a. Humidity is too high
    b. Temperature is too low
    c. Humidity is too low
    d. Temperature is too high

44. All of the following are outbred stocks of rats, except the
    a. Long–Evans
    b. Sprague–Dawley
    c. Lewis
    d. Wistar

45. Animals that are free of absolutely all microorganisms and parasites are called
    a. Specific-pathogen–free
    b. Conventional
    c. Microbially defined
    d. Axenic

46. To sanitize a large piece of equipment, such as a sheep transport cage, you would use
    a. Cabinet cage washer
    b. Rack cage washer
    c. Bottle washer
    d. Tunnel cage washer

47. What laboratory animal species is most sensitive to bright light?
    a. Syrian hamster
    b. Long–Evans rat
    c. BALB/C mouse
    d. Dutch rabbit

48. What zoonotic viral disease of primates produces a mild disease with ulcers on the mucous membranes and tongue in its natural host, the Macaca?
    a. Rabies
    b. Tuberculosis
    c. Measles
    d. Herpes B

49. What animal is covered by the Animal Welfare Act?
    a. Rat specifically bred for research
    b. Sheep used for wool-production experiments
    c. Wild mouse used in research
    d. Chicken used in egg-production experiments

50. The best type of caging system for a near-term pregnant rat is
    a. Shoebox
    b. Suspended
    c. Metabolism
    d. Squeeze

51. Four of five mice housed together have large areas of alopecia on their muzzles. The most likely problem is
    a. Barbering
    b. Lice infestation
    c. Mite infestation
    d. Fighting

52. A detailed description of the procedures to be used in a research project that is reviewed by an appointed committee is a
    a. Prospectus
    b. Report
    c. Protocol
    d. Summary

53. Which of these laboratory animal species hibernates?
    a. Rabbit
    b. Hamster
    c. Gerbil
    d. Guinea pig

54. Which of these is a zoonotic disease of sheep?
    a. Psittacosis
    b. Orf
    c. Shigellosis
    d. Yellow fever

55. The most accessible vein for blood collection in the rabbit is the
    a. Jugular
    b. Femoral
    c. Ear
    d. Orbital

56. The best method for euthanizing a large group of mice is
    a. Decapitation
    b. Carbon dioxide
    c. Cervical dislocation
    d. Lethal injection

57. Use of penicillin is contraindicated in the
    a. Rabbit
    b. Mouse
    c. Guinea pig
    d. Gerbil

58. The preferred temperature for most laboratory rodents is
    a. 21° C
    b. 15° C
    c. 24° C
    d. Any temperature

59. The preferred ratio of hours of light to darkness for most laboratory rodents is
    a. 14:10
    b. 10:14
    c. 12:12
    d. 20:4

60. The young of the altricial rodents generally have their hair and open their eyes at about
    a. 1 week of age for both
    b. 2 weeks of age for hair and 1 week of age for eyes
    c. 1 week of age for hair and 2 weeks of age for eyes
    d. Within a few days of birth for both

61. If the purpose of a breeding system is to decrease genetic variability, then one should
    a. Random breed
    b. Outbreed
    c. Not breed at all
    d. Inbreed

62. The species that does not have a fertile postpartum estrus is the
    a. Mouse
    b. Hamster
    c. Rat
    d. Gerbil

Correct answers are on pages 393-400.

63. Rodents practice coprophagy primarily to recover
    a. Water
    b. Vitamin A
    c. B-vitamin complex
    d. Fats and carbohydrates

64. The main function of brown fat tissue is to store
    a. Glycogen
    b. Vitamins
    c. Glucose
    d. Water

65. Sendai virus is a
    a. Coronavirus
    b. Rotavirus
    c. Reovirus
    d. Paramyxovirus

66. Tyzzer disease is caused by
    a. Coronavirus
    b. *Clostridium piliforme*
    c. *Syphacia obvelata*
    d. Paramyxovirus

67. It is difficult to accurately convert the drug dosage used for cats and dogs to lab animal species because the latter have a
    a. Low basal metabolic rate
    b. High basal metabolic rate relative to body surface area
    c. Low basal metabolic rate relative to body mass
    d. Higher core temperature

68. One of the main disadvantages to using wire mesh floor cages is that
    a. More cleaning is required.
    b. The animal is not in contact with its excreta.
    c. Enrichment devices cannot be used.
    d. The animal cannot create a microenvironment.

69. The respective gestation periods of a rabbit, guinea pig, and mouse are
    a. 30, 68, and 21 days
    b. 30, 42, and 21 days
    c. 24, 42, and 21 days
    d. 21, 68, and 30 days

70. Signs of pain in a rodent include all of the following, except
    a. Lack of appetite
    b. Change in attitude
    c. Abnormal posturing
    d. Malocclusion

71. The basis of restraint techniques for most animals is proper control of the
    a. Tail
    b. Head
    c. Torso
    d. Legs

72. A rat is all hunched up in front of you with dyspnea, inactivity, ruffled hair coat, wheezy-sounding lungs, and nasal and ocular discharge of slightly red color. There is no photophobia or a swollen neck. The veterinarian likely suspects
    a. Sendai virus
    b. Sialodacryoadenitis
    c. Murine respiratory mycoplasmosis (MRM)
    d. Either Sendai virus or MRM

73. What average weight do you expect your male adult mice and rats to be respectively?
    a. 20 g and 200 g
    b. 10 g and 200 g
    c. 25 g and 250 g
    d. 30 g and 500 g

74. Rats are primarily
    a. Diurnal
    b. Nocturnal
    c. Crepuscular
    d. Antisocial

75. The gland of mice and rats that secretes porphyrin in the tears is
    a. Hibernating gland
    b. Harderian gland
    c. Thymus gland
    d. Lacrimal gland

76. A small group of anestrus females come into heat when a male is introduced. This is known as the
    a. Whitten effect
    b. Bruce effect
    c. Lee Boot effect
    d. Facultative diapause

77. The Bruce effect in mice is when
    a. Anestrus females come into heat with the introduction of a male.
    b. Pregnant females are exposed to the urine of a strange male and abort.
    c. Females go into pseudopregnancy without being bred.
    d. Females that are bred at the postpartum estrus have an extended lactation.

78. Females that are bred at the postpartum estrus have an extended gestation period. This is known as the
   a. Whitten effect
   b. Bruce effect
   c. Lee Boot effect
   d. Facultative diapause

79. You want to do monogamous, nonintensive, timed breeding on mice. Which of the following statements is false?
   a. The female is best put in the male's cage in the evening until next morning.
   b. The copulatory plug will likely be found in the bedding the next morning.
   c. The breeding pair should be left together until after postpartum estrus.
   d. Vaginal smear signs should indicate large cornified cells.

80. Regarding the anatomy of mice and rats,
   a. Mice have five pairs of mammary glands and rats have six pairs.
   b. The aglandular section of the stomach is rich in histamine-producing cells.
   c. Mice and rats both pant and have sweat glands.
   d. Rats and mice have a gall bladder.

81. A cage of mice is in front of you in which some mice have facial hair missing around the nose. You are best to
   a. Individually separate all the mice with missing hair.
   b. Squirt with water every time you notice a problem.
   c. Treat them with ivermectin for mite infestation.
   d. Separate the mouse that does not have any missing hair.

82. You are to give a mouse fluids on recovery from anesthesia. The maximum amount of the warmed fluids that you should be giving IP at one dose is
   a. 0.5 to 1 ml
   b. 1 to 2 ml
   c. 2 to 3 ml
   d. 5 to 10 ml

83. A healthy adult rat recovers ___ from an episode of sialodacryoadenitis.
   a. In approximately 1 month
   b. In approximately 1 week
   c. Immediately
   d. Not at all

84. Murine respiratory mycoplasmosis is caused by
   a. *Clostridium piliforme*
   b. *Mycoplasma pulmonis*
   c. *Mycoplasma piliforme*
   d. Paramyxovirus

85. The most effective way to prevent ringtail in suckling rats is to keep the
   a. Humidity greater than 50%
   b. Humidity less than 50%
   c. Temperature greater than 80° F
   d. Temperature less than 15° C

86. Up to how much blood could you safely take from your 360-g rat when doing a venipuncture?
   a. 18 to 36 ml
   b. 1.8 to 3.5 ml
   c. 1.0 ml
   d. 0.35 ml

87. A useful venous site for blood collection without an anesthetic in mice is the
   a. Medial saphenous
   b. Jugular
   c. Retro-orbital
   d. Lateral saphenous

88. The normal dentition for the hamster is
   a. 1003/1003
   b. 2003/2003
   c. 1002/1002
   d. 2033/1023

89. The gestation period, estrous cycle, and average litter size of hamsters, respectively, are about
   a. 24 days, 4 to 5 days, and 4 to 5 young
   b. 21 days, 1 to 2 days, and 4 to 5 young
   c. 16 days, 4 to 5 days, and 5 to 9 young
   d. 16 days, 1 to 2 days, and 4 to 5 young

90. The gestation periods, estrous cycle, and litter size of gerbils, respectively, are about
   a. 24 days, 4 to 5 days, and 7 to 9 young
   b. 24 days, 4 to 5 days, and 4 to 5 young
   c. 21 days, 1 to 2 days, and 4 to 5 young
   d. 16 days, 4 to 5 days, and 4 to 5 young

91. A client calls and says that she thinks her 2-month-old hamster has that "common hamster disease" that you hear about in the pet store. The sign she notices is likely
   a. Constipation
   b. Red tears
   c. Vomiting
   d. Diarrhea

Correct answers are on pages 393-400.

92. A client wishes to get a pet hamster but wants to know how long it is expected to live. You tell her that the average life span for hamsters is about
    a. 1 year
    b. 2 years
    c. 3 years
    d. 4 years

93. A client wishes to get a pet gerbil. You tell him that the average life span for gerbils is
    a. 1 year
    b. 2 years
    c. 3 years
    d. 4 years

94. You notice that one of the gerbils in a cage of postpubertal young has some nasal hair loss with some erythema and scabbing. No other alopecia is noted. This is likely caused by
    a. Barbering
    b. Nasal dermatitis
    c. Putting its nose through the food bars
    d. *Demodex*

95. If a client asks whether it is okay to feed sunflower seeds to her gerbil, you suggest that the seeds
    a. Can be used as the main diet
    b. Should never be eaten
    c. Have increased vitamin C and calcium and decreased vitamin D
    d. Have increased fat and decreased calcium

96. You are to give a gerbil a combination of drugs before anesthetic induction in a chamber. Which of the following drugs should not be used?
    a. Diazepam
    b. Acepromazine
    c. Atropine
    d. Telazol

97. Interesting morphophysiologic characteristics of guinea pigs include all of these except
    a. Both sexes have two inguinal nipples.
    b. The urine is alkaline with ammonium phosphate crystals.
    c. They have a glandular and aglandular divided stomach.
    d. Their blood contains Foa-Kurloff cells.

98. With regard to the behavior of guinea pigs,
    a. They tend to be nocturnal animals.
    b. They dig and hibernate.
    c. They react to fear by stomping their feet.
    d. Secretions from the anal and supracaudal gland are used to mark territory.

99. Regarding the reproduction of guinea pigs,
    a. Breeding is best at about 4 to 5 months of age.
    b. Lordosis and a nonperforated vaginal membrane are found in estrus.
    c. The estrous cycle is 4 to 5 days.
    d. The dam does not pass antibodies in the milk.

100. A client says that she is worried because she has noticed that the four guinea pig pups that were born about 3 hours ago are not nursing at all, and she is positive she has been watching closely. You suggest that she
    a. Bring in the sow and pups so that the veterinarian can give oxytocin
    b. Give it Mamalac and begin to stimulate for urination and defecation
    c. Not worry because guinea pig pups do not nurse for the first 12 to 24 hours
    d. Not worry until the next one is born

101. A client is concerned that her guinea pig is not getting enough vitamin C in its diet, because she is not sure how old the food is. She would be best to
    a. Feed it rabbit chow
    b. Give it multivitamins for children (Flintstones variety is the type she has)
    c. Put enough ascorbic acid tablets in the water for 2 days
    d. Put some kale, cabbage, and red peppers in its food hopper

102. A young, inactive, ruffled-looking guinea pig with piloerection and dull eyes is brought into the clinic. The client reports that it has not eaten for a few days, is showing a shuffling gait, and is sore when touched at the joints. You notice it is dehydrated as well. The likely cause is
    a. Vitamin D deficiency
    b. Vitamin C deficiency
    c. Ketosis
    d. *Bordetella*

103. To differentiate between a male and female guinea pig, the
    a. Male has no break in the ridge between the anus and urethral orifice
    b. Anogenital space is greater in the male
    c. Female has a perforated vaginal membrane
    d. Female only has a pair of inguinal nipples

104. You are to give an IM injection to a guinea pig. What maximum volume should you use?
    a. 0.1 ml
    b. 0.3 ml
    c. 0.5 ml
    d. 1 ml

105. When doing daily examinations, you note that a rabbit has a glossy hair coat and no lumps, is defecating in one spot, and is passing liquid, cream-colored urine. You should
    a. Report the ill health to the veterinarian
    b. Note the abnormal signs on the chart
    c. Note on the chart that all is normal
    d. Immediately isolate the rabbit

106. The normal dentition for the rabbit is
    a. 1003/1003
    b. 2003/2003
    c. 1002/1002
    d. 2033/1023

107. A client is concerned because she has noticed that a recently lactating doe seems to be abandoning her babies. When she looks in the nest, the young jump like popcorn. You suggest that she
    a. Provide more heat for the young
    b. Start to feed them solid food
    c. Cross foster the young to another doe
    d. Not worry because the doe normally nurses once a day

108. *Pasteurellosis*
    a. Is a gram-positive coccobacillus
    b. Is passed directly only
    c. Can produce rhinitis, torticollis, abscesses, and vaginal discharge
    d. Is eliminated once signs are displayed

109. Snuffles in rabbits is most commonly caused by
    a. *Bordetella* sp.
    b. *Clostridium spiroforme*
    c. *Pasteurella multocida*
    d. *Eimeria* sp.

110. How much water does a 3.5-kg adult rabbit drink a day?
    a. 100 ml
    b. 350 ml
    c. 700 ml
    d. 1000 ml

111. Before inducing anesthesia in your rabbit you do a quick physical. You find the rabbit's temperature to be 39.0° C, the pulse to be 250 beats/min, and the respiration to be 40 breaths/min. These are all
    a. Normal
    b. Really high
    c. On the high side
    d. Low

112. Rabbits are
    a. Spontaneous ovulators
    b. Induced ovulators
    c. Cyclic ovulators
    d. Intensive ovulators

113. Monitoring reflexes of the rabbit for anesthesia would include all of the following except
    a. Tail pinch
    b. Ear pinch
    c. Palpebral
    d. Watching the third eyelid and pupil response

114. A male guinea pig is called a
    a. Buck
    b. Barrow
    c. Bull
    d. Boar

115. A female rabbit is called a
    a. Queen
    b. Sow
    c. Doe
    d. Bitch

116. Which of the following rodents has cheek pouches?
    a. Gerbil
    b. Mouse
    c. Rat
    d. Hamster

117. Which of the following species has a gestation period of 30 days?
    a. Rabbit
    b. Mouse
    c. Ferret
    d. Gerbil

118. The species that is often referred to as *cavies* is the
    a. Rat
    b. Guinea pig
    c. Hamster
    d. Rabbit

Correct answers are on pages 393-400.

119. *Mus musculus* is the scientific name of the
    a. Mouse
    b. Gerbil
    c. Hamster
    d. Rabbit

120. The scientific name of the rabbit ear mite is
    a. *Aspiculuris*
    b. *Otodectes*
    c. *Psoroptes*
    d. *Eimeria*

121. The species that gives birth to large, precocious young is the
    a. Ferret
    b. Rabbit
    c. Hamster
    d. Guinea pig

122. Estrogen toxicity that results from prolonged estrus is a common clinical problem in which of the following species?
    a. Ferret
    b. Rabbit
    c. Hamster
    d. Guinea pig

123. The type of mouse that has a deficiency in its immune system is
    a. Swiss
    b. Nude
    c. BALB/C
    d. DBA

124. The type of cage that is designed to separate urine and feces for specimen collection is
    a. Squeeze
    b. Front opening
    c. Microisolator
    d. Metabolism

125. Ferrets are susceptible to all diseases except
    a. Human influenza
    b. Rabies
    c. Heartworm
    d. Feline distemper

126. Rodents are generally fed *ad libitum,* which means
    a. Once daily
    b. Twice daily
    c. With water
    d. Free choice

127. When two inbred strains of mice are bred, the offspring are called
    a. Outbred
    b. Hybrid
    c. Knockout
    d. Transgenic

128. A spayed female ferret is called a
    a. Jill
    b. Hob
    c. Sprite
    d. Gib

129. The type of guinea pig that has short, coarse hair arranged in whorls or rosettes is the
    a. Peruvian
    b. Abyssinian
    c. English
    d. Dunkin–Hartley

130. Young mice and rats are
    a. Kits
    b. Pups
    c. Piglets
    d. Bunnies

131. The type of caging system that provides rodents with excellent containment and protection from disease organisms is
    a. Front-opening
    b. Shoebox
    c. Suspended
    d. Microisolator

132. An animal that results from the introduction of genetic material (DNA) from one animal into the fertilized egg of a different animal is
    a. Recombinant
    b. Knockout
    c. Transgenic
    d. Conisogenic

133. In rabbits, coccidiosis causes lesions in which of the following two main areas of the body?
    a. Liver and intestine
    b. Kidney and brain
    c. Intestine and kidney
    d. Brain and liver

134. The coccidia of rabbits is
    a. *Isospora*
    b. *Taenia*
    c. *Eimeria*
    d. *Toxocara*

135. The species that normally has cream-colored urine is the
    a. Rat
    b. Gerbil
    c. Mouse
    d. Hamster

136. The smallest hamster is the
    a. Dwarf
    b. European
    c. Syrian
    d. Chinese

137. A breeding system in which one male is placed with two or more females is
    a. Intensive
    b. Monogamous
    c. Polygamous
    d. Pair

138. Which of the following is classified as a lagomorph?
    a. Hamster
    b. Guinea pig
    c. Rabbit
    d. Gerbil

139. Animals in which certain disease-causing agents have been eliminated are
    a. Microbially defined
    b. Specific-pathogen–free
    c. Axenic
    d. Conventional

140. A healthy animal that is susceptible to certain diseases and is placed in a room with other animals as a means of detecting the presence of diseases-is-called
    a. SCID
    b. Conventional
    c. Transgenic
    d. Sentinel

141. HEPA is a type of
    a. Filter
    b. Cage washer
    c. Feeder
    d. Housing unit

142. The species that has air sacs and lungs is the
    a. Rabbit
    b. Pigeon
    c. Hamster
    d. Ferret

143. The 1985 amendment to the Animal Welfare Act provided standards for the exercise of
    a. Cats
    b. Hamsters
    c. Dogs
    d. Ferrets

144. A characteristic that distinguishes lagomorphs from rodents is
    a. Five toes on front and rear feet
    b. Large cecum
    c. Double pair of upper incisors
    d. Lengthy small intestine

145. Ulcerative pododermatitis in rabbits is commonly called
    a. Slobbers
    b. Lumps
    c. Foot slip
    d. Sore hocks

146. The species that is prone to nasal dermatitis initiated by its burrowing activity is the
    a. Hamster
    b. Gerbil
    c. Rat
    d. Mouse

147. Two species that are prone to trichobezoars are the cat and the
    a. Hamster
    b. Rabbit
    c. Ferret
    d. Dog

148. The species that is very susceptible to Tyzzer disease, caused by *Clostridium piliforme,* is the
    a. Hamster
    b. Rat
    c. Gerbil
    d. Mouse

149. A New World monkey commonly used in research is the
    a. Squirrel
    b. Baboon
    c. Chimpanzee
    d. Rhesus

150. Malocclusion in which of the following species involves elongated premolars and molars?
    a. Rabbit
    b. Ferret
    c. Rat
    d. Guinea pig

Correct answers are on pages 393-400.

151. Lymphocytic choriomeningitis, a viral disease with zoonotic potential, is associated with which of the following species?
    a. Rat
    b. Gerbil
    c. Hamster
    d. Mouse

152. Mice, rats, and hamsters are weaned at ___ days.
    a. 21
    b. 30
    c. 63
    d. 45

153. Pyrogen and Draize tests involve which of the following species?
    a. Guinea pig
    b. Rabbit
    c. Rat
    d. Mouse

154. Induced ovulators include
    a. Mouse and rat
    b. Gerbil and hamster
    c. Rabbit and ferret
    d. Hamster and rat

155. Which laboratory animal is monogamous and mates for life?
    a. Gerbil
    b. Hamster
    c. Rabbit
    d. Guinea pig

156. According to the Animal Welfare Act, which of these species must be provided with an environment adequate to promote their psychological well-being?
    a. Rabbit
    b. Guinea pig
    c. Ferret
    d. Nonhuman primate

157. Severe combined immunodeficient (SCID) mice lack
    a. B cells
    b. Null cells
    c. T cells
    d. B and T cells

158. Teratology involves the study of
    a. Abnormal fetal development
    b. Number of live births
    c. Reproductive organ maturation
    d. Deaths before delivery

159. What agency prepares standards and enforces the Animal Welfare Act?
    a. ACLAM
    b. USDI
    c. AVMA
    d. USDA

160. What organization certifies laboratory technicians and includes researchers and technicians in its membership?
    a. AALAS
    b. USDA
    c. AALAC
    d. ASLAP

161. Ringtail in rats is most commonly caused by what condition?
    a. *Streptococcus*
    b. Low humidity
    c. *Mycoplasma*
    d. Wet environment

162. A minimum of how many generations of brother–sister matings is necessary to create an inbred strain?
    a. 4
    b. 10
    c. 20
    d. 50

163. What viral disease carried by mice and other rodents is zoonotic?
    a. Salmonellosis
    b. Lymphocytic choriomeningitis
    c. Livim
    d. Mycoplasmosis

164. Weaning in mice, rats, and hamsters usually occurs at what age?
    a. 1 week
    b. 2 weeks
    c. 3 weeks
    d. 4 weeks

165. Which sex of rat, mouse, hamster, and gerbil has the longest anogenital distance?
    a. Female
    b. Male
    c. Not a valid indicator in these species
    d. Male in rat and hamster, female in mouse and gerbil

166. What is seen in chromodacryorrhea in rats?
    a. Diarrhea
    b. Hematuria
    c. Head tilt
    d. Red tears

167. Which of the following is not considered an ape?
   a. Baboon
   b. Orangutan
   c. Chimpanzee
   d. Gibbon

168. What problem is commonly associated with overfeeding pelleted feed to rabbits?
   a. Ketosis
   b. Urinary calculi
   c. Trichobezoars
   d. Malocclusion

169. In what species are the young precocious?
   a. *Oryctolagus cuniculus*
   b. *Cavia porcellus*
   c. *Mesocricetus auratus*
   d. *Meriones unguiculatus*

170. In taxonomy, what does the term *Rodentia* refer to?
   a. Phylum
   b. Class
   c. Family
   d. Order

171. The lab rat is known as *Rattus norvegicus*. What does *Rattus* refer to?
   a. Class
   b. Family
   c. Genus
   d. Species

172. Scurvy is most likely to be seen in what animal?
   a. Rabbit
   b. Gerbil
   c. Hamster
   d. Guinea pig

173. Which of the following has a prehensile tail?
   a. Spider monkey
   b. Common marmoset
   c. Rhesus macaque
   d. Chimpanzee

174. What is not one of the common syndromes seen in rabbits with pasteurellosis?
   a. Upper respiratory infection
   b. Diarrhea
   c. Torticollis
   d. Abscesses

175. Open-rooted molars are seen in which of the following animals?
   a. Gerbil
   b. Rat
   c. Guinea pig
   d. Hamster

176. Which of the following causes a proliferative otitis externa in rabbits?
   a. *Psoroptes cuniculi*
   b. *Cheyletiella parasitovorax*
   c. *Encephalitozoan cuniculi*
   d. *Cuterebra cuniculi*

177. What disease are nonhuman primates routinely tested for in the laboratory setting?
   a. Aspergillosis
   b. Tuberculosis
   c. Polio
   d. Pasteurellosis

178. What disorder is common in female rabbits older than 5 years?
   a. Uterine adenocarcinoma
   b. Mammary adenocarcinoma
   c. Adrenal adenoma
   d. Thyroid adenoma

179. What is the likely cause of vulval swelling in a spayed ferret?
   a. Insulinoma
   b. Hyperpituitarism
   c. Hyperadrenocorticism
   d. Hyperthyroidism

180. Which of the following is a small South American primate often used as a laboratory animal?
   a. Rhesus macaque
   b. Green monkey
   c. Woolly monkey
   d. Common marmoset

181. What is a common problem in ferrets whereby they become weak and may temporarily drag their rear legs?
   a. Disk disease
   b. Insulinoma
   c. Hypoadrenocorticism
   d. Saddle thrombus

182. Nude mice are used in research because they lack which of the following structures?
   a. Thyroid gland
   b. Thymus gland
   c. Gall bladder
   d. Spleen

183. What human viral disease is contagious to nonhuman primates?
   a. Measles
   b. Campylobacteriosis
   c. Herpes B
   d. Salmonellosis

Correct answers are on pages 393-400.

184. What is the earliest common clinical sign seen in ferrets or rabbits that are overheating?
    a. Sweating
    b. Panting
    c. Licking their front legs
    d. Vocalizations

185. Red leg is a common finding in what laboratory animal?
    a. Frogs
    b. Ferrets
    c. Mice
    d. Guinea pigs

186. Pregnancy toxemia is most commonly seen in which of the following animals?
    a. Rabbit
    b. Rat
    c. Gerbil
    d. Hamster

187. What occurs in an animal with pregnancy toxemia?
    a. Hyperglycemia
    b. Ketosis
    c. Hyperadrenocorticism
    d. Pyometra

188. What rat is also known as the *hooded rat*?
    a. Himalayan rat
    b. Wood rat
    c. Long-Evans rat
    d. Wistar rat

189. The armadillo is one of the few animal models of what human disease?
    a. Leprosy
    b. Muscular dystrophy
    c. Parkinson disease
    d. Graves disease

190. In addition to cats, the cat bag is a useful restraint device for what animal?
    a. Miniature swine
    b. Rhesus macaque
    c. Guinea pig
    d. Rabbit

191. What lab animal is best housed singly, because they often fight?
    a. Gerbil
    b. Rabbit
    c. Guinea pig
    d. Rat

192. The pigeon's crop is part of what structure?
    a. Esophagus
    b. Cecum
    c. Spleen
    d. Pancreas

193. How do pigeon blood cells differ from those of rabbits and rodents?
    a. There are no thrombocytes.
    b. There are no eosinophils.
    c. All of the mature blood cells are nucleated.
    d. Only the mature erythrocytes are nucleated.

194. Into what structure is the drug given when using a gavage needle in a rat?
    a. Muscle
    b. Urinary bladder
    c. Saphenous vein
    d. Stomach

195. What anatomic structure is similar in rodents and horses?
    a. Gall bladder
    b. Large cecum
    c. Carnassial teeth
    d. Rumen

196. What vein may readily be used for blood collection in mice and rats?
    a. Brachial vein
    b. Tail vein
    c. Jugular vein
    d. Ear vein

197. What is the usual approximate life span of mice, rats, and hamsters?
    a. 10 years
    b. 5 years
    c. 3 years
    d. 1 year

198. Which of the following is a common subclinical, contagious coronavirus seen in mice used in research?
    a. Mouse hepatitis virus
    b. Hantavirus
    c. Encephalomyocarditis virus
    d. Ectromelia

199. What is a common cause of gastric ulcers in ferrets?
    a. *Clostridium difficile*
    b. *Helicobacter mustelae*
    c. Herpes G virus
    d. Ferret coronavirus

200. Splenic hyperplasia is commonly seen in which of the following?
   a. Guinea pig
   b. Ferret
   c. Rabbit
   d. Gerbil

201. Tyzzer disease is most commonly seen in what animal?
   a. Sheep
   b. Cat
   c. Rodent
   d. Ferret

202. What is the causative agent of Tyzzer disease?
   a. Sin Nombre virus
   b. *Clostridium piliforme*
   c. *Salmonella tyzzer*
   d. Herpes T virus

203. *The Guide for the Care and Use of Laboratory Animals* is used by what organization in its voluntary accreditation of laboratory animal facilities?
   a. MISMR
   b. AAALAC
   c. AALAS
   d. NIH

204. Which of the following is an outbred strain of rat?
   a. Fisher
   b. Lewis
   c. Long–Evans
   d. Wistar Kyoto

205. Porphyrins are secreted by the ___ gland in rats.
   a. Harderian
   b. Chromolachrial
   c. Pituitary
   d. Ocular

206. *Cavia porcellus* is the scientific name for the
   a. Potbellied pigs
   b. Rabbit
   c. Guinea pig
   d. Yucatán pig

207. Kurloff corpuscles are a common finding in what species?
   a. *Rattus norvegicus*
   b. *Cricetulus griseus*
   c. *Mesocricetus auratus*
   d. *Cavia porcellus*

208. Which of the following species cannot synthesize vitamin C and needs to have it supplemented?
   a. Guinea pig
   b. Hamster
   c. Gerbil
   d. Rabbit

209. Pododermatitis affects what species?
   a. Guinea pig
   b. Hamster
   c. Gerbil
   d. Rat

210. What species is prone to trichobezoar formation?
   a. *Oryctolagus cuniculus*
   b. *Cricetulus griseus*
   c. *Gallus domesticus*
   d. *Cavia porcellus*

211. Tularemia is most commonly associated with what species?
   a. *Oryctolagus cuniculus*
   b. *Cricetulus griseus*
   c. *Gallus domesticus*
   d. *Cavia porcellus*

212. The department within the USDA that is responsible for administering the Animal Welfare Act is the
   a. Food and Drug Administration
   b. National Institutes of Health
   c. Animal Plant and Health Inspection Service
   d. Public Heath Service

213. Slobbers, or moist dermatitis, is a condition that occurs in
   a. Mice
   b. Rats
   c. Rabbits
   d. Guinea pigs

214. In what species is coprophagia a normal behavior?
   a. Rabbit
   b. Nonhuman primate
   c. Ferret
   d. Gerbil

215. The inguinal rings completely close in which of the following species?
   a. Nonhuman primate
   b. Rabbit
   c. Rat
   d. Mouse

Correct answers are on pages 393-400.

216. What species has ventral midline sebaceous glands that are more prominent in the male?
    a. Hamster
    b. Gerbil
    c. Rat
    d. Mouse

217. *IACUC* stands for
    a. International Animal Care and Utilization Committee
    b. Institutional Animal Care and Use Committee
    c. International Association for Compassion, Understanding, and Care
    d. Institutional Association for Compassion, Understanding, and Care

218. The maximum amount that can be safely administered to the rabbit by IM injection in one site is
    a. 1 cc
    b. 1.5 cc
    c. 0.5 cc
    d. 2 cc

219. Before inducing anesthesia, how long should a pet rat be fasted?
    a. 12 hours
    b. 6 hours
    c. Fasting is not indicated.
    d. 24 hours

220. Which of the following is a characteristic of New World monkeys?
    a. Prehensile tail
    b. Ischial callosities
    c. Cheek pouches
    d. Opposable thumbs

221. Which of the following nonhuman primates does not carry the herpes B virus?
    a. Pig-tailed macaque
    b. Rhesus
    c. Cebus
    d. Cynomolgus

222. Which of the following nonhuman primates is considered to be platyrrhine, or broad nosed?
    a. Saimiri
    b. Cynomolgus
    c. Stump-tailed macaque
    d. *Macaca arctoides*

223. *Gallus domesticus* is the scientific name for the
    a. Pigeon
    b. Duck
    c. Chicken
    d. Crow

224. What species has a uropygial gland?
    a. *Gallus domesticus*
    b. *Oryctolagus cuniculus*
    c. *Cricetulus griseus*
    d. *Cavia porcellus*

225. The glandular portion of the stomach in birds is referred to as the
    a. Diverticulum
    b. Ventriculus
    c. Proventriculus
    d. Cloaca

226. Bumblefoot is a bacterial infection that causes swollen feet in what species?
    a. *Gallus domesticus*
    b. *Oryctolagus cuniculus*
    c. *Cricetulus griseus*
    d. *Cavia porcellus*

227. Which of the following is not an induced ovulator?
    a. Rabbit
    b. Guinea pig
    c. Ferret
    d. Cat

228. Ferret young are called
    a. Pups
    b. Kids
    c. Jills
    d. Kits

229. The genus of the ferret ear mite is
    a. *Psoroptes*
    b. *Eimeria*
    c. *Aspiculuris*
    d. *Otodectes*

230. What species is prone to audiogenic seizures?
    a. *Meriones unguiculatus*
    b. *Oryctolagus cuniculus*
    c. *Cricetulus griseus*
    d. *Cavia porcellus*

231. The sex of a parrot is determined by
    a. Anogenital distance
    b. Blood test
    c. Palpation of the pelvic region
    d. Secondary sex characteristics

232. From what species might you obtain a cloacal sample?
    a. *Gallus domesticus*
    b. *Oryctolagus cuniculus*
    c. *Cricetulus griseus*
    d. *Cavia porcellus*

233. In what species would you expect to find a hemipenis?
    a. Rat
    b. Rabbit
    c. Lizard
    d. Pigeon

234. All adult amphibians are
    a. Omnivores
    b. Herbivores
    c. Carnivores
    d. Their dietary preference is unknown.

235. The coccidia of the rabbit is
    a. *Psoroptes*
    b. *Eimeria*
    c. *Aspiculuris*
    d. *Otodectes*

236. The female of what species exhibits the sexually dimorphic characteristic called the *dewlap*?
    a. *Meriones unguiculatus*
    b. *Oryctolagus cuniculus*
    c. *Cricetulus griseus*
    d. *Cavia porcellus*

237. Blood collection from the orbital sinus is common in what animal?
    a. Rabbit
    b. Mouse
    c. Lizard
    d. Pigeon

238. The sex of a juvenile chinchilla is determined by
    a. Anogenital distance
    b. Secondary sex characteristics
    c. Palpation of the pelvic region
    d. Blood test

239. The common mite of the hedgehog is
    a. *Sarcoptes*
    b. *Demodex*
    c. *Cheyletiella*
    d. *Caparinia*

240. Pole and collar restraint is used for what species?
    a. *Macaca mulatta*
    b. *Meriones unguiculatus*
    c. *Oryctolagus cuniculus*
    d. *Cricetulus griseus*

241. Which of the following is a zoonotic disease associated with birds?
    a. Hantavirus
    b. Ectromelia
    c. Chlamydiosis
    d. Encephalomyocarditis

242. On what animal would you expect to find wattles?
    a. Rabbit
    b. Amphibian
    c. Chicken
    d. Guinea pig

ANSWERS

1. a

2. b

3. c

4. d

5. a The penis may be manually prolapsed. The opening of the female is shaped like a Y, and the male is like a colon mark (:).

6. c

7. a

8. d Dystocia is a problem in guinea pigs, particularly those bred for the first time after age 6 months.

9. d The anogenital distance in male mice is twice that of female mice.

10. b

11. b

12. d

13. a A hamster has a 16-day gestation.

14. d

15. b Rabbits are lagomorphs, not rodents.

16. d Grasping the end of the gerbil's tail during restraint may separate the skin from the distal portion of the tail.

17. a

18. d

19. c

20. a

21. d

22. a

23. d

24. b

25. c

26. d

27. a

28. b

29. d

30. **b** Rabbits have delicate bones and can suffer vertebral fractures and dislocations just by kicking hard if they are improperly restrained.

31. a

32. d

33. d

34. **a** Nonhuman primates and guinea pigs require supplementation with vitamin C.

35. **d** Rabbits have moist night feces, which are reingested, and dry day feces.

36. a

37. **b** Squirrel monkeys are New World, nonhuman primates.

38. a

39. d

40. b

41. a

42. c

43. a

44. c

45. d

46. **b** A rack cage washer is the only one in which a cage of this size would fit.

47. **c** Retinal damage occurs in albino strains exposed to bright lights.

48. d

49. **c** Birds, mice, or rats bred specifically for research and sheep used for fiber or food are all exempt from the Animal Welfare Act.

50. **a** Shoebox caging offers a solid flooring with contact bedding.

51. **a** The mouse with no alopecia is the dominant animal and is chewing the hair and whiskers from the subordinate animals. This is called *barbering*.

52. c

53. b

54. b

55. c

56. b

57. c

58. **a** For most of the common laboratory species, the important thing is moderation with very minimal environmental fluctuations. Temperature is generally preferred to be about 21° C to 22° C, but ranges can be tolerated.

59. **c** For most laboratory species, 12 hours of light and darkness are usually best.

60. **c** There is a variation, but most of the common altricial rodents (rats, mice, hamsters, gerbils) are haired by 7 to 10 days with eyes open by 14 and 20 days.

61. **d** Inbreeding establishes genetically identical animals known as homozygotes. This is most common with mice. An inbred strain is established by breeding siblings or breeding parents with their own offspring for a minimum of 20 generations. Random breeding maintains a wide range of characteristics and maintains heterozygosity.

62. **b** Hamsters do not have a fertile postpartum estrus. The Syrian hamster comes into estrus 2 to 18 days after weaning, whereas Chinese

hamsters do so 4 days after weaning. Gerbils, rats, and mice have a postpartum estrus of about 24 hours.

63. **c** Fecal pellets often constitute a significant portion of what rodents consume. It is presumed that they provide nutrients, such as vitamin B, that are produced by the colonic bacteria.

64. **a** Young rodents have masses of brown fat in various cervical locations and between the scapulas. It is thought that the fat helps neonatal and cold-stressed rodents as a thermogenic material and metabolic regulator. The quantity and significance tends to diminish into puberty and adulthood.

65. **d** Sendai is a ribonucleic acid (RNA) paramyxovirus-parainfluenza type 1 virus.

66. **b** This is a bacterial disease that occurs in many rodents and other mammalian species. Stress is considered an important component.

67. **b** The metabolic rate of laboratory animals is rapid relative to their body surface area. The dose that lightly sedates one animal may heavily anesthetize a cage mate.

68. **d** Microenvironment is the environment that immediately surrounds the animal. If the caging is wire mesh, it is difficult to keep a constant humidity and temperature. The advantage of wire mesh flooring is that the animal is *not* in contact with its excreta.

69. **a** Rabbits have a gestation period of 28 to 35 days, guinea pigs gestate in 59 to 72 days, and mice in 19 to 21 days.

70. **d** Malocclusion or abnormal dentition is not a sign of pain.

71. **b** Once the head is properly controlled, it is usually easy to manage the rest of the animal.

72. **d** The Sendai virus and murine respiratory mycoplasmosis show respiratory signs. Sialodacryoadenitis (SDAV) does as well; however, common clinical signs of SDAV are photophobia and swollen neck (inflamed salivary glands, lacrimal glands, and lymph nodes). Actual signs for these three diseases depend on the immune status of the animal at the time of infection.

73. **d** Male rats average 450 to 550 g, whereas male mice are 30 to 40 g.

74. **b** Main activity of mice and rats occurs at night, although mice usually exhibit more daylight activity than rats. *Crepuscular* refers to increased activity during twilight. Rats are very social animals.

75. **b** The harderian gland is a red-brown gland found caudal to the eyeball and is larger than the eyeball. It secretes a lipid and red porphyrin-rich secretion that lubricates the eye and lids. It may help determine pineal diurnal rhythms in the neonate. When stressed or during illness, the red tears overflow and stain the face and nose.

76. **a** The Whitten effect is most common in mice. Group-caged female mice may be in a phase of continuous anestrus that is terminated on the introduction of a male or his odor. Synchronization of cycles occurs, with most of the females coming into estrus in about 72 hours.

77. **b** The Bruce effect is when a female bred within the past 24 hours is exposed to the pheromones or presence of a strange male and aborts the existing pregnancy.

78. **d** Facultative diapause, or delayed implantation, is when females bred at the postpartum estrus have an extended pregnancy.

79. **c** Intensive breeding refers to taking advantage of the postpartum estrus that occurs in mice within 24 hours of whelping. If the breeding pair is left together, this would not be nonintensive breeding. The other statements are true.

80. **a** This is true. The mammary tissue distributes extensively and includes areas as far dorsal as the shoulder blades along the length of the trunk. The nonglandular proximal forestomach does not secrete any enzymes or histamine. Neither species pants or has sweat glands, and it is only the rat that does not have a gall bladder.

81. **d** *Barbering* is the chewing off of hair patches so close that the area looks clean shaven. The dominant mouse is typically the only one not barbered. Removing this mouse usually solves the problem.

82. **c** It is suggested that no more than 2 to 3 ml be given intraperitoneally to mice. Rats can tolerate up to 5 to 10 ml.

83. **b** Healthy adults usually shed the sialodacryo-adenitis virus in about 1 week only and show a complete clinical recovery in 1 to 2 weeks. An adult may occasionally have permanent eye damage.

84. **b** The etiologic agent is *M. pulmonis.*

85. **a** Ringtail occurs mainly in young laboratory rats in a low-humidity environment and often in hanging cages. Humidity greater than 50% usually prevents the problem.

86. **b** The general rule of thumb is that 0.5% to 1% of the body weight can be safely taken. The lower range is safer. More specific rules apply for each species.

87. **d** An excellent site for rapid and repeated blood collection; 100 microliters can easily be taken with a simple prick to the vein. It can also be used in the rat, hamster, gerbil, guinea pig, ferret, and mink.

88. **a** The Muridae rodents (hamsters, mice, rats, and gerbils) all have a total of 16 teeth.

89. **c** The gestation period of hamsters is 16 days (the shortest among the Muridae rodents); the estrous cycle is typical at 4 to 5 days, and there are usually 5 to 9 young in a litter of Syrian hamsters.

90. **b** Gerbils have a gestation period of 24 days, an estrous cycle of 4 to 5 days, and an average litter size of 4 to 5, although they may have from 2 to 9 young in a litter.

91. **d** The client is most likely referring to "wet tail." This term is applied to hamsters with enteric disease, because the most frequent sign is the perineum covered with diarrhea. It is not uncommon in young pet store hamsters. This is not a single entity or disease but a clinical feature that has a variety of syndromes associated with it. Gastrointestinal disease is the most significant cause of morbidity and mortality in hamsters.

92. **b** Hamsters live an average of 18 to 24 months but can live as long as 3 years.

93. **c** Gerbil females average about 3 years, whereas males average about 2 and 3/4 years, but both sexes can live up to 4 years.

94. **b** It is most likely nasal dermatitis or "sore nose," especially at this age and in cases of overcrowding or high humidity. The harderian gland then secretes excessive porphyrin, which becomes an irritant. There is excessive grooming leading to self-traumatization. *Staphylococcus* infection often invades the area. Barbering, a dominance behavior, does not usually occur with gerbils. "Bald nose," which occurs when the animal aggressively puts its nose through the bar to get food, is not usually accompanied by scabbing or erythema.

95. **d** If gerbils eat sunflower seed to the detriment of other food, there will be a deficiency of calcium and other minerals as well as increased fat intake leading to obesity.

96. **b** Because certain strains of gerbils (20% to 40%) are prone to reflex, stereotypic, epileptiform seizures, and because acepromazine can lower the seizure threshold, it is better to avoid this as part of the preanesthetic protocol.

97. **c** Unlike the Muridae rodents, guinea pigs do not have an aglandular portion of the stomach. Foa-Kurloff cells protect the fetus from maternal rejection.

98. **d** Part of their hierarchy is maintained by these secretions and other displays. They are considered to be crepuscular but are active throughout the day and night. Fear is shown by scattering and immobility responses, and they do not dig or hibernate.

99. **a** Virgin guinea pigs are best bred at this age and definitely before 6 to 8 months, or there will be fusion of the symphysis pubis that will occlude the passage of a fetus through the birth canal. Lordosis is a typical estrus response, but the only time that the vaginal closure membrane is perforated is during the 3 to 4 days of proestrus and estrus and at parturition. The estrous cycle is 16 days. The sow does pass antibodies in the milk.

100. **c** Guinea pigs do not nurse for the first 12 to 24 hours. The young are born precocial.

101. **d** These vegetables are high in vitamin C and can be supplemented, provided that they are clean, fresh, and make up no more than 20 to 30 g of the daily diet. She is still best to feed a fresh pelleted diet that has been milled within the past 90 days. On a body weight basis, the daily requirement for vitamin C is 10 mg/kg. If added to the water, vitamin C

deteriorates within 24 hours. Rabbit food has no added vitamin C and has high levels of vitamin D. Multivitamins carry the risk of overdose of other vitamins.

102. b These are signs of scurvy or scorbutism that result from hypovitaminosis C. Overt signs of deficiency are shown within 14 days. If untreated, these guinea pigs usually die within 2 weeks of onset of clinical signs.

103. a The penis can also be palpated in the midline and digital pressure applied to this region to extrude the ensheathed penis. The anogenital space in males is greater in the Muridae rodents only. The female does have the relaxed membrane, which is seen as a U-shaped shallow crease between the anal and urethral openings, but it remains closed except during a few days at estrus and proestrus and at parturition. Both sexes have inguinal nipples, but only the female has mammary glandular tissue.

104. b The maximum volume suggested for an IM injection in a guinea pig is 0.3 ml.

105. c These are all normal. Normal urine does vary in color and consistency and can be white, turbid, pale yellow, dark yellow, bright orange, brown, and bright red. Excess of dietary calcium may be responsible for thick, white urine.

106. d A small second set of incisors called *peg teeth* sit just behind the larger upper incisors. Folds of skin behind the incisors and premolars limit visibility of the rest of the oral cavity. All teeth are open rooted (hypsodontic) and grow continuously through life.

107. d A doe typically nurses her young only once or twice a day. Normal, healthy young jump about in the nest.

108. c *Pasteurella multocida* is a gram-negative rod that can affect one or more body systems. The most common signs are nasal discharge and sneezing. The organism is transmitted through direct contact and via fomites and is difficult to eradicate.

109. c Snuffles, or upper respiratory disease (rhinitis, sinusitis, conjunctivitis, lacrimal duct infection), is caused by *P. multocida*. The most common forms are rhinitis and sinusitis with a typical white or yellowish mucopurulent discharge.

110. b Normal, nonlactating rabbits usually drink about 100 ml/kg of body weight. Thus a 3.5-kg rabbit drinks about 350 ml of water a day.

111. a These are all normal rabbit values.

112. b Like cats and ferrets, rabbits are induced ovulators.

113. a The other reflexes can be used to help determine the depth of anesthesia.

114. d A buck is a male rabbit, a barrow is a male pig, and a bull is a male bovine.

115. c A queen is a female cat, a sow is a female pig, and a bitch is a female dog.

116. d

117. a The mouse has a gestation of 21 days, the ferret 42 days, and the gerbil 24 days.

118. b Relates to the scientific name *Cavia porcellus*

119. a

120. c *Otodectes* is the ear mite of the dog.

121. d Young are well developed because of a long gestation period of 68 days.

122. a It is recommended that ferrets be spayed because of this potential problem.

123. b Nude mice are deficient in T cells and thus susceptible to infections.

124. d

125. d

126. d

127. b

128. c A *jill* is an intact female, a *hob* is an intact male, and a *gib* is a neutered male.

129. b

130. b

131. d

132. c

133. a

134. **c** *Isospora* is the coccidia of dogs and cats.

135. **d**

136. **a**

137. **c**

138. **c**

139. **b**

140. **d**

141. **a** A high-efficiency particulate air (HEPA) filter prevents airborne microorganisms from entering the animal room or workstation.

142. **b**

143. **c**

144. **c**

145. **d** Sore hocks actually involves the ventral metatarsal region rather than the hock; it is caused by poor husbandry or environmental pressures.

146. **b**

147. **b** Gastric hair balls can be a problem in rabbits, especially if they are obese or are not fed a high-fiber diet.

148. **c**

149. **a** The rhesus is commonly used in research; however, it is an Old World monkey.

150. **d** The guinea pig has open-rooted premolars and molars that continually grow. If the teeth are not aligned properly, they overgrow and irritate the gingiva, causing excessive salivation.

151. **c**

152. **a**

153. **b** The pyrogen test, used to check for the presence of bacterial toxins, and the Draize test, used to check for product toxicity and tissue irritation, use the rabbit.

154. **c**

155. **a**

156. **d** Psychological well-being of primates is covered in the 1985 amendment to the Animal Welfare Act.

157. **d** SCID mice lack both T and B cells.

158. **a**

159. **d** The United States Department of Agriculture is responsible for developing regulations and enforcing the Animal Welfare Act.

160. **a** The American Association for Laboratory Animal Science (AALAS) administers a program that certifies laboratory technicians and includes researchers and technicians in its membership.

161. **b** Ringtail, an avascular necrosis in rats, is caused by humidity less than 50%.

162. **c** Twenty generations of brother–sister matings are necessary to create an inbred strain.

163. **b** Lymphocytic choriomeningitis is a zoonotic viral disease carried by mice and other rodents. Salmonellosis is a bacterial zoonotic disease. Lethal intestinal viral infection in mice and mycoplasmosis is not zoonotic.

164. **c** Weaning in mice, rats, and hamsters usually occurs at 3 weeks.

165. **b** The male rat, mouse, hamster, and gerbil have an anogenital distance twice as long as the female's.

166. **d** Red tears from the harderian gland are seen in chromodacryorrhea.

167. **a** The baboon, a member of the genus *Papio*, is not considered an ape. The orangutan, chimpanzee, and gibbon are all anthropoids, or apes.

168. **c** Trichobezoars, or hair balls, are commonly associated with overfeeding pelleted feed to rabbits.

169. **b** The young of the guinea pig, *Cavia porcellus*, are born fully furred with their eyes open and the ability to move or run around. *Oryctolagus cuniculus*, the domestic rabbit; *Mesocricetus auratus*, the golden hamster; and *Meriones unguiculatus*, the Mongolian gerbil, all have young born hairless, with eyes closed, and the inability to run around.

170. **d** Rodentia is the largest order in the class Mammalia.

171. **c** *Rattus* is a genus within the order Rodentia.

172. **d** The guinea pig is unable to synthesize vitamin C like most other mammals and is thus susceptible to scurvy, a vitamin C deficiency.

173. **a** The spider monkey, a New World monkey, has a prehensile tail by which it can hang from branches.

174. **b** Diarrhea is not one of the common syndromes seen in rabbits with pasteurellosis. Those syndromes include upper respiratory infection, torticollis, abscesses, pneumonia, and septicemia.

175. **c** Open-rooted molars that grow continuously are seen in the guinea pig. All rodents have open-rooted incisors.

176. **a** *Psoroptes cuniculi,* an ear mite, causes a proliferative otitis externa in rabbits.

177. **b** Nonhuman primates are routinely tested for tuberculosis in the laboratory setting.

178. **a** Uterine adenocarcinoma is common in female rabbits older than 5 years.

179. **c** Hyperadrenocorticism produces estrogens, which commonly cause vulval swelling in ferrets.

180. **d** The common marmoset is a small South American primate often used as a laboratory animal. The rhesus macaque is the most commonly used primate in research but is from Asia. The green monkey, also used in research, is from Africa, and the woolly monkey, from South America, is rarely used in research.

181. **b** Ferrets often suffer from insulinomas, which cause them to become weak and temporarily drag their rear legs.

182. **b** Nude mice are used in research because they lack a thymus gland.

183. **a** Measles is a human viral disease that is contagious to nonhuman primates. Campylobacteriosis and salmonellosis are bacterial diseases, and herpes B is a deadly zoonotic virus carried by some nonhuman primates.

184. **c** Ferrets and rabbits have a limited ability to thermoregulate, because they cannot sweat or pant. When hot, they lose body heat by salivating and licking their front legs.

185. **a** Red leg is a sign of septicemia in frogs.

186. **a** Pregnancy toxemia is most commonly seen in rabbits.

187. **b** Ketosis occurs when an animal has pregnancy toxemia.

188. **c** The hooded rat, which has black or brown coloration over its head and shoulders, is also known as the *Long–Evans rat.*

189. **a** The armadillo is one of the few animal models for leprosy.

190. **d** In addition to cats, the cat bag is a useful restraint device for rabbits.

191. **b** Rabbits are best housed singly, because they often fight. Gerbils, guinea pigs, and rats are social and rarely fight.

192. **a** The pigeon's crop is a dilation of the esophagus located at the thoracic inlet.

193. **c** In pigeons, as in all birds, all of the blood cells are nucleated.

194. **d** A gavage needle, also known as a *dosing needle*, is placed in the stomach to deliver drugs to rodents.

195. **b** Horses and rodents have similar digestive tracts, with a large cecum.

196. **b** The tail vein may readily be used for blood collection in mice and rats.

197. **c** The usual life span of mice, rats, and hamsters is 3 years, although some may live slightly longer.

198. **a** Mouse hepatitis virus is a common subclinical, contagious coronavirus seen in mice that are used in research.

199. **b** *Helicobacter mustelae* is a common cause of gastric ulcers in ferrets.

200. **b** Ferrets often exhibit splenic hyperplasia.

201. **c** Tyzzer disease is most commonly seen in rodents.

202. **b** Tyzzer disease is caused by *C. piliforme.*

203. **b** The Association for Assessment and Accreditation of Laboratory Animal Care International is a voluntary accreditation body.

204. c All of the other rats listed are inbred.

205. a The harderian gland is responsible for keeping the eye moist and producing porphyrins.

206. c

207. d Guinea pigs commonly have Kurloff corpuscles.

208. a

209. a

210. a Rabbits are prone to trichobezoar, or hair ball, formation.

211. a Tularemia can be contracted by handling rabbit hides or carcasses.

212. c The Animal Plant and Health Inspection Service is the only division of the USDA listed; it administers the Animal Welfare Act, and the Regulator Enforcement and Animal Care division enforces the Animal Welfare Act.

213. c

214. a

215. a The inguinal rings close in the nonhuman primate to prevent the retraction of the testicles. The other species listed all have the ability to retract their testicles back into the abdominal cavity.

216. b

217. b

218. c

219. c Fasting is not indicated in rats, because the limiting ridge in the stomach prevents vomiting.

220. a New World monkeys have prehensile tails, but none of the other characteristics listed. Those all belong to Old World monkeys.

221. c New World monkeys do not carry the herpes B virus.

222. a New World monkeys are considered broad nosed. Only the Saimiri (squirrel monkey) is a New World monkey.

223. c

224. a The uropygial gland, or oil gland, produces an oil that is used to preen feathers.

225. c The diverticulum is the crop; the ventriculus is the gizzard, or the muscular portion of the stomach; and the cloaca is where urine and feces exit the body.

226. a

227. b

228. d

229. d

230. a Gerbils can have seizures due to auditory (sound) stimuli.

231. b Many parrots do not exhibit obvious signs of sexual dimorphism. A blood test or surgical sexing is the recommended method of determining gender.

232. a Birds have cloacas, the other species listed do not.

233. c

234. c

235. b

236. b Female rabbits have a dewlap.

237. b

238. a The clitoris in the chinchilla can be mistaken for a penis due to its size and shape. The male chinchilla lacks a scrotum, making it difficult to visualize the testicles. Therefore anogenital distance is used to determine the sex of juvenile chinchillas.

239. d

240. a A pole and collar restraint is used for rhesus monkeys.

241. c *Chlamydiosis* is also known as *psittacosis*.

242. c

Medical Nursing

Joann Colville

QUESTIONS

1. The most appropriate solution to use as an ear cleaner in an animal that does not have an intact tympanum is
   a. Commercial ceruminolytic
   b. Dilute povidone-iodine
   c. Physiologic saline
   d. Dilute chlorhexidine

2. The most critical factor to expedient healing of decubital sores is
   a. Regular rotation of the patient
   b. Application of antibiotics to prevent infection
   c. Administration of sedatives to keep the animal still
   d. Exposure to air so that the area remains dry

3. To calculate the quantity of food to administer at one feeding to a 2-day-old orphaned puppy, you would multiply the body weight in grams by
   a. 5%
   b. 10%
   c. 25%
   d. 50%

4. Which of the following values is a normal rectal temperature for a dog?
   a. 102° F
   b. 98° F
   c. 106° F
   d. 95° F

5. A pulse deficit occurs when
   a. The heart rate is faster than the pulse rate.
   b. The heart rate is slower than the pulse rate.
   c. The pulse rate is too thready to palpate.
   d. There is an absence of palpable pulse.

6. Sinus arrhythmia occurs when the
   a. Heart and pulse rates increase with inspiration and expiration.
   b. Heart and pulse rates decrease with inspiration and expiration.
   c. Heart and pulse rates increase with inspiration and decrease with expiration.
   d. Heart and pulse rates decrease with inspiration and increase with expiration.

7. If you are syringe-feeding a patient, the most appropriate positioning of the head would be
   a. A natural position
   b. Flexed upward 90 degrees
   c. Turned 90 degrees to one side
   d. Hanging over the edge of the table

8. Fluids administered via the subcutaneous route should be at
   a. Room temperature and hypertonic
   b. Body temperature and isotonic
   c. Body temperature and hypotonic
   d. Room temperature and hypotonic

9. The cages of immunocompromised animals should be cleaned
   a. Before cleaning the general nursing wards
   b. After cleaning the general nursing wards
   c. Only when they are dirty
   d. At least three times a day

10. Which of the following is not a symptom of hypostatic pneumonia?
    a. Fast and frequent shallow breathing
    b. Increased respiratory effort
    c. Moist noises when breathing
    d. Nonproductive cough

11. Which of the following is the least desirable method of warming a recumbent patient?
    a. Instant-heat pads
    b. Electric heating pad
    c. Wrapped hot water bottles
    d. Infrared lamps

12. What is the average length of gestation for a dog?
    a. 70 days
    b. 63 days
    c. 59 days
    d. 55 days

Correct answers are on pages 427-429.

13. Isosthenuria is best described as
    a. Urine with a specific gravity and osmolality similar to glomerular filtrate and plasma
    b. Urine with a specific gravity and osmolality greater than glomerular filtrate and plasma
    c. Urine with a specific gravity and osmolality less than glomerular filtrate and plasma
    d. Urine with a specific gravity greater than plasma but less than glomerular filtrate

14. Pinpoint hemorrhage of the mucous membranes and skin is termed
    a. Epiphora
    b. Petechiation
    c. Lichenification
    d. Cyanosis

15. The least desirable method of administering insulin is
    a. Intramuscular (IM)
    b. Subcutaneous
    c. Per os
    d. Intravenous (IV)

16. Milk fever is caused by a
    a. Raised blood calcium level
    b. Lowered blood calcium level
    c. Raised blood magnesium level
    d. Raised blood phosphorus level

17. Milk fever may have all of the following clinical signs except
    a. Staggering
    b. Ascending paralysis
    c. Neck kink
    d. Hypersalivation

18. The colloquial term for acetonemia in cattle is
    a. Milk fever
    b. Mastitis
    c. Ketosis
    d. Bloat

19. Q fever in sheep is caused by
    a. *Coxiella burnetii*
    b. *Clostridium chauvoei*
    c. *Chlamydia psittaci*
    d. *Campylobacter jejuni*

20. Which of the following diseases of sheep is not zoonotic?
    a. Rabies
    b. *Chlamydia* infection
    c. Toxoplasmosis
    d. Johne's

21. Hypocalcemia in dogs
    a. Does not occur
    b. Occurs most often at parturition
    c. Occurs most often in mid to late lactation
    d. Can occur at any time

22. Grass tetany in cattle
    a. Occurs in midsummer
    b. Is caused by a low blood calcium level
    c. Is caused by a low blood magnesium level
    d. Occurs in midwinter

23. Which of the following is not true of inactivated vaccines?
    a. A finite antigen mass at injection
    b. Provides cellular and mucosal immunity
    c. Requires adjuvant
    d. Relatively stable and safe

24. Which of the following is generally not a core vaccine for dogs?
    a. Distemper
    b. Adenovirus
    c. *Leptospira*
    d. Parvovirus

25. A client calls to say that her horse is sweated up, keeps looking at his belly, and is trying to roll; the veterinarian will most likely find that the horse is suffering from
    a. Tetanus
    b. Colic
    c. Strangles
    d. Epistaxis

26. Cheyne-Stokes respiration signifies a
    a. Vestibular problem
    b. Midbrain lesion
    c. Severe cortical injury
    d. Brainstem lesion

27. Increased carbon dioxide levels are detected by
    a. Chemoreceptors in the pulmonary artery
    b. Chemoreceptors at the bifurcation of the carotid arteries
    c. Chemoreceptors at the bifurcation of the jugular veins
    d. Chemoreceptors in the renal veins

28. The pulse of a horse is most conveniently palpated using the
    a. Femoral artery
    b. Dorsal pedal artery
    c. Coccygeal artery
    d. Facial artery

29. Abdominal palpation in large animals is correctly termed
    a. Percussion
    b. Ileus
    c. Ballottement
    d. Tympany

30. Cystocentesis is contraindicated in all of the following except
    a. Bleeding disorders
    b. Periparturient dams
    c. Pyometra
    d. Bladder tumors

31. The blood group of canines that is synonymous with the term *universal donor* is
    a. DEA 1.1 negative
    b. DEA 1.1 positive
    c. DEA 3 positive
    d. DEA 3 negative

32. Analgesia should be provided by a regimen that
    a. Requires a specified time to elapse between administrations
    b. Requires an interval of time to elapse that allows the animal to demonstrate the current level of pain
    c. Provides one administration of an analgesic agent every 24 hours
    d. Administers the analgesic before the onset of anticipated pain returns

33. Hospitalized patients that require nutritional support are those that have lost ___ of their body weight.
    a. 5%
    b. 10%
    c. 15%
    d. 20%

34. The vein of choice for blood sampling in horses is the
    a. Cephalic vein
    b. Saphenous vein
    c. Jugular vein
    d. Coccygeal vein

35. Blood sampling in cats is best achieved from the
    a. Cephalic vein
    b. Saphenous vein
    c. Cuticle bleed
    d. Jugular vein

36. A significant difference in IM injections in small animals compared to large animals is
    a. The muscles for injection are not comparable.
    b. The needle is first inserted into large animals before the syringe is attached.
    c. There is no preswabbing with an antiseptic.
    d. IM injections are avoided in large animals if possible.

37. When applying a tendon support bandage on a horse's front leg, the outer wrap may be secured by
    a. Tucking the end of the roll of bandage into the top of wrapped bandage
    b. Using adhesive tape and ensuring that the end of the tape overlaps
    c. Using adhesive tape and ensuring that the ends of the tape do not overlap
    d. Using a piece of twine wrapped completely around the leg

38. Rumen inoculation is
    a. Introducing a bacteria percutaneously to destroy a population explosion of ruminal microorganisms
    b. Drenching an antibiotic solution via an orogastric tube into the rumen
    c. Siphoning ruminal contents from a healthy animal and introducing them into the rumen of a debilitated animal
    d. Vaccinating against the many enteric pathogens of ruminants

39. Which of the following sites should not be used for blood sampling in rabbits?
    a. Cephalic vein
    b. Jugular vein
    c. Medial saphenous vein
    d. Ear vein

40. Which of the following statements is true as it pertains to clipping overgrown nails in a dog?
    a. The nails should be immediately clipped back to 1/4 inch in length.
    b. A Dremel-type instrument should be used to file each nail to 1/2 inch.
    c. The nails should be gradually trimmed back over the course of several weeks.
    d. The dog should be temporarily housed on concrete to encourage each nail to break at an appropriate length.

Correct answers are on pages 427-429.

41. If 1 hour after surgery, it is suspected that an animal is bleeding, and the packed cell volume (PCV) remains normal, it would be beneficial to evaluate the
    a. Hemoglobin
    b. Total protein
    c. Mean corpuscular hemoglobin concentration (MCHC)
    d. Red blood cell (RBC) count

42. Blood transfusion reactions that result from incompatibility are rarest in
    a. Dogs
    b. Cats
    c. Horses
    d. Cows

43. Which of the following lists the stages of wound healing in the correct order?
    a. Collagen, maturation, exudative
    b. Maturation, collagen, exudative
    c. Exudative, maturation, collagen
    d. Exudative, collagen, maturation

44. A Thomas splint is an example of a
    a. Coaptation splint
    b. Anchor splint
    c. Traction splint
    d. Reducing splint

45. Plaster of paris-type casting material can bear weight in approximately
    a. 2 hours
    b. 12 hours
    c. 24 hours
    d. 36 hours

46. The proper way to restrain and carry a rabbit is
    a. Grasp the ears with one hand, and put the other hand under the rabbit's abdomen.
    b. Hold the rabbit by the ears only.
    c. Hold the rabbit by the scruff with one hand, and grasp the hocks of the rabbit with the other.
    d. Place both hands under the rabbit's body and lift.

47. Which of the following is the best way to retrieve a parrot from a cage?
    a. Grasp the parrot's legs in one hand, the neck in the other hand, and pull out the parrot.
    b. Place a towel over the body, hold the wings tightly to its chest, and pull out the parrot.
    c. Grasp the tail near the base of the body with one hand, the wings with the other hand, and pull out the parrot.
    d. Place a towel over it, firmly hold its neck, hold the towel lightly wrapped around the wings and body, and pull out the parrot.

48. Which of the following is not an observable skin condition?
    a. Alopecia
    b. Seborrhea
    c. Hyphema
    d. Erythema

49. What does it mean when you hear *rales* on auscultation of the lungs of a foal?
    a. You hear moist congestion in the lungs.
    b. You hear a fast heart rate.
    c. A foreign object is trapped in the esophagus.
    d. The foal has a tracheal tear.

50. Which of the following is not done on a routine physical examination of a cat?
    a. Open the mouth and look at the teeth, tongue, and gums.
    b. Perform a rectal examination.
    c. Listen to the heart and lungs.
    d. Palpate the abdomen for masses.

51. Normal mucosal bleeding time in a dog is
    a. 30 to 90 seconds
    b. 20 to 30 minutes
    c. 5 to 10 seconds
    d. 600 to 1000 seconds

52. Which of the following heart rates would be considered abnormal for a healthy adult cat?
    a. 150 beats/min
    b. 175 beats/min
    c. 200 beats/min
    d. 250 beats/min

53. Which urine specific gravity would you expect to see in a dehydrated dog?
    a. 1.007
    b. 1.025
    c. 1.015
    d. 1.060

54. Which of these can be positive in the urine of a normal, healthy dog?
    a. Glucose
    b. Ketones
    c. Bilirubin
    d. Alanine aminotransferase (ALT)

55. The urine of a normal rabbit can be which of the following colors?
    a. Orange
    b. Black
    c. Green
    d. Turquoise

56. Which of the following is the best route to give epinephrine in an emergency if a vein is inaccessible?
    a. Intratracheal
    b. Subcutaneous
    c. Oral
    d. Drip under the tongue

57. What drug cannot be given IM?
    a. Penicillin G procaine, an antibiotic
    b. Doxorubicin hydrochloride (Adriamycin; chemotherapeutic drug)
    c. Polysulfated glycosaminoglycan (Adequan; arthritis treatment)
    d. Dexamethasone (Decadron Phosphate; antiinflammatory drug)

58. Which of these compounds can be safely given via IV?
    a. Metoclopramide (Reglan; antacid and antiemetic)
    b. Tap water
    c. Penicillin sodium succinate (antibiotic)
    d. Penicillin G procaine (antibiotic)

59. Which of these drugs comes in an oral form only?
    a. Enrofloxacin (Baytril; antibiotic)
    b. Metoclopramide (Reglan; antacid and antiemetic)
    c. Methimazole (Tapazole; hyperthyroidism treatment)
    d. Cimetidine (Tagamet; antihistamine)

60. Which of these catheters is best to use to draw multiple blood samples?
    a. 24-gauge femoral catheter
    b. 22-gauge cephalic catheter
    c. 18-gauge jugular catheter
    d. 24-gauge catheter in the lateral saphenous vein

61. Which of these compounds is not found in lactated Ringer solution?
    a. Sodium chloride
    b. Potassium chloride
    c. Magnesium chloride
    d. Calcium chloride

62. You are monitoring a patient under anesthesia. Fluid therapy helps
    a. Lower the blood pressure
    b. Raise the blood pressure
    c. Prevent bleeding
    d. Slow the heart rate

63. Which of these IV fluids would increase oncotic (osmotic) pressure?
    a. Lactated Ringer
    b. 5% dextrose in water
    c. Normal saline
    d. Hetastarch

64. An animal with what condition is more prone to fluid overload?
    a. Early renal disease
    b. Parvovirus infection
    c. Cardiac insufficiency
    d. Fractured humerus

65. A wet-to-dry bandage is best for what type of wounds?
    a. Deep lacerations
    b. Contaminated wounds that need to be debrided
    c. Abscesses
    d. Healing wounds with good granulation tissue

66. A fracture in what bone is least likely to be effectively immobilized with a splint?
    a. Tibia
    b. Metacarpal
    c. Humerus
    d. Ulna

67. What sling is used to stabilize the coxofemoral joint?
    a. Velpau
    b. Ehmer
    c. Arm
    d. Robert Jones

68. Which of these shows the correct order for placing a splint on the antebrachium?
    a. Place tape stirrups; place a contact layer on the wound, a layer of padding, a gauze conforming layer, and the splint; and attach stirrups to the gauze layer and wrap with protective tape.
    b. Place tape stirrups; then the splint, a layer of padding, and gauze to conform to the limb; and then wrap with protective tape.
    c. Apply a padded layer to the wound, place the splint, and then wrap with tape.
    d. Place the splint on the leg, secure it with a layer of gauze, and wrap with tape at the top of the leg.

Correct answers are on pages 427-429.

69. Which of the following is the maximum length of time that a compression bandage should be left on?
    a. 1/2 hour
    b. 4 hours
    c. 72 hours
    d. 1 week

70. Which of the following procedures would be chosen to allow a wound to heal by second intention?
    a. Two surgeries performed 1 week apart
    b. Wound closed surgically and a drain placed
    c. Wound left open and not closed surgically
    d. Three days after the injury, wound closed after a local antiseptic is applied

71. A contaminated wound differs from one that is infected in that
    a. The bacterial count is lower in a contaminated wound.
    b. An infected wound can never be closed.
    c. A contaminated wound should not be bandaged.
    d. A contaminated wound cannot become an infected wound.

72. Which of the following would delay wound healing?
    a. Moisture
    b. Dessication
    c. Antibiotics
    d. Drains

73. What fluid should you choose to lavage a deep traumatic wound?
    a. Warm sterile saline
    b. Undiluted Nolvasan
    c. 50% dextrose
    d. Hydrogen peroxide

74. What is true about a degloving injury in a dog?
    a. It commonly results from tight bandages.
    b. It is considered a clean wound.
    c. It results in skin loss.
    d. It can never be closed surgically.

75. Which of these dog breeds is sensitive to ivermectin?
    a. Husky
    b. German shepherd
    c. Pug
    d. Collie

76. Which of these pet birds is sexually dimorphic?
    a. Grey cockatiel
    b. Yellow-naped Amazon
    c. Green parakeet
    d. Blue and gold macaw

77. What species of reptile is venomous?
    a. King snake
    b. Iguana
    c. Water dragon
    d. Gila Monster

78. Which of these birds does not eat seeds?
    a. Finch
    b. Macaw
    c. Duck
    d. Parakeet

79. Which of these dog breeds is most likely to get hip dysplasia?
    a. Beagle
    b. Yorkshire terrier
    c. Borzoi
    d. Golden retriever

80. Which disease is the result of a blood parasite infection that causes anemia in cats?
    a. FIV
    b. FIA
    c. FIP
    d. Malaria

81. For which of the following are there no commercially available vaccines?
    a. Guinea pig
    b. Ferret
    c. Parrot
    d. Chicken

82. Which of the following is a virus that is not highly contagious and does not have a commercial vaccine available for non-human animals?
    a. Parvovirus
    b. Papillomavirus
    c. Distemper virus
    d. Coronavirus

83. What clinical sign is not associated with canine distemper?
    a. Seizures
    b. Coughing
    c. Limping
    d. Behavioral changes

84. What animal is a common reservoir for the rabies virus?
    a. Rabbit
    b. Rat
    c. Pig
    d. Skunk

85. Which statement is true about rabies?
    a. Contact with infected urine is the most common mode of transmission.
    b. Bites from suspected animals should be left untreated to prevent spreading the virus.
    c. Rural dogs develop natural immunity to rabies because of their exposure to wild animals.
    d. Dogs, cats, horses, and cows can transmit rabies, but rabbits, gerbils, hamster, and mice seldom do.

86. What bacterium that is pathogenic to humans is contracted from chickens, horses, and reptiles?
    a. *Proteus*
    b. *Salmonella*
    c. *Bordetella*
    d. *Pasteurella*

87. What is true about psittacosis (chlamydiosis)?
    a. Psittacosis is spread to humans only by direct contact with an infected bird.
    b. Testing live birds for psittacosis is easy and highly accurate.
    c. Psittacosis causes a severe rash on the hands and face in people.
    d. Psittacosis in birds is controlled by adding antibiotics to bird feed.

88. Which of the following causes diarrhea in dogs and humans?
    a. *Staphylococcus*
    b. *Streptococcus*
    c. *Pseudomonas*
    d. *Campylobacter*

89. Which statement about scabies is true?
    a. People cannot get scabies from dogs.
    b. Scabies is diagnosed by a fecal examination.
    c. Scabies is transmissible between dogs and humans.
    d. Scabies is incurable even with an adulticide treatment.

90. Mad cow disease (bovine spongiform encephalopathy) is thought to have originated in what species?
    a. Sheep
    b. Dogs
    c. Pigs
    d. Rodents

91. Which statement about anthrax is true?
    a. People cannot get anthrax from eating contaminated meat.
    b. Anthrax is caused by bacteria.
    c. Anthrax spores can survive outside of the host for a few hours only.
    d. Anthrax affects cattle and humans only.

92. Which of the following are potential side effects of chemotherapy?
    a. Anorexia, anemia, and alopecia
    b. Vomiting, constipation, and flatulence
    c. Anorexia, increased hair growth, and hyperactivity
    d. Aggression, drooling, and polyphagia

93. Which of these bandages should not be used on wounds with exudate?
    a. An occlusive bandage
    b. A dry-dry bandage
    c. A wet-dry bandage
    d. Wound lavage without a bandage

94. Failure of an organ or a part of an organ to grow to its full size is an example of
    a. Metaplasia
    b. Hypertrophy
    c. Hypoplasia
    d. Atrophy

95. Which of the following is not a primary skin lesion?
    a. Macule
    b. Vesicle
    c. Excoriation
    d. Wheal

96. A Wood's lamp can be used to detect what condition in the dog?
    a. Demodectic mange
    b. Scabies
    c. Ringworm
    d. Blastomycosis

97. Which of the following is the most aseptic technique for collecting urine for culture and sensitivity?
    a. Free catch
    b. Expression
    c. Cystocentesis
    d. Catheterization

98. The function of a Robert Jones bandage is to
    a. Support the shoulder joint after surgery
    b. Stabilize a fracture before surgery
    c. Support the hind limb after reduction of hip luxation
    d. Stabilize a fracture after surgery

Correct answers are on pages 427-429.

99. A client brings her new 7-week-old puppy into the clinic and is curious about the ideal vaccination schedule for her pet. You tell her that the ideal schedule is
    a. Distemper at 12, 16, and 20 weeks with rabies at 12+ weeks
    b. Distemper at 8, 12, and 16 weeks with rabies at 8 weeks
    c. Distemper at 8, 12, and 16 weeks with rabies at 12+ weeks
    d. Distemper at 8, 12, and 16 weeks with rabies at 1 year of age

100. How soon after a significant exposure to the feline leukemia virus will a cat have a positive result on a feline leukemia test (ELISA antigen test)?
    a. 4 to 8 months
    b. 4 to 8 weeks
    c. Within days
    d. Not before 1 year

101. Which of the following agents is not safe for cats?
    a. Halogens
    b. Coal tar
    c. Benzoyl peroxide
    d. Chlorhexidine

102. Subcutaneous fluids are contraindicated when
    a. The patient has mild dehydration.
    b. The patient requires 5% dextrose.
    c. The patient is very small.
    d. There is evidence of chronic heart failure.

103. When an animal has a sinus bradycardia, the heart rate
    a. Is too fast
    b. Has stopped
    c. Is normal
    d. Is too slow

104. To auscult the pulmonic, aortic, and mitral valves of the dog, you should place your stethoscope in
    a. Left intercostal spaces 4 to 6
    b. Right intercostal spaces 6 to 8
    c. Left intercostal spaces 3 to 5
    d. Right intercostal spaces 3 to 5

105. The term *pyrexia* refers to
    a. Weakness
    b. Fever
    c. Incoordination
    d. Paralysis

106. A Velpeau sling is used to
    a. Support the hind limb after reduction of hip luxation
    b. Prevent self-trauma
    c. Stabilize a fractured leg before surgery
    d. Support the shoulder joint after surgery

107. The term *pruritus* refers to
    a. Edema
    b. Alopecia
    c. Itching
    d. Dandruff

108. An irregular heart rhythm that results from variations in vagal nerve tone as a result of respiration in dogs is
    a. Normal sinus tachycardia
    b. Gallop rhythm
    c. Ectopic heart beat
    d. Normal sinus arrhythmia

109. The term *nystagmus* refers to
    a. The eyes being off center
    b. The eyes moving in a horizontal or vertical motion
    c. Abnormal protrusion of the eye
    d. Marked edema of the eyes

110. The purpose of the fluorescein dye test is to
    a. Evaluate for corneal abrasions/ulcerations
    b. Evaluate tear production ability
    c. Measure the pressure in the eye
    d. Clear the nasolacrimal ducts

111. When performing a wing clip on a bird, the wing should be grasped firmly at the
    a. Flight feathers
    b. Primary feathers
    c. Carpal joint
    d. Radius and ulna

112. When tube feeding a bird, the gavage tube should be passed into the crop by positioning the tube
    a. Over the tongue and to the right side of the mouth
    b. Over the tongue and to the left side of the mouth
    c. Over the tongue and in the middle of the mouth
    d. Over the tongue and into the trachea

113. In smaller birds (parakeets), the most accessible sites for IM injections are the
    a. Pectoral muscles
    b. Triceps muscle
    c. Biceps muscle
    d. Extensor carpi radialis

114. In the avian species, intraosseous fluid administration is performed by using the
    a. Proximal humerus
    b. Distal radius
    c. Distal femur
    d. Proximal tibia

115. Which phase of the electrocardiogram (ECG) represents the depolarization of the atria?
    a. P wave
    b. T wave
    c. P–R interval
    d. Q–T interval

116. Which phase of the ECG represents the repolarization phase of the ventricles?
    a. P wave
    b. T wave
    c. P–R interval
    d. Q–T interval

117. The principal intracellular cation that is commonly measured in a blood chemistry profile and that contributes to maintaining the acid–base balance is
    a. Sodium
    b. Chloride
    c. Potassium
    d. Bicarbonate

118. When a healthy animal's airway is obstructed, thereby decreasing its ability to properly ventilate, the most likely condition that will result is
    a. Respiratory acidosis
    b. Respiratory alkalosis
    c. Metabolic acidosis
    d. Metabolic alkalosis

119. With reference to the eyes, the abbreviation *OD (oculus dexter)* refers to
    a. Both eyes
    b. Left eye
    c. Right eye
    d. One eye at a time

120. In most cases of respiratory, cardiovascular, and musculoskeletal disorders, which of the following is contraindicated?
    a. Feeding
    b. Drinking
    c. Exercise
    d. Grooming

121. When planning the appropriate nutritional treatment for a patient, the caloric intake should
    a. Meet the metabolic requirements of the patient
    b. Slightly exceed the metabolic requirements of the patient
    c. Be slightly less than the metabolic requirements of the patient
    d. Greatly exceed the metabolic requirements of the patient

122. A pharyngostomy tube is used when a patient is
    a. Dyspneic
    b. Anemic
    c. Anuric
    d. Anorexic

123. Bleeding from a nail during a nail trim is frequently stopped by using
    a. Silver nitrate sticks
    b. Baking powder
    c. K-Y Jelly
    d. Ice packs

124. The two infectious agents most often involved in otitis externa in the dog are
    a. Viruses and protozoa
    b. Yeast and viruses
    c. Viruses and bacteria
    d. Yeast and bacteria

125. Flushing the external ear canal is contraindicated if
    a. A viral infection is suspected.
    b. The patient has floppy ears.
    c. The patient has previously been diagnosed with a bacterial infection.
    d. The tympanic membrane is ruptured.

126. The function of the anal glands is to
    a. Produce a scented, oily, sweaty material that serves no function
    b. Produce sweat that helps lower the body temperature
    c. Produce an oily substance to lubricate feces
    d. Produce a scented material used to mark territory

127. The opening of the anal sac ducts is on the rectum at the
    a. 4 and 8 o'clock positions
    b. 2 and 10 o'clock positions
    c. 12 and 6 o'clock positions
    d. 11 and 4 o'clock positions

Correct answers are on pages 427-429.

128. Decubital sores are
    a. Found in the ears in severe cases of otitis externa
    b. Found around the rectum in cases of anal sac problems
    c. Found on the skin because of urine scalding and pressure from lying in one position too long
    d. Found in the mouth as the result of prolonged anorexia

129. Ninety-five percent of the circulating antibodies in puppies younger than 48 hours old come from the
    a. Colostrum
    b. Placenta
    c. Puppies' bone marrow
    d. Environment

130. Passive antibodies
    a. Give temporary protection to the puppy
    b. Are the major protection source for the mother while she is pregnant
    c. Are produced by a series of vaccinations
    d. Last for most of the puppy's life

131. For canine distemper and hepatitis, the most commonly recommended time for the last vaccine in a puppy series is at
    a. 10 weeks of age
    b. 8 weeks of age
    c. 16 weeks of age
    d. 24 weeks of age

132. The two most common types of vaccines in common use today in veterinary practices are
    a. Killed (inactivated) and activated
    b. Modified live and killed
    c. Killed and reactivated
    d. Modified live and modified killed

133. Which statement about immunizations is true?
    a. Older animals have more effective immune systems and thus require less frequent vaccinations.
    b. Young animals have passive immunity, making vaccination unnecessary for the first year of life.
    c. Older animals can have reduced immune status and may require more frequent vaccination.
    d. Young animals should be given only killed vaccines because of the passive immunity they get from their mothers.

134. How long does a modified live vaccine remain effective after it is mixed, if it is left at room temperature?
    a. 2 to 3 hours
    b. 24 hours
    c. Several days
    d. 1 hour

135. Which of the following conditions is/are more common in geriatric patients?
    a. Arthritis and degenerative joint disease
    b. Viral and bacterial infections
    c. Lameness that results from accidents and muscle damage
    d. Gastric torsion and dilatation

136. When gavage is used to feed young puppies, vomiting immediately following the feeding is usually the result of
    a. Not giving enough formula
    b. Leaving some formula in the gavage tube
    c. Giving too much formula and overextending the stomach
    d. Holding the puppy in the wrong position while gavage is given

137. The feeding tube used in gavage is measured to equal a distance from the
    a. Mouth to the base of the trachea
    b. Lips to the eighth rib
    c. Lips to the last lumbar vertebra
    d. Lips to the end of the duodenum

138. The stomach capacity of puppies and kittens is approximately
    a. 20 ml/kg
    b. 30 ml/kg
    c. 1 ml/kg
    d. 9 ml/kg

139. Puppies are expected to gain
    a. 50% of their birth weight in the first week of life
    b. 10% to 20% of their birth weight in the first week of life
    c. 1 to 2 lb daily for the first week of life
    d. 1 to 2 lb in the first few weeks of life

140. A glass rectal thermometer has
    a. No constriction in the mercury to interfere with temperature taking
    b. An elongated bulb and a mercury constriction
    c. A round bulb and a mercury constriction
    d. A round bulb with no mercury constriction

141. When taking body temperature via the ear or the axilla, the temperature obtained is usually assumed to be
    a. 10 degrees lower than the rectal temperature
    b. 2 degrees lower than the rectal temperature
    c. The same as the rectal temperature
    d. Of no relation to the rectal temperature

142. The most common artery used in dogs and cats to obtain a pulse is the
    a. Femoral artery
    b. Saphenous artery
    c. Cephalic artery
    d. Coronary artery

143. For Doppler assessment of the pulse rate, the most commonly used arteries are the
    a. Femoral and plantar
    b. Palmar and plantar
    c. Saphenous and plantar
    d. Cephalic and palmar

144. A pulse deficit occurs when
    a. The pulse rate lags behind the heart rate.
    b. The pulse rate is higher than the heart rate.
    c. The blood pressure is lower than expected.
    d. There is an enlarged QRS wave on the electrocardiograph.

145. When taking a respiration rate,
    a. Count inspiration and expiration as two breaths.
    b. Count inspiration and expiration as one breath.
    c. Listen to the expirations only.
    d. Listen to the inspirations only.

146. Tachypnea is
    a. Rapid heart rate
    b. Rapid pulse
    c. Excessive coughing
    d. Rapid respiration rate

147. Dyspnea is
    a. Increased thirst
    b. A type of painful cough
    c. Painful breathing
    d. A slow heart rate

148. The tests that are very useful in assessing fluid loss in a patient are
    a. PCV, BUN, and ALT
    b. PCV, plasma protein, and urine specific gravity
    c. PCV and BUN
    d. PCV only

149. Besides skin tenting, one of the best physical signs to access fluid status is
    a. Heart rate
    b. Respiration
    c. Pulse
    d. Weight

150. For subcutaneous administration of fluids, the fluids are preferred to be
    a. Hypertonic
    b. Isotonic
    c. Hypotonic
    d. Supertonic

151. Subcutaneous fluids are usually absorbed in
    a. 48 hours
    b. 1 to 2 hours
    c. 5 to 8 hours
    d. 5 to 10 minutes

152. Which statement about intraperitoneal fluid therapy is true?
    a. It is not routinely used because of the slow rate of absorption.
    b. It is used commonly in veterinary practice when a vein cannot be accessed.
    c. It is used for shock therapy when there is venous collapse.
    d. It is used to administer nutrients and fluids because of its closeness to the stomach and intestine.

153. During fluid therapy, a low plasma protein combined with a decreased cardiac rate can easily result in
    a. Cardiac arrest
    b. Rapid rehydration and recovery from shock
    c. Pulmonary edema
    d. Seizures

154. Which statement about central venous pressure (CVP) is true?
    a. CVP is an indirect method of measuring blood pressure.
    b. CVP measures fluid pressure in the right atrium.
    c. CVP rises when the amount of circulating fluid falls.
    d. CVP falls when cardiac output rises.

155. The instrument used in measuring central venous pressure is called a
    a. Doppler
    b. Sphygmomanometer
    c. Manometer
    d. Pulse oximeter

Correct answers are on pages 427-429.

156. For accuracy, a central venous pressure reading should be taken at least
    a. 2 times
    b. 3 times
    c. 10 times
    d. 5 times

157. Normal central venous pressure readings for dogs are
    a. 8 to 10 cm
    b. 0 to 5 cm
    c. 10 to 20 cm
    d. 0 to 20 cm

158. Which statement about PCV measurement in acute blood loss is true?
    a. It is an accurate assessment of the condition, but only if combined with serum albumin determination.
    b. It is an accurate assessment of the condition, but only if combined with a BUN determination.
    c. It is an inaccurate assessment of the condition because of vasoconstriction and splenic contraction.
    d. It is an inaccurate assessment of the condition because of vasodilation and hepatic contraction.

159. How long do platelets survive in stored fresh blood?
    a. 24 hours
    b. 12 hours
    c. 2 hours
    d. 1 hour

160. Transfusions in cases of autoimmune hemolytic anemia are
    a. Recommended to replace lost platelets
    b. Recommended to replace lost RBCs
    c. Not recommended unless done very early in the condition
    d. Not recommended, because they may increase hemolysis

161. When a blood transfusion is to be administered, the blood
    a. Should be administered in a cooled state directly from the refrigerator to avoid blood component breakdown
    b. Should be administered after being allowed to warm slowly to room temperature
    c. Should be warmed to body temperature before administration
    d. Should be warmed to above body temperature to avoid cooling the patient down before administration

162. A delayed hemolytic reaction is indicated by a drop in PCV how many days posttransfusion?
    a. 2 to 20 days
    b. Only immediately following transfusion
    c. After 2 to 3 weeks
    d. Years later in the patient's life

163. When applying physical therapy to a patient, cold or hot compresses are usually applied for what time period?
    a. 1 hour
    b. 10 minutes
    c. 20 minutes
    d. 3 to 4 hours

164. When "clearing" a skin scraping in search of a dermatophyte infection, heat the slide after applying
    a. Alcohol
    b. Acetic acid
    c. Peroxide
    d. Potassium hydroxide

165. Before doing a skin scraping for a fungal culture, apply
    a. Alcohol
    b. Peroxide
    c. Tincture of iodine
    d. Potassium hydroxide

166. How deep should you scrape the skin for a fungal culture?
    a. Surface scraping only
    b. Deep scraping after surgical scrub
    c. Deep scraping with no skin preparation
    d. Surface scraping down to bleeding dermis with no skin preparation

167. On a deep skin scraping, sarcoptic mange mites are
    a. Easy to find, because they are so numerous on the patient
    b. Very difficult to find, because very few are often on the patient
    c. Never found, because they are temporary parasites
    d. More often found if you pinch the skin before doing the skin scraping

168. A benzoyl-peroxide shampoo is used to
    a. Clean and groom the dog on a regular basis
    b. Kill bacteria and flush the hair follicles
    c. Replace the oil in dogs with dry skin
    d. Remove heavy grease on dogs with Cushing disease

169. Long-handle neck tongs can be used to grasp a pig to apply a
   a. Harness
   b. Snout rope
   c. Dental speculum
   d. Halter

170. A struggling sheep rapidly becomes hyperthermic in hot weather, because its normal body temperature is
   a. 90° F (36.6° C)
   b. 98° F (38.3° C)
   c. 103° F (39.4° C)
   d. 107° F (40.5° C)

171. The easiest large domestic animal to handle is the
   a. Sheep
   b. Goat
   c. Cow
   d. Pig

172. What is the most important skill that a restrainer can develop?
   a. Hypnosis
   b. Firm voice
   c. Slow movements
   d. Self-confidence

173. One clinical sign of hyperthermia is
   a. Decreased heart rate
   b. Increased respiratory rate
   c. Decreased temperature
   d. Increased urine output

174. One clinical sign of hypothermia is
   a. Increased body temperature
   b. Increased cardiac output
   c. Decreased blood pressure
   d. Bright red mucous membrane

175. What is one clinical sign of shock?
   a. Increased blood pressure
   b. Pale mucous membranes
   c. Decreased heart rate
   d. Increased cardiac output

176. What is the best method of handling an extremely agitated cat?
   a. Apply firm restraint
   b. Use a cat bag
   c. Use a cat muzzle
   d. Back off and allow the cat to calm down

177. When restraining a domestic cat, the best rule to remember is
   a. Always wear gloves.
   b. Use the least amount of restraint possible for the procedure.
   c. Always grasp the cat with your fingers encircling its head.
   d. Always use a cat bag or towel.

178. When setting a sheep up on its haunches, you should never
   a. Lift the head over the neck
   b. Grasp the flank area
   c. Twist the sheep's head to the side
   d. Try to set the animal up if it weighs more than 200 lb

179. Pigs naturally pull back when pressure is applied around their
   a. Lower jaw (mandible)
   b. Tail
   c. Midsection
   d. Upper jaw (maxilla)

180. The first concern when dealing with any animal should be the
   a. Safety of the animal
   b. Safety of the handlers
   c. Protection of the equipment
   d. Time the procedure will take

181. The normal temperature, pulse rate, and respiration rate (TPR) of swine are
   a. 102° F to 103.6° F, 60 to 80/min, 8 to 18/min
   b. 99.5° F to 101.5° F, 28 to 45/min, 8 to 16/min
   c. 101.5° F, 110 to 140/min, 26/min
   d. 99.5° F, 66 to 114/min, 330 to 480/min

182. The normal rectal temperature of an adult cat is
   a. 94° F to 96° F
   b. 96° F to 98° F
   c. 98° F to 100° F
   d. 100° F to 102° F

183. What are the normal temperature, pulse rate, and respiration rate of a cow?
   a. 100° F, 30/min, 50/min
   b. 101.5° F, 60/min, 20/min
   c. 102.5° F, 30/min, 50/min
   d. 102.5° F, 60/min, 20/min

Correct answers are on pages 427-429.

184. Causing an animal to lie on its side with pressure exerted its muscles and nerves by a series of carefully placed and tightened ropes is called
    a. Casting
    b. Chuting
    c. Haltering
    d. Hog tying

185. From what area is it best to approach a horse?
    a. Rear
    b. Directly in the front
    c. At a 45-degree angle from the left shoulder
    d. Any direction is okay

186. What is the basic tool of restraint for the horse?
    a. Leg hobbles
    b. Nose twitch
    c. Casting
    d. Halter

187. What is the normal capillary refill time in a dog?
    a. 1 to 2 seconds
    b. 5 to 6 seconds
    c. 1 minute
    d. 10 minutes

188. Which is not a route of injection?
    a. IV
    b. Anteroposterior
    c. IM
    d. Subcutaneous

189. Which of these needles has the largest interior diameter?
    a. 18-gauge
    b. 27-gauge
    c. 22-gauge
    d. 16-gauge

190. Which of these veins is not used to collect blood in a dog?
    a. Saphenous
    b. Cephalic
    c. Tail
    d. Jugular

191. Which of these veins is found on the lateral aspect of the back leg?
    a. Saphenous
    b. Cephalic
    c. Femoral
    d. Jugular

192. Which of these veins is located on the cranial (dorsal) surface of the front leg?
    a. Saphenous
    b. Cephalic
    c. Femoral
    d. Jugular

193. Which of these agents should not be used to control blood flow from a nail that was cut too short?
    a. Styptic powder
    b. Alcohol
    c. Silver nitrate
    d. Cornstarch

194. What are the normal temperature, pulse rate, and respiration rate of a dog?
    a. 101.5° F, 90/min, 20/min
    b. 101.5° F, 180/min, 25/min
    c. 100° F, 90/min, 20/min
    d. 100° F, 180/min, 25/min

195. Which lymph node may be palpated caudal to the stifle?
    a. Axillary
    b. Inguinal
    c. Popliteal
    d. Mandibular

196. Which of these instruments is used to examine the ear canal?
    a. Ophthalmoscope
    b. Fluoroscope
    c. Microscope
    d. Otoscope

197. An animal in sternal recumbency is
    a. On its side
    b. Sitting on its rump
    c. Positioned with its back on the table or floor
    d. Positioned with its abdomen on the table or floor

198. When collecting blood using a needle and syringe, how should the bevel of the needle be positioned?
    a. Up
    b. Down
    c. Pointing to the medial side
    d. Pointing to the lateral side

199. When giving an IM injection, it is good practice to withdraw the syringe plunger after the needle is inserted to
    a. Draw air into the syringe
    b. See whether the needle has been inserted into a blood vessel
    c. Make the plunger easier to depress
    d. Provide stability to the syringe

200. When using isopropyl alcohol as a disinfectant, what is the recommended concentration?
    a. 25%
    b. 50%
    c. 70%
    d. 99%

201. What muscle located cranial to the femur can be used for IM injections?
    a. Quadriceps
    b. Triceps brachii
    c. Semitendinosus
    d. Trapezius

202. What type of preparation is a biologic?
    a. Antibiotic
    b. Vaccine
    c. Anesthetic
    d. IV fluid

203. What does a tonometer measure?
    a. Venous pressure
    b. Arterial blood flow
    c. Intraocular pressure
    d. Speed of capillary refill

204. Where are the anal sacs located?
    a. Ventral to the mandible
    b. Cranial to the scapula
    c. In the inguinal area
    d. In the perianal area

205. When examining a patient, you count 7 pulses in 10 seconds. How should you record this animal's pulse rate?
    a. 7 beats/min
    b. 42 beats/min
    c. 28 beats/min
    d. 70 beats/min

206. When using a mercury thermometer to measure rectal temperature, what is the minimum time the thermometer should be left in the rectum?
    a. 10 seconds
    b. 60 seconds
    c. 2 minutes
    d. 5 minutes

207. The blood smear of a normal dog should have what percentage of eosinophils?
    a. 60% to 77%
    b. 35% to 75%
    c. 2% to 10%
    d. 12% to 30%

208. The blood smear of a normal dog should have what percentage of lymphocytes?
    a. 12% to 30%
    b. 60% to 70%
    c. 2% to 8%
    d. 25% to 60%

209. The PCV of a normal adult dog is
    a. 10% to 21%
    b. 37% to 55%
    c. 10 to 21 g/dl
    d. 35 to 55 g/dl

210. The total white blood cell count of a normal adult dog is
    a. 1000 to 3000/μl
    b. 30,000 to 50,000/μl
    c. 4000 to 10,000/μl
    d. 6000 to 17,000/μl

211. The hemoglobin level of a normal adult dog is
    a. 12% to 18%
    b. 12 to 18 g/dl
    c. 100 to 120 g/dl
    d. 20% to 80%

212. The total RBC count of a normal dog is
    a. 5.5 to 8.5 $\times$ 10^6/μl
    b. 3000 to 5000/μl
    c. 1.1 to 6.4 $\times$ 10^6/μl
    d. 10,000 to 20,000/μl

213. The blood urea nitrogen of a normal dog is
    a. 10 to 28 mg/dl
    b. 1 to 2 mg/dl
    c. 10% to 28%
    d. 1% to 2%

214. The serum creatinine level of a normal dog is
    a. 55% to 93%
    b. 1 to 2 mg/dl
    c. 10 to 30 mg/dl
    d. 1% to 2%

215. The blood glucose level of a normal dog is
    a. 45 to 70 mg/dl
    b. 1000 to 2000 mg/dl
    c. 70 to 100 mg/dl
    d. 10 to 30 g/dl

Correct answers are on pages 427-429.

216. The total plasma protein level of a normal dog is
    a. 6 to 7 g/dl
    b. 10% to 40%
    c. 10 to 30 g/dl
    d. 1 to 2 g/dl

217. Which of the following would not be seen in a peripheral blood smear from a normal dog?
    a. Erythrocytes
    b. Platelets
    c. Leukocytes
    d. Megakaryocytes

218. The normal mean corpuscular volume (MCV) of a dog is
    a. 300 to 345 fl (femtoliter)
    b. 1 to 2 fl
    c. 60 to 77 fl
    d. 103 to 400 fl

219. The normal MCHC of a dog is
    a. 32 to 36 g/dl
    b. 1 to 2 g/dl
    c. 135 to 234 g/dl
    d. 60 to 98 g/dl

220. The normal PCV of a horse is
    a. 20% to 39%
    b. 48% to 58%
    c. 12% to 30%
    d. 32% to 52%

221. The normal white blood cell count of a horse is
    a. 5000 to 12,500/µl
    b. 10,000 to 20,000/µl
    c. 4000 to 5000/µl
    d. 10,500 to 30,000/µl

222. How much urine does an average dog normally produce in 24 hours?
    a. 5 ml/kg
    b. 15 ml/kg
    c. 30 ml/kg
    d. 45 ml/kg

223. How much urine does an average adult cat normally produce in 24 hours?
    a. 5 ml/kg
    b. 15 ml/kg
    c. 30 ml/kg
    d. 45 ml/kg

224. How many white blood cells per high-power field are considered normal in typical canine urine?
    a. 0 to 3
    b. 2 to 8
    c. 10 to 14
    d. 1 to 8

225. The most common type of leukocyte found in the peripheral blood of dogs is the
    a. Monocyte
    b. Basophil
    c. Eosinophil
    d. Neutrophil

226. Which of the following are both agranulocytes?
    a. Monocytes and neutrophils
    b. Lymphocytes and monocytes
    c. Eosinophils and basophils
    d. Lymphocytes and eosinophils

227. Which route of drug administration produces the fastest onset of action?
    a. Topical
    b. Oral
    c. IM
    d. IV

228. Which of the following is not a parenteral route of drug administration?
    a. Subcutaneous
    b. IM
    c. Oral
    d. IV

229. Agents used to induce vomiting are called
    a. Pyrethrins
    b. Emetics
    c. Sulfonamides
    d. Diuretics

230. Another term for a laxative is
    a. Relaxant
    b. Diuretic
    c. Adjuvant
    d. Cathartic

231. What drug is used as an anthelmintic?
    a. Penicillin
    b. Piperazine
    c. Pyrethrin
    d. Streptomycin

232. What drug is not an antibiotic?
    a. Chloramphenicol
    b. Amoxicillin
    c. Tetracycline
    d. Furosemide

233. What type of drug is used to stimulate urine production?
    a. Depressant
    b. Relaxant
    c. Emetic
    d. Diuretic

234. How often should controlled substances be inventoried?
    a. Monthly
    b. Continuously, with use
    c. Annually
    d. Every other month

235. An intra–articular injection is given into a/the
    a. Blood vessel
    b. Eye
    c. Skin
    d. Joint

236. The accepted abbreviation for the intracardiac route of drug administration is
    a. PO
    b. IC
    c. IV
    d. IM

237. The accepted abbreviation for the intramuscular route of drug administration is
    a. PO
    b. IC
    c. IV
    d. IM

238. The accepted abbreviation for the intravenous route of drug administration is
    a. PO
    b. IC
    c. IV
    d. IM

239. The accepted abbreviation for the oral route of drug administration is
    a. PO
    b. IC
    c. IV
    d. PM

240. The abbreviation meaning "treatment" is
    a. q
    b. prn
    c. Rx
    d. dd

241. The abbreviation meaning "divided" is
    a. q
    b. prn
    c. Rx
    d. dd

242. The abbreviation meaning "every" is
    a. q
    b. prn
    c. Rx
    d. dd

243. The abbreviation meaning "as needed" is
    a. q
    b. prn
    c. Rx
    d. dd

244. The higher the hematocrit and total protein values, the greater the degree of
    a. Anemia
    b. Hypoglycemia
    c. Dehydration
    d. Hyperkalemia

245. What is the approximate degree of dehydration in a patient that shows increased skin turgor, prolonged capillary refill time, dry mucous membranes, and eyes sunken into the orbits?
    a. 0.5% to 1%
    b. 10% to 12%
    c. 2% to 3%
    d. 5% to 6%

246. Which of the following is not a sign of fluid volume overload?
    a. Restlessness
    b. Hyperpnea
    c. Serous nasal discharge
    d. Dry mucous membranes

247. What is the best route of fluid administration for a slightly dehydrated patient that can drink water and is not vomiting?
    a. Oral
    b. IV
    c. Intraosseous
    d. IM

Correct answers are on pages 427-429.

248. Use of a cephalic catheter for IV fluid administration is usually limited to
    a. 2 to 4 hours
    b. 7 to 14 days
    c. 48 to 72 hours
    d. 30 days

249. Normal daily water maintenance requirements for a typical adult dog and cat are approximately
    a. 10 to 15 ml/kg
    b. 50 to 100 ml/kg
    c. 100 to 300 ml/kg
    d. 500 to 600 ml/kg

250. Which statement concerning subcutaneous administration of fluids is true?
    a. Fluids should be infused with a large-bore needle.
    b. Fluids should be first warmed to above body temperature.
    c. A 9% saline solution can safely be administered subcutaneously.
    d. A 50% dextrose solution cannot safely be administered subcutaneously.

251. Isotonic solutions
    a. Must be given IV only
    b. Must be given subcutaneously only
    c. May be given intraperitoneally or subcutaneously
    d. May be given IV, subcutaneously, or intraperitoneally

252. Hypertonic solutions
    a. Must be given IV only
    b. Must be given subcutaneously only
    c. May be given intraperitoneally or subcutaneously
    d. May be given IV, subcutaneously, or intraperitoneally

253. The principal cation in extracellular fluid is
    a. Na^+
    b. Mg^{++}
    c. K^+
    d. Fe^{++}

254. The principal anion in extracellular fluid is
    a. SO_4^-
    b. NO_3^-
    c. Cl^-
    d. HCO_3^-

255. Lactated Ringer solution is
    a. Equitonic
    b. Hypertonic
    c. Hypotonic
    d. Isotonic

256. Sterile water is
    a. Hypotonic
    b. Isotonic
    c. Hypertonic
    d. Equitonic

257. Bandaging provides all of the following except
    a. Keeping the wound warm
    b. Promoting an alkaline environment
    c. Minimizing postoperative edema
    d. Absorbing wound exudates

258. Bandaging promotes wound healing by all of the following except
    a. Protecting the wound from additional trauma and contamination
    b. Preventing desiccation
    c. Immobilizing the wound to prevent cellular disruption
    d. Decreasing oxygen availability

259. Fiberglass cast materials have all of the following advantages except
    a. Slow setting time
    b. Lightweight
    c. Good ventilation
    d. Extreme rigidity

260. What bandage is most commonly used for temporary immobilization of fractures distal to the elbow or stifle before surgery?
    a. Full-leg stack
    b. Robert Jones
    c. Modified Robert Jones
    d. Military field

261. How frequently should splints be adjusted on foals?
    a. Once a day
    b. Twice a day
    c. Every other day
    d. Three times a day

262. The major functions of a stent bandage include all of the following, except
    a. Works in regions that are difficult to cover
    b. Applies direct pressure and decreases motion
    c. Reduces the tension on the primary incision line
    d. Provides good absorption of exudates

263. The equine joint that is never splinted is the
    a. Carpus
    b. Hock
    c. Fetlock
    d. Stifle

264. Failure to use adequate padding in bandages on limbs can produce any of the following except
    a. Tendonitis
    b. Pressure sores
    c. Severe edema
    d. Instability

265. The ties of the many-tailed spider bandage are positioned on which aspect of the affected limb?
    a. Dorsal
    b. Palmar/plantar
    c. Medial
    d. Lateral

266. What splint is used on simple, closed fractures of the radius and ulna or tibia and fibula in young dogs and occasionally on large animals (mostly the rear limbs of cattle)?
    a. Kimzey
    b. Schroeder-Thomas
    c. Board
    d. Plastic (PVC)

267. The Robert Jones bandage is not appropriate for stabilizing fractures of the
    a. Femur or humerus
    b. Radius or carpus
    c. Tibia or third metacarpal bone
    d. Third metacarpal bone

268. The toes of a bandaged limb should be monitored daily for all of the following except
    a. Warmth
    b. Sensitivity
    c. Color
    d. Swelling

269. A compression bandage used to immobilize a structure aids in all of the following except
    a. Controlling swelling
    b. Reducing movement
    c. Supporting damaged structures
    d. Containing an infectious inflammatory condition

270. A chest or abdominal bandage, when applied firmly for compression, should not remain in place on a small animal for longer than
    a. 4 hours
    b. 1 hour
    c. 6 hours
    d. 8 hours

271. What is the correct order for the processes of wound healing?
    a. Inflammation, debridement, repair, maturation
    b. Maturation, debridement, repair, inflammation
    c. Debridement, inflammation, maturation, repair
    d. Repair, inflammation, maturation, debridement

272. What phase of healing begins immediately after tissue injury?
    a. Debridement
    b. Repair
    c. Inflammation
    d. Maturation

273. What phase of healing begins approximately 6 hours after tissue injury?
    a. Debridement
    b. Repair
    c. Inflammation
    d. Maturation

274. What phase of healing begins 3 to 5 days after tissue injury?
    a. Debridement
    b. Repair
    c. Inflammation
    d. Maturation

275. The breed of dog that is considered naturally barkless is the
    a. Pug
    b. Basenji
    c. Pomeranian
    d. Lhasa apso

276. The breed of cat known for its normally stubby tail is the
    a. Persian
    b. Maine Coon
    c. Siamese
    d. Manx

277. The breed of dog that frequently has urate crystals in its urine is the
    a. Dalmatian
    b. German shepherd
    c. Chihuahua
    d. Cocker spaniel

278. The breed of dog most likely to be affected by hip dysplasia is the
    a. Wirehaired fox terrier
    b. Brittany spaniel
    c. Whippet
    d. Labrador retriever

Correct answers are on pages 427-429.

279. The breed of goat with long, wide, pendulous ears and a Roman nose is the
    a. Toggenburg
    b. Nubian
    c. Saanen
    d. French alpine

280. The breed of goat with almost no external ears is the
    a. Oberhasli
    b. French alpine
    c. LaMancha
    d. Saanen

281. The all-white breed of goat is the
    a. Saanen
    b. French alpine
    c. LaMancha
    d. Toggenburg

282. The breed of pig that is red is the
    a. Berkshire
    b. Duroc
    c. Yorkshire
    d. Landrace

283. The breed of dog that requires a smaller dose of thiobarbiturate anesthetic per pound than that calculated by its weight is the
    a. Whippet
    b. Labrador retriever
    c. Collie
    d. Newfoundland

284. The breed of pig that is white and has erect ears is the
    a. Landrace
    b. Hampshire
    c. Yorkshire
    d. Berkshire

285. The breed of dairy cow whose milk contains the highest percentage of butterfat is the
    a. Holstein
    b. Ayrshire
    c. Guernsey
    d. Jersey

286. The breed of dairy cow that is usually black and white is the
    a. Holstein
    b. Guernsey
    c. Ayrshire
    d. Jersey

287. Of the breeds listed, the breed of dog most commonly affected with intervertebral disk disease is the
    a. Dalmatian
    b. Dachshund
    c. Great Dane
    d. Irish setter

288. Of the breeds listed, the breed of dog most commonly affected with gastric dilatation/volvulus (bloat) is the
    a. Pug
    b. Saint Bernard
    c. Lhasa apso
    d. Shar-Pei

289. The breed of dog frequently exhibiting inherited idiopathic epilepsy is the
    a. Great Dane
    b. Miniature schnauzer
    c. Miniature poodle
    d. Siberian husky

290. The breed of chicken known for its white eggs is the
    a. Rhode Island red
    b. Leghorn
    c. White Plymouth rock
    d. New Hampshire

291. The breed of dog frequently affected by entropion is the
    a. Basset hound
    b. Samoyed
    c. Shar-Pei
    d. Saint Bernard

292. The breed of dog that is brachycephalic is the
    a. Pekingese
    b. Collie
    c. Greyhound
    d. Malamute

293. The breed of dog that commonly has its tail docked is the
    a. Dachshund
    b. Siberian husky
    c. Newfoundland
    d. Old English sheepdog

294. The breed of dog that commonly has its ears cropped is the
    a. Borzoi
    b. Keeshond
    c. Doberman pinscher
    d. Cocker spaniel

295. Which breed of cattle is a beef breed?
  a. Guernsey
  b. Holstein
  c. Jersey
  d. Angus

296. A long-coated guinea pig is the
  a. Peruvian
  b. Abyssinian
  c. American
  d. Crested

297. What breed of guinea pig has a rough hair coat?
  a. Crested
  b. American
  c. Peruvian
  d. Abyssinian

298. What breed of rabbit is most commonly used in research?
  a. Angora
  b. Mini Lop
  c. Netherland dwarf
  d. New Zealand white

299. The long-haired breed of cat that resembles the Siamese in color is the
  a. Manx
  b. Burmese
  c. Himalayan
  d. Persian

300. The breed of beef cattle that is black and polled is the
  a. Limousin
  b. Angus
  c. Charolais
  d. Hereford

301. The breed of cat that frequently has crossed eyes and a kinked tail is the
  a. Siamese
  b. Himalayan
  c. Persian
  d. Maine Coon

302. The breed of dog known for its ability to track scents is the
  a. Boston terrier
  b. Welsh corgi
  c. Bedlington terrier
  d. Bloodhound

303. An ideal breed of dog to be kept as a blood donor is the
  a. Greyhound
  b. Basset hound
  c. Dachshund
  d. Chihuahua

304. The breed of cat with uniquely folded (bent over) ears is the
  a. Persian
  b. Burmese
  c. English flop
  d. Scottish fold

305. What breed of sheep is used predominantly for meat?
  a. Merino
  b. Romney marsh
  c. Suffolk
  d. Karakul

306. What type of cat is most likely to be deaf?
  a. Calico
  b. Orange tiger
  c. Tortoiseshell
  d. White

307. The breed of dog particularly prone to parvoviral infection after 4 months of age is the
  a. German short-haired pointer
  b. Rottweiler
  c. Yorkshire terrier
  d. Afghan hound

308. The breed of dog known for its predisposition to retinal problems is the
  a. Pekingese
  b. Dalmatian
  c. Doberman pinscher
  d. Collie

309. The dairy breed with the highest average milk yield is the
  a. Holstein
  b. Guernsey
  c. Jersey
  d. Ayrshire

310. The breed of dog prized for its lack of shedding is the
  a. Collie
  b. Labrador retriever
  c. Poodle
  d. Pug

Correct answers are on pages 427-429.

311. What breed of cat is most likely to develop hairballs?
    a. Domestic shorthair
    b. Burmese
    c. Persian
    d. Siamese

312. Of the following horse breeds, which is in the pony class?
    a. Arabian
    b. Welsh
    c. Morgan
    d. Appaloosa

313. What horse breed is considered a draft horse?
    a. Clydesdale
    b. Standardbred
    c. Thoroughbred
    d. American saddlebred

314. What horse breed is used for harness racing?
    a. Standardbred
    b. Thoroughbred
    c. Percheron
    d. Palomino

315. What dog breed would probably require the smallest amount of thiobarbiturate anesthetic per pound of body weight?
    a. Jack Russell terrier
    b. Lhasa apso
    c. Great Pyrenees
    d. Keeshond

316. What breed of dog is particularly susceptible to heat stroke?
    a. Beagle
    b. English bulldog
    c. Italian greyhound
    d. Schipperke

317. What breed of dog is more commonly born by cesarean section?
    a. Collie
    b. Beagle
    c. Pomeranian
    d. Boston terrier

318. The breed of beef cattle noted for its heat tolerance is the
    a. Angus
    b. Longhorn
    c. Hereford
    d. Brahman

319. The breed of dog born with no tail is the
    a. Old English sheepdog
    b. Schipperke
    c. Miniature poodle
    d. Miniature schnauzer

320. What dog breed is considered to have the greatest tendency to exhibit destructive behavior?
    a. Chihuahua
    b. Pomeranian
    c. Malamute
    d. Shih Tzu

321. What dog breed is considered to have the greatest tendency to exhibit aggressive behavior?
    a. Irish setter
    b. Labrador retriever
    c. Saint Bernard
    d. Chow Chow

322. The breed of chicken bred for meat is the
    a. Cornish
    b. Leghorn
    c. Rhode Island red
    d. Wyandotte

323. What dog breed has Scottish ancestry?
    a. Brittany spaniel
    b. Wheaten terrier
    c. Rough collie
    d. Pembroke corgi

324. High mountain or brisket disease of cattle is caused by
    a. Parasitic infection of the lung
    b. *Pasteurella* infection
    c. Hypoxia from low oxygen pressure
    d. Cardiotoxic plants

325. A previously nonvaccinated mature horse that receives a traumatic wound that becomes contaminated should be given
    a. Tetanus antitoxin only
    b. Tetanus toxoid only
    c. Both tetanus antitoxin and tetanus toxoid
    d. Local wound therapy only

326. Colostrum is important for the newborn because it provides
    a. Passive immunity from the dam
    b. Protection against internal parasites
    c. Protection against hypothermia
    d. Active immunity from the sire

327. Which statement concerning newborn foals is true?
- **a.** Equine encephalitis vaccine should never be given to a newborn foal.
- **b.** An injection of tetanus antitoxin is recommended.
- **c.** Newborn foals should be kept in lateral recumbency for at least 2 hours.
- **d.** The umbilical cord should be severed.

328. The scientific name for heaves in horses is
- **a.** Chronic obstructive pulmonary disease
- **b.** Acute bronchopneumonia
- **c.** Tracheobronchitis
- **d.** Pulmonary embolism

329. Equine infectious anemia is diagnosed by
- **a.** Fecal examination
- **b.** Coggins test
- **c.** Blood culture
- **d.** Bangs test

330. The term *sleeping sickness* in horses refers to
- **a.** Strangles
- **b.** Distemper
- **c.** Encephalitis
- **d.** Tetanus

331. Scours in calves
- **a.** Is caused by *E. coli* only
- **b.** Requires treatment to replenish fluids
- **c.** Usually occurs at about 3 months of age
- **d.** Is seldom fatal

332. What area of the bovine body does hardware disease affect?
- **a.** Foot
- **b.** Abomasum
- **c.** Reticulum
- **d.** Intestine

333. Signs of snuffles in rabbits include
- **a.** Vomiting
- **b.** Diarrhea
- **c.** Splayed legs
- **d.** Chronic rhinitis

334. Contagious ecthyma (orf) is an infectious viral dermatitis of
- **a.** Swine
- **b.** Horses
- **c.** Cattle
- **d.** Sheep

335. Blue eye, or corneal edema, can occur with what canine disease or after vaccination against that disease?
- **a.** Toxocariasis
- **b.** Canine adenovirus infection
- **c.** Kennel cough
- **d.** Rabies

336. Two of the most common viral infections of dogs include
- **a.** Rickets and scurvy
- **b.** Pasteurellosis and staphylococcosis
- **c.** Canine distemper and canine hepatitis
- **d.** Toxoplasmosis and coccidioidomycosis

337. Feline infectious peritonitis is caused by a
- **a.** Bacterium
- **b.** *Rickettsia*
- **c.** Fungus
- **d.** Virus

338. Which of the following is not an infectious disease of small animals?
- **a.** Distemper
- **b.** Leptospirosis
- **c.** Patent ductus arteriosus
- **d.** Pneumonitis

339. What canine bacterial disease can be transmitted through the air by aerosolization of urine?
- **a.** Infectious hepatitis
- **b.** Leptospirosis
- **c.** Parvovirus infection
- **d.** Salmonellosis

340. What disease of monkeys that causes small sores in and around the mouth can be fatal to people?
- **a.** Tuberculosis
- **b.** B-virus encephalitis
- **c.** Salmonellosis
- **d.** Coccidiosis

341. Which of these animals is most likely to transmit the rabies virus to people?
- **a.** Marmot
- **b.** Fox
- **c.** Mule deer
- **d.** Bear

342. At what age should a dog or cat be first vaccinated against rabies?
- **a.** 3 weeks
- **b.** 10 weeks
- **c.** 12 weeks
- **d.** 16 weeks

Correct answers are on pages 427-429.

343. Against what disease should ferrets be
     vaccinated?
     a. Feline panleukopenia
     b. Feline rhinotracheitis
     c. Canine distemper
     d. Canine parvovirus infection

344. What organism causes diamond skin disease
     in pigs?
     a. Transmissible gastroenteritis virus
     b. *Erysipelothrix rhusiopathiae*
     c. *Haemophilus suis*
     d. *Bordetella bronchiseptica*

345. What disease is most dangerous in a herd of
     breeding horses?
     a. Influenza
     b. Strangles
     c. Rhinopneumonitis
     d. Chronic obstructive pulmonary disease

346. Which canine disease responds to antibiotic
     therapy?
     a. Canine distemper
     b. Parvovirus infection
     c. Canine adenovirus infection
     d. *Bordetella bronchiseptica* infection

347. What respiratory disease of cats causes
     ulcerative stomatitis?
     a. Rhinotracheitis
     b. Calicivirus infection
     c. Pneumonitis
     d. Distemper

348. Purpura hemorrhagica is a complication of
     what disease in horses?
     a. Rhinopneumonitis
     b. Infectious anemia
     c. Influenza
     d. Strangles

349. Which disinfectant is most effective against
     parvovirus?
     a. Chlorhexidine
     b. Povidone iodine
     c. Alcohol
     d. Sodium hypochlorite

350. Why are intranasal vaccines so effective
     against respiratory diseases?
     a. They kill all viruses as they are inhaled.
     b. Immunoglobulin A is produced at the site of
        virus entry.
     c. Given intranasally, they work with nasal
        mucus to increase protection.
     d. It is much easier to give them intranasally
        than subcutaneously or IM.

351. What disease of cats interferes with
     production of immunoglobulins during
     vaccination?
     a. *Toxascaris leonina* infection
     b. Cheyletiellosis
     c. Feline leukemia virus infection
     d. Coccidiosis

352. Bacterins are commonly used to vaccinate
     animals against all of the following except
     a. Blackleg
     b. Feline distemper
     c. Leptospirosis
     d. Borreliosis

353. What tissue is the preferred tissue to be
     submitted for rabies diagnosis?
     a. Heart
     b. Lung
     c. Brain
     d. Lymph node

354. What disease of cattle cannot be prevented by
     vaccination?
     a. Blackleg
     b. Botulism
     c. Malignant edema
     d. Brucellosis

355. *Campylobacter fetus*, which can cause abortion
     in cattle, is transmitted by
     a. Oral ingestion
     b. Inhalation
     c. Venereal contact
     d. Penetrating wounds

356. For what disease is the Coggins test used in
     diagnosis?
     a. Brucellosis
     b. Equine infectious anemia
     c. Tuberculosis
     d. Bovine leukemia

357. The rabies virus introduced by a bite from an
     infected animal travels from the bite area to
     the brain via
     a. Venous blood
     b. Lymph vessels
     c. Tissue diffusion
     d. Peripheral nerves

358. Probably the most prevalent serious viral
     infection of cats is
     a. Feline panleukopenia
     b. Leptospirosis
     c. Toxoplasmosis
     d. Cat-scratch fever

359. The two most common agents involved in feline respiratory disease complex for which vaccines exist are
a. Papovavirus and reovirus
b. Herpesvirus and calicivirus
c. Calicivirus and myxovirus
d. Herpesvirus and myxovirus

360. Infertility and abortion in cattle can be caused by
a. *Staphylococcus aureus*
b. Foot and mouth disease
c. *Campylobacter fetus*
d. Coronavirus diarrhea of calves

361. Which is the most common sign of ear mite infestation in cats?
a. Purulent discharge from the ear
b. Serosanguineous discharge from the ear
c. Ear flap hematomas
d. Persistent head shaking

362. Which of the following could be a symptom/sign of toxoplasmosis in people?
a. Subcutaneous, red tracts
b. Chronic cough
c. Abortion during first trimester
d. Chronic diarrhea

363. *Yersinia pestis* is most pathogenic to
a. Dogs
b. Cattle
c. Horses
d. Humans

364. What vaccine is used to vaccinate people against rabies?
a. Modified-live canine virus
b. Bacterin from monkeys
c. Human diploid cell vaccine
d. Killed chimpanzee virus

365. Rabbits can transmit what disease to people?
a. Syphilis
b. Herpesvirus infection
c. Leukemia
d. Tularemia

366. Which statement concerning zoonotic diseases is true?
a. Cat-scratch fever produces high fever in affected cats.
b. Ringworm is not transmitted from cats to people.
c. Human pinworms are not found in dogs or cats.
d. Rabies does not affect horses.

367. Which statement concerning zoonotic diseases is true?
a. Tuberculosis is never transmitted from dogs to people.
b. Histoplasmosis is seldom transmitted from dogs to people.
c. Animals with toxoplasmosis are always visibly ill.
d. Blastomycosis occurs in reptiles and amphibians only.

368. The incidence of trichinosis in people is decreased by
a. Feeding cooked garbage to hogs
b. Applying hydrated lime to the premises
c. Smoking meat before eating it
d. Eliminating rabbits from the farm

369. Which of the following is considered a potential vector for Lyme disease (borreliosis), which can cause severe human illness?
a. Flea
b. Mite
c. Tick
d. Louse

370. Which of these is an example of a disease transmitted by an arthropod vector?
a. Lice infestation transmitted by community use of a saddle blanket
b. Toxoplasmosis transmitted by contact with infective cat feces
c. Malaria transmitted from one person to another by a mosquito
d. Ascariasis transmitted by eating contaminated dirt

371. What condition is produced by a migrating *Toxocara canis* larva if it moves into a human brain?
a. Encephalitis
b. Elephantiasis
c. Strabismus
d. Brain tumor

372. A person who ingests *Toxocara canis* ova is most likely to develop
a. Visceral larva migrans
b. Cutaneous larva migrans
c. Creeping eruption
d. Anal pruritus

373. What area of the human body does creeping eruption affect?
a. Skin
b. Eye
c. Liver
d. Lung

Correct answers are on pages 427-429.

374. Which of these tapeworms uses people as its definitive host?
   a. *Dipylidium caninum*
   b. *Echinococcus granulosus*
   c. *Taenia pisiformis*
   d. *Taenia solium*

375. Which of these tapeworms uses people as intermediate hosts and causes the disease known as *hydatid disease*?
   a. *Taenia pisiformis*
   b. *Echinococcus granulosus*
   c. *Dipylidium caninum*
   d. *Taenia solium*

376. What defect can be produced in a human fetus exposed to *Toxoplasma gonii*?
   a. Hydrocephalus
   b. Down syndrome
   c. Spina bifida
   d. Dwarfism

377. If you are advising a pregnant woman to avoid *Toxoplasma gondii*, which of the following would you tell her?
   a. Store cat feces in an open container.
   b. Wear gloves while gardening to avoid contact with cat feces.
   c. Wash your hands after handling your dog.
   d. Avoid procedures involving horses.

378. How are people commonly exposed to *Giardia* from wild or domestic animals?
   a. Undercooked beef
   b. Infected feces
   c. Infected water supplies
   d. Infected animal blood

379. What condition must be reported to the Department of Health?
   a. Toxocariasis
   b. Ancylostomiasis
   c. Strongylosis
   d. Echinococcosis

380. People infected with *Dirofilaria immitis* via a mosquito could develop lesions in the
   a. Myocardium
   b. Glomeruli
   c. Alveoli of the lungs
   d. Cerebral cortex

381. Which statement concerning parasitism is true?
   a. Demodex is the tapeworm of people.
   b. Equine pinworms have major significance in people.
   c. *Toxocara canis* larvae can eat blood from the human intestine.
   d. *Echinococcus multilocularis* can use people as intermediate hosts.

382. What canine parasite can cause the disease called *visceral larva migrans* in children?
   a. *Toxocara canis*
   b. *Isospora*
   c. *Toxascaris leonina*
   d. *Trichuris vulpis*

383. People who own cats can be exposed to *Toxoplasma* oocysts from cat feces in a litter box. After being passed in the feces, the oocyst is
   a. Infectious immediately
   b. Infectious after 2 to 4 days
   c. Infectious after 24 hours
   d. Infectious after 1 to 5 hours

384. What disease can cause cyclic fever in people and can be contracted from cattle?
   a. Borreliosis
   b. Brucellosis
   c. Tetanus
   d. Malignant edema

385. Bubonic or pneumonic plague (*Yersinia pestis*) can be transmitted to people by the bite of
   a. Mosquitoes
   b. Rodent fleas
   c. Biting flies
   d. Ticks

386. Erysipeloid of people, caused by *Erysipelothrix rhusiopathiae*, is the result of wound infection with contaminated material. What farm animal is most likely to carry this organism?
   a. Horses
   b. Cattle
   c. Sheep
   d. Pigs

387. Psittacosis (ornithosis) is a chlamydial disease that people can develop from contact with infected animals. What species is most likely to transmit psittacosis to people?
   a. Ferret
   b. Cockatiel
   c. Llama
   d. Horse

388. People can contract tetanus, caused by *Clostridium tetani*, by
    a. Contact with sheep
    b. Wound infection from fecal contaminated soil
    c. Performing a necropsy on a hawk
    d. Performing a fecal examination on a dog

389. What fungus can cause ringworm in people?
    a. *Malassezia*
    b. *Cryptococcus*
    c. *Microsporum*
    d. *Brucella*

390. Tularemia, caused by *Francisella tularensis*, could infect people who perform which activity?
    a. Examining cat feces
    b. Vaccinating cattle
    c. Deworming horses
    d. Skinning rabbits

391. How can a person develop sarcocystosis?
    a. Eating contaminated beef
    b. Contact with avian blood samples
    c. Contact with llama saliva
    d. Bite by an infected mosquito

392. What species is the most likely source of tuberculosis (*Mycobacterium tuberculosis*) for people?
    a. Sheep
    b. Parrots
    c. Nonhuman primates
    d. Dogs

393. What disease is transmissible from horses to humans?
    a. Toxoplasmosis
    b. Leptospirosis
    c. Cryptococcosis
    d. Brucellosis

394. Eating raw or partially cooked salmon can infect people with what tapeworm?
    a. *Taenia*
    b. *Echinococcus*
    c. *Dipylidium*
    d. *Diphyllobothrium*

395. Eating raw or rare meat from which wild animal can cause trichinosis in people?
    a. Deer
    b. Bear
    c. Squirrel
    d. Antelope

396. Equine encephalomyelitis (EEE, WEE, VEE) is a viral disease that can be transmitted to people by the bite of an infected
    a. Tick
    b. Mite
    c. Louse
    d. Mosquito

397. What animal is the most likely reservoir for infectious hepatitis A for people contacting the animal's feces?
    a. Dog
    b. Horse
    c. Monkey
    d. Snake

398. Rabies is a fatal viral disease that is most likely to be transmitted to people by the bite of a
    a. Guinea pig
    b. Macaw
    c. Rhesus monkey
    d. Bat

399. What disease causes abortions in cattle, fistulous withers in horses, and undulant fever in people?
    a. Campylobacteriosis
    b. Leptospirosis
    c. Erysipelas
    d. Brucellosis

400. What coccidian is most likely to infect people who drink contaminated water?
    a. *Sarcocystis*
    b. *Eimeria*
    c. *Cryptosporidium*
    d. *Isospora*

ANSWERS

1. c If the tympanic membrane is ruptured, or a rupture is suspected, it would be harmful to the animal to place any type of antiseptic or cleaner into the tympanic cavity.

2. d Once decubital sores are present, they should be kept dry, because a moist environment only aids secondary bacterial infections and not healing.

3. **a** The question asks for quantity at one feeding, not over 24 hours, therefore 5%.

4. **a**

5. **a** As the name implies, there is a deficit or "downfall" of the pulse to accurately represent the pumping of the heart.

6. **c**

7. **a** Aspiration pneumonia is a risk with syringe feeding, but this risk can be minimized by ensuring that the animal's head is in a natural position and that the animal swallows each bolus.

8. **b** Isotonic fluids have an osmotic pressure approximately equal to that of extracellular fluid, and at body temperature, they are better assimilated into the body.

9. **a** Immunocompromised animals are highly susceptible to contracting diseases because of their altered immune state, therefore first cleaning these animals' cages, and following good isolation procedures, will minimize the risk to these already at-risk patients.

10. **d** Hypostatic pneumonia is the pooling of blood and a consequent decrease in the viability of the dependent lung. Most at risk are the old and sick patients in lateral recumbency.

11. **b** Electrical heating pads are not recommended unless the animal is to be under constant, dedicated supervision, because burns from pressure points and electrical fluctuations may occur.

12. **b**

13. **a** *Iso*, "to be in balance"; animal is unable to concentrate urine.

14. **b**

15. **c** Insulin is not absorbed efficiently via the gastrointestinal system.

16. **b** Milk fever is a common occurrence in dairy cattle (sometimes beef), which is generally associated with a high-producing cow after calving, when the calcium demands are highest; colostrum has twice the amount of calcium as regular milk. Calcium is "shifted" from muscle tissue to try to help demand.

17. **d** Hypersalivation is not a clinical sign associated with milk fever.

18. **c** Ketosis is when the cow is unable to meet her energy demands after calving and mobilizes stored energy, the catabolism of which produces ketones.

19. **a**

20. **d**

21. **c** Hypocalcemia occurs when the bitch is at peak lactation, generally around her fifth week of lactation; but depending on litter size and individual animals, it may occur earlier.

22. **c**

23. **b** Inactivated vaccines provide little to no cellular and mucosal immunity.

24. **c** *Leptospira*, although becoming increasingly more frequent as an administered vaccine, is currently not a core vaccine. Core vaccines are based on (1) severity of disease, (2) transmissibility, and (3) zoonotic potential.

25. **b** Colic has many causative factors, but it usually always manifests in some form of mild to severe abdominal pain.

26. **c** Cheyne-Stokes respiration is the rhythmic waxing and waning of respiration and is indicative of injury to the higher brain centers responsible for control of respiration.

27. **b**

28. **d** The facial artery is the most easily palpated and best accepted by the horse. Although the dorsal pedal artery is also fairly easily palpated, it is not considered the most accurate.

29. **c** Ballottement is usually performed in large animals, using the fist.

30. **b** All of the other choices have inherent risks associated with them because of the status of the animal; a pregnant dog or cat may easily have a cystocentesis, because this poses no risk to her or the fetuses.

31. **a**

32. **d** Pain relief is a basic right of any animal. Healing, whether it is medical or surgical, is greatly facilitated by the preemptive alleviation of painful stimuli.

33. **b**

34. **c** Routine blood sampling of horses is nearly always done from a jugular vein.

35. **d** Cat veins are smaller and more fragile than other species; the jugular vein provides a large vessel with easy access and minimal discomfort to the animal, and the sample is retrieved more efficiently from this vein than from the cephalic.

36. **b** In large animal IM injections, the needle is inserted first into the tissue without being attached to the syringe, in case the animal kicks or reacts adversely.

37. **c** Adhesive tape is perfectly acceptable to secure the bandage. However, because it has no elasticity to it (no give), if it completes 360 degrees, it can make a pressure point on the caudal (and to a lesser degree, the cranial) aspect of the bandage.

38. **c**

39. **c** Medial saphenous vein is generally not a vein used for sampling in any species, but in the rabbit, it is difficult, because the animal resists the restraint required. When other veins are still intact, they should always be chosen first.

40. **c** Clipping back overgrown nails should be done gradually so that the ("quick") ungual vein responds to the shortening of the nail and gradually regresses.

41. **b** PCV may be normal because of compensatory vasoconstriction and splenic contraction. Blood loss includes protein loss, for which there are no immediate compensatory mechanisms.

42. **b** All cats are considered to be of the same blood group.

43. **d** Stages of wound healing tend to overlap; however, for successful healing, it follows this route.

44. **c**

45. **b**

46. **c** Rabbits should not be held by the ears, and their backs should be supported.

47. **d** Birds need to expand their chest to breathe. It is safer to hold a bird's neck than a mammal's neck, because birds have complete tracheal rings.

48. **c** *Hyphema* means "blood in the eye."

49. **a**

50. **b** Rectal examinations are performed for special reasons and are not done on all patients.

51. **a**

52. **d** Cats can have normal heart rates up to 220 beats/min.

53. **d** Urine is concentrated (high specific gravity) in dehydrated animals.

54. **c** A small amount of bilirubin can be normal in dog urine.

55. **a** Porphyrins cause the urine of rabbits to look orange.

56. **a** Absorption in the lungs is quicker than in the mouth or under the skin.

57. **b** Adriamycin is caustic to tissues.

58. **c** The succinate (clear liquid solution) form of penicillin can be given IV.

59. **c** Tapazole comes in an oral form or can be compounded into a transdermal gel.

60. **c** Multiple blood samples can be obtained from a jugular catheter.

61. **c** Magnesium chloride is not a constituent of lactated Ringer solution.

62. **b** Fluids raise the blood pressure by increasing the volume of blood.

63. **d** Hetastarch has a higher molecular weight than the other fluids.

64. **c** Fluid overload increases the volume and workload on the heart.

65. **b** Wet-to-dry bandages debride necrotic tissue and do not disrupt delicate granulation tissue.

66. **c** A splint should stabilize the joint above and below a fracture. The shoulder joint is difficult to stabilize with a splint, because it tends to slip.

67. **b**

68. a

69. b After 4 hours, venous return will be compromised.

70. c *Second intention* means that the wound is allowed to contract on its own.

71. a Bacterial numbers are the main distinguishing factor in contaminated versus infected wounds.

72. a Wounds heal better in a dry rather than a moist environment, because bacteria grow better in moisture.

73. a Saline is closest to body fluids and therefore less irritating.

74. c A degloving wound has the skin removed from the bone and soft tissues.

75. d

76. a Male cockatiels have larger orange cheek patches and yellow heads; females have mostly gray heads.

77. d

78. c Finches, macaws, and parakeets eat different sizes of seeds.

79. d

80. b *Haemobartonella* is the parasite that causes feline infectious anemia (FIA).

81. a Parrots can be vaccinated for Pacheco disease and poxviruses. Chickens are vaccinated for Newcastle disease. Ferrets are vaccinated for distemper and rabies.

82. b Papillomavirus causes oral warts.

83. c Seizures and behavioral changes are the hallmark of canine distemper, but it can start with coughing.

84. d Skunks can carry rabies for long periods without showing signs of the disease.

85. d

86. b

87. d The tests for psittacosis are not very sensitive or specific. Only liver histopathology is diagnostic.

88. d

89. c Scabies is caused by host-specific mites. Canine mites live only a short time on humans.

90. a Cows developed bovine spongiform encephalopathy (BSE) after eating the offal of sheep with a similar disease, called *scrapie*. The offal was added to their diet as a protein source.

91. b Anthrax is caused by a bacteria that sporulates.

92. a Chemotherapy affects the fast-growing cells of the body, such as those in the gastrointestinal (GI) tract, bone marrow, and hair follicles.

93. a An occlusive bandage holds the exudate to the wound, causing more necrosis.

94. c Hypoplasia is the incomplete or less than normal development of an organ or tissue or cell.

95. c Excoriation is a secondary, self-induced lesion. A primary lesion is a lesion caused directly by disease.

96. c The Wood's lamp detects (fluoresces) certain species of *Microsporum canis*.

97. c Cystocentesis is the most sterile technique to obtain urine for culture and sensitivity.

98. b It is used for immobilization of fractures distal to the elbow or stifle before surgery. It stabilizes a fracture before surgery with its several layers of rolled cotton compressed tightly and therefore prevents constriction of the limb.

99. c Distemper vaccinations are started at 8 weeks with boosters 3 to 4 weeks apart. A killed rabies vaccine can be given at 12 weeks.

100. b An animal exposed to FeLV usually tests positive within 4 to 8 weeks following exposure. If the test is positive, a follow-up FeLV test should be done in 3 to 4 weeks. If it is still positive, a Hardy test/immunofluorescent assay (IFA) should be done.

101. b Coal tar causes toxicity in cats and is irritating to the tissue.

102. b Dextrose is an unbalanced hypotonic solution and may cause sloughing.

103. d *Bradycardia* means "slow heart rate."

104. **c** The pulmonic valve is at the left third inter-costal space, the aortic valve at the left fourth intercostal space, and the mitral valve at the left fifth intercostal space.

105. **b** *Pyrexia* is a medical term for "fever."

106. **d** A Velpeau sling is used to support the shoulder joint after surgery.

107. **c**

108. **d** Normal sinus arrhythmia is a nonpathologic arrhythmia.

109. **b** Nystagmus is an involuntary, constant movement of the eye in a horizontal or vertical motion.

110. **a** The fluorescein dye test is a diagnostic test to detect corneal injury by placing dye onto the surface of the cornea.

111. **c** Grasping the carpal joint prevents injury to the bird.

112. **a** The esophagus deviates to the right and down the neck. At the thoracic inlet, its ventral wall expands to form the crop, which bulges to the right.

113. **a** The pectoral muscles are located on either side of the keel.

114. **d** The proximal tibial bone is used for intraosseous administration of fluids and some medications.

115. **a** The P wave is the first deflection, representing excitation or depolarization of the atria.

116. **b** The T wave results from recovery or repolarization of the ventricles.

117. **c** Potassium is an intracellular cation, and there is no constancy of relationships between extracellular and intracellular potassium. With acidosis, cells tend to take in hydrogen and give up potassium.

118. **a** The animal becomes acidotic because of problems with respiration (poor ventilation) that cause an increase in blood PCO_2 with a resulting decrease in blood pH (acidosis).

119. **c** *OD* means right eye, *OS* means left eye, and *OU* means both eyes.

120. **c** Exercise is usually detrimental to these conditions, because it places unneeded strain on the systems mentioned.

121. **b** Metabolic requirements of the patient should be exceeded to give the patient an energy reserve to fight the current disease, but excessive calories would increase the stress on the systems to dispose of the excess and may lead to obesity.

122. **d** Pharyngostomy tubes are used to force-feed a patient.

123. **a** Silver nitrate is a simple, effective, and inexpensive method to cauterize a broken nail.

124. **d** Most otitis externa cases have clinical signs that are the result of bacteria or yeast infections or both.

125. **d** Flushing the ear when the tympanic membrane is ruptured can lead to the extension of the infection to the middle ear.

126. **d** The anal sacs store secretions that are produced by the anal gland.

127. **a** Four o'clock and 8 o'clock positions are the normal positions for the openings of the anal sacs.

128. **c** Decubital ulcers are bedsores that result from pressure or prolonged exposure to urine contamination combined with pressure.

129. **a** The colostrum is the major source of antibodies in young puppies.

130. **a** Passive antibodies are passed from the mother to the puppy and provide temporary protection to the puppy in the first few weeks to months of its life.

131. **c** Most vaccine manufacturers recommend a final vaccination for canine distemper and hepatitis at 16 weeks of age to prevent maternal antibody interference.

132. **b** Most modern vaccines are either modified live or killed (inactivated).

133. **c** Older animals often have compromised immune systems, and vaccine procedures should not be reduced unless titers are taken to establish immune status.

134. **d** Mixed vaccines are viable for 1 hour at room temperature if they are kept in the dark, away from ultraviolet light.

135. **a** Degenerative joint disease is most often diagnosed in older patients.

136. **c** Overextension of the stomach results in vomition immediately following gavage.

137. **b** This distance places the tip of the feeding tube in the stomach.

138. **d** Most formula amounts are calculated based on a volume of 9 ml/kg stomach capacity for puppies and kittens.

139. **b** Puppies should gain 10% to 20% of their birth weight in the first week of life.

140. **c** Rectal thermometers have a round bulb and a mercury constriction to stop the mercury from falling until the thermometer can be read.

141. **b** Rectal temperature is considered to be 2 degrees higher than peripheral body temperature.

142. **a** The easiest and most convenient artery for discerning pulse rate is the femoral, located on the medial side of the hind leg, mid thigh.

143. **b** Palmar and plantar arteries are convenient to tape the Doppler sensors to, and, because these vessels are close to the surface, they give good arterial sounds.

144. **a** A *deficit* means to lag behind and refers to the pulse rate lagging behind the actual heartbeat.

145. **b** Inspiration and expiration should be monitored and counted together as one breath.

146. **d** *Tachypnea* is a rapid respiration rate.

147. **c** *Dyspnea* means painful, difficult breathing.

148. **b** PCV, plasma protein, and urine specific gravity, when taken together, give a good picture of the patient's fluid status.

149. **d** Weight can give a rough assessment of fluids retained.

150. **b** Only isotonic solutions can be properly absorbed when given subcutaneously.

151. **c** Subcutaneous fluids are absorbed in 5 to 8 hours and are often administered three times daily.

152. **a** Intraperitoneal route for fluid therapy is the poorest and slowest route for absorption and the route most likely to result in secondary medical problems.

153. **c** Low osmotic pressure in the plasma combined with slow movement of the blood results in pooling of the blood in the lungs and pulmonary edema.

154. **b** Central venous pressure measures fluid pressure in the right atrium or anterior vena cava.

155. **c** A manometer is used to measure the pressure in the catheter during the central venous pressure procedure.

156. **b** Three readings are taken and averaged for the final central venous pressure measurement.

157. **b** Normal canine central venous pressure readings are in the range of 0 to 5 cm of H_2O.

158. **c** PCV can be inaccurate in assessing blood loss early in acute hemorrhage because of vasoconstriction and a large influx of RBCs resulting from splenic contraction.

159. **b** Platelets survive in stored blood for up to 12 hours.

160. **d** Increased hemolysis may be the result of a transfusion in cases of autoimmune hemolytic anemia. Transfusion is used in life-threatening situations only, and only absolute minimal numbers of RBCs are used.

161. **c** Blood transfusions are given at body temperature, and prolonged warming is not recommended.

162. **a** Delayed reactions usually occur in the first 2 to 20 days after transfusion.

163. **c** Hot or cold compresses are applied for 20-minute intervals with frequent rewarming or cooling changes during this time period.

164. **d** Potassium hydroxide clears the hair and allows the ringworm spores to be visualized.

165. **a** Alcohol kills bacteria in the area that may inhibit fungal culture attempts.

166. **b** Surgical scrub removes surface contaminants, and a deep scraping limits culturing of surface contaminants.

167. **b** Multiple scrapings are often necessary to find a single sarcoptic mite.

168. **b** Benzoyl-peroxide shampoo is too harsh for regular grooming but does flush organisms out of the hair follicles. Tar shampoos are preferred for their degreasing attributes.

169. **b** Long-handle neck tongs can be used to help apply a snout rope, which is a better means of restraint.

170. **c** The normal body temperature of a sheep is about 103° F, with a range of 102° to 104° F.

171. **a** The sheep is usually the easiest to handle, because it is less aggressive than the others listed.

172. **d** Although all are good skills, self-confidence is the most important.

173. **b** The other signs indicate hypothermia.

174. **c** The other signs indicate hyperthermia.

175. **b**

176. **d** Attempts to control an extremely agitated cat often end with injury to the cat through use of excessive force.

177. **b** Cats respond best when the least amount of restraint is applied to the extent necessary for the procedure being performed.

178. **a** Lifting the head over the neck may cause injury, whereas turning the head to the side helps set the animal on its haunches.

179. **d** When pressure is applied to the upper jaw, a pig will pull back, which can be used to guide the animal.

180. **b** Safety of the people working on the animal should always be the primary concern, although the safety of the animal must also be taken into consideration.

181. **a** b: Horse, c: Cat, d: Rat

182. **d** The normal rectal temperature of an adult cat is 100° to 102° F.

183. **b**

184. **a** Casting is a means of restraint by applying ropes to pull the animal down on its side and is used mainly when a chute is not available.

185. **c** It is best to approach the horse at a 45-degree angle from the left shoulder, because this is what most horses are accustomed to.

186. **d** A halter is the most common horse restraint and the first tool usually used; the others may be used if more restraint is needed to perform a procedure.

187. **a** Normal capillary refill time is 1 to 3 seconds for a dog.

188. **b**

189. **d** Needle circumference decreases as the gauge number increases.

190. **c** The tail vein is rarely used to draw blood from a dog.

191. **a** The saphenous vein is found lateral to the hock.

192. **b** The cephalic is found on the front leg.

193. **b** Alcohol prolongs bleeding time.

194. **a**

195. **c** The popliteal lymph node is located behind the stifle.

196. **d** An otoscope is used to examine ears.

197. **d** In sternal recumbency, the animal's chest and abdomen are adjacent to the table.

198. **a** The bevel of the needle should be pointed upward.

199. **b** Before administering any injection, you should aspirate to check for blood.

200. **c**

201. **a** The quadriceps muscle is a good choice for IM injections.

202. **b**

203. **c**

204. d

205. b

206. b 60 seconds is the minimum, or until the mercury stops rising.

207. c

208. a

209. b

210. d

211. b

212. a

213. a

214. b

215. a

216. c

217. d Megakaryocytes are multinucleated bone marrow cells that produce platelets by breaking off pieces of cytoplasm.

218. c

219. a

220. d

221. a

222. c

223. b

224. a

225. d

226. b

227. d

228. c

229. b

230. d

231. b

232. d

233. d

234. b

235. d

236. b

237. d

238. c

239. a

240. c

241. d

242. a

243. b

244. c

245. b

246. d Dry mucous membranes are a sign of dehydration.

247. a Oral fluid administration is the preferred method because of reduced expense, ease of administration, and safety.

248. c Beyond 3 days, the patency of the catheter decreases, and the risk of infection increases.

249. b

250. d A dextrose solution with a concentration greater than 2.5% given subcutaneously could cause sloughing of skin and abscess formation.

251. d

252. a

253. a

254. c

255. d

256. a

257. **b** Bandaging promotes an acidic environment at the wound surface by preventing carbon dioxide loss and absorbing ammonia produced by bacteria.

258. **d** Covering a wound provides an acidic environment, which increases oxygen dissociation from hemoglobin and thus increases oxygen availability in the wound.

259. **a** Fiberglass is known for its rapid setting time.

260. **b** A Robert Jones bandage provides stability through compression of many cotton layers; a modified Robert Jones is less bulky and provides little or no splinting capabilities.

261. **b**

262. **d**

263. **d** The hock is angled and therefore more difficult to splint. The carpus and fetlock would be more easily splinted, because they have no angulation. Stifles are never splinted.

264. **d**

265. **d**

266. **b**

267. **a**

268. **b**

269. **d** If the infection is not under control, a compression bandage may force bacteria and associated toxic products deeper into the tissues.

270. **a**

271. **a**

272. **c**

273. **a**

274. **b**

275. **b** A Basenji can make a sound, but that sound is not considered a bark.

276. **d** Manx; all of the other breeds listed have a long tail.

277. **a** Urate crystals are seen more abundantly in the urine of Dalmatians than of other breeds.

278. **d** Hip dysplasia is most commonly seen in dogs whose mature weight is greater than 40 pounds.

279. **b** The Nubian has long, wide, pendulous ears and a Roman nose.

280. **c** The LaMancha has almost no external ears (*gopher ears*) or extremely short ears (*elf ears*).

281. **a** The Saanen is a large, all-white breed of goat.

282. **b**

283. **a** The whippet and other thin breeds of dog require much less thiobarbiturate because they lack body fat.

284. **c**

285. **d** The Jersey produces milk with an average butterfat content of 4.73%.

286. **a**

287. **b** The dachshund, a chondroplastic breed, is commonly affected with intervertebral disk disease.

288. **b** The Saint Bernard, a large, deep-chested breed, is highly susceptible to gastric dilatation and torsion (bloat).

289. **c** The miniature poodle is frequently affected by inherited idiopathic epilepsy.

290. **b** The Leghorn lays white eggs, whereas the other three breeds lay brown eggs.

291. **c** Entropion, or infolding of the eyelid, is frequently seen in the Shar-Pei.

292. **a** The Pekingese is a brachycephalic or short-nose breed.

293. **d** Of the four breeds listed, only the Old English sheepdog has its tail docked.

294. **c** Of the breeds listed, only the Doberman pinscher has its ears cropped.

295. **d** The Angus is a breed of beef cattle. All others are breeds of dairy cattle.

296. **a** The Peruvian guinea pig is long coated; all others are short coated.

297. **d** The Abyssinian is the only rough-coated breed of guinea pig.

298. **d**

299. **c** The Himalayan has the full coat of the Persian with the pale coloring and darker parts of the Siamese.

300. **b** The Limousin is gold, the Charolais is white, and the Hereford is red with a white face.

301. **a** The Siamese frequently has genetically induced crossed eyes and a bend at the distal end of the tail.

302. **d** The bloodhound is frequently used in tracking.

303. **a** The greyhound makes an ideal blood donor because of its short hair and long straight veins and because most lack the A factor.

304. **d** The Scottish fold first appeared in Scotland as a result of a spontaneous mutation in the 1960s. It has folded ears, a short nose, and large round eyes.

305. **c** The Suffolk is a meat breed, whereas the others are used for their wool or pelt.

306. **d** The dominant gene for a white coat also predisposes to deafness.

307. **b**

308. **d** The collie has a high incidence of an underdeveloped retina.

309. **a** The Holstein has an average milk yield of over 20,000 lb per year.

310. **c** The poodle, while shedding, retains loose hair within its hair coat, which predisposes it to mat formation.

311. **c** The Persian cat, as a result of its long hair, is most likely to develop hairballs.

312. **b** The Welsh is a pony.

313. **a** The Clydesdale is a draft horse used for pulling.

314. **a**

315. **c** The larger the animal, the lower its basal metabolic rate and, consequently, the anesthetic agent is more slowly metabolized.

316. **b** The English bulldog, because of respiratory difficulty, is especially prone to heat stroke.

317. **d** The Boston terrier, because of its large head, is frequently born by cesarean section.

318. **d**

319. **b**

320. **c** The malamute and other northern breeds are considered to have the greatest tendency to exhibit destructive behavior.

321. **d**

322. **a** The Cornish is a meat breed, whereas the others are bred primarily for eggs.

323. **c** The collie descended from Scottish herding dogs.

324. **c** Hypoxia from low oxygen pressure is seen in cattle that live at high altitudes.

325. **c** Tetanus antitoxin and tetanus toxoid are given together. The antitoxin immediately supplies immunoglobulins against tetanus; the toxoid causes the equine lymphocytes to produce immunoglobulin for long-term protection.

326. **a** Passive immunity from the dam protects the newborn against diseases to which the dam has developed immunity.

327. **b** Tetanus toxoid is given at 4 months. Encephalitis vaccine is given at 6 to 8 months. Never sever an umbilical cord, because it will keep hemorrhaging and could exsanguinate (bleed out) the foal.

328. **a**

329. **b**

330. **c** a: Bacterial respiratory infection, b: Viral infection, d: Causes rigidity and convulsions

331. **b** Electrolytes are used to treat scours from almost any cause. Specific treatment for bacterial infection and supportive treatment for viral scours are also needed.

332. **c** Metal objects can lodge in the reticulum and penetrate to the liver and pericardium of ruminants, especially cattle.

333. **d** Snuffles is an acute, subacute, or chronic inflammation of the nasal passages of rabbits. It is caused by *Pasteurella*.

334. **d**

335. **b** Canine adenovirus infection (infectious canine hepatitis) or vaccination with a modified-live virus can result in corneal edema.

336. **c**

337. **d** Feline infectious peritonitis is caused by a virus but is also associated with immunodeficiencies caused by feline leukemia virus or feline immunodeficiency virus infection.

338. **c** Patent ductus arteriosus is a congenital cardiac abnormality.

339. **b** Leptospirosis is a renal disease. The bacteria are found in the urine of an infected animal.

340. **b** B-virus of monkeys can cause encephalitis in people.

341. **b** Foxes, bats, raccoons, and skunks are the most common wild animals involved in transmission of the rabies virus.

342. **c** Killed rabies vaccine is given at 12 weeks or older in dogs and cats.

343. **c**

344. **b** Diamond skin disease of swine, including potbellied pigs, is caused by the bacterium *Erysipelothrix*.

345. **c** Rhinopneumonitis in horses can cause pregnant mares to abort and induces upper respiratory tract disease.

346. **d** *Bordetella bronchiseptica* is a bacterial pathogen that should respond to antibiotics. The other choices are viral diseases, which do not respond to antibiotics.

347. **b** Calicivirus infections in cats cause ulcers of the mouth.

348. **d** Strangles, caused by *Streptococcus equi*, can result in purpura.

349. **d** Sodium hypochlorite (Clorox bleach) is the most effective disinfectant against parvovirus.

350. **b** Immunoglobulin A is formed in the mucous membranes of the nasal passages; as a result, it quickly produces immunity.

351. **c** Leukemia virus infection causes immunodepression, which prevents lymphocytes from producing immunoglobulin after vaccination.

352. **b** Feline distemper is a parvoviral disease; the others are bacterial diseases, which can be prevented by using a bacterin.

353. **c** Rabies virus causes Negri bodies to form in the brain, and these can be used to diagnose the disease in the laboratory.

354. **b** Vaccines are available for blackleg, malignant edema, and brucellosis, but not for botulism.

355. **c** The venereal route is the usual means of transmission for *Campylobacter* infection.

356. **b** Equine infectious anemia is diagnosed by blood samples and the Coggins test.

357. **d**

358. **a** Feline panleukopenia (feline distemper) is the most serious viral disease of those listed. *Leptospira* is a bacterial spirochete. Cat-scratch fever is caused by a gram-negative bacterium; it occurs in people, not in cats.

359. **b** Herpesvirus and calicivirus are the most common agents associated with feline respiratory diseases.

360. **c** *Campylobacter* (Vibrio) can cause infertility and abortion in cattle.

361. **c** *Otodectes cynotis* can cause irritation in the ear canal, which may result in a hematoma when the cat tries to scratch the ear.

362. **c**

363. **d** Of the species listed, *Yersinia pestis* (plague) occurs most often in people.

364. **c**

365. **d** Tularemia, caused by the bacterium *Francisella tularensis*, is a zoonotic disease.

366. **c** Human pinworms (*Enterobius*) are not found in dogs or cats.

367. **b** Histoplasmosis is seldom transmitted from dogs to people.

368. **a** Cooking kills *Trichinella* larvae in the garbage. Cooking meat to 158° F before eating also kills the larvae. Smoking the meat does not affect the larvae.

369. **c** *Ixodes* and other ticks can transmit *Borrelia* from deer to mice to people and dogs.

370. **c** An arthropod vector involves transmission of disease from animal to animal or from animal to person via an insect.

371. **a** Migrating ascarid larvae in people can cause encephalitis.

372. **a** Visceral larva migrans occurs in people when *Toxocara canis* larvae enter the human body by ingestion.

373. **a** *Ancylostoma caninum* larvae can burrow through intact skin, including human skin, and cause intense pruritus.

374. **d** The larval and adult stages of *Taenia solium*, the beef tapeworm, can live in people or cattle; therefore, it is a zoonotic disease.

375. **b** *Echinococcus granulosus* is a tapeworm that can infect people who ingest the ova. The person becomes the intermediate host, and the cysts that form can cause space-occupying lesions that can be fatal.

376. **a** *Toxoplasma gondii* that is ingested by a pregnant woman can result in hydrocephalus (water on the brain) in the developing fetus.

377. **b** Cats can transmit *Toxoplasma gondii* to people. Cats defecate in gardens, and the woman might come into contact with the feces while gardening.

378. **c** Water-borne *Giardia* is the most common method of transmitting the parasite to people.

379. **d** *Echinococcus granulosus* and *Echinococcus multilocularis* can infect people and cause severe or fatal disease; therefore, infected animals should be reported to prevent human disease.

380. **c** *Dirofilaria immitis* in people can cause coin lesions on radiographic examination of the lungs, because this is the capillary bed where the microfilariae are trapped.

381. **d** *Echinococcus multilocularis* ova ingested by people can cause cysts in the lungs.

382. **a** *Toxocara canis* larvae migrate in the human body if ingested and can cause multiple lesions, including retinitis and blindness.

383. **b** Oocysts are not infectious until they sporulate, which takes 2 to 4 days after they are passed in feces.

384. **b** Brucellosis in people is called *undulant fever*.

385. **b** The rodent flea is the most common source of plague transmitted from animals to people. People can also become infected by inhaling the organism.

386. **d** Pigs get diamond skin disease from *Erysipelothrix*, which can become a wound contaminant in people who contact an infected pig.

387. **b** Psittacosis is primarily an avian respiratory disease, but it can also infect people.

388. **b** Wound infection is the most common method of tetanus infection in people.

389. **c** *Microsporum* and *Trichophyton* are dermatophytes of animals that can cause the skin lesions or ringworm in people.

390. **d** Wound contact with infected rabbits can cause tularemia in people.

391. **a** *Sarcocystis* is a protozoan parasite that can infect people who eat raw or undercooked beef, pork, or lamb.

392. **c** Monkeys with tuberculosis cough up the organism, and people may inhale the bacteria and develop the disease.

393. **b** *Leptospira* infection (Leptospirosis) is a bacterial disease associated with dogs, livestock (including horses), rodents, and wildlife.

394. **d** *Diphyllobothrium* is the broad fish tapeworm. People contract the parasite by eating raw salmon. This can occur when improperly prepared sushi is served.

395. **b** Bears that eat from garbage dumps may develop trichinosis.

396. d The mosquito is the major vector of equine encephalomyelitis. People bitten by infected mosquitoes can develop the disease, which can be fatal.

397. c Nonhuman primates are the most common source of zoonotic infections.

398. d Bats are one of the most common animals to become rabid, and they can infect people by biting.

399. d *Brucella abortus* causes disease in cattle, horses, and people.

400. c *Cryptosporidium* is a protozoan parasite of cattle and other animals that can contaminate water supplies and infect people who drink the water.

Diagnostic Imaging

Joann Colville

Questions

1. Which of the following is a physical property of x-rays?
   a. Travel in straight lines
   b. Refract and reflect similar to visible light
   c. Are visible in the dark
   d. May be deflected by magnets

2. As the wavelength of x-ray photons shortens, the energy of the x-ray beam will
   a. Stay the same
   b. Lengthen
   c. Decrease
   d. Increase

3. The kVp setting on an x-ray machine controls the
   a. Quality of the x-ray beam
   b. Quantity of x-ray beams
   c. Number of electrons emitted
   d. Focal spot size

4. The milliampere-seconds (mAs) setting on an x-ray machine controls the
   a. Quality of the beam
   b. Quantity of x-rays emitted
   c. Speed of electrons emitted
   d. Wavelength of the beam

5. During an exposure, electrons in the x-ray tube travel from the
   a. Anode to the cathode
   b. Anode to the target
   c. Cathode to the anode
   d. Cathode to the filament

6. To produce x-rays, a great deal of energy in an x-ray tube is converted into heat. The ratio of heat generated to x-ray production is generally considered to be
   a. 1%:99%
   b. 99%:1%
   c. 50%:50%
   d. 75%:25%

7. The acceleration of the electrons and their ultimate striking energy is determined by the
   a. Milliamperage (mA)
   b. Kilovoltage (kVp)
   c. Milliamperage-seconds (mAs)
   d. Exposure time (Time)

8. When depressing the "prep" switch on a rotating anode x-ray machine, you are effectively
   a. Determining the acceleration of the electrons
   b. Taking the exposure
   c. Heating up the focal spot and spinning the rotating anode
   d. Heating up the filament and spinning the rotating anode

9. Regarding the production of x-rays in the x-ray tube, the
   a. Purpose of the anode is to provide a source of electrons
   b. Target and focal spot are provided by the cathode
   c. Cathode side of the tube is positively charged, and the anode is negatively charged
   d. Cathode includes the filament and the focusing cup

10. What transformer in an x-ray machine controls the temperature of the filament?
    a. Step-up transformer
    b. Step-down transformer
    c. Autotransformer
    d. Self-rectifying transformer

11. The heel effect is going to be more noticeable with
    a. Larger film, longer focal-film distance, and higher kVp
    b. Larger film, shorter focal-film distance, and lower kVp
    c. Smaller film, shorter focal-film distance, and higher kVp
    d. Smaller film, longer focal-film distance, and lower kVp

441

Correct answers are on pages 465-478.

12. *Full-wave rectification* means that
    a. The bottom half of alternating current is not used.
    b. The machine performs its own rectification.
    c. 60 pulses of x-rays are produced per second.
    d. 120 pulses of x-rays are produced per second.

13. What is the minimum distance in feet that a safelight in the darkroom should be away from the work site?
    a. 2
    b. 3
    c. 4
    d. 5

14. If using both blue- and green-sensitive films, what type of safelight should you use?
    a. Amber
    b. Blue
    c. Green
    d. Red

15. The main purpose of the x-ray developer is to
    a. Clear away the unexposed, undeveloped silver halide crystals
    b. Convert the exposed silver halide crystals into black metallic silver
    c. Reduce the unexposed silver halide crystals into black metallic silver
    d. Swell and soften the emulsion

16. The main purpose of the x-ray fixer is to
    a. Clear away the unexposed, undeveloped silver halide crystals
    b. Convert the exposed silver halide crystals into black metallic silver
    c. Reduce the unexposed silver halide crystals into black metallic silver
    d. Swell and soften the emulsion

17. A safelight illumination test was performed in the darkroom. On processing the film, you see various gradations of blackness on your film. The area exposed for the longest period of time is
    a. Green
    b. Clear
    c. Slightly gray
    d. Darkest

18. After you manually process a film, you notice that there is a green area of about 1/2 inch along one narrow edge of the film. This is due to the area not being
    a. Developed
    b. Fixed
    c. Developed or fixed
    d. Exposed to radiation

19. You notice that there is a clear line at the top of the shorter edge of a radiograph that you have manually processed. This is due to the area not being
    a. Developed
    b. Fixed
    c. Developed or fixed
    d. Collimated

20. You are looking at a film that is totally clear except for a bit of black that you notice along the edges. Your film has not been
    a. Developed
    b. Fixed
    c. Developed or fixed
    d. Exposed to radiation

21. You have a film in front of you that has a relatively clear edge all the way around the radiograph. This is because of
    a. A light leak
    b. Collimation
    c. Not being developed or fixed
    d. Overexposure to radiation

22. The remaining silver halide crystals from exposed x-ray film are removed in the
    a. Fixer
    b. Developer
    c. Wash water
    d. Storage envelope

23. Which of the following would cause the image on a processed x-ray film to be fogged?
    a. Two films in the same cassette
    b. kVp too low
    c. Film stored in an area of high room temperature
    d. Focal-film distance too long

24. What should be the maximum intensity of the bulb in a safelight in developing rooms?
    a. 2.5 watts
    b. 7.5 watts
    c. 15 watts
    d. 60 watts

25. A bullet fragment on a film appears as a
    a. Black mark
    b. Diffuse greenish gray area
    c. Clear mark
    d. White mark

26. A crease in the film after exposure but before processing will likely appear as a
    a. Black crescent mark
    b. White crescent mark
    c. Clear crescent mark
    d. Diffuse grayish black area

27. Safelight fogging on a radiograph appears as a
    a. Black mark
    b. White mark
    c. Clear mark
    d. Diffuse grayish area

28. The cells that are most susceptible to the hazards of ionizing radiation are
    a. The rapidly dividing cells of the intestinal lining, neoplastic cells, and gonad cells
    b. The connective tissue cells of bone, cartilage, and tendons
    c. The rapidly dividing cells of bone, lymphatics, and skin and leukocytes and hemopoietic cells
    d. All of the cells of the body

29. A sievert (Sv) is the
    a. Film badge that contains lithium fluoride compounds
    b. Radiation that occurs when the primary beam interacts with matter
    c. Unit of radiation dose equivalent to the absorbed dose in tissue
    d. Unit of absorbed dose imparted by ionizing radiation

30. A radiation film badge worn at the collar level
    a. Determines the type of radiation exposure
    b. Monitors exposure of the thyroid gland and lenses of the eyes
    c. Monitors primary beam exposure
    d. Informs everyone you are radiographing an animal

31. When taking radiographs, you should whenever possible use
    a. Increased exposure time, decreased distance from radiation sources, and increased shielding
    b. Increased exposure time, increased distance from radiation sources, and increased shielding
    c. Decreased exposure time, increased distance from radiation sources, and increased shielding
    d. Decreased exposure time, increased distance from radiation sources, and decreased shielding

32. There is a gloved hand visible on a radiograph. This is
    a. Not a problem, because shielding protects you from primary radiation
    b. Not a problem, because shielding protects you from secondary radiation
    c. An interesting artifact that appears black
    d. A real concern, because the hand has been exposed to radiation

33. A small filament produces an image of
    a. Equal detail to a large filament
    b. Lesser detail to a large filament
    c. Greater detail than a large filament
    d. Greater intensity than a large filament

34. You are preparing to take a radiograph, and you want to confirm that you have set the correct mAs of 15. Which of the following scenarios will give you 15 mAs?
    a. 300 mA and 1/10 sec
    b. 300 mA and 1/20 sec
    c. 150 mA and 1/15 sec
    d. 150 mA and 1/20 sec

35. If you were going to decrease the focal-film distance from 100 cm to 50 cm, what should your new mAs be if the old mAs was 16?
    a. 2.0 mAs
    b. 4.0 mAs
    c. 8 mAs
    d. 32 mAs

36. Scatter radiation on a film is more noticeable if there is
    a. Lower kVp, thicker patient, and larger field size
    b. Lower kVp, thinner patient, and smaller field size
    c. Higher kVp, thicker patient, and smaller field size
    d. Higher kVp, thicker patient, and larger field size

37. To get more density on a film, you should do what to the kVp and mAs?
    a. Decrease one and increase the other
    b. Decrease both
    c. Increase either or both
    d. Only increase kVp, because mAs does not affect density

38. Sante's rule states that when setting up a technique chart, you should use what base kVp for the abdomen?
    a. (2 × thickness [cm]) + 100
    b. (2 × thickness [cm]) + 40
    c. (2 × thickness [in]) + 100
    d. (2 × thickness [in]) + 40

39. Because of the relationship between milliamp (mA) and mAs, as you increase the mA, you can
    a. Decrease the length of the exposure, so that there is less chance of movement
    b. Decrease the length of the exposure, so that there is more chance of movement
    c. Increase the length of the exposure, so that there is more chance of movement
    d. Increase the kVp, which means no change in density

Correct answers are on pages 465-478.

40. The crystals of high-speed screens, as compared to similar types of par screens, are
    a. Bigger, and there is less detail
    b. Bigger, and there is more detail
    c. Smaller, and there is more detail
    d. Smaller, and there is less detail

41. The main advantage of fast-speed screens and films is that
    a. The films can be processed more quickly.
    b. X-rays can directly affect the film without fluorescing the screens.
    c. Lower exposure factors can be used, which can allow use of a smaller focal spot.
    d. The system is not as costly.

42. If using rare-earth screens, what spectrum of light must the film be sensitive to?
    a. Blue range
    b. Green range
    c. Violet range
    d. Red range

43. You are looking at a radiograph that appears gray overall. This is best described as a
    a. High-contrast film with few steps but large changes between each step
    b. High-contrast film with many steps but small changes between each step
    c. Low-contrast film with few steps but large changes between each step
    d. Low-contrast film with many steps but few changes between each step

44. A radiograph in front of you appears dark. You note that the bones are gray. You are best to do what for the next radiograph?
    a. Decrease kVp
    b. Decrease mAs
    c. It really does not matter which setting you decrease.
    d. Increase kVp or mAs

45. *Grid cutoff* can be described as
    a. The improvement of scatter noted with the use of one grid over another
    b. Not using the grid when exposing a tabletop radiograph
    c. Incorrect use of the grid, so that the grid absorbs more radiation than it should
    d. Incorrect use of the grid, so that the grid absorbs less radiation than it should

46. You have taken a radiograph using 10 mAs and 60 kVp. To double the radiographic density for a second film, you should use
    a. 100 mA, 1/5 sec, 66 kVp
    b. 150 mA, 1/10 sec, 60 kVp
    c. 200 mA 1/10 sec, 60 kVp
    d. 300 mA, 1/10 sec, 60 kVp

47. You want to set up an abdominal radiography technique chart. All of the following factors should be standardized except
    a. Whether to use a grid
    b. The type of film used
    c. Focal-film distance
    d. The kVp used

48. Low mAs, high kVp techniques are recommended for abdominal radiography in dogs, because they
    a. Produce radiographs with higher contrast
    b. Produce radiographs with lower contrast
    c. Require increased exposure times
    d. Do not necessitate use of a grid

49. A grid with a ratio of 10:1 absorbs
    a. Less scatter radiation and requires less exposure factors than a 5:1 grid
    b. Less scatter radiation and requires greater exposure factors than a 5:1 grid
    c. More scatter radiation and requires greater exposure factors than a 5:1 grid
    d. More scatter radiation and requires less exposure factors than a 5:1 grid

50. A dog is lying in left lateral recumbency for a pelvis radiograph. The right femur will be
    a. Less magnified because of increased focal-film distance and decreased object-film distance
    b. Less magnified because of decreased focal-film distance and increased object-film distance
    c. More magnified because of decreased focal-film distance and increased object-film distance
    d. More magnified because of increased focal-film distance and decreased object-film distance

51. In a lateral pelvic projection, the affected limb should be
    a. Closest to the film and pulled slightly caudally
    b. Closest to the film and pulled slightly cranially
    c. Farthest from the film and pulled slightly cranially
    d. Farthest from the film and pulled slightly caudally

52. The term *dorsomedial-plantarolateral oblique* is in reference to the
    a. Metatarsus
    b. Stifle
    c. Metatarsus and stifle
    d. Carpus

53. The term *dorsomedial-plantarolateral oblique* means that the x-ray beam is directed at the
    a. Dorsal limb aspect, and the film is against the medial side of the limb
    b. Dorsal limb aspect, and the film is against the lateral side of the limb
    c. Plantar limb aspect, and the film is against the medial side of the limb
    d. Plantar limb aspect, and the film is against the lateral side of the limb

54. For proper radiographic exposure, a radiograph should be taken during maximum
    a. Expiration for the abdomen and inspiration for the thorax
    b. Expiration for the thorax and inspiration for the abdomen
    c. Expiration for thorax and abdomen
    d. Inspiration for thorax and abdomen

55. The best view of the elbow is
    a. Dorsopalmar
    b. Palmarodorsal
    c. Caudocranial
    d. Craniocaudal

56. The peripheral borders for an elbow radiograph are
    a. 1/3 of the radius/ulna and 1/3 of the humerus
    b. 1/3 of the tibia/fibula and 1/3 of the femur
    c. 2/3 of the bones distal and proximal
    d. The carpus and the shoulder joint

57. The cranial and caudal borders for a lateral abdomen should be
    a. The thirteenth rib and the cranial aspect of the wings of the ilium
    b. The eighth rib and femoral head
    c. The scapulohumeral articulation and L7
    d. The last rib and the first coccygeal vertebra

58. The best view for tympanic bullae is
    a. Lateral
    b. Open-mouthed ventrodorsal
    c. Open-mouthed rostrocaudal
    d. Dorsoventral oblique

59. For a Dorsoventral (DV) view of the entire skull, you should center the primary beam
    a. At the medial canthi on the bridge of the nose
    b. Between the ears
    c. At the highest point of the zygomatic arch
    d. Between lateral canthi on sagittal crest

60. To ensure that your DV radiograph for the skull is parallel and perpendicular, you should try to have
    a. An imaginary line drawn between the medial canthi parallel to the film
    b. An imaginary line drawn between the medial canthi perpendicular to the film
    c. The nose pointing to the front of the cassette
    d. The ears parallel with each other

61. You are required to take intraoral radiographs of the teeth of a Labrador. You are to use your regular x-ray machine, because you do not have a dental unit in the facility. The animal is anesthetized. You should use
    a. Nonscreen film
    b. Hi-plus screens
    c. Rare-earth screens
    d. An increased object-film distance

62. For cervical studies you should center the primary beam at
    a. C7 to C8
    b. The atlas
    c. The axis
    d. C3 to C4

63. The femurs in a hip dysplasia view appear fore-shortened. This is likely due to not having the
    a. Femurs kept stationary
    b. Tube head perpendicular to the cassette and the femurs
    c. Femurs perpendicular to the cassette
    d. Femurs parallel to the cassette

64. Positive contrast media are considered to be
    a. Radiopaque, which means it will be white on a processed film
    b. Radiopaque, which means it will be dark on a processed film
    c. Radiolucent, which means it will be white on a processed film
    d. Radiolucent, which means it will be dark on a processed film

---

Correct answers are on pages 465-478.

65. The triiodinated compound that is least irritating to the gastrointestinal (GI) tissues and has less toxicity is the
    a. Sodium diatrizoic salt
    b. Sodium metrizoic salt
    c. Meglumine diatrizoic salt
    d. Oily iodine solution

66. The positive contrast compound that does not influence the movement of fluid through the intestinal wall is
    a. Barium sulfate preparation
    b. High osmolar triiodinated compound
    c. Meglumine diatrizoic salt
    d. Sodium diatrizoic salt

67. The veterinarian suspects a perforation of the small bowel in a 9-year-old lethargic German shepherd and wishes to confirm her diagnosis via a special positive contrast study. What positive contrast media would you use because it is the least irritating to the peritoneum?
    a. Barium sulfate
    b. Triiodinated compound
    c. Carbon dioxide
    d. Room air

68. Angiography consists of a bolus injection of iodinated contrast media into the
    a. Lymphatic system
    b. Biliary system
    c. Respiratory system
    d. Vascular system

69. An intravenous pyelogram (IVP) is also referred to as a(n)
    a. Cystogram
    b. Gastrogram
    c. Excretory urogram
    d. Esophagram

70. An upper GI study is performed to evaluate
    a. Esophagus and stomach
    b. Stomach and small intestine
    c. Large intestine
    d. Stomach only

71. The film-focal distance for a dental radiograph machine is ___ inches.
    a. 16
    b. 25
    c. 36
    d. 40

72. Which of the following is a false statement regarding portable x-ray units?
    a. Commonly used in large animal practice
    b. Can be carried easily from one location to another
    c. Use long exposure times because of low mA capability
    d. Have a rotating anode tube and single focal spot

73. The exposure factor that is responsible for accelerating the electrons from the cathode to the anode is
    a. Film-focal distance
    b. Time
    c. kVp
    d. mA

74. The temperature of the cathode filament is controlled by which of the following exposure factors?
    a. Film-focal distance
    b. Time
    c. kVp
    d. mA

75. The nine-penny test is a quality control test for
    a. View box uniformity
    b. Light field/x-ray field alignment
    c. Screen-film contact
    d. Source-image distance marks

76. Elongation and foreshortening of anatomic structure are associated with
    a. Radiographic definition
    b. Geometric unsharpness
    c. Radiographic detail
    d. Geometric distortion

77. A tabletop (nongrid) technique is used to radiograph the
    a. Thorax
    b. Abdomen
    c. Extremity
    d. Pelvis

78. Sante's rule is used to calculate
    a. Time
    b. Focal-film distance
    c. mA
    d. kVp

79. If the mA is set at 300, and the time is set at 1/60, the mAs is
    a. 50
    b. 20
    c. 7.5
    d. 5

80. A special study that involves use of a negative contrast media is
    a. Myelography
    b. Pneumocystogram
    c. Nephrogram
    d. Arthrography

81. The field of view of the pelvis for the Orthopedic Foundation for Animals (OFA) includes
    a. Pelvis, femurs, and stifles
    b. Femurs and stifles
    c. Lumbar 7, pelvis, and femurs
    d. Pelvis and femurs

82. The standing lateral view of the thorax with a horizontal beam is used to confirm the presence of
    a. Diaphragmatic hernia
    b. Foreign body
    c. Fluid or free air
    d. Megaesophagus

83. A skyline view is used to radiograph what part of a horse's anatomy?
    a. Carpus
    b. Guttural pouch
    c. Elbow
    d. Shoulder

84. Which of the following is a false statement regarding positioning for a lateral view of the shoulder?
    a. Patient is placed in lateral recumbency.
    b. Shoulder of interest is closest to the cassette.
    c. Leg of interest is extended cranial and ventral to sternum.
    d. Opposite limb is pulled in a craniodorsal position.

85. The bisecting angle technique is associated with taking an x-ray of the
    a. Thorax
    b. Teeth
    c. Spine
    d. Hip

86. To determine whether an animal had an ununited anconeal process, the veterinarian would want you to x-ray the
    a. Femur
    b. Humerus
    c. Elbow
    d. Stifle

87. The pH of the fixer chemicals is
    a. Strongly alkaline
    b. Neutral
    c. Acidic
    d. Slightly alkaline

88. The ideal temperature of the chemicals for manual radiograph processing is
    a. 68° F
    b. 75° F
    c. 39° C
    d. 25° C

89. Which of the following is a false statement regarding film storage?
    a. Boxes should be stored flat, in a horizontal position.
    b. Film should be away from chemicals and sources of ionizing radiation.
    c. Storage areas should be cool, 10° C to 15° C.
    d. Storage areas should have a relative humidity of 40% to 60%.

90. Nonscreen film would most likely be used to take what type of radiograph?
    a. Thoracic
    b. Abdominal
    c. Hip dysplasia
    d. Dental

91. An x-ray film exposed to visible light and developed would appear
    a. White
    b. Black
    c. Green
    d. Clear

92. An x-ray film accidentally developed before exposure to radiation appears
    a. White
    b. Black
    c. Green
    d. Clear

93. A new x-ray film taken directly from the box appears
    a. White
    b. Black
    c. Green
    d. Clear

94. A black "tree" pattern artifact on the film is caused by
    a. Static electrical charge
    b. Chemical splash
    c. Dirt in the cassette
    d. Bending the film

95. All artifacts appear as clear or white marks on film except
    a. Scratches in film emulsion
    b. Hair in the cassette
    c. Contrast media on the table
    d. Crimping or folding of the film

Correct answers are on pages 465-478.

96. Heavy lines on a processed radiograph are most likely due to
    a. Too high kVp
    b. Light leaking into the cassette
    c. Roller marks from an automatic processor
    d. Too low mA

97. All are true statements regarding fast film, except
    a. Has large silver halide crystals
    b. Requires more exposure by x-rays
    c. Produces a grainier image that lacks definition
    d. Has less latitude in exposure factors

98. If a radiograph is too light, and the image appears underpenetrated, you should
    a. Increase mAs 30% to 50%
    b. Decrease kVp 10% to 15%
    c. Decrease mAs 30% to 50%
    d. Increase kVp 10% to 15%

99. If a radiograph is too dark, but the image shows adequate penetration, you should
    a. Increase mAs 30% to 50%
    b. Decrease kVp 10% to 15%
    c. Decrease mAs 30% to 50%
    d. Increase kVp 10% to 15%

100. If a film is too light, but the image shows adequate penetration, you should
    a. Increase mAs 30% to 50%
    b. Decrease kVp 10% to 15%
    c. Decrease mAs 30% to 50%
    d. Increase kVp 10% to 15%

101. If a film is too dark and the image appears overpenetrated, you should
    a. Increase mAs 30% to 50%
    b. Decrease kVp 10% to 15%
    c. Decrease mAs 30% to 50%
    d. Increase kVp 10% to 15%

102. The exposure factors from a standard technique chart should be modified by decreasing the mAs by 50% for which of the following patients?
    a. Heavily muscled
    b. Obese
    c. Plaster cast on leg
    d. Neonatal dog

103. The technique chart should be modified by increasing the mAs by 50% for which of the following patients?
    a. A kitten
    b. Excessively thin animals
    c. Animals with ascites
    d. Animals with pneumothorax

104. Mitchell markers are primarily used in standing radiography of the equine head to assist in identifying
    a. Right or left side
    b. Fluid levels in paranasal sinuses
    c. Patient being radiographed
    d. Tooth in question

105. The unit of absorbed ionizing radiation dose is
    a. Maximum permissible
    b. Gray (Gy)
    c. Sievert (Sv)
    d. Rem

106. The workplace program that has been developed to ensure radiation exposures are kept as low as possible is
    a. ALARA
    b. MPD
    c. NCRP
    d. NIOSH

107. If cracks are present in protective apparel, they appear ___ when radiographed.
    a. Gray
    b. White
    c. Black
    d. Clear

108. The minimum age, in years, for a person to be involved in radiographic procedures is
    a. 14
    b. 16
    c. 18
    d. 21

109. One sievert (Sv) equals
    a. 1 rem
    b. 100 rad
    c. 1 rad
    d. 100 rem

110. Which of the following is a false statement regarding scatter radiation?
    a. The main source of radiation exposure to the veterinary technician comes from the area of patient that is exposed during radiography.
    b. Scatter radiation is of concern, because it decreases film quality and increases radiation exposure to the person taking the radiograph.
    c. Scatter radiation is composed of high-energy x-ray photons that have undergone a change in direction after interacting with structures in the patient's body.
    d. The best way to decrease radiation exposure is to use beam-limiting devices and pay close attention to technical factors to avoid retakes.

111. A noninvasive imaging procedure that uses a small amount of radioactive material administered intravenously is
    a. Ultrasound
    b. Tomography
    c. Magnetic resonance
    d. Scintigraphy

112. The imaging technique that involves a piezoelectric crystal within a transducer is
    a. Ultrasound
    b. Tomography
    c. Magnetic resonance
    d. Scintigraphy

113. Images are displayed in real time in which of the following?
    a. Ultrasound and fluoroscopy
    b. CT and MRI
    c. Scintigraphy
    d. PET scan

114. The ultrasound term that refers to few echoes detected, and the area is a low-level gray compared with the surrounding tissue, is
    a. Anechoic
    b. Hyperechoic
    c. Echoic
    d. Hypoechoic

115. The imaging technique that uses x-rays and computers to produce images that show anatomy in a cross section is
    a. Scintigraphy
    b. CT
    c. MRI
    d. Fluoroscopy

116. Which of the following involves no ionizing radiation to create the image?
    a. Scintigraphy
    b. CT
    c. MRI
    d. Fluoroscopy

117. Assume that you are going to produce a technique chart by holding mAs constant while varying kVp. Use Sante's rule to calculate the trial kVp that you would use for a canine thorax using the following parameters: thorax measurement = 16 cm, assume no grid is to be used, and focal-film distance = 40 in.
    a. 72 kVp
    b. 82 kVp
    c. 160 kVp
    d. 40 kVp

118. The maximum permissible dose (MPD) for whole-body radiation per year in sieverts is
    a. 0.05
    b. 0.50
    c. 5.0
    d. Not established

119. Which of the following is the best definition for *ionizing radiation dose equivalent*?
    a. Quantity of energy from ionizing radiation per unit mass of tissue
    b. The quantity of radiation per unit mass, taking into consideration the biologic effect on specific tissue types
    c. The number of grays of exposure per year
    d. The number of rads of exposure per year

120. In which of the following scenarios does the activity not increase the likelihood of personnel exposure to scatter radiation?
    a. Inability to collimate
    b. Personnel are leaning across the x-ray table to reach a patient
    c. Use of a fast screen/fast film combination
    d. Increase in kVp setting

121. The primary difference between an OFA and a PennHIP evaluation is that
    a. PennHIP focuses on the degree of joint laxity using three views.
    b. OFA focuses on the degree of joint laxity using three views.
    c. OFA provides specific parameters for various breeds of dogs.
    d. PennHIP does not require special training of personnel.

122. To prevent geometric distortion when performing radiographs, which of the following guidelines should be followed?
    a. The primary x-ray beam should be perpendicular to the object of interest, and the patient should be positioned parallel to the film.
    b. The primary x-ray beam should be parallel to the object of interest, and the patient should be positioned parallel to the film.
    c. There is no magnification or distortion that can occur if the patient is located close to the film.
    d. Geometric distortion can occur in very large-breed animals only.

Correct answers are on pages 465-478.

123. Tabletop exposures can usually be made under which of the following circumstances?
    a. When the area of interest (or the entire patient) is less than 10 cm thick
    b. When the patient is very cooperative and does not move, regardless of thickness
    c. When a fast screen and film combination is used
    d. Only when a grid is not available

124. Lateral thoracic radiographs are taken
    a. At peak inspiration
    b. At peak expiration
    c. In between breaths
    d. At midexpiration

125. Which views must be taken to properly perform a thoracic metastasis check on a patient with mammary adenocarcinoma?
    a. Right or left lateral view and a VD view
    b. Right and a left lateral view only
    c. Right and left lateral views and a VD or a DV view
    d. DV or a VD view only

126. Which lung field is best visualized in an animal that is in left lateral recumbency?
    a. Right lung field
    b. Left lung field
    c. Cranial lung field
    d. Caudal lung field

127. A veterinarian is performing a radiographic survey of a cat's skull to evaluate the trabecular bone in the nasal cavity for a nasal tumor (producing asymmetry). Knowing that ultra fine detail is needed, which of the following equipment would best allow for a diagnostic study?
    a. Fast screen and film combination
    b. Slow screen and film combination
    c. Fast screen and slow film combination
    d. Slow screen and fast film combination

128. When discerning the possible source of artifacts on film, a veterinary technician might attribute a yellowing of radiographic films to
    a. A light leak in the darkroom
    b. Incomplete washing of processing chemicals
    c. Grid out of focal range
    d. Pitted anode

129. A technician notes that there are equally spaced, heavy lines on a radiographic film. What is most likely to have caused this artifact?
    a. Grid out of focal range
    b. Pitted anode
    c. Light leak in darkroom
    d. Nail scratches

130. Which of the following would not result in poor detail on a radiographic film?
    a. Patient motion
    b. Fast film and screen combination
    c. Double exposure
    d. Light leak in x-ray room

131. To take advantage of the "heel effect," a veterinary technician would do which of the following when positioning an animal for a study?
    a. Place the thickest part of the patient toward the cathode side of the x-ray tube.
    b. Place the thickest part of the patient toward the anode side of the x-ray tube.
    c. Place the thickest part of the patient parallel to the primary beam.
    d. Place the thickest part of the patient centered on the primary beam.

132. When evaluating a film, you note that the film is too light. You then determine that the film does not have adequate penetration, because you cannot discern the various forms in the abdomen. The best adjustment to make when repeating the film would be to
    a. Increase the mAs
    b. Increase the kVp
    c. Decrease the mAs
    d. Decrease the kVp

133. When altering mAs or kVp settings to improve a radiograph, which of the following guidelines regarding incremental changes are appropriate when making adjustments?
    a. kVp should be changed 10% to 15% and mAs should be changed 30% to 50%
    b. kVp should be changed 30% to 50% and mAs should be changed 10% to 15%
    c. kVp and mAs should be changed 5%
    d. kVp and mAs should be changed 75%

134. A veterinary technician notes that a film is too dark, and there is minimal contrast (everything is gray). What is the most appropriate adjustment to be made to improve the quality of the repeat film?
    a. Increase kVp
    b. Increase mAs
    c. Decrease kVp
    d. Decrease mAs

135. The *palmar* surface of the forelimb refers to
    a. The caudal surface of the forelimb proximal to the carpus
    b. The caudal surface of the forelimb distal to the carpus
    c. The cranial surface of the forelimb proximal to the carpus
    d. The cranial surface of the forelimb distal to the carpus

136. When naming a radiographic view, which of the following best describes a DPaMLO of the carpus?
    a. The beam enters the dorsal/medial surface of the carpus and exits the palmar/lateral surface.
    b. The beam enters the palmar/lateral surface and exits the dorsal/medial surface.
    c. This is a dorsal/ventral view of the carpus.
    d. This is a lateral/medial view of the carpus.

137. What information can a barium-impregnated polyethylene spheres (BIPS) study provide?
    a. Information about the mucosal surface of the small intestine
    b. Information about gastric transit time
    c. Information about a relatively minor obstruction in the colon
    d. Information about gastric ulceration

138. A veterinarian expresses concern when trying to decide whether to perform a double-contrast study of a cat's bladder. Because of the presence of hematuria, she decides not to perform the study. What would be the most probable factor to influence her decision?
    a. She is concerned about vascular integrity and absorption of the positive contrast agent.
    b. She is concerned about vascular integrity and resultant air embolism with the negative contrast agent.
    c. She is concerned because the hematuria makes the patient a poor anesthetic risk.
    d. The hematuria interferes with the contrast agents.

139. The information yielded with nuclear scintigraphy includes which of the following?
    a. Anatomic detail of the organ being studied
    b. Mucosal detail of the organ being studied
    c. Physiologic information about the function of the organ under study
    d. Prognosis with respect to a malignant or nonmalignant status

140. Common uses of technetium-99 nuclear scintigraphy include all but which of the following types of studies?
    a. Scan of the thyroid gland to detect hyperthyroidism in cats
    b. Bone scan for undiagnosed lameness in horses
    c. Insulin regulation for a diabetic dog
    d. Detection of a portosystemic shunt in the liver of a dog

141. A Newfoundland dog is presented to the clinic for an upper GI study. The veterinarian suspects an intramural tumor in the small intestine and wants excellent mucosal detail on the films. What contrast agent will the veterinarian most likely choose?
    a. Ionic iodinated compounds
    b. Nonionic iodinated compounds
    c. Barium sulfate
    d. Negative contrast agents

142. A pit bull is presented to the clinic for a GI study, because she consumed four sewing needles. Given her depression, anorexia, and abdominal tenderness, the doctor suspects that she has an intestinal perforation. You are asked to perform a positive contrast study. Which of the following contrast agents is contraindicated in this circumstance?
    a. Ionic iodinated compounds
    b. Nonionic iodinated compounds
    c. Barium sulfate
    d. BIPS

143. Hypoechoic tissues have which of the following characteristics in an ultrasonic study?
    a. Reflect few echoes that result in low-level grays on the screen
    b. Reflect many echoes that result in bright white areas on the screen
    c. Reflect few to no echoes that result in black areas on the screen
    d. Reflect few echoes that result in bright white areas on the screen

144. Which of the following best describes a high-frequency ultrasound unit transducer?
    a. Decreases resolution and decreases penetration
    b. Increases resolution and increases penetration
    c. Decreases resolution and increases penetration
    d. Increases resolution and decreases penetration

Correct answers are on pages 465-478.

145. A bladder stone is hyperechoic. What type of image does this project on the ultrasound monitor?
    a. Bright white image
    b. Black image
    c. Nondetectable
    d. Gray image

146. A urine-filled bladder is usually best classified as
    a. Hyperechoic
    b. Anechoic
    c. Hypoechoic
    d. Attenuated

147. The tungsten plate (target) is located where on the x-ray machine?
    a. Anode
    b. Cathode
    c. Collimator
    d. Bucky

148. In an x-ray tube, x-rays are formed on the
    a. Tungsten target on the anode
    b. Tungsten target on the cathode
    c. Copper target on the anode
    d. Copper target on the cathode

149. Anyone working with, or in the near vicinity of, an x-ray machine should use
    a. Lead-lined gloves
    b. A dosimetry badge
    c. An abdominal shield
    d. Polarized glasses

150. The distance between the x-ray tube and the film is the
    a. Primary beam distance
    b. Tube-table distance
    c. Focal-film distance
    d. Cathode-screen distance

151. The focal spot is
    a. The center of the x-ray beam
    b. The spot on the tungsten target that the electron beam is aimed at
    c. The lighted area of the beam
    d. The spot on your uniform where you put your dosimetry badge

152. The unit of radiation exposure *rad* stands for
    a. Radiation absorbed dose
    b. Radiation accessory device
    c. Roentgen absorbed dose
    d. Roentgen advisory dosage

153. What can cause a series of parallel white lines on the developed radiograph?
    a. The collimator is collimated to the area to be radiographed
    b. A poorly functioning focusing cup
    c. The bucky
    d. The grid

154. When positioning an animal for radiographs, it is best to place the thicker portion of the patient toward ___ of the tube to produce a radiograph with uniform density.
    a. Either end
    b. The anode end
    c. The cathode end
    d. The center

155. Most x-ray film cassettes now have what kind of screens that glow when irradiated?
    a. Glow screens
    b. Intensifying screens
    c. Iridescent screens
    d. High-density screens

156. High kVp produces
    a. A long scale of contrast
    b. The best bone radiographs
    c. Good radiographs of distal extremities
    d. Minimal grays

157. Low kVp produces
    a. Lots of shades of gray
    b. A short scale of contrast
    c. A good abdominal study
    d. A good chest film study

158. The annual maximum permissible dose (MPD) standard of radiation for anyone working with radiation is
    a. 5 rem
    b. 0.5 rem
    c. 50 rad
    d. 15 rad

159. Which of the following would do the most to minimize scatter radiation?
    a. kVp is low
    b. mAs is high
    c. The collimator is open.
    d. The collimator is narrowed.

160. If the finished radiograph is too light, a probable cause is
    a. The kVp/mAs is too high.
    b. Light leaked into the film cassette.
    c. Focal-film distance is too long.
    d. The fixer is exhausted.

161. You have accidentally put two sheets of x-ray film in a cassette. You did not notice this until after you have taken a very difficult shot. Without having to take a second shot, what is the best option for the veterinarian to successfully evaluate the radiograph?
    a. Develop both films and pick the best one for the veterinarian to evaluate.
    b. Develop both films and overlay them for the veterinarian to evaluate.
    c. Develop the film that was closest to the patient.
    d. Develop the film that was closest to the x-ray tube.

162. If the finished radiograph has white splotches on it, the most likely cause is
    a. Motion
    b. Spots of fixer on the film
    c. Gridlines
    d. Static electricity

163. Clear edges on a finished radiograph may be caused by
    a. A misaligned Bucky tray
    b. Motion
    c. A light leak in the cassette
    d. Gridlines

164. A focal-film distance that is too short causes the radiographed image to
    a. Appear larger
    b. Appear too light
    c. Appear too dark
    d. Appear smaller

165. When radiographing a distal extremity, a ___ scale of contrast is best.
    a. Long
    b. Short
    c. Medium
    d. It does not matter

166. Dosimetry badges should be
    a. Worn on the collar outside the apron
    b. Removed from the x-ray room
    c. Changed annually
    d. Optional for personnel using the x-ray machine only occasionally

167. How often should chemical (drug) restraint be used during radiologic procedures?
    a. Rarely
    b. For long procedures only
    c. As often as possible
    d. Only if the patient is going straight to surgery

168. The minimum lead equivalence for protective radiographic aprons and gloves is
    a. 5 mm
    b. 0.05 mm
    c. 0.5 mm
    d. 0.5 cm

169. Personnel of what age should not be actively working within an x-ray–producing area?
    a. Older than 62 years
    b. Younger than 18 years
    c. Younger than 21 years
    d. Older than 70 years

170. When taking radiographs, the veterinary technician should
    a. Maximize distance between herself or himself and x-ray sources
    b. Maintain at least 2 feet of separation between herself or himself and x-ray sources
    c. Wear lead gloves and aprons only if a dosimeter is not available
    d. Wear lead gloves only if hands will be in the x-ray beam

171. Abdominal radiographs are best taken when the
    a. Animal is under anesthesia
    b. Animal exhales
    c. Animal inhales
    d. Animal is at peak inspiration

172. When taking a lateral thoracic radiograph, the veterinary technician should
    a. Center the beam at the tenth rib
    b. Position the forelegs cranially
    c. Take the film on complete exhalation
    d. Measure at the fifth rib

173. When taking a lateral thoracic radiograph, you should make sure the spine and sternum are
    a. Perpendicular to the table
    b. Obliqued slightly to the table
    c. Equidistant from the table
    d. Lying on the table

174. When taking a VD thoracic radiograph, you should measure at the level
    a. Of the twelfth rib
    b. Just caudal to the thirteenth rib
    c. Between the fourth and fifth ribs
    d. Anywhere

Correct answers are on pages 465-478.

175. The collimation field for a lateral abdominal radiograph is from the
    a. Shoulder to the hip
    b. Caudal-most rib to the hip
    c. Xyphoid process to the hip
    d. Manubrium to the hip

176. Extremity radiographs should be taken with the film cassette
    a. In the Bucky
    b. In the Bucky and the focal-film distance decreased
    c. On the tabletop
    d. On the tabletop with the kVp increased

177. When radiographing extremities, the beam should be centered
    a. Midway on the shaft of the bone of choice
    b. At the thickest portion of the extremity
    c. At the larger joint end
    d. Wherever the collimator allows inclusion of the entire extremity

178. Radiographs of the lateral pelvis should be measured over the
    a. Ileal points
    b. Ischial points
    c. Hip joints
    d. Ileal points

179. Positioning the lateral pelvis should include the
    a. Hip joints superimposed
    b. Ilia rotated slightly, so you can see both on the radiograph
    c. Hind legs positioned caudally
    d. Lower leg perpendicular to the body, and the upper leg positioned caudally

180. A VD view of the pelvis for hip dysplasia evaluation should not show which of the following?
    a. An anesthetized animal
    b. A sedated patient
    c. Patellae on top of the patellar grooves
    d. Stifles rotated laterally

181. A lateral skull radiograph should be
    a. Done on awake patients only
    b. Done on anesthetized patients only
    c. Always done without an endotracheal tube
    d. Taken from the zygomatic arch to the sagittal crest

182. An open-mouth, end-on radiograph highlights the
    a. Nasal turbinates
    b. Pinnae
    c. Temporomandibular joint
    d. Tympanic bullae

183. When taking cervical radiographs, one should measure at
    a. C1
    b. C2
    c. C3
    d. C4

184. An important radiographic aid used during lateral cervical radiographs is a
    a. Sandbag under the midcervical region
    b. Radiolucent positioner under the midcervical region
    c. Sandbag over the midcervical region
    d. No aid needed

185. For VD thoracic spine radiographs, you would measure at
    a. T5
    b. T13
    c. T11
    d. T10

186. Thoracic vertebral radiographic series should be
    a. Centered and measured at the cranial border of the scapula
    b. Centered and measured at the caudal border of the scapula
    c. Centered and measured at the level of C2
    d. Centered and measured at the level of L2

187. Cervical VD radiographs should be
    a. Just ahead of shoulders
    b. Just behind shoulders
    c. Measured at the level of the umbilicus
    d. Measured at the level of the xyphoid

188. The mA selector
    a. Controls the number of electrons produced by the filament
    b. Controls the duration of exposure
    c. Determines the penetrating power of the x-ray beam
    d. Determines the energy of the x-ray beam

189. Which of these ratio grids requires the highest mAs to obtain the desired density on a finished radiographic film?
    a. 8:1
    b. 12:1
    c. 10:1
    d. 5:1

190. Which of these ratio grids is most efficient?
    a. 8:1 with 102 lines/inch
    b. 5:1 with 80 lines/inch
    c. 10:1 with 103 lines/inch
    d. 12:1 with 113 lines/inch

191. How does milliamperage affect the electrons in an x-ray beam?
    a. Increasing the milliamperage increases the number of electrons produced and increases the number of x-rays produced per unit of time.
    b. Increasing the milliamperage increases the speed at which the electrons hit the anode, which increases the penetrating power of the x-ray beam.
    c. Decreasing the milliamperage increases the number of electrons generated and decreases the number of x-rays produced per unit of time.
    d. Decreasing the milliamperage decreases the speed at which the electrons hit the anode, which decreases the number of x-rays available.

192. What type of x-ray machine allows for faster time and more output?
    a. Half-wave rectified, single phase
    b. Full-wave rectified, single phase
    c. Full-wave rectified, three phase
    d. Self-rectified

193. Which of the following controls radiographic contrast?
    a. kVp
    b. mAs
    c. Focal-film distance
    d. Object-film distance

194. Which of the following does not affect radiographic density?
    a. kVp
    b. mAs
    c. Focal-film distance
    d. Object-film distance

195. The focusing cup of an x-ray machine is a
    a. Small depression where the filament is placed
    b. Negative electrode
    c. Tungsten coil that emits electrons when heated
    d. Positive electrode

196. The target of an x-ray machine is a/an
    a. Tungsten coil that emits electrons when heated
    b. Small depression where the filament is placed
    c. Area of the anode struck by electrons during an exposure
    d. Positive electrode

197. The filament of an x-ray tube is the
    a. Negative electrode
    b. Positive electrode
    c. Area of the anode struck by electrons during an exposure
    d. Tungsten coil that emits electrons when heated

198. When a spinning-top test is performed on a full-wave rectified machine, how many dots should you see in 1/60 seconds?
    a. 6
    b. 2
    c. 1
    d. 12

199. If you suspect that your machine is not producing x-radiation, what would be the easiest and fastest test you could perform to confirm this?
    a. Spinning-top
    b. Film/screen contact
    c. Step wedge
    d. Screen fluorescence

200. Tube saturation can occur with a
    a. Too-high kVp reading
    b. Too-high mA reading
    c. Too-low kVp reading
    d. Too-low mA reading

201. Which of the following absorbs the most x-rays?
    a. Fat
    b. Air
    c. Metal
    d. Bone

202. What direction should a grid move in relation to the grid lines in order to blur the lines?
    a. Same direction as the grid lines
    b. Perpendicular to the grid lines
    c. Always stationary
    d. Moves in both directions

203. If the focal-film distance is increased by a factor of 2, how must the mA be adjusted to maintain density?
    a. Increased by a factor of 4
    b. Increased by a factor of 2
    c. Decreased by a factor of 4
    d. Decreased by a factor of 2

204. If a radiographic film appears overexposed, is it too light or too dark? Would you increase or decrease the exposure to improve the quality?
    a. Too dark; exposure should be increased
    b. Too light; exposure should be increased
    c. Too dark; exposure should be decreased
    d. Too light; exposure should be decreased

Correct answers are on pages 465-478.

205. How does kVp affect the electrons and the x-ray beam?
    a. Increasing it increases the number of electrons produced and also increases the penetrating power of the x-ray beam.
    b. Decreasing it decreases the number of electrons produced and also decreases the number of x-rays produced.
    c. Increasing it increases the speed at which electrons are pulled across to the anode and also increases the penetrating power of the x-ray beam.
    d. Increasing it increases the speed at which electrons are pulled across to the anode and lengthens the wavelength of the x-rays produced, making them more penetrating.

206. A radiographic film is underexposed. It does not appear to be properly penetrated. The technique used to make the film was 5 mAs and 60 kVp. Which of the following techniques might be chosen to increase the density and penetration of the radiographic film?
    a. 10 mAs and 60 kVp
    b. 5 mAs and 70 kVp
    c. 2.5 mAs and 70 kVp
    d. 10 mAs and 50 kVp

207. An abdominal radiographic film is made at 12 mAs and 68 kVp. It is now necessary to halve the radiographic density. Which of the following techniques would you use?
    a. 6 mAs and 34 kVp
    b. 12 mAs and 82 kVp
    c. 6 mAs and 68 kVp
    d. 10 mAs and 68 kVp

208. Tube overload occurs with
    a. Too-high kVp and mAs
    b. Too-low kVp and mAs
    c. Too-high kVp
    d. Too-low mAs

209. What effect does doubling the mAs have on radiographic density?
    a. It doubles it.
    b. It halves it.
    c. Density is the same.
    d. Radiographic film is blackened.

210. The electron cloud is generated at the
    a. Anode
    b. Cathode
    c. Focal spot
    d. Effective focal spot

211. Which of the following techniques produces the image with the most radiographic density?
    a. 100 mA, 1/10 sec
    b. 150 mA, 1/30 sec
    c. 200 mA, 1/20 sec
    d. 200 mA, 1/10 sec

212. Which of these contrast studies best demonstrates a diaphragmatic hernia?
    a. Pneumocystography
    b. Pneumoperitoneography
    c. Double-contrast cystography
    d. Celiography

213. Which contrast medium listed is considered negative contrast?
    a. Water-soluble organic iodide
    b. Barium sulfate
    c. Air
    d. Organic iodide

214. Which contrast procedure listed generally uses both positive and negative contrast media?
    a. Barium enema
    b. Urethrography
    c. Excretory urogram
    d. Myelography

215. Which contrast medium listed is contraindicated if a rupture or perforation of the bowel is suspected?
    a. Diatrizoate (Gastrografin)
    b. Barium sulfate
    c. Water-soluble organic iodide
    d. Air

216. Which contrast study listed requires the patient's head to be elevated after injection of contrast medium?
    a. Arthrography
    b. Fistulography
    c. Myelography
    d. Pneumoperitoneography

217. Which contrast medium listed is considered positive contrast?
    a. Nitrous oxide
    b. Air
    c. Barium sulfate
    d. Oxygen

218. Which contrast study listed is used to evaluate the kidneys, ureters, and urinary bladder?
    a. Urethrography
    b. Positive-contrast cystography
    c. Double-contrast cystography
    d. Excretory urography

219. Which contrast medium listed appears radiolucent on the finished radiographic film?
    a. Barium sulfate
    b. Metrizamide
    c. Air
    d. Water-soluble organic iodide

220. Which contrast study of the GI tract is monitored until contrast medium reaches the colon?
    a. Gastrography
    b. Upper GI series
    c. Barium enema
    d. Esophagography

221. Which of the following is not a reason that survey radiographic films should always be made before administering contrast medium?
    a. To establish proper exposure technique
    b. To establish proper patient preparation
    c. To make a diagnosis
    d. To help determine the dosage of contrast medium

222. Which contrast medium appears radiopaque on a radiographic film?
    a. Air
    b. Nitrous oxide
    c. Oxygen
    d. Barium sulfate

223. Which contrast study listed is indicated if a draining tract is present?
    a. Arthrography
    b. Celiography
    c. Fistulography
    d. Myelography

224. Which contrast study listed is used to detect ectopic ureters?
    a. Excretory urogram
    b. Urethrography
    c. Vaginography
    d. Positive-contrast cystography

225. With the heel effect, the x-ray beam intensity is greater toward the
    a. Anode
    b. Collimator
    c. Cathode
    d. Tube window

226. Which of these factors does not affect the amount of penumbra on a radiographic film and does not contribute to the penumbra?
    a. Object-film distance
    b. kVp
    c. Focal-film distance
    d. Focal-spot size

227. The spinning-top test is performed when you suspect a problem with the
    a. mA stations
    b. X-ray tube
    c. Timer
    d. kVp

228. A good layout of a darkroom should include dry-bench and wet-bench areas separate from each other. Select the area where each task should be performed from the two choices given.
    Loading and unloading cassettes
    a. Wet bench
    b. Dry bench

229. A good layout of a darkroom should include dry-bench and wet-bench areas separate from each other. Select the area where each task should be performed from the two choices given.
    Drying washed films
    a. Wet bench
    b. Dry bench

230. A good layout of a darkroom should include dry-bench and wet-bench areas separate from each other. Select the area where each task should be performed from the two choices given.
    Film storage
    a. Wet bench
    b. Dry bench

231. A good layout of a darkroom should include dry-bench and wet-bench areas separate from each other. Select the area where each task should be performed from the two choices given.
    Film processing
    a. Wet bench
    b. Dry bench

232. How do low-grade light leaks in the darkroom affect film quality?
    a. They have no effect on the film quality.
    b. They increase film quality by decreasing scatter radiation.
    c. They decrease film quality by increasing overall fog of the film.
    d. They decrease film quality by decreasing radiographic density.

Correct answers are on pages 465-478.

233. When must radiographs be labeled for certification organizations and for legal purposes?
    a. Before exposure and after processing
    b. During or after exposure but before processing
    c. After exposure and after processing
    d. Before filing or mailing

234. What is the total time the film should be placed in the fixer?
    a. Two times the developing time
    b. Three times the developing time
    c. The same as the developing time
    d. 30 seconds

235. A radiographic film of a dog's thorax is made. What occurs when the film is placed in the developer?
    a. The sensitized silver halide crystals are changed into black metallic silver.
    b. The potassium bromide crystals are changed into black metallic silver.
    c. The silver halide crystals are cleared from the film.
    d. All of the silver halide crystals are changed into black metallic silver.

236. When manually processing films, there are two methods for maintaining the tanks: the *exhausted method* and the *replenishing method*. Match the method with the statement given.
    Allows chemicals to drain from the film back into their respective tanks
    a. Exhausted method
    b. Replenishing method

237. When manually processing films, there are two methods for maintaining the tanks: the *exhausted method* and the *replenishing method*. Match the method with the statement given. This method allows chemicals to drain into the wash tank only.
    a. Exhausted method
    b. Replenishing method

238. When manually processing films, there are two methods for maintaining the tanks: the *exhausted method* and the *replenishing method*. Match the method with the statement given. Periodically, chemicals are added to bring chemical levels back up to the top of the tanks.
    a. Exhausted method
    b. Replenishing method

239. How often should the manual processing tanks be drained and cleaned and old chemicals replaced with fresh chemicals?
    a. Once a day
    b. Once a week
    c. At least every 3 months
    d. Once a year

240. What would happen if exposed film were accidentally placed in the fixer before being placed in the developer?
    a. The radiographic film turns black.
    b. The radiographic film becomes clear.
    c. If the mistake is detected soon enough, the image can be spared.
    d. The radiographic film appears underexposed.

241. The pH of the developer chemicals is
    a. Strongly acidic
    b. Neutral
    c. Alkaline
    d. Slightly acidic

242. When reconstituting the powder form of processing chemicals, what is the most important factor to remember?
    a. Always reconstitute the chemicals in the darkroom.
    b. Always reconstitute the chemicals under bright lights.
    c. Always use sterile saline to reconstitute the chemicals.
    d. Never reconstitute the chemicals in the darkroom.

243. A radiographic film of a cat's thorax is made. When viewing the film, you note a decrease in radiographic density and a gray swirly appearance of the background. What caused this problem?
    a. Processing chemicals were too hot.
    b. Film was not left in the fixer long enough.
    c. Processing chemicals were too cold.
    d. Film was not washed for 30 minutes after processing.

244. Radiographic films made 5 years earlier have turned brown. What was the cause?
    a. Too long in the developer
    b. Too long in the fixer
    c. Incomplete development
    d. Incomplete final wash

245. When using a direct safelight system, the distance from the workbench should be at least
    a. 20 inches
    b. 30 inches
    c. 48 inches
    d. 72 inches

246. Lateral and ventrodorsal projections of a dog's abdomen are made and manually processed at the same time. However, both radiographic films have identical areas of decreased radiographic density that appear to be artifacts. What could have caused this artifact on both films?
    a. They stuck together in the fixer.
    b. They stuck together in the developer.
    c. They stuck together in the wash tank.
    d. They were overexposed.

247. What is a *latent* image?
    a. An image on the film after processing
    b. Calcium tungstate crystals in the film's emulsion that have been exposed to radiant energy before processing
    c. Silver halide crystals in the film's emulsion that have been exposed to radiant energy before processing
    d. An image on the film before exposure

248. Screen-type film
    a. Is most sensitive to light produced by the intensifying screen
    b. Is most sensitive to direct x-ray beams
    c. Requires a longer exposure time than direct-exposure film
    d. Can be processed manually only

249. Some direct-exposure film cannot be processed in an automatic processor because
    a. It tends to scratch too easily.
    b. The emulsion is too thick.
    c. It cannot tolerate high temperatures.
    d. It is too sensitive to safelights.

250. Direct-exposure film differs from screen-type film in that it requires a
    a. Lower mAs
    b. Higher mAs
    c. Higher kVp
    d. Lower kVp

251. Film is most sensitive
    a. Before exposure and processing
    b. Before exposure but after processing
    c. After exposure but before processing
    d. After exposure and processing

252. High-speed film has
    a. Larger silver halide crystals than slow-speed film, which increases the detail on the finished radiographic film
    b. Larger silver halide crystals than slow-speed film, which decreases the detail on the finished radiographic film
    c. Smaller silver halide crystals than slow-speed film, which increases the detail on the finished radiographic film
    d. The same size silver halide crystals as slow-speed film

253. Long-latitude film
    a. Produces a short scale of contrast
    b. Produces a long scale of contrast
    c. Has large calcium tungstate crystals
    d. Cannot be processed manually

254. Which statement concerning film storage and handling is least accurate?
    a. Unexposed film should be stored in a cool, dry place.
    b. A base fog can occur if film is stored in adverse conditions.
    c. Film should be stored in boxes stacked on end, not flat on their sides.
    d. Strong chemical fumes have no effect on unexposed film.

255. Radiographic films must be permanently labeled. Which of the following does not need to appear as part of the permanent identification on a radiographic film?
    a. Clinic's name
    b. Owner's name
    c. Patient's date of birth
    d. Owner's telephone number

256. What is the purpose of an oblique projection?
    a. To delineate an area that is normally superimposed over another
    b. To image areas toward the median plane
    c. To decrease detail on the finished radiographic film
    d. To image the coccygeal vertebrae

257. What are the topographic landmarks of the thorax?
    a. Cranial landmark, second cervical vertebra; caudal landmark, fifth thoracic vertebra
    b. Cranial landmark, manubrium sterni; caudal landmark, halfway between the xiphoid and last rib
    c. Cranial landmark, three rib spaces cranial to the xiphoid; caudal landmark, greater trochanter
    d. Cranial landmark, manubrium sterni; caudal landmark, greater trochanter

Correct answers are on pages 465-478.

258. What are the topographic landmarks of the abdomen?
    a. Cranial landmark, second cervical vertebra; caudal landmark, fifth thoracic vertebra
    b. Cranial landmark, manubrium sterni; caudal landmark, halfway between the xiphoid and last rib
    c. Cranial landmark, three rib spaces cranial to the xiphoid; caudal landmark, greater trochanter
    d. Cranial landmark, manubrium sterni; caudal landmark, greater trochanter

259. When radiographing a long bone, it is important to
    a. Include as much of the abdomen as possible.
    b. Include the joint proximal and the joint distal.
    c. Measure over the thinnest area for the kilovoltage peak.
    d. Include the long bone only, not the joints.

260. When radiographing the skull in the dorsoventral position, it is important to
    a. Position the animal so the tympanic bullae are superimposed over one another
    b. Position the animal so the hard palate is perpendicular to the cassette
    c. Remove the endotracheal tube before making the exposure
    d. Place the animal in left lateral recumbency

261. Foreshortening occurs when radiographing a long bone, and the
    a. Bone is not parallel to the cassette
    b. Bone is not perpendicular to the cassette
    c. Cassette is of the wrong speed
    d. Exposure technique is incorrect

262. When radiographing a joint, why is it important to center the primary beam on the joint?
    a. To decrease scatter radiation
    b. To decrease exposure
    c. To maximize joint space and minimize false narrowing
    d. To minimize the joint space and maximize false narrowing

263. A lateral projection of a dog's shoulder is made. On the finished radiographic film, the manubrium and the trachea are superimposed over the joint space. How can the animal be repositioned to correct this?
    a. Extend the head cranioventrally, and relax the caudal extension of the contralateral limb.
    b. Extend the head caudodorsally, and draw the contralateral limb farther caudally.
    c. Pull the limb being imaged farther caudally.
    d. Nothing; the shoulder cannot be repositioned without superimposing other structures over it.

264. The plantar surface is the
    a. Caudal aspect of the rear limb, distal to the tarsocrural joint
    b. Caudal aspect of the front limb, distal to the antebrachiocarpal joint
    c. Cranial aspect of the rear limb, proximal to the tarsal joint
    d. Cranial aspect of the front limb, proximal to the carpal joint

265. *Cranial* describes a location toward the
    a. Tail
    b. Head
    c. Underside on a quadruped
    d. Point of attachment

266. An area on the distal limb is
    a. Toward the tail
    b. Away from the point of attachment
    c. Toward the head
    d. Toward the point of attachment

267. *Ventral* describes a location toward the
    a. Underside on a quadruped
    b. Back on a quadruped
    c. Head
    d. Point of attachment

268. *Rostral* describes a location
    a. Away from the median plane
    b. Toward the tail
    c. Toward the nose
    d. Toward the ears

269. *Medial* describes a location
    a. Toward the median plane
    b. Toward the tail
    c. Away from the median plane
    d. Away from the point of attachment

270. A dorsopalmar-lateromedial oblique projection of a horse's fetlock is made. Which sesamoid listed is clearly delineated with this film?
    a. Medial
    b. Lateral
    c. Interdigital
    d. Distal

271. What landmarks should be included when radiographing the humerus?
    a. Proximal landmark, elbow; distal landmark, carpus
    b. Proximal landmark, shoulder joint; distal landmark, elbow
    c. Proximal landmark, shoulder joint; distal landmark, carpus
    d. Proximal landmark, stifle joint; distal landmark, tarsocrural joint

272. A left 20-degree ventral/right dorsal oblique projection of a dog's skull is made. Which tympanic bulla would be more ventral on this film?
    a. Left
    b. Right
    c. Neither; they would be superimposed over one another.
    d. Neither; they are not imaged with this projection.

273. What procedure must be followed to take advantage of the heel effect when obtaining a radiographic film?
    a. Place the distal part of the patient toward the anode.
    b. Place the thick or dense part of the patient toward the cathode.
    c. Place the thick or dense part of the patient toward the anode.
    d. Place the heavy or dense part of the patient in the middle of the beam.

274. What information must be included on a radiographic film for proper identification?
    a. Name and address of the hospital; date (day, month, year); name of the client and patient; age, sex, and breed of the patient
    b. Name of the hospital; date (day, month, year); name of the client and patient
    c. Name and phone number of the hospital; date (day, month, year); name of the client
    d. Name of the hospital; date (day, month, year); name of person taking the radiographic film

275. Where should the primary beam be centered when radiographing the canine lumbar spine in a ventrodorsal projection?
    a. L2
    b. L3
    c. L4
    d. L5

276. Where should the primary beam be centered for a lateral view of the canine thoracic spine?
    a. T3
    b. T5
    c. T7
    d. T9

277. What is the purpose of the collimator on an x-ray machine?
    a. Reduces the exposure time
    b. Increases the detail of the x-ray film
    c. Compensates for movement
    d. Limits the primary beam size

278. If mA = 100 and s = 1/10, what is the mAs of the x-ray exposure technique?
    a. 1
    b. 10
    c. 100
    d. 1000

279. What x-ray intensifying screen provides the least detail on the developed film?
    a. Low speed
    b. Par speed
    c. High speed
    d. Rare earth

280. What setting on the x-ray machine adjusts the penetrating ability of the x-ray beam?
    a. mA
    b. kVp
    c. Time
    d. Collimation

281. What is the term used to describe the tube-to-film distance?
    a. Focal-film distance
    b. Focal-object distance
    c. Focal-skin distance
    d. Focal spot

282. When the object-to-film distance is increased, the image is
    a. Distorted
    b. Magnified
    c. Darkened
    d. Lightened

283. What piece of equipment helps reduce exposure time?
    a. Collimator
    b. Grid
    c. Rare-earth screens
    d. Rotating anode

284. What is the proper order of manual processing of x-ray film?
    a. Develop, rinse, fix, wash, dry
    b. Rinse, fix, dry, wash, develop
    c. Wash, develop, rinse, fix, dry
    d. Fix, wash, develop, dry, rinse

285. Subject contrast on a radiographic film depends on what two variables?
    a. Focal-film and object-film distance
    b. mAs and kVp
    c. Age and species of the subject
    d. Thickness and density of the anatomic part

Correct answers are on pages 465-478.

286. What is the primary source of scatter radiation?
    a. Target anode
    b. Cassette
    c. Patient
    d. Primary beam

287. Which of these techniques causes a major increase in scatter radiation?
    a. Increasing the kVp
    b. Increasing the mA
    c. Increasing the time
    d. Increasing the focal-film distance

288. What happens when a focused x-ray grid is placed outside of the grid-focus distance recommended by the manufacturer?
    a. Decreased grid efficiency
    b. Grid cutoff
    c. Increased grid ratio
    d. Decreased grid factor

289. Calcium tungstate in the intensifying screens of an x-ray cassette emits what color of light when bombarded by an x-ray beam?
    a. Red
    b. Blue
    c. Green
    d. Yellow

290. An intensifying screen that contains large crystals of calcium tungstate produces which of the following characteristics?
    a. Slow screens, less detail, low grain
    b. Slow screens, more detail, low grain
    c. Fast screens, more detail, high grain
    d. Fast screens, less detail, high grain

291. One disadvantage of the rare-earth intensifying screen is the resultant density variation that can occur on a uniform exposed radiographic film as a result of the fewer x-rays required. What is the name of this spotty radiographic artifact?
    a. Latent image
    b. Film latitude
    c. Afterglow
    d. Quantum mottle

292. What is the name of the process for visualizing motion radiographic films?
    a. Radioscopy
    b. Endoscopy
    c. Fluoroscopy
    d. Computed tomography

293. What is the light-sensitive chemical impregnated into an x-ray film?
    a. Silver halide
    b. Polyester base
    c. Gelatin emulsion
    d. Supercoat

294. Nonscreen x-ray film is more sensitive than screen film to what form of energy?
    a. Light
    b. X-ray
    c. Magnetic
    d. Electron

295. What type of x-ray film produces the greatest detail?
    a. Nonscreen
    b. Low speed
    c. High speed
    d. Rare earth

296. What x-ray film has the greatest latitude, or significant variation in exposure factors, without great change in density?
    a. Fast
    b. Medium
    c. Slow
    d. Rare earth

297. What is the correct interpretation of the statement, "The technician must know the film-speed system to produce quality radiographs"?
    a. Different speeds of film can be used with different speeds of screens.
    b. The matching film speed and cassette speed combination produces a higher quality system.
    c. The system required for good radiographic films is independent of film or cassette speed.
    d. To systematically improve the quality of radiographic films, more expensive film and cassettes are needed.

298. A light leak in the darkroom produces a type of artifact on the final radiographic film. The image will appear
    a. Light
    b. Fogged, with a dark cast
    c. Markedly contrasted
    d. Underdeveloped

299. What is the most common color of the safelight used in a darkroom for processing blue-light–sensitive film?
    a. Dark red
    b. Brown
    c. Dark green
    d. Blue

300. What is the most common filter color of the safelight used in the darkroom for processing green-light–sensitive film?
    a. Brown
    b. Dark red
    c. Blue
    d. Dark green

301. What consideration is most important when splitting an x-ray cassette into two separate images?
    a. Position the animal so that all views are facing the same direction.
    b. Position the animal so that separate views are in opposite directions.
    c. Position the animal so each view parallels the next.
    d. Alter the position so the views mirror each other.

302. What can be done to prevent processed x-ray film from turning yellow over time?
    a. Increase the initial exposure time.
    b. Make sure the film is fixed properly.
    c. Decrease the developing time.
    d. Use quality x-ray film only.

303. What is the maximum recommended grid ratio for a 90-kVp x-ray machine for veterinary practice?
    a. 5:1
    b. 8:1
    c. 12:1
    d. 16:1

304. What is the cause of a dark lightning streak across developed x-ray film?
    a. Too-rapid development
    b. Light exposure before development
    c. Static electrical discharge during film removal from the cassette
    d. Electrical short in the automatic film developer

305. What is the advantage of using screen x-ray film over nonscreen film?
    a. Screen film costs less.
    b. Screen film requires shorter exposure time.
    c. Nonscreen film takes longer to develop.
    d. Screen film produces better detail.

306. A grid is indicated when the body part exceeds what thickness?
    a. 6 cm
    b. 7 cm
    c. 8 cm
    d. 10 cm

307. Why are intensifying screens added to an x-ray cassette?
    a. To allow even x-ray distribution over the film
    b. To reduce scatter inside the cassette
    c. To cause light exposure of the film
    d. To change blue-sensitive to green-sensitive film

308. Fog on the unexposed area of a processed radiographic film indicates
    a. Overexposure
    b. Underexposure
    c. No exposure
    d. Exposure to extraneous light

309. What is a common cause for streaks and stains on the film from an automatic film processor?
    a. Not enough time in the fix
    b. Not enough wash
    c. Oversupply of developer
    d. Dirty rollers

310. Which of these terms describes a unit of absorbed dose of x-radiation?
    a. Rad
    b. Roentgen
    c. Rem
    d. Radon

311. The biologic effect of x-radiation is measured in
    a. Roentgens
    b. Rads
    c. Rems
    d. LD50

312. What device worn by an individual making radiographic films measures the actual amount of any ionizing radiation received?
    a. Film badge
    b. Dosimeter
    c. Ring badge
    d. Pocket ionization chamber

313. What is the maximum allowable whole-body occupational dose of x-ray beams in rems per calendar year?
    a. 1.25
    b. 5
    c. 7.5
    d. 9

314. How many millirems are in 7.5 rems of radiation exposure?
    a. 75
    b. 750
    c. 7500
    d. 75,000

Correct answers are on pages 465-478.

315. Where is the most effective place to wear an x-ray film badge?
    a. On the belt
    b. On the shirt collar outside of the apron
    c. On the hand
    d. In the area of anatomic risk

316. What is the minimum aluminum filter equivalent for x-ray machines with an output greater than 70 kVp?
    a. 1 mm
    b. 1.5 mm
    c. 2.5 mm
    d. 5 mm

317. Aluminum filters remove what part of the x-ray beam?
    a. High energy
    b. Low energy
    c. Gamma rays
    d. Infrared rays

318. When is it permissible to have a part of your body in the primary beam during an x-ray procedure?
    a. When it is difficult to restrain the patient
    b. When the hands are protected by lead-lined gloves
    c. When holding a cassette for a large animal
    d. Never; you should not expose any part of your body to the primary beam.

319. The minimum standard of lead equivalent for protective aprons and gloves is
    a. 0.25 mm
    b. 0.3 mm
    c. 0.4 mm
    d. 0.5 mm

320. If an operator can increase the distance from the primary beam by a factor of 2, what would be the resultant dose of radiation?
    a. 1/3
    b. 1/2
    c. 1/4
    d. 1/10

321. Which of the following substantially reduces the amount of radiation needed to produce diagnostic radiographic films?
    a. Chemical restraint
    b. Mobile leaded shields
    c. Collimators
    d. Rare-earth screens

322. Which of the following increases the chance of exposure to ionizing radiation?
    a. High line voltage
    b. Retakes (repeated exposures)
    c. Increased focal-film distance
    d. Failure to check tank developing temperature

323. What safety feature on x-ray machines limits the size of the primary beam and reduces secondary x-ray exposure to the operator?
    a. Filter
    b. Collimator
    c. Leaded glass
    d. Dead-man switch

324. Which statement is supportive of the importance of good technique in radiation safety?
    a. Good technique requires higher energy radiation.
    b. Good technique usually requires two people for restraint.
    c. Images produced with longer exposures are necessary for good technique.
    d. Good technique results in fewer repeated exposures of radiographic films.

325. What patient restraint is recommended for the greatest safety from radiation exposure?
    a. Chemical restraint without holding the patient
    b. Gauze ties held at a distance
    c. Open-mit leaded gloves held out of the beam
    d. Full-leaded gloves and apron

326. How often are radiation-monitoring film-badge reports usually submitted?
    a. Weekly
    b. Monthly
    c. Semiannually
    d. Annually

327. Exposure of personnel to radiation should be monitored if there is a reasonable possibility that individuals will be exposed to what fraction of the MPD?
    a. 1/4
    b. 1/2
    c. 1/3
    d. Equal to the MPD

328. What device offers technicians the least protection from x-radiation?
    a. Leaded apron
    b. Leaded glasses
    c. Dosimeter badge
    d. Cassette holder

329. What is the international unit of ionizing radiation exposure, abbreviated as R?
   a. Rem
   b. Rad
   c. Roentgen
   d. Radon

330. Which of these barriers is the most effective for protection against x-ray exposure?
   a. Plate glass window
   b. Fiberglass
   c. Plaster wall
   d. 6 feet of distance from radiation source

331. The nonoccupational maximum permissible radiation dose for an individual is what proportion of the occupational dose?
   a. 5%
   b. 10%
   c. 15%
   d. 20%

ANSWERS

1. **a** Travel of x-ray photons is in a straight line, until there is interaction with matter. The direction of the primary beam is then altered. Photons possess no electrical charge and are not affected by either magnetic or electric fields, and they cannot be refracted or reflected as per visible light.

2. **d** As with other forms of electromagnetic radiation, as the wavelength becomes shorter, the frequency of the x-ray beam increases. Frequency is measured by the number of cycles that pass a stationary point per second. The higher the frequency, the greater the energy and penetrating power.

3. **a** Kilovoltage peak, or kVp, determines the peak energy of the x-rays, which determines the penetrating power, a quality of the x-ray beam.

4. **b** Milliampere seconds, or mAs, determines the amount of the electrical energy applied to the filament per second and determines the number of x-rays produced during the exposure.

5. **c** The cathode provides the source of the electrons at the filament, and the kilovoltage directs the electrons to the anode during the exposure.

6. **b** Ninety-nine times more heat than actual x-rays is produced in an x-ray tube. Part of this is the heat of the cathode filament, and part is produced when the electron beam strikes the focal spot on the anode target. Modern x-ray tubes are designed to prevent this large amount of heat from destroying the x-ray tube.

7. **b** The kilovoltage peak (kVp) determines the maximum speed of the electrons flowing across the x-ray tube. This determines the maximum energy of the x-ray photons produced and thus their penetrating power.

8. **d** Before the electrons can be boiled off, the filament has to be at a proper temperature, and the anode must be rotating at the correct speed in preparation for the electrons and subsequent heat. The focal spot, choice **c**, is that area on the target that receives the electrons. The kVp determines the acceleration, choice **a**, and the exposure is not made until the exposure button is depressed, choice **b**.

9. **d** The x-ray tube provides the source of the electrons, a method of accelerating them, a target for the interaction of the electrons to change into x-ray photons and heat, a method of heat dissipation, and a glass envelope to maintain the evacuated path for the accelerated electrons to travel. The negatively charged cathode provides the source of electrons through the heated filament, the focusing cup helps direct the path, and the kVp provides the method of acceleration. The anode provides the target and focal spot.

10. **b** Minimum energy is needed for heating the tungsten filament, so a step-down transformer is placed between the cathode filament and the power supply to the x-ray machine. The extreme incoming voltage of 110 to 220 volts would cause instant evaporation of the filament. The step-down transformer decreases the incoming voltage to 10 V. A step-up transformer, choice **a**, is necessary for increasing the incoming voltage to kilovoltage to transport the electrons at a fast enough speed to produce x-rays.

11. **b** Because of the angle of the anode, there is a greater intensity of the x-ray beam toward the cathode side. As with beams of light, there is increasing spread of the beam from the source. The divergent effects are more noticeable with larger film, because a greater percentage of the

beam is affected. The full effect of the beam, and the variation in intensity, are more noticeable with shorter focal-film distance. At lower kVp there is a greater variation in the intensity of the beam as compared to higher kVp, which leads to a more noticeable heel effect.

12. **d** Rectification is the process of changing alternating current into direct current. By adding four valve tubes or silicon rectifiers, the negative portion of the wave is converted into a positive wave, and an almost constant electrical potential is created across the tube at all times. The electrical current pulses at 120 times per second. Pulsation of 60 times per second occurs when two valve tubes are added to create half-wave rectification.

13. **c** It is suggested that, to prevent safelight fogging, direct safelight should be a minimum of 4 feet away from the exposed film. Indirect lighting, in which the safelight shines on the ceiling or wall rather than on the workbench, is also suggested.

14. **d** A red safelight has a light emission toward the red end of the spectrum (greater than 600 nm) and does not expose either blue-sensitive or green-sensitive film. An amber safelight emits at about 500 nm and does not expose blue-sensitive film but exposes green-sensitive film.

15. **b** The main function of the developer is for the reducing agents to convert the exposed silver halide crystals to elemental black metallic silver ($Ag^+ + e^- = Ag$). If the crystals are not exposed, they cannot turn black with proper developing. Swelling and softening of the emulsion also occurs, but it is not the primary purpose.

16. **a** Sodium or ammonium thiosulfate in the fixer converts the undeveloped and unexposed silver halide crystals into soluble compounds and dissolves them away, leaving a clear or white image.

17. **d** A safelight illumination test often consists of covering various parts of an unexposed film for various time periods and exposing them to the safelight. The film is then processed. The length of time that the radiograph is exposed to safelight should be less than the time that you note any grayness on the blank film, otherwise your radiograph will show evidence of fogging. Because the developer's main purpose is to convert the exposed silver halide crystals to black, the more exposed the crystals, the darker the image.

18. **c** The green is the original color of blue-sensitive film, which indicates that neither of the solutions has touched the film at this point.

19. **a** If a radiograph is not placed into the developer, any crystals that are exposed will not be turned to black. The fixer will clear away the undeveloped crystals, leaving no image in that area. Collimation, choice **d**, is more likely to be evidenced on all sides, and, because of scatter radiation, leaving an image that does not usually show up as totally clear.

20. **d** The black area along the edges likely indicates a light leak, which demonstrates that the film must have been processed correctly. The film has not been exposed to any radiation, because there are no exposed silver halide crystals to be converted to black.

21. **b** Collimation limits the field size and prevents the primary beam from exposing that area, so that no crystals are exposed. Any slight exposure outside of this area will be due to scatter radiation. Both a light leak and overexposure appear as black.

22. **a** The fixer removes the silver halide crystals into soluble compounds and dissolves them away. Silver can be recovered from the fixer.

23. **c** High room temperature degrades the quality of the film, so that the film contrast is minimized. There are fewer white or transparent areas. A low kVp, a long source-image distance, and two films in the cassette would cause a lighter image.

24. **c** It is suggested that a bulb of no greater than 15 watts be used. It is also important to ensure that the correct filter is used depending on the film type used.

25. **d** A bullet, which is composed of lead, has a higher atomic number than bone. This means that it absorbs even more x-rays than bone and prevents them from reaching the film. Thus, the image appears white.

26. **a** A crescent-shaped crease such as this is usually made when taking the film out of the cassette just before processing. The crystals are further compressed, leaving a darker image at that spot.

27. **d** Safelight fogging causes unwanted exposure to a part of or all of the film. The increased amount of silver deposited means that there

will be greater darkness on the radiograph and less contrast.

28. **a** All living cells are susceptible to ionizing radiation, but the cells most sensitive to radiation are the rapidly dividing, metabolically active cells.

29. **c** A sievert (Sv) accounts for the fact that different tissues absorb radiation differently. It is the dose of radiation equivalent to the absorbed dose in tissue (1 sievert equals 100 rem).

30. **b** The film badge worn at the collar indicates that you are monitoring the degree of exposure to the neck and head region. In this area, the degree of exposure to the thyroid and lens of the eye is important to monitor.

31. **c** To ensure maximum safety, your goal with every radiograph should be whenever possible to decrease the time exposed to radiation, to increase the distance from the primary beam, and to shield yourself with proper equipment. The inverse square law says that as you double your distance from a radiation source, the exposure level you receive is only 1/4 as much. Protection should include at least 0.5 mm lead equivalent for gloves, thyroid collar, and apron and 0.35 mm for glasses.

32. **d** Consider the analogy of wearing dark colored sunglasses. You are not totally protected from the sun and simply reduce the amount of rays that get through. Every time a body part is in the field of x-rays, it is exposed to radiation, regardless of whether protective lead is worn. It is even worse if gloves are placed over the top of the hands rather than wearing them directly. The secondary radiation from the patient, table, and cassette still creates ionization and biologic changes in the hands.

33. **c** The small filament on the cathode means that a smaller focal spot will be used. A small focal spot means that the electron beam is narrowed to a smaller area, which means that the projected image will be sharper or have less penumbra as compared to a larger focal spot.

34. **b** Milliamp times seconds (mA $\times$ s = mAs) gives you the number of milliamperes per second. If you are given the mAs, multiply the mA by the time to arrive at the appropriate mAs. 300 $\times$ 1/20 sec = 15 mAs.

35. **b** The inverse square law says that as you decrease the distance from the radiation source, the intensity of the beam must be reduced. The intensity of the beam varies inversely according to the square of the distance. Thus, as you decrease your distance by one half, to compensate for being closer to the source, you must decrease the exposure by $(1/2)^2$ or by 1/4. The adjustment is usually made to the mAs. 1/4 $\times$ 16 = 4 mAs. You could also calculate the change in mAs through the formula old mAs $\times$ (new focal-film distance^2/old focal-film distance^2) = new mAs, or 16 mAs $\times$ [(50 cm)^2/(100 cm)^2] = 16 $\times$ 4 = 4 mAs.

36. **d** Scatter, or that radiation that occurs because of the interaction of the primary beam with tissue or matter, travels in a different direction and is composed of lower energy. It is more noticeable as the kVp is increased (the primary beam has more penetrating power to interact with matter), the patient thickness and density increases (more tissue and matter for the photons to interact with), and as the field size is larger (more photons bombarding a larger area, so there is more matter to interact with).

37. **c** The mAs and kVp affect density or the degree of blackness on the film. As you increase either exposure factor, more crystals will be affected, and the film will be blacker. But mAs does not appreciably alter contrast or the variation in degree of blackness, because all areas are affected equally, and kVp does affect contrast. As you increase kVp, there will be less contrast, because more photons are at the same energy level. More radiation is penetrated, and less is absorbed by the body part, so there will be more grayness on the radiograph, which is less contrast.

38. **b** Sante's rule states that when determining the kVp setting to use, you should multiply your tissue measurement in centimeters by 2, and add this to the source-image distance (focal-film distance), which is usually 40 inches. (Note: measure in centimeters, but use the focal-film distance in inches.)

39. **a** mA times exposure time in seconds gives you mAs (mA $\times$ s = mAs). Mathematically, this says that to get the same mAs as you increase the mA, you must invert or decrease the exposure time; thus, as you increase the mA, you must decrease the length of the exposure. The advantage of the shorter time is that blurring due to movement is less likely to occur.

40. **a** High-speed screens have larger phosphor crystals. Because one photon will affect a whole crystal, less exposure will be needed to cause the whole area to fluoresce, emitting a larger source of light. The larger crystals also mean that the image will be grainier and less detailed.

41. **c** Faster screens mean that less exposure is needed to create fluorescence and an image. If you use less exposure, then a lower mAs can be used, which often means a faster time and the use of the lower mA or smaller focal-spot size. The smaller focal-spot size helps increase the detail.

42. **b** The rare-earth phosphors have peak wavelengths at 420 to 540 nm, with most occurring at 540 nm, which is the green range. Calcium tungstate crystals emit a wavelength of 360 to 435 nm, which is the ultraviolet to blue-violet range.

43. **d** A film that has low contrast has very little difference in optical densities between different portions of the radiograph. There are a lot of grays that are considered to have many steps, but the change between each variation is minimal. This is also expressed as a long scale of contrast.

44. **a** To tell which exposure factor you should change, you first need to tell whether it is too dark or too light (use a toast analogy—is the toast burnt or not dark enough?). In this case, it is too dark, so you need to decrease exposure factors. To determine which exposure factor, first rule out kVp. This you can determine by looking at the contrast. For dark radiographs, look at the bones. If the bones are gray, there has been too much penetration, so you should decrease the kVp by about 10% to 15%. If the bones are dark, but still appear to have some contrast as compared with the surrounding soft tissue, they have not been overpenetrated, and the problem is too-high mAs. If the radiograph is too light, look at the organs. If you cannot clearly see the organs, the area has not had enough penetration, so you need to increase your kVp by about 10% to 15% so that density and contrast can be improved. If the organs are discernible, penetration has not been a problem, so increase mAs to increase the density or blackness on the radiograph.

45. **c** *Grid cutoff* is defined as the loss of the primary beam that occurs when the grid is used incorrectly. Because the grid is normally oriented in such a way that most of the primary beam passes through the grid, while the scatter radiation is absorbed, any misuse of the grid means increased primary beam absorption. Problems include using the grid upside down, not having the central beam perpendicular to the center of the grid, not having the grid within the focusing range, having a tilted grid, or having any combination of these problems.

46. **c** To increase the density on the film, either increase the mAs by 50% to 100% or the kVp by about 10% to 15%. Settings of 200 mA and 1/10 sec will give you 20 mAs, which is double the density. If you increase kVp and mAs, you will quadruple the density.

47. **d** When setting up a technique chart, standardize as many factors as possible, including grid use, film and screen type and speed, focal-film distance, processing time, and temperature. kVp will change depending on the thickness of the tissue.

48. **b** Low mAs and high kVp means that there is less contrast or more shades of gray, which is more desirable for soft tissue, to see all of the various steps or tissue changes.

49. **c** The grid ratio is the relation of the height of lead strips in a grid to the distance between them. A grid ratio of 10:1 means that the lead strip is 10 times higher than the width of the interspace. As the grid ratio increases, the grid becomes more efficient in absorbing the scatter radiation, but it will also absorb more of the primary beam. To compensate for absorption of the primary beam, exposure factors need to be increased, otherwise the image will appear lighter with the higher ratio.

50. **c** There will be increased magnification and distortion as the object-film distance is increased and the focal-film distance is decreased. On the radiograph, the limb nearest to the film will appear closer in size to the actual body part and will have more distinct edges. Because the right femur is further from the film and closer to the source of radiation, it will be more magnified.

51. **b** The affected area of interest should normally be placed against the film, so that a truer image is projected, with less distortion. It is best that the affected limb be pulled cranially, so that there is minimal joint interference.

52. **a** Following proper anatomic nomenclature, this term is in reference to the portion of the limb distal to or including the tarsus. The terminology for the stifle is *craniomedial-caudolateral oblique*. The carpus is *dorsomedial-palmarolateral oblique*.

53. **b** Positioning terminology describes the path of the x-ray beam through the body – where it enters the body forms the first part of the term and where it exits forms the second part. In an oblique view, the beam is directed about 45 degrees from the midsagittal plane. A dorsomedial view means that this oblique beam is directed toward the dorsal and medial aspect of the limb while it exits at the plantar and lateral limb side, which is also against the film.

54. **a** For an abdomen, exposures are best made during the pause at the end of expiration, so that the diaphragm is cranially displaced, and the body wall is relaxed. This prevents crowding of the abdominal contents and also ensures enough time to make the exposure without possible blurring, resulting from respiratory movements. This also maximizes kidney separation in lateral projection. For the thorax, exposures are best made at maximum inspiration to enhance the contrast between the radiolucent and the radiodense structures. If one can observe the patient's breathing before the exposure and breathe with the animal, the proper phase can more accurately be determined.

55. **d** For limbs distal to and including the elbow and stifle, the patient is best placed in sternal recumbency. For the front limb, the beam then enters from the cranial aspect of the limb and exits at the caudal aspect, where the film is also placed. Distal to and including the carpus, the terminology becomes *dorsopalmar,* choice **a**.

56. **a** One-third of the long bones distal and proximal to the joint should be included, and, because this is the front limb, portions of the radius and ulna should also be radiographed.

57. **b** If interested in the whole abdomen, it is important to include the area from the diaphragm to the pubis. For larger patients, separate radiographs of the cranial and caudal abdomen may need to be taken.

58. **c** The patient would be placed in dorsal recumbency, so that the head and nose are pointing upward. Gauze can be placed around the upper canine teeth and pulled rostrally, and gauze around the lower canine teeth should be pulled caudally. The vertically directed beam will be perpendicular to the tabletop to bisect the angle created by the open-mouth. This view is sometimes referred to as a *basilar view* and also permits evaluation of the odontoid process. A true lateral would cause superimposition. If an oblique view is desired, the ventrodorsal (not DV oblique) should be used.

59. **d** For a full skull, the vertically directed beam should be placed midway between the eyes at the level of the lateral canthi of the eyes. If the interest is in the rostral part of the skull, the beam should be centered just rostrally to the eyes.

60. **a** If one draws an imaginary line between the medial canthus of each eye, and ensures that this line is parallel to the film and table, as noticed when looking at the patient from the front and at eye level, the resulting radiographic image should be perfectly positioned.

61. **a** Nonscreen film gives you the greatest detail and is also easiest to position in the mouth.

62. **d** There are seven cervical vertebrae, and the beam should always be centered in the middle of the area of interest.

63. **d** To prevent image distortion, it is important that the area of interest always be parallel to the film. In this case, the proximal and/or distal portions of the femurs were not properly extended and thus not parallel to the table. Elongation would occur if the femurs and film were not perpendicular to the tube head.

64. **a** *Positive* means it is radiopaque and absorbs radiation, and thus it appears as a white image on the film.

65. **c** Meglumine triiodinated salt is less toxic because of the lower sodium content.

66. **a** The iodine compounds become diluted by fluid drawn into the GI tract.

67. **b** Iodine does not irritate the peritoneum, whereas barium is irritative and can cause a granuloma. Air and carbon dioxide are negative contrast agents.

68. **d**

69. **c**

70. **b** An esophagram is used to study the esophagus, and a barium enema is used to study the large intestine.

71. **a**

72. **d**

73. **c** kVp, the voltage difference between the anode and cathode in the x-ray tube, controls the speed of the electron beam.

74. **d** Milliamperage controls how hot the filament gets, and this determines the number of electrons flowing from it.

75. **b**

76. **d**

77. **c** Nongrid technique is normally used to radiograph extremities, the skull, or other body parts less than 10-cm thick.

78. **d**

79. **d**

80. **b**

81. **a**

82. **c**

83. **a** The skyline view is used to reduce superimposition of the carpal bones.

84. **d** The opposite limb is pulled in a caudodorsal direction to rotate the sternum slightly away from the shoulder joint.

85. **b** Use of the bisecting-angle technique prevents elongation or foreshortening of the tooth when taking intraoral radiographs.

86. **c**

87. **c**

88. **a**

89. **a** Boxes should be stored on end in a vertical position. If stored in a horizontal position for an extended period, pressure on the emulsion of the film can show up after processing as a fogging artifact.

90. **d** Nonscreen film would produce a high-detail image that would allow detection of subtle tooth and jaw changes.

91. **b**

92. **d**

93. **c**

94. **a**

95. **d** Bend marks appear as half-moon-shaped black artifacts.

96. **c** Light leaks appear as black areas, not generalized heavy lines.

97. **b** Fast film requires less exposure by x-rays.

98. **d**

99. **c**

100. **a**

101. **b**

102. **d**

103. **c**

104. **b**

105. **b**

106. **a** *ALARA* stands for "as low as reasonably achievable," which means to use a technique to keep exposure levels to a minimum yet take a diagnostic quality film.

107. **c**

108. **c** Persons under 18 years of age should not be involved in radiographic procedures.

109. **d**

110. **c** Scatter radiation has lower energy than the primary beam that produced it.

111. **d** Nuclear scintigraphy is a noninvasive imaging technique used primarily in horses.

112. **a**

113. **a**

114. **d**

115. **b**

116. **c**

117. **a** Sante's rule allows one to calculate kVp using the following formula:
kVp = 2 × thickness measurement (cm) + 40

118. **a** The MPD for personnel is 0.05 sieverts per year of whole-body radiation.

119. **b** The quantity of ionizing radiation per unit of body mass best defines absorbed dose of radiation. Dose equivalent measurements take into account the variable biologic effect of this ionizing radiation across tissue types. It better represents the functional effect of the radiation on various tissue types. Grays are a unit of measurement for absorbed dose estimates and have replaced the unit formally used, called a *rad.*

120. **c** Lack of collimation, increased contact with the x-ray table, and high kVp settings all result in increased scatter and personnel exposure. The use of a fast screen and fast film provide for shorter exposure times and do not increase the level of scatter radiation.

121. **a** Three views are taken for a PennHIP evaluation, and the primary predictor of susceptibility to hip dysplasia is the degree of joint laxity. Specific parameters are published for various breeds of dogs based on a large database. Veterinary staff must receive special training before performing the PennHIP procedure as a diagnostic tool.

122. **a** Geometric distortion, such as foreshortening, can occur when the beam is not directed perpendicularly to the object of interest and/or when the patient is not parallel to the film.

123. **a** Tabletop films are desirable for small patients, thin body parts, and most exotics.

124. **a** Ideally, lateral thoracic radiographs are taken at peak inspiration, when the lungs have achieved their maximum inflation.

125. **c** Three views should be taken to adequately visualize the lung fields. A right and left lateral view are taken in addition to a VD or a DV view as well. Anything less than this is considered incomplete by a veterinary oncologist.

126. **a** The nonrecumbent (noncompressed) lung is best visualized when performing a lateral thoracic radiograph.

127. **b** Slow screen and slow film combinations require longer exposure times (and higher levels of ionizing radiation), yet they are able to provide better detail. This degree of detail is required for this type of study. Fast screen and fast film combinations provide rapid exposure times yet may provide a grainy, mottled image, precluding evaluation of the lacy trabecular bone in the nasal sinuses. To combine fast screens with slow film speeds and vice versa prevents one from gaining the benefit of either; therefore, this type of mixing of film and screen speeds is not routinely done.

128. **b** When processing chemicals are incompletely washed from a radiograph, the resulting image rapidly develops a yellowish tinge.

129. **a** When a focused grid is used out of its focal range (because of inappropriate focal-film distance), lines may appear on the resultant film.

130. **d** Motion, graininess that results from fast film and fast screens, and a double exposure all result in a film with poor detail.

131. **a** The heel effect occurs because of the anode target angle that results in a stronger beam on the cathode side of the x-ray beam. To take advantage of this variation, one would place the thicker part of the animal or body part on that side.

132. **b** The film is too light, thereby suggesting that the exposure settings should be increased. The lack of penetration can be remedied by increasing the kVp setting.

133. **a** Incremental changes of 10% to 15% in kVp settings are noticeable, and changes of 30% to 50% in mAs are detectable.

134. **c** Exposure settings must be decreased, because the film is too dark. If there is little distinction in scale between bone and soft tissue (i.e., all tissue is gray), it indicates that the contrast may be improved by decreasing kVp.

135. **b**

136. **a** The view is named by where the beam enters (first) and then exits the animal (last). For oblique views, one must provide more detail (i.e., dorsal vs. palmar and lateral vs. medial surface).

137. **b** BIPS are inert, radiopaque beads that are fed to an animal, and then sequential radiographs are taken. They primarily provide information about GI transit time. They provide no information about the intestinal mucosa.

138. **b** Negative contrast using room air is contraindicated for a double-contrast study of the bladder when there is excessive hematuria. The risk of air embolism is increased.

139. **c** Nuclear scintigraphy is an imaging modality in which a small amount of radioactive material is administered. The uptake of these materials provides indirect information regarding the physiologic function of the organs in question. Anatomic detail is not provided.

140. **c** Technetium-99 is a labeled compound that is used alone or tagged to other compounds. It is then absorbed by the target organ in question, and some evaluation of function can be made.

141. **c** Barium provides excellent mucosal detail, and unlike the water-soluble iodinated compounds, it does not absorb water from the GI tract (because of hypertonicity) and become diluted.

142. **c** Barium is contraindicated, because if it passed through a perforation into the abdominal cavity, it would not be absorbed by the animal; instead it would remain there where it could result in an inflammatory response.

143. **a** There is minimal contrast, because few echoes are reflected, and the resulting image contains gray areas that blend with surrounding tissues.

144. **d** Higher energy transducers provide improved resolution but sacrifice penetration. There is a trade-off between resolution and penetration ability. A 7.5-mHz transducer is usually used on cats, and a 5.0-mHz transducer is used on large dogs.

145. **a** Hyperechoic objects or tissues reflect bright white echoes.

146. **b** Anechoic objects and tissues reflect few to no echoes and thus present a black image on the ultrasound monitor.

147. **a** The tungsten plate is located in the anode within the x-ray tube.

148. **a** When the high-speed electrons hit the tungsten target on the anode, the x-rays are formed.

149. **b** Anyone who takes radiographs should use a thyroid shield and lead glasses, but anyone in the vicinity of the x-ray unit (especially if it is not in a separate room) should wear a dosimetry badge to monitor the amount of radiation exposure.

150. **c**

151. **b** The electron beam is aimed at the target and centered on the focal spot.

152. **a**

153. **d** The grid is used to decrease scatter radiation and increase the contrast on the radiation. It is made of radiodense strips of lead and is placed between the patient and the film. Grids can cause thin white lines to form.

154. **c** This is due to the anode heel effect, which is the unequal distribution of the x-ray beam intensity. The higher intensity is at the cathode side of the beam and can better penetrate thicker objects.

155. **b** Intensifying screens have been great assets to radiography, because they enhance the effects of the radiation and create a clearer and deeper scale of contrast.

156. **a** Higher kVp is needed in thicker objects to penetrate the density, resulting in more shades of gray, also known as *longer scale of contrast.*

157. **b** Low kVp has a low penetration into the subject and thus creates an image with less shades of gray. This is known as *increased overall contrast* and *shorter scale of contrast.*

158. **a** The National Council on Radiation Protection and Measurements sets this standard for occupationally exposed individuals.

159. **d** The collimator adjustment is one means of minimizing radiation scatter.

160. **c** This is due to the inverse square law that states that the intensity of the x-ray beam is inversely proportional to the square of the distance from the source of the x-ray.

161. **b** The two films will have to be viewed exactly overlapping each other to get a satisfactory radiograph. Each film separately will not be a good film.

162. **b** Splotching may occur if film-developing guidelines are not followed. Chemicals may splatter, affecting the final radiograph. Motion causes a blurred image, gridlines cause white lines, and static electricity creates a dark "tree-like" artifact.

163. **a** Misaligned Bucky trays cut off x-rays to edges of the film, so when developed, there is no change to the silver halide, and it is thus washed clean.

164. **c** The closer the target is to the film, the denser the radiation dose is to the film, and therefore the denser (darker) the radiograph.

165. **b** Distal extremities are relatively thin structures with different minimal densities in them (skin, muscle, bone), so a short scale of contrast (higher overall contrast) is best.

166. **a** Dosimetry badges should always be worn in the x-ray room, should be changed at least monthly, and should be worn by all personnel using x-ray machinery.

167. **c** This helps minimize motion by the patient, gives the technicians time to properly position the animal to minimize the number of retakes, and can permit the radiographers to use adjunct equipment, so that they may leave the near vicinity of the x-ray beam when the picture is taken.

168. **c** The 0.5-mm lead equivalence is a standard from the National Council on Radiation Protection and Measurements.

169. **b** Because the young adult body is still growing, people younger than 18 years should not be allowed to work with x-radiation to minimize effects on rapidly growing cells.

170. **a** The inverse law says that the more distance that is placed between the handler and the x-ray source, the less the exposure to radiation.

171. **b** To see the entire abdominal field, the film should be taken at peak expiration.

172. **b** Positioning the forelegs cranially moves the muscle bellies of the foreleg in front of the heart and a majority of the cranial chest, allowing for better visualization of the thoracic contents.

173. **c** Proper positioning for a lateral thoracic view should include the spine and sternum being equidistant from the table.

174. **a** The twelfth rib is generally the widest and largest part of the thorax, the best place to measure.

175. **c** The abdomen extends from the tip of the diaphragm to the hip. The xiphoid process is the external landmark closest to the position of the tip of the diaphragm.

176. **c** Tabletop radiographs are preferred for object thickness up to about 10 cm. The increased kVp needed to penetrate greater thickness causes greater scatter, so a grid is needed.

177. **a** Unless there is a specific spot that the veterinarian wants to view, radiographs of extremities should be on the midshaft of the bone with a joint included on either end.

178. **c** The hip joints are the widest and densest part of the pelvis.

179. **d** This positioning allows differentiation between the upper and lower leg. The affected leg should always be "down," closest to the film, to minimize distortion.

180. **d** For proper pelvic positioning, the patellae should be riding atop the patellar grooves.

181. **b** It is very difficult to get proper positioning of the skull in an awake patient.

182. **d** This position enables the tympanic bullae to be viewed without obstruction.

183. **c** C3 is the best place to measure for a standard cervical film.

184. **b** When lying laterally, the cervical region has a tendency to dip toward the film. A radiolucent positioner can alleviate that dip and minimize false positives for narrowed intervertebral disk spaces.

185. **b** The T13 site is the tallest spot, to get the best exposure through the lungs and cranial abdomen.

186. **b** The caudal border of the scapula rests over the approximate midway point of the thoracic vertebrae.

187. **a**

188. **a** The mA selector controls the number of electrons produced at the filament.

189. **b** With a 12:1 ratio grid, more x-rays are absorbed, requiring more x-rays to be produced, or a higher mAs.

190. **d** A 12:1 ratio grid with 113 lines per inch absorbs more scatter, producing an image with better contrast and less fogging on the finished radiographic film.

191. **a**

192. **c** A full-wave, rectified three phase allows for more positive potential across the terminals of the tube, producing a higher energy of electrons and a more constant energy x-ray beam.

193. **a** The kVp controls radiographic contrast by increasing or decreasing the shades of gray. The higher the kVp, the longer the scale of contrast. (More grays can be seen.)

194. **d** The object-film distance does not influence radiographic density.

195. **a** The focusing cup focuses the beam of electrons on the focal spot of the anode.

196. **c** The target of an x-ray machine is the area of the anode struck by electrons during an exposure.

197. **d**

198. **b** A full-wave rectified x-ray machine produces 120 pulses of x-rays per second, or 2 pulses per 1/60 second.

199. **d** A cassette with intensifying screens can be placed open under the x-ray beam and a low exposure made. If x-radiation is being produced, the screen will fluoresce.

200. **c** Tube saturation occurs when there is not enough positive potential (voltage) between the cathode and anode to pull all of the electrons across the tube. The extra electrons accumulate on the glass envelope and can crack the tube.

201. **c** Metal has the highest x-ray absorption, because it is the densest.

202. **b** A grid must move at right angles to the grid lines. This blurs the lines so that they are not visible on the radiographic film.

203. **a** The inverse square law states that the intensity of the x-ray beam is inversely proportional to the square of the distance from the source of the x-rays. The same number of x-rays must diverge, covering an area that is four times as large.

204. **c**

205. **c**

206. **b** Increasing the kVp 20% doubles the radiographic density and increases the penetration.

207. **c** Because mAs controls the number of x-rays produced, reducing the mAs reduces radiographic density. Reducing the kVp would decrease the shades of gray, because it also affects image contrast.

208. **a** When kVp and mAs are too high for the machine, too much heat is created, causing the anode to crack.

209. **a** The mAs controls the number of x-rays produced. If the mAs is doubled, this doubles the density on the radiographic film.

210. **b** The cathode holds the filament. When current is applied to the filament, electrons boil off, producing an electron cloud.

211. **d** 200 mA, 110 seconds = 20 mAs. This is the highest mAs, which produces the most x-rays.

212. **d** Celiography is useful when studying the abdominal cavity and the integrity of the diaphragm.

213. **c** Air appears black on a radiographic film.

214. **a** A barium enema generally uses positive- and negative-contrast media to evaluate the large intestine.

215. **b** Barium sulfate is very irritating to the peritoneum.

216. **c** The head is elevated after injection for a myelogram to decrease the chance of seizure.

217. **c** Barium sulfate has a high atomic number and appears white on a radiographic film.

218. **d** Excretory urography provides information relative to renal function and the structure of the kidneys, ureters, and bladder.

219. **c** Air appears radiolucent (black) on a radiographic film.

220. **b** This contrast study is used to evaluate the stomach and small intestine. The contrast medium is administered orally, and films are made during transit of the contrast medium through the stomach and small bowel into the colon.

221. **d** The dose of contrast medium is calculated using the weight of the animal.

222. **d** Barium sulfate appears radiopaque (white) on a radiographic film.

223. **c** Fistulography is a contrast study that delineates the extent and possibly the origin of fistulous tracts.

224. **a** An excretory urogram identifies the size, shape, location, and margination of the kidneys and ureters. It also shows where the ureters terminate.

225. **c** The cathode end of the x-ray beam has the higher x-ray beam intensity because of the angle of the target on the anode.

226. **b** The kVp controls the penetration power and scale of contrast on the film; it has no effect on penumbra, which causes a loss of detail. There are three main factors in the amount of penumbra on a radiographic film; these are *focal-film distance, object-film distance,* and *focal-spot size.*

227. **c** The spinning top shows the number of dots produced during the exposure. This represents the number of x-ray pulses produced during that exposure time. If the number of dots is incorrect, there is a problem with the timer.

228. **b**

229. **a**

230. **b**

231. **a**

232. **c** When film is exposed to low-grade light leaks, a base fog decreases the overall quality of the finished radiographic film, decreasing contrast and detail.

233. **b** For radiographic films to be legal in court, and for the certification organizations to accept them, they must be permanently identified. This can be done during the exposure with lead letters or radiopaque tape or after the exposure, but the film should be identified before the film is processed with manual or photo labelers.

234. **a** The total time the film must be in the fixer is double the time it was in the developer. The film can be viewed on a view box after the film has been in the fixer for 30 seconds only; however, it must be placed back into the fixer for the remaining time to complete the process.

235. **a**

236. **a**

237. **b**

238. **b**

239. **c** The fluids in manual processing tanks should be changed at least every 3 months. In busy practices, the frequency may need to be increased to maintain the quality of the radiographic film.

240. **b** The radiographic film is clear, because the fixer removes all of the silver halide crystals that remain after being in the developer. If the film has not been placed in the developer, the sensitized silver halide crystals have not yet been changed into black metallic silver. The fixer then removes all of the silver halide crystals, clearing the film of any image.

241. **c** Developer chemicals are kept at an alkaline pH, usually 9.8 to 11.4. Developer chemicals cannot function in a neutral or acid solution.

242. **d** The chemicals should be mixed in a bucket outside of the darkroom to prevent the chemical dust from contaminating unprotected films, thus causing artifacts.

243. **c** The processing chemicals should be at least 60° F to be efficient.

244. **d** If the films were not completely washed, the fixer that remained in the emulsion would oxidize, turning them a brownish color.

245. **c** A direct system shines the safelight directly toward the workbench. To prevent possible fogging of the film, the safelight should be placed at least 48 inches from the workbench.

246. **b** Because both had identical areas of decreased density, this means the films were stuck together in the developer. The density is decreased, because the developer was not able to change the sensitized silver halide crystals into black metallic silver; consequently, the fixer cleared the remaining silver halide crystals. This left areas of decreased density.

247. **c** A latent image is the silver halide crystals in the film's emulsion that have been exposed to radiant energy, causing them to become susceptible to chemical change.

248. **a** Screen-type film is more sensitive to the light from intensifying screens than it is to direct x-ray exposure.

249. **b** The emulsion is too thick for some types of direct-exposure film to be automatically processed. The processing chemicals cannot reach all of the silver halide crystals in the time that they take to automatically process.

250. **b** Direct-exposure film requires that more x-rays be generated to expose it, because it does not use the intensifying effect of screens.

251. **c** Film is most sensitive after it has been exposed but before it is processed. Care must be taken when handling the film after it has been exposed.

252. **b** The crystal size in high-speed film is larger, allowing a decrease in mAs; however, the detail is decreased compared with that of slow-speed film.

253. **b** Long-latitude film can produce a long scale of contrast.

254. **d** Film should be stored away from strong chemical fumes to prevent a base fog on the film.

255. **d** When identifying films, the label should include the clinic's name; the date; the client's and patient's names; and the species, sex, and age of the patient.

256. **a** An oblique projection is used to delineate an area that would normally be superimposed over another (e.g., the right and left sides of the mandible on a lateral projection of the skull).

257. **b** To include the entire thorax on a radiographic film, the cranial landmark is the manubrium sterni, and the caudal landmark is halfway between the xiphoid and the last rib.

258. **c** To include the entire abdomen on a radiographic film, the cranial landmark is three rib spaces cranial to the xiphoid, and the caudal landmark is the greater trochanter.

259. **b**

260. **c** The endotracheal tube is removed to prevent superimposition over the main bony structures.

261. **a** Foreshortening occurs when the long bone is not parallel to the cassette, causing the bone to appear shorter than it actually is.

262. **c** Centering the beam on the joint maximizes the size of the joint space and minimizes the amount of false narrowing that can occur, as the center of the primary beam is moved away from the joint.

263. **b** Extending the head caudodorsally moves the trachea off of the shoulder joint; extending the contralateral limb farther caudally moves the manubrium away from the shoulder joint.

264. **a**

265. **b**

266. **b**

267. **a**

268. **c**

269. **a**

270. **b** With a dorsopalmar-lateromedial oblique projection, the lateral sesamoid is imaged without superimposition of any other bones.

271. **b**

272. **b** With a left 20-degree ventral/right dorsal oblique projection of the skull, the right tympanic bulla is delineated from the left.

273. **b** Placing the thick part of the patient toward the cathode of the x-ray tube produces a more uniform density on the radiographic film.

274. **a** Radiographic films are legal medical records and must contain all of the information found in answer choice **a**.

275. **c** L4 is midway between the pubis and the xiphoid cartilage in a dog lying in the ventrodorsal position.

276. **c** T7 is approximately midway between the 1st and 13th rib.

277. **d** To reduce the divergent x-ray energy beam, a restriction device can focus the column of energy on the cassette.

278. **b** mA × time (in seconds) = mAs

279. **c** The larger the crystal size, the more light is produced. High-speed screens have larger crystals, even bigger than the rare-earth crystals.

280. **b** Change in kVp changes the energy level of the x-ray beam.

281. **a** The distance between the source of an x-ray (focal spot) and the image receptor (x-ray film) is called *focal-film distance.*

282. **b** If the object being x-rayed is farther from the receptor, the image formed on the film is magnified, because the x-ray beam strikes the object farther from the projected shadow.

283. **c** X-rays are more efficiently converted to light by rare-earth phosphors than by calcium tungstate, a major factor in reducing exposure time. All of the other items have no effect on exposure-time reduction.

284. **a**

285. **d** The area of contrast is dependent upon the density and mass of the tissue or subject.

286. **c** Scatter radiation originates from the patient as the primary beam strikes the first solid object and produces secondary radiation.

287. **a** Increasing kVp causes increased scatter radiation. As a result of the increase in energy, more x-rays penetrate farther into the patient and increase the opportunity for scatter radiation.

288. **b** If a grid is used outside of the specified range, grid cutoff may occur. This produces a progressive decrease in transmitted x-ray intensity near the edges of the grid.

289. **b** Calcium tungstate emits light in the blue and ultraviolet regions of the spectrum when struck by an x-ray beam.

290. **d** The larger the crystals, the faster the screen, the less the detail, and the grainier the appearance of the image.

291. **d** Increased film speed leads to a radiographic artifact known as *quantum mottle.* This can occur because the faster screens are sensitive to radiation; as a result, the reduced energy levels of the settings do not produce the desired uniformity of density.

292. **c** The crystals of a fluoroscopy unit emit green light, to which the human eye is sensitive. Motion radiographic films can be seen because conventional film is substituted for the fluoroscopy screen.

293. **a** Silver halide is a compound of silver and bromine, chlorine, or iodine that forms a latent image when ionized by light or radiation.

294. **b** Ionizing radiation causes latent images to be formed on nonscreen film without intensifying screens.

295. **a** Radiographs made with nonscreen film have greater detail compared with other speed film, because there is no loss of detail from intensifying screens.

296. **c** The very small silver halide crystals in the emulsion of slow x-ray film produce less change in radiographic density with changes in exposure factors.

297. **b** A processing system must be compatible with the film speed and the type of cassette to produce high-quality radiographic films.

298. **b** Light exposes the radiographic film unevenly, and the image on the film appears darkened, commonly known as *fogged.*

299. **b** The lightbulb is commonly filtered with brown for blue-light–sensitive film.

300. **b** The filter commonly used for the safelight when using green-light–sensitive film is dark red.

301. **a** If a lateral view of the tarsus was exposed with the toes of the patient facing to the right side of the cassette, the craniocaudal view should have the toes facing the same side of the cassette.

302. **b** If the fixer is exhausted, or time in the fixer is too short, the film does not harden properly, and the emulsion turns yellow.

303. **b** The 8:1 grid ratio is adequate for the average patient.

304. **c** Static electricity causes dark images as a result of the light produced over the unexposed film.

305. **b** Because x-ray film is more sensitive to light than to radiation, the use of fluorescent intensifying screens dramatically decreases the amount of radiation needed; therefore, much lower mAs settings and shorter exposure times can be used.

306. **d** Scatter radiation increases with an increase in the thickness of the body part, therefore a better image results if scatter is reduced by absorbing the nonparallel x-rays with a grid. Body parts thicker than 10 cm scatter enough radiation to cause distortion of the image.

307. **c** Crystals in the screens fluoresce or emit light during exposure to x-rays.

308. **d** Light leakage in a darkroom, from any source, adds to the overall darkness of the image, fogging the radiographic film.

309. **d** Crossover roller dirt is the most common cause of streaks and stains on automatically processed film.

310. **a** Radiation absorbed dose (rad) is the quantity of energy imparted to matter by ionizing radiation.

311. **c** Roentgen equivalent man (rem) measures ionizing radiation absorbed by tissue.

312. **b** The dosimeter measures the actual amount of ionizing radiation, whereas the other monitoring devices indicate exposure.

313. **b** For people over 18 years of age, the upper limit is 5 rem.

314. **c** 7.5 rems × 1000 millirems/rem = 7500 millirems

315. **b**

316. **c** All states have one safety code in common. It requires that at least 2.5 mm of aluminum filtration of the primary beam be used in any diagnostic machine with a capacity over 70 kVp.

317. **b** The filter eliminates the less penetrating or "soft" x-rays, which have low energy.

318. **d** At no time should any part of your body be exposed to the primary beam, even when shielded with protective covering.

319. **d** Regulations in veterinary radiography require 0.5 mm of lead equivalent in the aprons and gloves, because the restrainer is often very close to the primary beam.

320. **c** The intensity of the primary x-ray beam is inversely proportional to the source-image distance. At twice the distance, the beam intensity is 1/4 of the original intensity.

321. **d** The reduced radiation needed for diagnostic x-rays with rare-earth intensifying screens considerably reduces the exposure risk to the technician.

322. **b** When more radiographs are made, there is more chance of exposure to ionizing radiation.

323. **b** Careful collimation reduces the amount of secondary scatter and therefore reduces exposure of the operator.

324. **d** Good technique results in less exposure because of fewer repeats.

325. **a** Chemical (drug) restraint should be used when possible, so the technician does not have to be in the room with the animal during the exposure.

326. **b** Film-badge reports are usually submitted monthly.

327. **a** Radiation protection is regulated by the National Committee on Radiation Protection and Measurements. Their recommendation is to supply monitoring badges at a potential level of 1/4 MPD.

328. **c** The dosimeter badge does not protect from radiation; it detects radiation.

329. **c** Exposure units are physical amounts of radiation known as *roentgens*. Absorbed units are rads, and the measurement of biologic effect is a rem measurement. Radon is a radioactive gas.

330. **d** Increased distance from the primary beam greatly reduces the risk of exposure, as compared with that provided by any of the devices positioned next to the primary beam.

331. **b** Nonoccupationally exposed persons can receive 10% of the occupational dose. The maximum permissible dose (MPD) for the general public is set at a much lower level, because the public is not monitored and is untrained to recognize and avoid exposure.

Anesthesiology

Thomas Colville

QUESTIONS

1. The drug xylazine is best described as an
   a. Antiinflammatory
   b. Analgesic and sedative
   c. Antiemetic
   d. Anesthetic

2. Detomidine is approved for use in
   a. Dogs
   b. Cats
   c. Horses
   d. Cattle

3. Butorphanol is best described as a/an
   a. Antiinflammatory
   b. Analgesic
   c. Anesthetic
   d. Diuretic

4. Diazepam is considered to be a good choice in patients when which body system is compromised?
   a. Hepatic
   b. Renal
   c. Cardiovascular
   d. All body systems

5. In the United States, xylazine is not approved for use in
   a. Dogs
   b. Cats
   c. Horses
   d. Cattle

6. Guaifenesin is most often used in horses and cattle to provide
   a. Analgesia
   b. Muscle relaxation
   c. Anesthesia
   d. Diuresis

7. The combination of xylazine and butorphanol is used to
   a. Provide greater analgesia and muscle relaxation than either drug can alone
   b. Cause central nervous system (CNS) excitement
   c. Increase the dose of butorphanol
   d. Increase the dose of xylazine

8. Which drug is the most potent sedative?
   a. Xylazine
   b. Detomidine
   c. Acepromazine
   d. Diazepam

9. Which drug is most likely to cause hypotension in normal doses?
   a. Diazepam
   b. Butorphanol
   c. Acepromazine
   d. Flunixin meglumine

10. The combination drug Telazol contains
    a. Diazepam and ketamine
    b. Diazepam and xylazine
    c. Zolazepam and tiletamine
    d. Xylazine and tiletamine

11. Epidural techniques are used in many species, but the primary disadvantage in animals is
    a. High cost
    b. Difficulty of administration
    c. Poor analgesia
    d. Movement of the patient

12. Which inhalant anesthetic drug is most likely to cause cardiac arrhythmias in dogs?
    a. Isoflurane
    b. Halothane
    c. Sevoflurane
    d. Nitrous oxide

479

Correct answers are on pages 503-514.

13. Which inhalant anesthetic drug is biotrans-formed to the greatest extent in the animal body?
    a. Isoflurane
    b. Halothane
    c. Sevoflurane
    d. Nitrous oxide

14. All of the following cross the placental barrier in significant amounts except
    a. Acepromazine
    b. Diazepam
    c. Isoflurane
    d. Neuromuscular blocking agents

15. Which drug is not classified as a barbiturate?
    a. Phenobarbital
    b. Thiopental
    c. Pentobarbital
    d. Propofol

16. Glycopyrrolate is an anticholinergic with all of the following advantages over atropine except
    a. Longer duration of action
    b. Crosses the placental barrier
    c. Less likely to cause cardiac arrhythmias
    d. Smaller dose volume

17. At normal doses, what effect does atropine have on the heart rate?
    a. Decreases
    b. No effect
    c. Increases
    d. Prevents a decrease

18. Opioid drugs are used in anesthetic protocols primarily as
    a. Anesthetics
    b. Analgesics
    c. Antiinflammatories
    d. Antihistamines

19. The advantage of xylazine over acepromazine is that it
    a. Does not cause cardiac arrhythmias
    b. Produces a short period of analgesia
    c. Has antiemetic properties
    d. Is an antiinflammatory

20. Routine use of atropine in horses should be avoided, because it may
    a. Cause colic
    b. Slow the heart rate
    c. Cause excitement
    d. Increase salivation

21. Which drug should be avoided in the stallion because it may cause permanent prolapse of the penis?
    a. Glycopyrrolate
    b. Acepromazine
    c. Xylazine
    d. Diazepam

22. Which drug is a narcotic antagonist?
    a. Naloxone
    b. Atropine
    c. Pancuronium
    d. Droperidol

23. A 10% solution of thiopental sodium for anes-thetic induction contains
    a. 10 mg/ml
    b. 100 mg/ml
    c. 20 mg/ml
    d. 40 mg/ml

24. Depressant preanesthetic medication may have what effect on the anesthesia procedure?
    a. Shorten the recovery time
    b. Prolong the recovery time
    c. Leave the recovery time unaltered
    d. Necessitate increasing the dose of induction agent

25. Which drug is an antagonist of xylazine?
    a. Butorphanol
    b. Detomidine
    c. Yohimbine
    d. Pentazocine

26. Diazepam is used to produce
    a. Analgesia
    b. Hypnosis
    c. Muscle relaxation
    d. Vomiting

27. Epinephrine
    a. Increases the heart rate
    b. Decreases the heart rate
    c. Decreases the blood pressure
    d. Should be used to reverse the effects of acepromazine

28. Use of nitrous oxide in anesthesia
    a. Increases the amount of inhalation anesthetic required
    b. Decreases the amount of inhalation anesthetic required
    c. Slows the induction process
    d. Has no effect on the time or amount of anesthetic required

29. A disadvantage of breathing 50% nitrous oxide is that it
    a. Decreases the arterial PaO_2
    b. Increases the arterial PaO_2
    c. Slows the induction time
    d. Prolongs the recovery time

30. How many milligrams per milliliter (mg/ml) does a 2% lidocaine solution contain?
    a. 5
    b. 10
    c. 20
    d. 30

31. What volume of thiopental sodium should be administered intravenously to a 500-kg horse for induction of anesthesia? The dosage is 8 mg/kg, and you are using a 10% solution.
    a. 24 ml
    b. 40 ml
    c. 60 ml
    d. 65 ml

32. Apneustic breathing patterns are frequently seen in cats with use of
    a. Pentobarbital
    b. Thiamylal
    c. Ketamine
    d. Guaifenesin

33. Which of the following is not a good reason to use a preanesthetic?
    a. Calms the patient
    b. Minimizes the dose of induction agent needed
    c. Smoothes induction and recovery
    d. Increases vagal activity

34. If 180 ml of a 5% solution of guaifenesin is administered to a 150-kg foal, how many mg/kg would be administered?
    a. 30
    b. 60
    c. 90
    d. 15

35. Caudal epidural administration of lidocaine in the dog is
    a. Useful to prevent movement
    b. Not to be used for cesarean section
    c. An excellent caudal analgesic
    d. An old procedure with little value in veterinary anesthesia today

36. Mask inductions are
    a. Best used in dogs and cats with airway obstruction
    b. Best used in aggressive dogs and cats
    c. Absolutely the best way to induce anesthesia in all dogs and cats
    d. More appropriately used in calm dogs and cats

37. Which of the following is not an effect associated with atropine administration?
    a. Tachycardia
    b. Excessive salivation
    c. Mydriasis
    d. Decreased gastrointestinal motility

38. The dosage of acepromazine is 0.1 mg/kg, and the maximum dose is 4 mg. How many milligrams would you administer to a 60-kg dog?
    a. 2
    b. 4
    c. 6
    d. 8

39. Halothane concentrations of 1% to 2% may produce any of the following except
    a. Hypotension
    b. Hypoventilation
    c. Hypothermia
    d. Increased cardiac output

40. The adverse effects of anesthetic compounds are
    a. Nothing to worry about
    b. Never present with smaller doses
    c. Dose dependent
    d. Not dose dependent

41. The most reliable sign of inadequate anesthetic depth is
    a. Increased heart rate
    b. Increased respiratory rate
    c. Active palpebral reflex
    d. Responsive movement

42. Propofol is a/an
    a. Xylazine antagonist
    b. Ultrashort-acting barbiturate
    c. Ketamine-like dissociative
    d. Nonbarbiturate, intravenous anesthetic with hypotensive potential

Correct answers are on pages 503-514.

43. Acepromazine should be avoided in
    a. Patients with a history of seizures
    b. Aggressive patients
    c. All old dogs
    d. All Dobermans

44. In dogs, normal doses of opioids generally produce all of the following except
    a. Respiratory depression
    b. Decreased heart rate
    c. Analgesia
    d. Excitement

45. When comparing inhalation anesthetics, you should use the minimum alveolar concentration (MAC) as a guide in assessing
    a. Respiratory depression
    b. Potency of the agent
    c. Cardiovascular effects
    d. Solubility coefficients

46. Which drug is a dissociative anesthetic?
    a. Thiopental sodium
    b. Ketamine
    c. Xylazine
    d. Acepromazine

47. Which inhalant anesthetic is associated with the longest induction and recovery times?
    a. Nitrous oxide
    b. Isoflurane
    c. Halothane
    d. Sevoflurane

48. In rabbits, intravenous anesthetics should be injected into which of the following veins?
    a. Femoral
    b. Jugular
    c. Auricular
    d. Cephalic

49. The oxygen flow rate necessary to prevent rebreathing of exhaled gases with an Ayre's T piece is
    a. 0.5 L/min
    b. 1 L/min
    c. 2 L/min
    d. Greater than 1.5 times the minute ventilation

50. A half-full tank of nitrous oxide gas has a pressure of
    a. 375 psi
    b. 2200 psi
    c. 750 psi
    d. 50 psi

51. When inflating lungs with the thoracic cavity open to the atmosphere, be sure that the pressure reached on the manometer is
    a. 10 cm H_2O
    b. 20 cm H_2O
    c. 60 cm H_2O
    d. 70 cm H_2O

52. Precision vaporizers, such as those used for isoflurane, work correctly when placed
    a. In the circle
    b. Out of the circle
    c. Either in or out of the circle
    d. In the high-pressure portion of the anesthetic system

53. If the unidirectional valves are missing from an anesthetic machine, it is
    a. Okay to use the machine until you find them
    b. Okay to use the machine if soda lime is new
    c. Okay to use the machine with the pop-off valve closed
    d. Definitely not okay to use the machine, except with a nonrebreathing circuit

54. The oxygen flush valve
    a. Allows oxygen to flow into the breathing system without going through the vaporizer
    b. Increases the anesthetic concentration within the circuit
    c. Causes the patient to breathe deeper
    d. Is used primarily to keep the reservoir bag deflated

55. The advantages of a nonrebreathing system, as compared with a circle breathing system, include all of the following, except
    a. Reduced resistance to breathing
    b. Greater potential for hypothermia caused by high flows needed
    c. Reduced mechanical dead space
    d. No soda lime required

56. The minimum fresh gas flow in a semiclosed system is correctly determined by the
    a. Patient's metabolic rate
    b. Patient's respiratory rate
    c. Drugs used for premedication
    d. Size of the soda lime canister

57. All inhalant anesthetic machines should have
    a. A nitrous oxide flowmeter
    b. Blood pressure monitors
    c. Respiratory monitors
    d. An anesthetic waste gas scavenging system

58. Vaporizers may be classified according to all of the following, except the
    a. Method of regulating output
    b. Method of vaporization
    c. Location in the anesthetic circuit
    d. Type of breathing circuit with which they can be used

59. An intravenous catheter should be
    a. Large enough to allow adequate fluid delivery, if cardiac arrest occurs
    b. As small as possible to avoid pain
    c. Placed in critically ill patients only
    d. Left in place for at least 3 days after surgery

60. The volume of the rebreathing bag on an anesthetic machine should be at least
    a. The same as the patient's tidal volume
    b. Three times the patient's tidal volume
    c. Six times the patient's tidal volume
    d. Nine times the patient's tidal volume

61. Pulse oximetry monitoring devices give an estimate of
    a. Respiratory rate
    b. Cardiac output
    c. Percentage of hemoglobin saturation with oxygen in arterial blood
    d. Oxygen content of arterial blood

62. Which statement concerning soda lime is least accurate?
    a. It removes carbon dioxide from the breathing circuit.
    b. Its capacity should be at least one to two times the patient's tidal volume.
    c. It can be nonfunctional and still maintain its original color.
    d. It should be changed once a month.

63. If the rebreathing bag is empty during anesthesia, all of the following may be the cause, except
    a. The oxygen flow may be too high.
    b. The oxygen flow may be too low.
    c. There may be a leak in the system.
    d. The waste gas scavenging system is not working properly.

64. Nitrous oxide cylinders are painted what color?
    a. Green
    b. Gray
    c. Blue
    d. Brown

65. The approximate volume of oxygen in an E cylinder is
    a. 70 L
    b. 700 L
    c. 7000 L
    d. 2200 L

66. The approximate volume of oxygen in an H cylinder is
    a. 70 L
    b. 700 L
    c. 7000 L
    d. 2200 L

67. The pressure of gas that enters the flowmeter of an inhalant anesthetic machine is
    a. 20 to 30 psi
    b. 50 to 60 psi
    c. 100 to 120 psi
    d. 2200 psi

68. Which statement concerning the pressure manometer in an inhalant anesthetic circuit is least accurate?
    a. It is calibrated in centimeters of water or millimeters of mercury.
    b. It is helpful when ventilating patients.
    c. It is related to the pressure in the patient's airway.
    d. It measures oxygen partial pressure.

69. Activated charcoal devices absorb all inhalation agents except
    a. Isoflurane
    b. Halothane
    c. Sevoflurane
    d. Nitrous oxide

70. According to the National Institute for Occupational Safety and Health (NIOSH), the maximum recommended level of exposure of people to volatile anesthetic agents in the environment is
    a. 2 ppm
    b. 4 ppm
    c. 6 ppm
    d. 8 ppm

71. There is evidence of increased health risks among people exposed chronically to trace levels of inhalant anesthetic gases. All of the following conditions have been associated with such exposure except
    a. Abortion and congenital abnormalities
    b. Hepatic and renal disease
    c. CNS dysfunction
    d. Insomnia

Correct answers are on pages 503-514.

72. All of the following are methods that reduce waste gas levels except
    a. Scavenging systems
    b. Elimination of breathing circuit leaks
    c. Careful filling of vaporizers to avoid spillage
    d. Chamber and mask inductions

73. When inflating the cuff on an endotracheal tube, you should change to a larger diameter tube if cuff inflation requires injection of more than what volume of air?
    a. 2 ml
    b. 5 ml
    c. 7 ml
    d. 10 ml

74. Ideally an endotracheal tube should be inserted so that
    a. Its tip is midway between the thoracic inlet and the larynx.
    b. The adaptor is just caudal to the incisors.
    c. It is deep enough to prevent backing out.
    d. Its tip just reaches the third rib.

75. When an endotracheal tube is being inserted in a horse, the animal should be placed in
    a. Sternal recumbency with its head at a 90-degree angle to the neck
    b. Sternal recumbency with its head and neck extended
    c. Lateral recumbency with its head at a 90-degree angle to the neck
    d. Lateral recumbency with its head, neck, and back extended

76. Which of the following is not an advantage for endotracheal intubation?
    a. Ensures a patent airway
    b. Increases dead space and allows for more efficient ventilation
    c. Prevents aspiration pneumonitis
    d. Improves oxygenation of arterial blood

77. Which animal is most likely to experience laryngospasm during endotracheal intubation?
    a. Thoroughbred mare
    b. Hereford cow
    c. Persian cat
    d. Dalmatian dog

78. Which of the following is the most common complication of endotracheal intubation?
    a. Placement of the tube in the esophagus
    b. Physical damage to the teeth and oral mucous membranes
    c. Overinflated cuff injuring the trachea
    d. Underinflated cuff collapsing the trachea

79. The best method for determining the proper inflation of an endotracheal tube cuff is
    a. Use 1 ml of air for each millimeter of internal diameter of the tube.
    b. Inject air while applying pressure from the reservoir bag until no air escapes around the tube.
    c. Inject air until the bulb on the cuff tubing is too hard to collapse.
    d. Use a 12-ml syringe and inject 12 ml of air into the cuff.

80. The preferred method for treating a cat with laryngospasm is to
    a. Use a sharp stylet to wedge the endotracheal tube between the vocal cords.
    b. Return the animal to its cage, and wait 20 minutes before trying again.
    c. Place a drop of a topical anesthetic in the laryngeal area, wait a few minutes, and then intubate the animal.
    d. Use a stiffer endotracheal tube that can force the vocal cords open.

81. Which of the following is not an advantage of using an endotracheal tube?
    a. Prevents atelectasis of lung alveoli
    b. Encourages proper examination of the animal's mouth, pharynx, and larynx
    c. Provides a means for treating respiratory and cardiac arrest
    d. Increases the chances of airway obstruction

82. In a Siamese cat, the endotracheal tube should be removed
    a. As soon as the surgery or diagnostic technique is completed
    b. Only after the animal is fully conscious and able to maintain a free airway
    c. When the animal is taken off of the anesthesia machine
    d. As soon as the animal begins to swallow and cough

83. In a pug, the endotracheal tube should be removed
    a. As soon as the surgery or diagnostic technique is completed
    b. Only after the animal is fully conscious and able to maintain a free airway
    c. When the animal is taken off of the anesthesia machine
    d. As soon as the animal begins to swallow and cough

84. What is the best technique to secure an endotracheal tube to an animal?
   a. It is best not to secure the tube to the animal, so that it can move freely if the animal starts to wake up.
   b. It should be secured by gauze strips around the head in cats and brachycephalic dogs and caudal to the upper canines in other breeds of dogs.
   c. It can be secured by several wraps of cloth and tape around the animal's nose and the tube.
   d. A rubber band can be looped tightly around the tube and the animal's nose.

85. Which statement concerning use of intravenous anesthesia in large animals is least accurate?
   a. It is routinely used for cast applications, castrations, and umbilical hernias.
   b. It works well on procedures that require complete immobilization of the patient.
   c. It should not be used on procedures that require more than 45 to 50 minutes to complete.
   d. It requires use of a preanesthetic for sedation and a barbiturate.

86. When monitoring the vital signs of an anesthetized patient, you must observe and record all of the following, except
   a. Mucous membrane color and capillary refill time
   b. Heart rate and respiratory rate and depth
   c. Reflexes
   d. Pulse quality and strength

87. The responsibilities of the anesthetist during a surgical procedure include continuous monitoring of the patient's vital signs and recording observations at approximately
   a. 10-minute intervals
   b. 5-minute intervals
   c. 2-minute intervals
   d. 15-second intervals

88. Adequate oxygen may be evaluated subjectively during anesthesia by the
   a. Heart rate
   b. Respiratory rate
   c. Mucous membrane color and capillary refill time
   d. Pulse pressure

89. Hypoventilation that occurs in the anesthetized patient is characterized by
   a. Decreased oxygen levels and increased carbon dioxide levels
   b. Decreased carbon dioxide levels and decreased oxygen levels
   c. Increased oxygen levels and decreased carbon dioxide levels
   d. Increased oxygen levels and increased carbon dioxide levels

90. In nonbrachycephalic breeds of dogs recovering from anesthesia, the endotracheal tube should be removed when the
   a. Palpebral reflex returns
   b. Swallowing reflex returns
   c. Pupils resume a central position
   d. Animal shows voluntary movement of the limbs

91. Concerning physical stimulation of the recovering anesthetized patient, which statement is least accurate?
   a. Stimulation should not include rubbing the chest, because it may interfere with respiration.
   b. Stimulation can include talking to the patient, moving the limbs, or pinching the toes.
   c. Stimulation increases the flow of information to the reticular activation center of the brain.
   d. A lack of stimulation may cause drowsiness in the conscious animal.

92. It is advisable to turn the anesthetized patient from side to side during the recovery period of anesthesia. Concerning this, which statement is least accurate?
   a. Turn the patient every 10 to 15 minutes until it regains consciousness.
   b. Turning the patient prevents pooling of blood in the dependent parts of the body.
   c. It is advisable to turn all animals dorsally, rather than sternally, to prevent gastric torsion.
   d. Turning the patient helps stimulate respiration and consciousness.

93. Once extubated, all animals should be placed in
   a. Right lateral recumbency with the neck extended
   b. Left lateral recumbency with the neck in a normal, flexed position
   c. Sternal recumbency with the neck extended
   d. Whatever position is most comfortable for the patient

Correct answers are on pages 503-514.

94. Following discontinuation of the anesthetic gas, periodic bagging of the patient with pure oxygen is advisable, because it
    a. Helps reinflate collapsed alveoli
    b. Allows for a faster recovery
    c. Helps flush anesthetic gas out of the hoses
    d. Allows expired waste gas to be evacuated by the scavenger system

95. In the anesthetized surgical patient, pale mucous membranes can indicate all of the following except
    a. Inadequate oxygen levels
    b. Cyanosis
    c. Excessive blood loss
    d. Decreased tissue perfusion

96. In patients with which of the following characteristics is it recommended to wait a longer period before extubation because of the likelihood of vomiting or airway obstruction?
    a. Dolichocephalic
    b. Undershot mandible
    c. Brachycephalic
    d. Cleft palate

97. Providing good nursing care for the recovering anesthetized patient is the duty of the attending anesthetist. Which of the following is not advisable for a patient immediately following surgery?
    a. Providing ample bedding to prevent heat loss and increase comfort
    b. Providing fresh food and water once the animal is conscious
    c. Providing a source of heat in hypothermia cases
    d. Administering postoperative analgesics as directed by the veterinarian

98. The minimum acceptable heart rate (beats per minute) for an anesthetized medium-sized dog is
    a. 40 bpm
    b. 60 bpm
    c. 80 bpm
    d. 100 bpm

99. It is cause for concern if an anesthetized cat's heart rate falls below
    a. 160 bpm
    b. 120 bpm
    c. 100 bpm
    d. 140 bpm

100. An anesthetist should be aware of the effects of anesthetic agents on the patient. When used as preanesthetics, atropine and acepromazine can cause all of the following, except
    a. Prolapse of the nictitating membrane
    b. Respiratory depression
    c. Reduced salivation and tear production
    d. Pupil dilatation in cats

101. A capillary refill time that is over 2 seconds indicates
    a. Congestive heart failure
    b. Decreased peripheral blood perfusion
    c. Decreased ventilation
    d. Hypertension

102. Use of an indwelling catheter in an artery to monitor blood pressure is termed
    a. Direct monitoring
    b. Central venous pressure
    c. Indirect monitoring
    d. Peripheral venous pressure

103. When monitoring the mucous membrane color of an anesthetized patient with pigmented gingivae, you could use each of the following alternative sites except
    a. Pinnae
    b. Tongue
    c. Buccal mucous membranes
    d. Membranes lining the prepuce or vulva

104. During the maintenance period of anesthesia in a cat or dog, respiratory rates lower than how many breaths/min may indicate excessive anesthetic depth that should be reported to the veterinarian?
    a. 5
    b. 8
    c. 10
    d. 12

105. Some anesthetists routinely bag the patient under inhalation anesthesia once every 5 minutes to help prevent
    a. Apnea
    b. Mydriasis
    c. Hypercapnia
    d. Atelectasis

106. The causes of true hyperventilation and tachypnea during anesthesia may include all of the following except
    a. Progression from light to moderate anesthesia
    b. Response to metabolic acidosis
    c. Response to a mild surgical stimulus
    d. Presence of pulmonary edema

107. If the rectum of a patient is covered by a surgical drape or is otherwise inaccessible to the anesthetist, a rough estimate of body temperature can be obtained by
    a. Touching the patient's nose or tail
    b. Touching the patient's feet or ears
    c. Touching the patient's tongue or mucous membranes
    d. Feeling the temperature of exhaled air

108. Throughout anesthesia, the animal's temperature should be maintained as close to normal as possible. Hypothermia can be prevented by all of the following measures except
    a. Warming the stainless-steel V trough before using it
    b. Administering warm intravenous fluids
    c. Use of a circulating warm-water heating pad
    d. Providing a comfortable air temperature in the surgery room

109. Malignant hyperthermia is a potentially fatal syndrome to the anesthetized patient. Which of these species is most prone to this condition?
    a. Cattle
    b. Pigs
    c. Dogs
    d. Goats

110. Use of succinylcholine in combination with general anesthetics may be advantageous to the surgeon during certain procedures, but it gives the anesthetist one less measure with which to monitor anesthetic depth. What measure would be of no use in monitoring patients given succinylcholine?
    a. Eye position and pupil size
    b. Heart rate
    c. Jaw muscle tone
    d. Respiratory rate

111. Using ketamine as an anesthetic agent diminishes the value of what measure in assessing anesthetic depth?
    a. Pinna reflex
    b. Pedal reflex
    c. Jaw muscle tone
    d. Eye position

112. Which statement concerning eye position, pupil size, and responsiveness to light as indicators of anesthetic depth is least accurate?
    a. In stage III, plane 3 of anesthesia, the eyes are usually central to slightly eccentric, with normal pupils that are responsive to light.
    b. In stage III, plane 2 of anesthesia, the eyes are usually rotated ventrally with slightly dilated pupils.
    c. In stage II of anesthesia, the eyes are usually central, and the pupils may be dilated and responsive to light.
    d. In stage IV of anesthesia, the eyes are central with widely dilated pupils that are unresponsive to light.

113. The presence or absence of salivary and lacrimal secretions may give clues regarding anesthetic depth. In an animal that has not received an anticholinergic, which statement concerning observance of these secretions is most accurate?
    a. Production of tears and saliva increases with increasing anesthetic depth.
    b. Production of tears and saliva is totally absent in light anesthesia.
    c. Tear and saliva production diminishes as anesthetic depth is increased.
    d. Tear and saliva production increases in all stages of anesthesia in the absence of anticholinergics.

114. The anesthetized patient may respond to surgical stimulation if the anesthetic depth is inadequate. Response to a painful stimulus may be indicated by all of the following except
    a. A considerable increase in heart rate and an increase in blood pressure
    b. A decrease in lacrimation and salivation
    c. An increase in respiratory rate
    d. Sweating on the foot pads

115. A 10-year-old dog has been anesthetized for removal of a skin tumor and is now maintained on 2% isoflurane. The anesthetist observes that its respirations are 8/min and shallow, its heart rate is 80 beats/min, its pupils are centrally positioned, its jaw tone is slack, and all of its reflexes are absent. This animal is in what stage and plane of anesthesia?
    a. Stage III, plane 2
    b. Stage III, plane 3
    c. Stage III, plane 4
    d. Stage IV, plane 1

Correct answers are on pages 503-514.

116. A 10-year-old dog has been anesthetized for removal of a skin tumor and is now maintained on 2% isoflurane. The anesthetist observes that its respirations are 8/min and shallow, its heart rate is 80 beats/min, its pupils are centrally positioned, its jaw tone is slack, and all of its reflexes are absent. What should be your response or actions to the condition of this animal?
    a. It is adequately anesthetized; no adjustments are necessary.
    b. You should try to stimulate the animal, to lighten the plane of anesthesia.
    c. You should notify the veterinarian of the dog's condition but not be alarmed.
    d. You should reduce the vaporizer setting to 1.5% isoflurane and continue to monitor for signs of decreased depth.

117. What stage of anesthesia may be characterized by vocalization, struggling, and breath holding?
    a. Stage I
    b. Stage II
    c. Stage III, plane 1
    d. Stage III, plane 2

118. A dog received intramuscularly the correct dose of xylazine. Second-degree heart block and bradycardia developed. Based on the most common cause of this adverse reaction, what would be the best therapy?
    a. No treatment is required.
    b. Yohimbine
    c. Glycopyrrolate
    d. Doxapram

119. An abnormally elevated central venous pressure that develops during anesthesia and surgery in an animal receiving intravenous fluids may indicate
    a. Intravenous fluid overload
    b. Increased cardiac output
    c. Dehydration
    d. Liver disease

120. A 1:10,000 dilution of epinephrine contains how much epinephrine per milliliter?
    a. 1 mg
    b. 0.01 mg
    c. 1 mg
    d. 0.1 mg

121. Cardiac arrhythmias that occur during anesthesia are commonly associated with all of the following except
    a. Normocapnia
    b. Excessive halothane concentration
    c. Hypoxemia
    d. Myocardial ischemia

122. Mean arterial blood pressure of the isoflurane-anesthetized horse
    a. Can be used as an indication of anesthetic depth
    b. Is not important
    c. Is not practical to monitor
    d. Is important for long procedures only

123. Surgical evaluation of a dog hit by a car revealed a PCV of 18% and plasma protein below 2.5 g/dl. All of the following are true, except the
    a. Patient is predisposed to pulmonary edema.
    b. Fluid administration rates should be watched closely.
    c. Patient should receive plasma or whole blood before surgery.
    d. Patient should not receive fluid before surgery.

124. The estimated blood volume in dogs is
    a. 25 ml/kg
    b. 50 ml/kg
    c. 75 ml/kg
    d. 100 ml/kg

125. The volume of blood administered to a patient is determined by all of the following except
    a. PCV of the donor
    b. PCV of the recipient
    c. Desired PCV
    d. Age of the recipient

126. While monitoring a horse during inhalation anesthesia, you note that the heart rate suddenly increases to 80 beats/min. Your most appropriate response is to
    a. Increase the delivered anesthetic concentration
    b. Administer intravenously 10 mg of butorphanol
    c. Evaluate the peripheral pulse, mucous membranes, and other vital organ function before responding
    d. Not be concerned, because the horse is not moving

127. While monitoring a horse receiving oxygen at the rate of 8 L/min, isoflurane 2.5%, and fluids at the rate of 10 ml/kg/hr, you note that the blood pressure suddenly falls to 60 mm Hg, and the peripheral pulse becomes weak. Your first response should be to
    a. Administer a vasoactive agent
    b. Lower the isoflurane concentration and increase fluid delivery rate
    c. Turn down the oxygen flow
    d. Not be concerned

128. Whole blood should be administered in which of the following presurgical situations?
    a. PCV 30%
    b. PCV 14%
    c. Von Willebrand positive
    d. Chronic anemia, PCV 25%

129. A 10-kg dog with a ventricular arrhythmia is treated with an IV lidocaine drip at 50 μg/kg/min. How many drops per minute from a minidrip infusion set (60 drops/ml) are necessary if the concentration of lidocaine is 1 mg/ml?
    a. 3
    b. 5
    c. 30
    d. 50

130. The most common arrhythmia associated with use of thiobarbiturates in dogs during induction of anesthesia is
    a. Atrial fibrillation
    b. Ventricular tachycardia
    c. Bigeminy
    d. Second-degree atrioventricular block

131. Tachycardia in an anesthetized patient may be an indication of any of the following except
    a. Hypotension
    b. Pain
    c. Light plane of anesthesia
    d. Xylazine overdose

132. A cardiac rhythm disturbance detected shortly after induction of anesthesia may be the result of any of the following except
    a. The induction agent
    b. Difficulty intubating
    c. Hypoxemia
    d. Breathing oxygen-enriched air

133. Hypothermia has become significant in a 4-kg anesthetized cat. The best way to restore body heat is
    a. With a warm-water blanket
    b. To submerge the animal in warm water
    c. With a heat lamp
    d. To warm the air in the breathing circuit by some method

134. In a cat that is too deeply anesthetized, all of the following may be present except
    a. Pale mucous membranes
    b. Tachycardia
    c. Bradycardia
    d. Voluntary movement

135. An isoflurane-anesthetized cat suddenly begins breathing 30 times a minute during a surgical procedure. Your first response should be to
    a. Turn down the oxygen flow rate
    b. Immediately begin to bag the patient
    c. Turn up the anesthetic concentration
    d. Evaluate vital organ function and endotracheal tube placement and make necessary adjustments

136. If a dog is too deeply anesthetized, all of the following may be seen except
    a. Tachycardia
    b. Bradycardia
    c. Pale mucous membranes
    d. Increased jaw muscle tone

137. A dog anesthetized with halothane in 99% oxygen develops ventricular tachycardia. What is the drug of choice for therapy?
    a. Propranolol
    b. Quinidine
    c. Lidocaine
    d. Atropine

138. Dobutamine is used in emergency anesthetic and clinical situations to
    a. Increase the respiratory rate
    b. Increase cardiac output
    c. Correct cardiac arrhythmias
    d. Decrease the heart rate

139. During cardiopulmonary resuscitation (CPR) in a medium-sized dog, you should maintain a ventilation rate of how many breaths per minute?
    a. 5
    b. 12
    c. 20
    d. 30

140. During CPR, adequate cardiac massage is present when
    a. The electrocardiogram (ECG) is normal.
    b. The heart rate is 60 beats/min.
    c. A peripheral pulse can be palpated.
    d. The mucous membranes are pink.

141. The only accurate way to evaluate the effectiveness of respiration is by
    a. Observing abdominal and chest movements during respiration
    b. Counting the respiratory rate
    c. Feeling air move through the endotracheal tube or nostrils
    d. Measuring the arterial blood oxygen and carbon dioxide partial pressures

Correct answers are on pages 503-514.

142. Dehydration greater than 10% is
    a. A seriously morbid state
    b. Nothing to worry about
    c. Not something that affects skin turgor
    d. Not associated with depression

143. Patients that have water withheld for long periods before surgery and general anesthesia may be prone to
    a. Vomiting during induction
    b. Dehydration and hypotension
    c. Nothing more than other patients
    d. Respiratory depression

144. When xylazine is used to induce vomiting before surgery,
    a. There is nothing to worry about.
    b. Do not place an endotracheal tube.
    c. Examine the airway for gastric contents before placing the endotracheal tube.
    d. Do not administer atropine.

145. Immediately after tracheal intubation in a 3-kg cat you notice extreme respiratory distress. The most likely cause is
    a. Light plane of anesthesia
    b. Hypoxemia
    c. Nothing; this is normal.
    d. Bronchial intubation

146. After placing, lubricating, and inflating the cuff of the endotracheal tube, you note a sudden decrease in heart rate. The most likely cause is
    a. Low oxygen flow
    b. Too deep a plane of anesthesia
    c. Cuff is underinflated
    d. Cuff may be overinflated, producing vagal-induced bradycardia

147. During CPR, 2% lidocaine is used to treat ventricular arrhythmias. A complication that may occur after intravenous infusion of lidocaine is
    a. Bradycardia
    b. Coughing
    c. Tachycardia
    d. Vomiting

148. Indications of poor cardiac function include all of the following except
    a. Cyanosis in patients with a PCV of 45%
    b. Poor perfusion
    c. Cardiac arrhythmias
    d. Normal pulse

149. Intravenous sodium bicarbonate is used to
    a. Treat cardiac arrhythmias
    b. Produce positive inotropic effects
    c. Stimulate respiration
    d. Combat acidosis

150. Doxapram may produce all of the following except
    a. CNS excitement
    b. Increased ventilation rate
    c. Respiratory alkalosis
    d. Hypoventilation

151. Obesity delays elimination of what drug because of its high lipid solubility?
    a. Propofol
    b. Xylazine
    c. Thiopental
    d. Guaifenesin

152. ___ is commonly used along with ketamine or thiopental as an induction agent for adult horses.
    a. Propofol
    b. Phenobarbital
    c. Guaifenesin
    d. Isoflurane

153. ___ can cause convulsions when administered alone at high doses.
    a. Dissociative anesthetics
    b. Barbiturates
    c. Benzodiazepine tranquilizers
    d. Propofol

154. ___ is an analgesic and a sedative.
    a. Acepromazine
    b. Atropine
    c. Diazepam
    d. Xylazine

155. All of the following drugs predispose the animal to bloat, except
    a. Atropine
    b. Medetomidine
    c. Glycopyrrolate
    d. Midazolam

156. A drug is considered an ___ if its action at the receptor is to stimulate.
    a. Agonist
    b. Antagonist
    c. Anarchist
    d. Antitussive

157. What drugs will not slow the heart rate?
    a. Anticholinergics
    b. Phenothiazine tranquilizers
    c. Alpha-2 agonists
    d. Gas anesthetics

158. Phenothiazine tranquilizers
    a. Cause nausea
    b. Increase the seizure threshold
    c. Cause vasoconstriction
    d. Suppress the sympathetic nervous system

159. An overdose of a barbiturate anesthetic can be appropriately treated with all of the following except
    a. Respiratory stimulant
    b. Fluid therapy
    c. Ventilator support
    d. An increase in the concentration of isoflurane

160. The following general anesthetic agents can be delivered to effect except
    a. Isoflurane
    b. Telazole given IM
    c. Ketamine/diazepam IV
    d. Thiopental IV

161. No more than ___ nitrous oxide should be delivered to an anesthetized patient.
    a. 40%
    b. 50%
    c. 60%
    d. 70%

162. Never use nitrous oxide
    a. In a closed anesthesia circuit
    b. In cats
    c. With rubber tubes on the anesthesia machine
    d. With isoflurane

163. ___ is a concern when recovering a patient from anesthesia if nitrous oxide has been used.
    a. Solubility
    b. Diffusion hypoxia
    c. Biotransformation
    d. Inflammation

164. Recovery from barbiturate anesthesia is prolonged by all of the following except
    a. Increased blood glucose concentration
    b. Sight hounds
    c. Liver disease
    d. Elevated cardiac output

165. ___ may occur because of rapid recovery from isoflurane anesthesia.
    a. Diffusion hypoxia
    b. Second gas effect
    c. Biotransformation
    d. Emergence delirium

166. ___ should not be used as part of the anesthetic plan if the patient has an intestinal obstruction.
    a. Isoflurane
    b. Acepromazine
    c. Nitrous oxide
    d. Atropine

167. Pediatric patients younger than 3 months that undergo general anesthesia are at higher risk than adult patients for all of the following except
    a. Having a fluid overdose
    b. Developing hypothermia
    c. Developing hypoglycemia
    d. Biting the endotracheal tube in half

168. Which of the following would not cause pale mucous membranes?
    a. Stress causing catecholamine release leading to vasoconstriction
    b. Anemia
    c. Hyperthermia
    d. Hypotension

169. The effect of intravenous administration of any anesthetic drug is usually detected in
    a. 30 to 60 seconds
    b. 3 to 5 minutes
    c. 15 to 20 minutes
    d. 1 hour

170. Kidney function can be assessed by the following preanesthetic screening tests except
    a. BUN
    b. ALT
    c. Urinalysis
    d. Creatinine

171. The oxygen-carrying capacity of the blood can be assessed by measuring all of the following except
    a. PCV
    b. Hematocrit
    c. Total solids
    d. Hemoglobin

Correct answers are on pages 503-514.

172. A patient's hydration status can be assessed by all the following except
    a. Respiratory rate
    b. PCV
    c. Total solids
    d. Skin turgor

173. Measures that help decrease waste anesthetic gas exposure include all except
    a. Frequent changing of the soda lime canister
    b. Properly fitting endotracheal tube cuffs
    c. Avoiding use of masks or induction chambers
    d. Leak testing the anesthesia machine

174. Charcoal canisters attached to the exhaust of the anesthesia machine
    a. Absorb carbon dioxide
    b. Remove all gas anesthetic agents
    c. Remove all gas anesthetic agents except nitrous oxide
    d. Change color when the canister must be changed

175. Daily preanesthesia check of the anesthesia machine should include all of these except
    a. Leak testing
    b. Weighing the charcoal canister
    c. Calibrating the vaporizer
    d. Filling the vaporizer with anesthetic gas agent

176. When cleaning up a gas anesthetic spill, you should do all of the following except
    a. Open windows
    b. Turn on any venting fans
    c. Soak up the agent in absorbent material
    d. Dispose of in a paper bag in the trash in the surgical area

177. Which of the following statements about neuromuscular blocking agents is false?
    a. Neuromuscular blocking agents cause profound muscle relaxation.
    b. Neuromuscular blocking agents interfere with acetylcholine activity.
    c. Neuromuscular blocking agents work at the neuromuscular junction (NMJ).
    d. Neuromuscular blocking agents must be injected around the nerve.

178. When given a neuromuscular blocking agent, the last muscle(s) to become paralyzed is/are the
    a. Muscles of the tail
    b. Diaphragm
    c. Abdominal muscles
    d. Muscle in to which the drug was injected

179. Neuromuscular blocking agents
    a. Cause increased release of inhibitory neurotransmitters
    b. Interfere with transmission of the electrical impulse along the nerve fiber
    c. Disrupt nerve impulse transmission at the NMJ
    d. Block catecholamine release

180. Local anesthetics
    a. Cause increased release of inhibitory neurotransmitters
    b. Interfere with transmission of the impulse along the nerve fiber
    c. Disrupt nerve impulse transmission at the NMJ
    d. Block catecholamine release

181. The MAC of an anesthetic agent will change for all of the following reasons except
    a. Preanesthetic drug administration
    b. Patient's age
    c. Patient's breed
    d. Anemia

182. Inhalant anesthetics with low ___ have short induction and recovery periods.
    a. Toxicity
    b. Solubility coefficient
    c. Vapor pressure
    d. Biotransformation

183. Highly volatile anesthetics are best suited for
    a. IV administration
    b. Precision vaporizers
    c. Draw-over vaporizers
    d. Open-drop or cone systems

184. Recovery from a volatile anesthetic will be prolonged because of all of the following, except when
    a. The animal is under for several hours.
    b. A high percent of the anesthetic is biotransformed.
    c. The solubility coefficient is high.
    d. The MAC is high.

185. Which volatile anesthetic agent is the most potent?
    a. One with a 1 MAC value of 0.59
    b. One with a 1 MAC value of 1.2
    c. One with a 1 MAC value of 5.3
    d. One with a 1 MAC value of 0.09

Agent	MAC	Solubility	Vapor pressure
A	0.76	2.3	30%
B	1.2	1.4	30%
C	0.16	13.00	4%
D	101.00	0.49	100%

For questions 186 to 188, use the information in the table above to answer the questions.

186. Which agent has the shortest induction and recovery time?
    a. A
    b. B
    c. C
    d. D

187. Which agent can maintain the patient under anesthesia at the lowest alveolar concentration?
    a. A
    b. B
    c. C
    d. D

188. Which agent has the longest induction and recovery time?
    a. A
    b. B
    c. C
    d. D

189. Weaning off of a ventilator should include all of the following except
    a. Reversal of the neuromuscular blocking drug
    b. Increase rate of ventilating breaths
    c. Decrease anesthetic gas concentration delivered
    d. Respiratory stimulant drugs

190. A/an ___ in the blood stimulates the animal to take a breath.
    a. Decrease in oxygen saturation
    b. Decrease in carbon dioxide
    c. Increase in carbon dioxide
    d. Increase in pH

191. The active phase of normal breathing is
    a. Shorter in duration than the passive phase
    b. The same duration as the passive phase
    c. Longer in duration than the passive phase
    d. Variable in duration sometimes shorter, sometimes longer

192. Overinflation of the lungs during artificial ventilation
    a. Is of little concern, except during open-chest surgery
    b. May cause emphysema
    c. May cause oxygen toxicity
    d. May cause the endotracheal tube to disconnect from the anesthesia machine

193. Neuromuscular blocking agents
    a. Provide analgesia
    b. Provide sedation
    c. Paralyze all skeletal muscles except the diaphragm
    d. Do not cross the blood–brain barrier

194. Neuromuscular blocking agents
    a. Paralyze skeletal muscles, but all reflexes are maintained
    b. Are also known as *peripheral muscle relaxants*
    c. Slow gut motility and predispose the patient to bloat
    d. First paralyze the diaphragm

195. Neuromuscular blocking agents are used for all of the following except
    a. Analgesia
    b. Facilitation of fracture reduction
    c. Facilitation of ocular surgery to immobilize the eye
    d. Prevention of spontaneous inspiratory efforts by the patient

196. Acetylcholinesterase inhibitors
    a. Are reversal agents for depolarizing neuromuscular blockers
    b. Are reversal agents for nondepolarizing neuromuscular blockers
    c. Decrease the concentration of acetylcholine in the NMJ
    d. Increase the breakdown of acetylcholine in the NMJ

197. Local anesthetics
    a. Are readily absorbed through intact skin
    b. Prevent nerve cell depolarization
    c. Are combined with vasodilators to prolong their activity
    d. Are injected directly into the nerve

198. ___ pain originates from internal organs.
    a. Somatic
    b. Preemptive
    c. Visceral
    d. Referred

Correct answers are on pages 503-514.

199. ___ analgesia is the administration of an analgesic before the pain develops.
    a. Somatic
    b. Preemptive
    c. Visceral
    d. Referred

200. To quickly lighten the depth of anesthesia in a patient under inhalant anesthesia, the anesthetist should
    a. Suck all of the anesthetic gas from the lungs
    b. Increase the flow of oxygen
    c. Turn the vaporizer setting off or down
    d. Prevent the patient from taking a breath

201. The patient is in an excessively deep plane of anesthesia. Which answer would not be an explanation?
    a. The vaporizer is set at a high concentration.
    b. The IV induction agent was given too quickly.
    c. The pet has a low body temperature.
    d. The endotracheal tube is kinked.

202. The patient is under anesthesia and in shock. Which of the following symptoms would you observe?
    a. Bradycardia
    b. Hypertension
    c. Cyanotic mucous membranes
    d. Excessively long capillary refill time

203. If the soda lime canister is exhausted, the patient may become
    a. Cyanotic
    b. Too light under anesthesia
    c. Hypercapnic
    d. Hyperthermic

204. You have just completed filling the cuff on the endotracheal tube. The pressure relief valve is stuck in the closed position. Your best option is to
    a. Turn up the oxygen flow rate
    b. Start bagging the pet
    c. Disconnect the patient from the anesthesia machine
    d. Continue prepping the pet for surgery, and fix the valve release knob after the surgery is finished

205. A small animal patient's systolic blood pressure was measured at 50 mm Hg. What is your best course of action?
    a. Turn up the oxygen flow rate.
    b. Turn up the concentration of gas anesthetic.
    c. Close the pop-off valve.
    d. Increase the drip rate of the IV fluids.

206. The patient is dyspneic. You should do all of the following except
    a. Turn down the vaporizer
    b. Check the oxygen flow
    c. Check the endotracheal tube
    d. Disconnect the pet from the anesthesia machine

207. A dog under anesthesia has a heart rate of 230 beats/min. Which of the following is the best explanation?
    a. This is normal.
    b. The patient is in too deep a plane of anesthesia.
    c. The patient is in too light a plane of anesthesia.
    d. The patient is hypothermic.

208. The patient is in shock. Which of these symptoms would not be expected?
    a. Tachycardia
    b. Hypertension
    c. Prolonged capillary refill time
    d. Pale mucous membranes

209. The patient is in respiratory arrest. Which of the following is the correct action and reason?
    a. Check the heart, because if the patient is not breathing, then the heart is not beating.
    b. Start ventilating breaths, because arrest is obviously due to an obstructed endotracheal tube.
    c. Tell the surgeon because he or she will be angry.
    d. Turn off the vaporizer, because chances are the patient is too deep, and you need to begin ventilating breaths with oxygen alone.

210. A patient in ASA class I physical status is
    a. A normal patient with no organic disease
    b. A moribund patient
    c. An adult animal with no signs of evident disease on physical examination
    d. In absolutely no danger while under anesthesia

211. Ways to minimize exposure to waste anesthetic gas include
    a. Use loose-fitting masks
    b. Properly inflate the endotracheal tube cuff
    c. Immediately disconnect the patient from the anesthesia machine once the procedure is completed
    d. Connect the patient to the breathing circuit after both the oxygen and isoflurane are turned on

212. Treatment for hypotension during anesthesia includes
    a. Turning up the anesthetic gas
    b. Increasing the drip rate of the IV fluids
    c. Increasing the flow of oxygen
    d. Giving ventilating breaths

213. Hypothermia
    a. Prolongs anesthetic induction
    b. Prolongs anesthetic recovery
    c. Is common in obese patients
    d. Is of no concern in neonatal patients

214. Isoflurane is mainly eliminated from the body by the
    a. Renal system
    b. GI system
    c. Respiratory system
    d. Hepatic system

215. It is generally safe to extubate the patient when the patient
    a. Vocalizes
    b. Swallows
    c. Stands
    d. Can rest in a sternal position

216. Which of the following is not a valid reason for administering a preanesthetic medication?
    a. It reduces the amount of general anesthetic for induction.
    b. It may calm an excited animal.
    c. It may reduce possible noxious side effects from the general anesthesia.
    d. It increases patient safety by allowing the animal to stay under the general anesthetic for a longer time.

217. An epidural agent would be administered where in a dog?
    a. Between L7 and the sacrum
    b. Just cranial to C1
    c. Immediately caudal to T13
    d. Directly into the spinal cord at T1

218. The epidural space is located
    a. Just below the supraspinous ligament
    b. In the subarachnoid area
    c. Between the dura mater and the vertebrae
    d. Immediately above the spinal cord

219. Epidural anesthesia could be appropriately used for all procedures except
    a. Tail amputation
    b. Cesarean section
    c. Eye enucleation
    d. Perianal surgery

220. The drug used for epidural anesthesia is
    a. Thiopental
    b. Ketamine
    c. Propofol
    d. Lidocaine

221. Perivascular injection of a barbiturate solution, such as thiopental, can cause
    a. Local anesthesia
    b. Tissue slough
    c. Increased blood pressure
    d. Respiratory acidosis

222. The barbiturate anesthetic drug that can be used in sight hounds for its ability to produce faster anesthetic recovery is
    a. Ketamine
    b. Thiopental
    c. Pentobarbital
    d. Methohexital

223. Sevoflurane is primarily eliminated from the body by
    a. Respiration
    b. Liver metabolism
    c. Feces
    d. Kidney excretion

224. The usual induction vaporizer setting for sevoflurane is
    a. 2% to 6%
    b. 1% to 4%
    c. 5% to 7%
    d. Up to 3%

225. The usual vaporizer maintenance setting for sevoflurane is
    a. 0.25% to 1%
    b. 3.3% to 4%
    c. 0.5% to 2%
    d. 1% to 3%

226. Which of these is a cyclohexamine agent?
    a. Ketamine
    b. Acetylpromazine
    c. Xylazine
    d. Propofol

227. Acepromazine is classified as a(an)
    a. Anticholinergic
    b. Phenothiazine
    c. Benzodiazepine
    d. Thiazine derivative

228. The preanesthetic mix abbreviated *BAA* contains
    a. Buprenorphine, atropine, acepromazine
    b. Butorphanol, atipamezole, atropine
    c. Buprenorphine, atropine, atipamezole
    d. Butorphanol, acepromazine, atropine

Correct answers are on pages 503-514.

229. What drug is an antagonist of medetomidine (Domitor)?
    a. Yohimbine
    b. Dopram
    c. Atipamezole
    d. Naloxone

230. Naloxone is classified as a(an) opioid
    a. Agonist
    b. Mixed agonist/antagonist
    c. Mu and kappa blocker
    d. Antagonist

231. Which of the following is a neuromuscular blocking agent?
    a. Succinylcholine
    b. Lidocaine
    c. Morphine
    d. Yohimbine

232. Which of the following is the anesthetic with the lowest blood/gas coefficient?
    a. Halothane
    b. Isoflurane
    c. Nitrous oxide
    d. Sevoflurane

233. All are traits of sevoflurane except
    a. Low lipid solubility
    b. Smooth recovery
    c. Nonpungent odor
    d. Severe heart depression

234. All are controlled substances except
    a. Acepromazine
    b. Ketamine
    c. Fentanyl
    d. Diazepam

235. Nonsteroidal antiinflammatory drugs used to control mild postoperative pain include
    a. Aspirin and xylazine
    b. Diazepam and acetaminophen
    c. Carprofen and ketoprofen
    d. Acetylpromazine and ibuprofen

236. All are true statements regarding transdermal use of fentanyl except
    a. Analgesic effect is immediate on placement of the patch.
    b. Patch should be applied to clipped skin.
    c. Patch is normally left in place for 3 to 5 days.
    d. Excessive amounts of drug can be released if the patch is heated.

237. The false statement regarding postsurgical pain is
    a. The pain serves a useful purpose by preventing activity that could cause further tissue injury.
    b. An animal that experiences postoperative pain is more likely to have a poor anesthetic recovery.
    c. Inhalation anesthetics currently used in small-animal practice do not provide significant postoperative pain control.
    d. If a procedure is known to be painful in humans, it should be regarded as such in animal patients.

238. The fundamental principle of administering analgesics before the animal has an awareness of pain is
    a. Windup
    b. Preemptive analgesia
    c. Referred pain
    d. Balanced analgesia

239. The drug that has the longest duration of effect after one injection is
    a. Butorphanol
    b. Morphine
    c. Buprenorphine
    d. Oxymorphone

240. Which of the following anesthetic agents may provide some analgesia in the postoperative period?
    a. Propofol
    b. Sevoflurane
    c. Ketamine
    d. Isoflurane

241. The local anesthetic agent that has the longest duration of action is
    a. Lidocaine
    b. Mepivacaine
    c. Tetracaine
    d. Bupivacaine

242. An alpha-2 agonist that provides sedation, muscle relaxation, and analgesia is
    a. Acepromazine
    b. Xylazine
    c. Diazepam
    d. Ketamine

243. A capnograph measures
    a. Central venous pressure
    b. Expired CO_2
    c. Arterial oxygen
    d. Blood pressure

244. Gas cylinders that are a part of the anesthetic machine are attached to it by a
    a. Y piece
    b. Vaporizer
    c. Yoke
    d. Reducing valve

245. The type of nonrebreathing system that consists of inner tubing surrounded by larger corrugated tubing is
    a. Mapleson A
    b. Ayres T
    c. Norman mask elbow
    d. Baines

246. Nonrebreathing systems are generally recommended for patients that weigh
    a. More than 15 lb
    b. Less than 7 kg
    c. Greater than 7 kg
    d. Less than 25 lb

247. The false statement regarding nonrebreathing systems is
    a. They must have a CO_2 absorber.
    b. They allow quick changes of depth of anesthesia.
    c. High amounts of waste gas are produced.
    d. They use high oxygen flow rates.

248. Medical oxygen cylinders are colored
    a. Blue
    b. Gray
    c. Green
    d. Orange

249. The pressure in a full cylinder of compressed oxygen is ___ psi.
    a. 1000
    b. 750
    c. 500
    d. 2000

250. The recommended carrier gas flow rate for chamber induction of a small animal is ___ L/min.
    a. 2
    b. 5
    c. 1
    d. 3

251. The false statement regarding scavenging systems is
    a. Waste gases can be safely vented to the floor.
    b. Active systems use a vacuum pump to draw gas into the scavenger.
    c. Passive systems use positive pressure of the gas to push gas into the system.
    d. Waste gas should be collected from the anesthetic machine and conducted to a disposal point.

252. High-pressure system tests of the anesthetic machine check for
    a. Escape of anesthetic gas from the machine
    b. Leaks between flowmeter and patient
    c. Oxygen or nitrous oxide leakage
    d. Leaks within the anesthetic circuit and attachments

253. Soda lime granules in the CO_2 absorber canister should be checked for color change
    a. Immediately before a starting a procedure
    b. Three to 6 hours after the procedure
    c. One hour before starting the procedure
    d. During and upon completing the procedure

254. For a given inhalation anesthetic agent, a vaporizer setting of ___ times MAC will produce a surgical depth of anesthesia.
    a. 2
    b. 0.5
    c. 1
    d. 1.5

255. When using a mechanical ventilator, the animal's chest is under
    a. Continuous pressure
    b. Negative pressure
    c. Positive pressure
    d. No pressure

256. To intubate a 45-lb dog, you should select an endotracheal tube with an internal diameter of ___ mm.
    a. 5
    b. 8
    c. 11
    d. 15

257. The piece of equipment that facilitates intubating a patient is the
    a. Esophageal stethoscope
    b. Laryngoscope
    c. Ophthalmoscope
    d. Otoscope

Correct answers are on pages 503-514.

258. A noncuffed endotracheal tube would most likely be used in a
   a. Newborn kitten
   b. Calf
   c. Lamb
   d. Newborn foal

259. An anesthetized animal should receive sigh breaths every ___ minutes.
   a. 15 to 20
   b. 3 to 5
   c. 10 to 15
   d. 5 to 10

260. A dog in an appropriate plane of anesthesia under isoflurane would be expected to have a pulse oximeter reading of
   a. 97
   b. 120
   c. 85
   d. 90

261. The pulse oximeter probe is generally placed on the
   a. Tongue
   b. Chest
   c. Tail
   d. Nose

262. An esophageal stethoscope can be used to monitor
   a. Direct blood pressure
   b. Oxygen saturation
   c. Heart and respiratory rates
   d. Carbon dioxide levels

263. If IV access is difficult, emergency drugs can be administered safely and effectively by the ___ route.
   a. Intracardiac
   b. Intraperitoneal
   c. Intratracheal
   d. Intramuscular

264. Puppies or kittens delivered by cesarean section that have reduced respiratory function can be given this drug underneath their tongue to stimulate respiration.
   a. Atropine
   b. Doxapram
   c. Epinephrine
   d. Lidocaine

265. Which of the following is least commonly used in cattle to perform procedures?
   a. Sedation
   b. Restraint
   c. General anesthesia
   d. Local analgesics

266. Before administering a general anesthetic, which of the following is the least important part of an animal's history?
   a. When the animal last ate
   b. When the animal was last vaccinated
   c. Whether the animal has a concurrent disease
   d. Prior anesthetic history

267. With dogs and cats, food is most commonly withheld before anesthesia for
   a. 1 to 2 hours
   b. 3 to 5 hours
   c. 6 to 8 hours
   d. 10 to 12 hours

268. Which of the following can activate the sympathetic portion of the autonomic nervous system?
   a. Intubation
   b. Handling viscera
   c. Administration of opioids
   d. Painful stimuli

269. All of the following are appropriate uses of anticholinergic drugs except
   a. As an antidote for organophosphate poisoning
   b. As an agent to increase intestinal peristalsis
   c. As an aid in the treatment of corneal ulcers
   d. As treatment for bradycardia

270. The values of the PCV/TP may indicate that all of the following are present except
   a. Anemia
   b. Hypoproteinemia
   c. Dehydration
   d. Infection

271. Which of the following is not an opioid drug?
   a. Diazepam
   b. Fentanyl
   c. Meperidine
   d. Butorphanol

272. Which of the following statements is incorrect?
   a. Phenothiazine tranquilizers may make an animal more aggressive.
   b. Obese animals are often underdosed.
   c. Brachycephalic animals are prone to respiratory complications.
   d. Isoflurane is more respiratory depressive than halothane.

273. Which of the following statements is incorrect?
   a. Diazepam is a potent sedative.
   b. Xylazine can cause bloat in deep-chested dogs.
   c. Atropine does not have to be administered with butorphanol.
   d. Opioids can be given by the epidural route.

274. Which of the following is least likely to cause hypotension after administration?
    a. Propofol
    b. Thiopental
    c. Acepromazine
    d. Ketamine

275. Which of the following is not seen when ketamine is administered IV rather than IM?
    a. Lower dose rate used
    b. Quicker onset of effects
    c. Longer duration of effects
    d. Less pain on injection

276. Why is apnea sometimes prolonged after barbiturates are administered too rapidly?
    a. Apnea is part of the excitement phase.
    b. Apnea is part of the parasympathetic nervous system stimulation.
    c. Barbiturates cause hypotension.
    d. Barbiturates suppress the respiratory center, making it less sensitive to carbon dioxide.

277. For which of the following species is ketamine use approved?
    a. Cats
    b. Birds
    c. Horses
    d. Dogs

278. Which of the following is (are) not characteristic(s) of propofol?
    a. Rapid induction and recovery
    b. Absence of "hangover effect" with repeated injections
    c. Good post anesthesia analgesia
    d. Smooth recoveries

279. Which of the following is not characteristic of ketamine anesthesia?
    a. Increased muscle tone
    b. Tachycardia
    c. Tachypnea
    d. Central pupils

280. Which of the following is least likely to be a result of administering barbiturates perivascularly?
    a. An excitement phase
    b. Pain
    c. Tissue sloughing
    d. Transient apnea

281. Which of the following statements is incorrect?
    a. Barbiturates are not active when protein-bound.
    b. Barbiturates are less potent in their unbound (free) form.
    c. Methohexital can be safely used in sight hounds.
    d. Barbiturates may cause hypotension when administered too quickly.

282. By which route can short-acting barbiturate drugs be safely administered to induce general anesthesia?
    a. IV
    b. IM
    c. Oral
    d. SQ

283. Advantages of inhalant anesthetics over injectable anesthetics include all of the following except
    a. The ability to quickly change the anesthetic concentration
    b. Less toxic effects on various body systems
    c. Less expensive
    d. Relatively rapid anesthetic induction and recovery

284. When inducing anesthesia with intravenous barbiturates,
    a. Give the full dose over 10 seconds.
    b. Give slowly to effect.
    c. Give the full dose over 5 seconds.
    d. Give 1/2 of the dose quickly, the rest to effect.

285. What is the maximum effective length for a scavenger hose used with a passive system?
    a. 5 feet
    b. 10 feet
    c. 15 feet
    d. 20 feet

286. Which of the following is least useful for detecting the proper placement of an endotracheal tube?
    a. Observing condensation in the tube with each breath
    b. Detecting one rigid tube, rather than two, in the neck area
    c. Feeling air come out of the tube when pressing on the chest
    d. Seeing the rebreathing bag move with respirations

Correct answers are on pages 503-514.

287. What is the standard color of medical nitrous oxide cylinders, and what is the pressure in a full cylinder?
    a. Green; 750 psi
    b. Blue; 750 psi
    c. Green; 2000 psi
    d. Blue; 2000 psi

288. Mask induction of anesthesia using inhalation agents is
    a. The best way to induce anesthesia in a patient with upper airway obstruction
    b. Best accomplished using a volatile anesthetic that is more soluble in body fluids, such as halothane
    c. Less expensive than routine parenteral induction
    d. Best accomplished using a volatile anesthetic that is relatively insoluble in body fluids, such as isoflurane

289. Postanesthetic myositis is most likely to occur in
    a. Pigs
    b. Horses
    c. Ruminants
    d. Rabbits

290. Malignant hyperthermia associated with inhalant anesthesia is most likely to be encountered in
    a. Dogs
    b. Rabbits
    c. Pigs
    d. Sheep

291. What agent is usually avoided when anesthetizing horses?
    a. Xylazine
    b. Atropine
    c. Guaifenesin
    d. Thiopental

292. When using a gas flowmeter with a spherical (floating ball) indicator, the flow should be read
    a. At the top of the indicator
    b. At the bottom of the indicator
    c. At the center of the indicator
    d. Spherical indicators are not in common use.

293. A 10% solution of thiopental contains the drug at a concentration of
    a. 0.1 mg/ml
    b. 1 mg/ml
    c. 10 mg/ml
    d. 100 mg/ml

294. Which of the following is not a potential toxic effect of commonly used local anesthetics?
    a. Arrhythmias
    b. Neurologic damage if injected into a nerve
    c. Seizures
    d. Acidosis

295. An animal that was hit by a car yesterday is having its diaphragmatic hernia repaired. Which of the following anesthetics would be the least desirable?
    a. Isoflurane
    b. Sevoflurane
    c. Nitrous oxide and halothane
    d. Continuous infusion of propofol

296. Balanced anesthesia commonly includes all of the following agents, except
    a. Nitrous oxide and an inhalant anesthetic
    b. Muscle-paralyzing agents
    c. Thiobarbiturates
    d. Dissociative agents

297. The ideal inhalant anesthetic should have all of the following characteristics except
    a. Low vapor pressure
    b. High solubility coefficient
    c. Low MAC
    d. Provide good muscle relaxation

298. Which of the following is associated with diffusion hypoxia?
    a. Isoflurane
    b. Halothane
    c. Sevoflurane
    d. Nitrous oxide

299. Which of the following statements regarding MAC is incorrect?
    a. The MAC expresses the potency of an anesthetic.
    b. A patient at the MAC value is at a surgical plane of anesthesia.
    c. Patient factors, such as pregnancy and disease, may influence the MAC.
    d. Isoflurane has a lower MAC than sevoflurane.

300. How much halothane is biotransformed in the body?
    a. About 1%
    b. About 12%
    c. About 20%
    d. About 50%

301. The ideal inhalant anesthetic would have
    a. Low vapor pressure, low MAC, high solubility coefficient
    b. Low vapor pressure, high MAC, low solubility coefficient
    c. High vapor pressure, low MAC, high solubility coefficient
    d. Low vapor pressure, low MAC, low solubility coefficient

302. What is included as a preservative in halothane?
    a. Thiamylal
    b. Thiopental
    c. Thymol
    d. Theophylline

303. Which of the following is not normally present in stage IV of general anesthesia?
    a. Cool extremities
    b. Weak pulse
    c. Constricted pupils
    d. Bradycardia

304. Which of the following cannot be used to detect blood pressure?
    a. Oscillometer
    b. Doppler
    c. Sphygmomanometer
    d. Pulse oximeter

305. What reflex may still be present under a light surgical plane of anesthesia?
    a. Patellar
    b. Palpebral
    c. Pinnal
    d. Pharyngeal

306. The optimal plane of anesthesia for most surgery is
    a. Stage 3, plane 1
    b. Stage 3, plane 2
    c. Stage 2, plane 2
    d. Stage 2, plane 3

307. Which of the following does not describe a true reflex response?
    a. Blink
    b. Toe pinch
    c. Jaw tone
    d. Ear flick

308. Which of the following is not likely to result in a patient demonstrating stage II of anesthesia?
    a. Masking an animal with an inhalant anesthetic
    b. Injecting an anesthetic agent IV too rapidly
    c. During recovery, when a premed has not been given
    d. Partial perivascular injection of a barbiturate while inducing anesthesia

309. Ideally, in a patient under anesthesia,
    a. The PaO_2 should be high, and the $PaCO_2$ should be low.
    b. The PaO_2 should be high, and the $PaCO_2$ should be high.
    c. The PaO_2 should be low, and the $PaCO_2$ should be low.
    d. The PaO_2 should be low, and the $PaCO_2$ should be high.

310. Which of the following monitoring devices is invasive?
    a. Pulse oximeter
    b. Central venous pressure manometer
    c. Doppler blood pressure monitor
    d. Oscillometric blood pressure monitor

311. Which of the following drugs is useful in the treatment of prolonged anesthetic recoveries?
    a. Diazepam
    b. Doxapram
    c. Dopamine
    d. Digoxin

312. Which of the following statements regarding brachycephalic breeds is incorrect?
    a. They may have stenotic nares.
    b. Brachycephalics have a hypoplastic trachea.
    c. A long, floppy soft palate may occlude the trachea.
    d. Brachycephalics often suffer from laryngospasm.

313. The pressure in a full medical O_2 tank is
    a. 500 psi
    b. 1000 psi
    c. 1500 psi
    d. 2000 psi

314. For which of the following agents can a nonprecision vaporizer be safely used?
    a. Halothane
    b. Isoflurane
    c. Sevoflurane
    d. None of the above

Correct answers are on pages 503-514.

315. For which of the following can a vaporizer not be compensated?
    a. Back pressure
    b. Temperature
    c. Solubility coefficient
    d. Flow rate

316. Which of the following is a component of a Bain anesthetic circuit?
    a. Reservoir bag
    b. Unidirectional valves
    c. Oxygen flush valve
    d. Carbon dioxide absorber

317. A half-full nitrous oxide cylinder should be
    a. Green, with a pressure of 2000 psi
    b. Blue, with a pressure of 750 psi
    c. Green, with a pressure of 1000 psi
    d. Blue, with a pressure of 375 psi

318. Pin indexing on inhalant anesthetic machines is used to
    a. Blow air out of connections
    b. Check for leaks
    c. Prevent oxygen and nitrous oxide cylinders from being exchanged
    d. Ensure that the oldest tanks are used first

319. Which of these species is most prone to developing malignant hyperthermia?
    a. Equine
    b. Porcine
    c. Ovine
    d. Feline

320. To minimize waste anesthetic exposure in the surgical suite, a realistic goal is to have the level of halothane no higher than
    a. 2 ppm
    b. 50 ppm
    c. 100 ppm
    d. 1000 ppm

321. Which is the incorrect statement regarding bovine anesthesia?
    a. Nitrous oxide is not suitable for bovine anesthesia.
    b. Cattle should be placed in lateral recumbency during recovery.
    c. The palpebral reflex is still present in cattle at a surgical plane of anesthesia.
    d. Atropine may cause bloat and thus should be avoided in cattle.

322. Which is the preferred order of administering emergency drugs?
    a. IC, IT, IV
    b. IV, IC, IT
    c. IT, IV, IC
    d. IV, IT, IC

323. Which of the following has not been associated with long-term exposure to waste anesthetic gases?
    a. Carcinogenic effects
    b. Hepatotoxicity
    c. Decline in short-term memory
    d. Increased incidence of miscarriages

324. Which of the following statements regarding avian anesthesia is incorrect?
    a. IM injections should be given in the pectoral muscle only.
    b. A cuffed tube should be used to maintain inhalant anesthesia.
    c. A nonrebreathing circuit should be used in birds.
    d. Ketamine is not effective in birds.

325. For a large dog receiving CPR, compressions and respirations should be administered at
    a. 60 compressions/minute; respirations every 1 to 3 seconds
    b. 60 compressions/minute; respirations every 3 to 5 seconds
    c. 120 compressions/minute; respirations every 15 seconds
    d. 120 compressions/minute; respirations every 3 to 5 seconds

326. Which of the following statements is incorrect?
    a. Furosemide may be used to treat pulmonary edema.
    b. Dopamine is an analeptic stimulant.
    c. When giving medications by the IT route, the dosage rate should be doubled from the IV dose.
    d. Doxapram is a respiratory stimulant.

327. Which of the following statements is incorrect?
    a. Neostigmine reverses the effects of succinylcholine.
    b. Succinylcholine is an example of a depolarizing type of muscle-paralyzing agent.
    c. Muscle cells are polarized at rest.
    d. Muscle-paralyzing agents should not be used if an animal has been given an aminoglycoside antibiotic.

328. What agent should be avoided in geriatric patients?
     a. Atropine
     b. Xylazine
     c. Ketamine
     d. Diazepam

329. What agent is excreted largely intact by the cat kidney?
     a. Atropine
     b. Ketamine
     c. Halothane
     d. Acetylpromazine

330. In cattle, an epidural block is performed by inserting the needle between
     a. T13 and L1
     b. L7 and the sacrum
     c. The sacrum and C1
     d. Cy1 and Cy2

331. For which patients should mask induction with isoflurane be avoided?
     a. Patients undergoing cesarean sections
     b. Patients with impaired cardiac function
     c. Patients with impaired respiratory function
     d. Patients with impaired gastrointestinal function

Answers

1. **b** Xylazine does not have antiinflammatory, antiemetic, or anesthetic properties.

2. **c** Although only approved for use in horses, detomidine is used clinically in other species.

3. **b** Butorphanol does not have antiinflammatory, anesthetic, or diuretic properties.

4. **c** Diazepam is an ideal drug for use in the cardiovascular-compromised patient. In patients with impaired renal or hepatic function, recovery may be significantly prolonged as a result of the metabolic requirements of diazepam.

5. **d** Although not approved for use in cattle, xylazine is sometimes used clinically in that species.

6. **b** Guaifenesin is a muscle relaxant drug used along with other general anesthetics in horses and cattle.

7. **a** The combination of xylazine and butorphanol provides greater analgesia and muscle relaxation, with the effects of both drugs being enhanced. One benefit of this combination is that the dose of each drug is reduced, minimizing side effects and maximizing therapeutic effects.

8. **b** Detomidine is a much more potent sedative on a volume-per-volume basis.

9. **c** Acepromazine is an alpha blocker with significant potential to produce hypotension; however, this is rarely a problem in healthy, normovolemic patients.

10. **c** Zolazepam is a benzodiazepine tranquilizer, and tiletamine is a dissociative anesthetic.

11. **d** Although epidural anesthetics are used to provide analgesia, patient movement is still of concern and prevents their use for many surgical procedures.

12. **b** Halothane sensitizes the myocardium to catecholamines such as epinephrine, which may lead to arrhythmias. Isoflurane and sevoflurane do not sensitize the myocardium to catecholamines. Nitrous oxide has little effect on cardiac function and is an inhalant analgesic, not an anesthetic.

13. **d** Halothane is biotransformed to a much greater extent than isoflurane or sevoflurane. Nitrous oxide is an inhalant analgesic, not an anesthetic.

14. **d** All drugs listed, except neuromuscular-blocking agents, cross the placental barrier in significant amounts, depressing the fetus. Neuromuscular-blocking agents are highly ionized and have high molecular weights, minimizing placental transfer.

15. **d** Propofol is an alkylphenol, nonbarbiturate, highly lipid-soluble hypnotic agent used to produce short-term anesthesia.

16. **b** Glycopyrrolate, a quaternary ammonium drug with anticholinergic properties, has fewer side effects than atropine and does not cross the placental barrier.

17. **d** Atropine is often used to prevent drug or parasympathetic nervous system–induced bradycardia in anesthetized animals.

18. **b** Opioids are often referred to as *narcotic analgesic* drugs.

19. **b** Acepromazine has no analgesic effect.

20. **a** The anticholinergic effects of atropine on the intestinal tract of horses may include ileus, intestinal distention, and colic. Atropine use in horses should be limited to treatment of bradycardia caused by increases in vagal tone.

21. **b** The phenothiazine tranquilizers all have the potential to produce paralysis of the penis in stallions.

22. **a** Naloxone is a pure narcotic antagonist with no agonist actions of its own.

23. **b** A 10% solution contains 10 g of solute (drug) in 100 ml of solvent (water). 10 g = 10,000 mg, so there are 10,000 mg of drug per 100 ml, or 100 mg per 1 ml (100 mg/ml)

24. **b** The addition of depressant premedication to an anesthetic protocol may prolong the recovery time because of anesthetic drug enhancement.

25. **c** Yohimbine antagonizes the depressant effects of xylazine.

26. **c** Diazepam does not have analgesic, hypnotic, or emetic properties.

27. **a** The adrenergic (sympathetic) effects of epinephrine increase heart rate.

28. **b** Because nitrous oxide is an inhalant analgesic, when it is used along with potent inhalant anesthetic drugs, it allows lower levels of the more potent drugs to be used to achieve appropriate levels of general anesthesia.

29. **a** The partial pressure of oxygen in arterial blood should be approximately five times the percent of inspired oxygen. Breathing 100% oxygen would then yield a PaO_2 of 500 mm Hg. Oxygen at 50% + N_2O at 50% would yield a PaO_2 of 250 mm Hg. In some patients this might not be desirable.

30. **c** A 2% solution contains 2 g of solute (drug) in 100 ml of solvent (water); 2 g = 2000 mg, so there are 2000 mg of drug per 100 ml, or 20 mg per 1 ml (20 mg/ml).

31. **b** 500 kg × 8 mg/kg = 4000 mg total dose; 10% thiopental = 100 mg/ml; 4000 mg/100 mg/ml = 40 ml

32. **c** Apneustic respirations are characterized by an inspiratory hold and rapid expiration.

33. **d** Premedication agents are used to minimize undesirable autonomic effects.

34. **b** 5% = 50 mg/ml × 180 ml = 9000 mg/150 kg = 60 mg/kg

35. **c** Epidural lidocaine can be used to provide analgesia preoperatively and postoperatively for surgical procedures that involve the rear limbs and anal area.

36. **d** Mask inductions in aggressive patients can be so stressful that they offset the benefit of avoiding premedication and induction agents.

37. **b** Atropine decreases salivation.

38. **b** 0.1 mg/kg × 60 kg = 6 mg. The maximum dose is still 4 mg.

39. **d** All inhalation anesthetics are expected to decrease cardiac output at working concentrations.

40. **c** The more anesthetic agent administered, the greater the adverse effect.

41. **d** Increased heart rate, increased respiratory rate, and active palpebral reflex may be indications of light planes of anesthesia, but patient movement as a result of painful stimuli is a clear indicator that the depth of anesthesia is not adequate.

42. **d** Propofol has none of the other characteristics.

43. **a** Acepromazine lowers the seizure threshold and should not be used in animals with a history of seizures. Old dogs with adequate liver function tolerate acepromazine quite well in proper doses.

44. **d** Opioids in the dog are commonly associated with respiratory depression, bradycardia, and analgesic activity. Excitement is rare.

45. **b** The MAC is the concentration in percent at 1 atmosphere that prevents gross, purposeful skeletal muscle movement in response to a noxious stimulus in 50% of patients. It is an expression of the potency of the drug.

46. **b** None of the other drugs have dissociative effects.

47. **c** Halothane is more soluble in body tissues than isoflurane or sevoflurane. Nitrous oxide is an inhalant analgesic, not an anesthetic.

48. **c** Provides easy access and adequate vessel size

49. **d** Oxygen flows less than 1.5 times the minute ventilation allows rebreathing of carbon dioxide.

50. **c** The pressure in the cylinder begins to drop when all of the liquid nitrous oxide has been vaporized, and the gas loses pressure. No change in full pressure (750 psi) takes place until that time.

51. **b** Adequate inflation of the normal lung requires approximately 20 cm H_2O.

52. **b** Precision vaporizers produce indicated concentrations of anesthetic agents only when located outside of the anesthetic circle system.

53. **d** The absence of unidirectional valves allows rebreathing of carbon dioxide. Because the attachment of a nonrebreathing device to the fresh gas port bypasses the circuit, it can be used.

54. **a** The oxygen flush valve allows a burst of oxygen to be added to the breathing system without adding additional amounts of anesthetic agent.

55. **b** The potential for hypothermia production is a disadvantage of nonrebreathing system use.

56. **a** Metabolic rate determines the minimum oxygen requirement.

57. **d** Waste anesthetic gases may pose a health risk to workers who inhale them.

58. **d** All vaporizers can be used with any breathing circuit.

59. **a**

60. **b** The rebreathing bag should be at least three times the patient's tidal volume to ensure an adequate volume of gases for patient needs.

61. **c** Variations in the transmission or reflection of the red–light beam is interpreted by a computer in the pulse oximeter as the percentage of saturation of arterial hemoglobin with oxygen.

62. **d** Soda lime should be changed on the basis of hours of use.

63. **a** An oxygen flow that is too high would cause the rebreathing bag to overinflate, not underinflate.

64. **c** Blue is the standard color for medical nitrous oxide cylinders.

65. **b**

66. **c**

67. **b**

68. **d**

69. **d**

70. **a**

71. **d**

72. **d** Chamber and mask inductions cause increased waste anesthetic gas exposures to personnel involved.

73. **b** If more than 5 ml of air are required to properly fill the cuff, the diameter of the endotracheal tube is too small. This restricts patient ventilation and can cause pressure damage to the tracheal lining.

74. **a** To reduce deadspace and prevent endobronchial intubation, you should premeasure and mark the tip of the tube so it can be placed midway between the thoracic inlet and the larynx.

75. **d** In this position, a horse's long, soft palate will usually guide the tube into the larynx.

76. **b** The endotracheal tube, when properly fitted and placed, should decrease, not increase, the dead space.

77. **c** Cats are more likely to experience laryngospasm than the other species listed.

78. **a** All of the choices are complications involved in placing an endotracheal tube. However, misplacement of the tube into the esophagus occurs more frequently than the others.

79. **b** The ideal method for inflating a cuff is to compress the rebreathing bag, or an Ambu bag, while adding air to the cuff. This method should prevent overinflation and tracheal necrosis.

80. **c** The safest way to treat laryngospasm is to apply 1 or 2 drops of lidocaine and wait a few minutes to allow the larynx to relax before proceeding.

81. **d** The endotracheal tube is specifically used to decrease the chances of having airway obstruction.

82. **d** In nonbrachycephalic animals, the endotracheal tube should be removed as soon as the animal is able to swallow and cough and at the first sign that it can chew on the tube. This must be done before the animal has had a chance to puncture the tube or injure itself on the tube.

83. **b** In brachycephalic breeds, the chances of respiratory complications are greater than in other animals. Therefore, the endotracheal tube should be left in place until the animal is conscious and able to maintain a patent airway.

84. **b** Although tape and rubber bands are used in some clinics, they are not recommended. The rubber bands may become tangled in the hair, and, if applied too tightly, can cause pressure necrosis. Tape will stick to the hair and may be difficult to remove in an emergency.

85. **b** Intravenous anesthesia alone (sedative plus a short-acting barbiturate) may not completely immobilize large animals and should not be used for procedures that require such control of movement.

86. **c** The term *vital sign* refers to measures that indicate the response of the animal's homeostatic mechanisms to anesthesia. These include heart rate, blood pressure, capillary refill time (CRT), central venous pressure, mucous membrane color, blood loss, respiratory rate, blood gases, and temperature. *Reflex* refers to an involuntary response to a stimulus.

87. **b** Continuous monitoring of the anesthetized patient may be impractical in many veterinary clinics. However, an attempt should be made to observe and evaluate an anesthetized animal at least once every 3 to 5 minutes.

88. **c** The color of mucous membranes and CRT are both used to evaluate oxygen levels in tissue. Pink mucous membranes suggest adequate oxygen levels, whereas bluish mucous membranes indicate cyanosis. A CRT of greater than 2 seconds indicates poor tissue perfusion with oxygenated blood.

89. **a** Every patient given an anesthetic drug is hypoventilating. During hypoventilation periods, oxygen levels decrease, and carbon dioxide levels increase.

90. **b** Although some of the other reflexes may be present (e.g., palpebral, pedal), the appearance of the swallowing reflex is most often cited as the appropriate time to remove the endotracheal tube, because return of this reflex will help protect the animal from aspirating vomitus. In brachycephalic breeds, the airway should be protected by leaving the tube in until the patient begins to choke on it.

91. **a** Patient recovery may be hastened by gentle stimulation, which includes talking to the animal, gently pinching the toes, opening the mouth, gently moving the limbs, and rubbing the chest.

92. **c** It is advisable to turn all animals sternally (the feet are moved under a dog as it is turned, rather than rolling the patient onto its back) to lessen the chance of gastric torsion, especially in deep-chested animals.

93. **c** Once extubated, all animals should be placed in sternal recumbency with the neck extended, because this position helps maintain a patent airway.

94. **a** Periodic bagging with pure oxygen is advisable for as long as the recovering patient is connected to the anesthetic machine, because it helps reinflate collapsed alveoli.

95. **b** Cyanosis is indicated by bluish coloring of the mucous membranes.

96. **c** Because of the structure of their nasal passages and palate, brachycephalic breeds are more prone to vomiting and possible airway obstruction after anesthesia.

97. **b** Food and water should not be offered immediately after consciousness is regained, because many animals experience periods of nausea and vomiting after anesthesia.

98. **b**

99. **c**

100. **b** Phenothiazine drugs, such as acepromazine, do not cause respiratory depression and are considered to have a wide margin of safety.

101. **b** Adequate perfusion of peripheral blood vessels results in a CRT of less than 2 seconds.

102. **a** *Direct monitoring* refers to the measuring of arterial blood pressure through use of an indwelling catheter placed in the femoral or dorsal pedal artery. *Indirect monitoring* refers to the use of external devices when recording blood pressure.

103. **a** Alternative sites for monitoring mucous membrane color include the tongue, buccal mucous membranes, conjunctivae of the lower eyelids, and lining of the prepuce or vulva.

104. **b**

105. **d** Atelectasis is a respiratory condition characterized by partially collapsed alveoli. It may be the result of shallow breathing, which causes a decrease in tidal volume. Bagging the patient helps prevent atelectasis by gently forcing air into the patient's breathing passages.

106. **a** Hyperventilation and tachypnea may be observed in animals that progress from moderate to light anesthesia.

107. **b** Feeling the temperature of the extremities, such as the paws and ears, can give an indication of the animal's body temperature.

108. **a** It is impractical and often impossible in many hospitals to prewarm the stainless-steel V trough before its use in surgery; the metal does not retain heat. Lining the trough with towels or newspapers would be a more practical way of keeping the animal away from the cold stainless steel.

109. **b** Although hyperthermia may occasionally be seen in dogs anesthetized with ketamine or halothane, pigs are more susceptible to this condition.

110. **c** Succinylcholine is a muscle-paralyzing agent that may be used to achieve pronounced muscle relaxation for certain procedures, but you will not have the degree of muscle relaxation as an indicator of anesthetic depth.

111. **d** Ketamine does not cause eye rotation, even at moderate depths of anesthesia.

112. **a** In stage III, plane 3 of anesthesia, the eye is usually central to slightly rotated, and the pupils are moderately dilated and respond slowly to light or not at all.

113. **c** Production of tears and saliva diminishes with increasing depth of anesthesia and is totally absent in deep surgical anesthesia. Ophthalmic solutions and ointments are used to prevent corneal drying.

114. **b** A light plane of anesthesia may be indicated by increasing lacrimation and salivation.

115. **b** Stage III, plane 3 is the indicated depth of anesthesia with the signs listed.

116. **d** The anesthetic plane is probably too deep for the given procedure. The age of the animal is also a risk factor. You should try to lighten the plane of anesthesia by adjusting the vaporizer setting to 1.5% and watch for signs of lightening, such as increased heart rate and respiratory rate, lacrimation, sweat on the foot pads, and movement. Maintain anesthesia on a setting that will permit the surgery without pain.

117. **b** Stage II is characterized as the "excitement stage" with the signs listed. This stage should be avoided by giving a bolus of injectable anesthetic to take the animal past this phase of excitement.

118. **c** The anticholinergic effects of glycopyrrolate block the vagal-induced bradycardia and second-degree heart block commonly associated with xylazine.

119. **a**

120. **d** 1/10,000 = 0.01/100 = 0.01% = 0.1 mg/ml

121. **a** Normal carbon dioxide levels do not induce arrhythmias.

122. **a** Arterial pressure in the horse is a more accurate indicator of anesthetic depth than heart rate.

123. **d** The patient needs fluids to help compensate for blood loss indicated by its low PCV and plasma protein values.

124. **c**

125. **d**

126. **c**

127. **b** Falling blood pressure indicates increasing depth of anesthesia in the horse. Lowering the isoflurane concentration will lighten the anesthetic depth. Increasing the fluid delivery rate will help increase the blood pressure.

128. **b**

129. **c** 10 kg × 50 g/kg/min = 500 g/min;
500 g = 0.5 mg = 0.5 ml = 30 drops/min

130. **c**

131. **d** A xylazine overdose would cause bradycardia.

132. **d**

133. **d** It is difficult to warm the patient by surface application of warm objects.

134. **d** Voluntary movement would indicate the cat was too light, not too deep.

135. **d**

136. **d** Increased jaw muscle tone would indicate the dog was too light, not too deep.

137. **c**

138. **b**

139. **b**

140. **c**

141. **d**

142. **a**

143. **b**

144. **c**

145. **d** Intubation of one bronchus prevents ventilation of the other lung.

146. **d**

147. **a**

148. **d**

149. **d**

150. **d**

151. **c** Barbiturates such as thiopental are lipophilic and highly soluble in fat tissue. Thus these drugs are stored in fat and slowly released to be metabolized and excreted. The fatter an animal, the more the storage capacity. The drugs are then stored before metabolism and excretion.

152. **c** Guaifenesin is a muscle relaxant that is commonly used in horse anesthesia, along with other induction agents. It ensures an excitement-free induction and recovery. Masking down with isoflurane is impossible due to lack of ability to control the animal during the excitement stage. Long-acting barbiturates such as phenobarbital are not used as induction agents. Propofol is not used in horses.

153. **a** Barbiturates, propofol, and benzodiazepine tranquilizers are all anticonvulsant drugs.

154. **d** Xylazine is an alpha-2 agonist drug with sedative and analgesic properties. Atropine is not a sedative. Acepromazine and diazepam are not analgesics.

155. **d** Midazolam is a benzodiazepine tranquilizer that does not affect GI motility.

156. **a** Antagonists block receptors. Agonists stimulate receptors. Antitussives inhibit the cough reflex.

157. **a** Anticholinergic drugs prevent bradycardia by blocking the parasympathetic response. The other three drugs can cause bradycardia.

158. **d** Phenothiazine tranquilizers are antiemetics; they cause vasodilation and decrease the seizure threshold.

159. **d** You would not increase the concentration or delivery of an anesthetic agent such as isoflurane to counteract an overdose of another anesthetic agent.

160. **b** Induction agents given by the IM route have to be calculated on the basis of weight and take 10 to 20 minutes to show maximal effect.

161. **d** You want to deliver no less than 30% oxygen with nitrous oxide to prevent hypoxia.

162. **a** As the animal consumes the oxygen in the closed system, the nitrous oxide may increase to a dangerous level.

163. **b** Diffusion hypoxia is a phenomenon seen when a patient has been breathing nitrous oxide. When nitrous oxide administration is stopped, the gas floods into the lung alveoli from the bloodstream. If the patient is breathing room air (21% oxygen), the nitrous oxide can dilute the oxygen concentration in alveoli to the point that the patient

can become hypoxic. This is called *diffusion hypoxia*. To prevent it, have the patient breathe 100% oxygen for at least 5 minutes after the nitrous oxide gas has been turned off.

164. **d** Sight hounds lack fat stores to which barbiturates can redistribute. Liver disease slows down the metabolism and excretion of barbiturates. Administration of 50% glucose will prolong the anesthetic effect of barbiturates.

165. **d** Animals will recover very quickly from isoflurane anesthesia because of its low solubility coefficient. Animals that have tranquilizers and other sedatives "on board" recover more slowly and smoothly.

166. **c** Nitrous oxide accumulates in areas of the body where gas is trapped. Because the nitrous oxide will diffuse into the area very rapidly, the pressure in this area can rapidly increase and cause distention.

167. **d** Overhydration, hypothermia, and hypoglycemia are concerns to guard against when anesthetizing a pediatric animal.

168. **c** Hyperthermia would most likely present with red mucous membranes.

169. **a** IV administration delivers the drug quickly and primarily to the brain, because the brain receives 30% of the cardiac output and is a vessel-rich tissue.

170. **b** ALT is a liver enzyme. Abnormal ALT levels indicate liver problems.

171. **c** Total solids are a measure of the protein content of the blood.

172. **a** Respiratory rate will not change with hydration status change.

173. **a** Soda lime absorbs carbon dioxide, not anesthetic gas.

174. **c** Nitrous oxide and carbon dioxide are not absorbed by charcoal. The canister must be changed when it has gained approximately 20% of its original weight.

175. **c** Calibration of the vaporizer must be done by professionals.

176. **d** A paper bag will allow the volatile gas anesthetic to escape into the ambient air.

The material used to pick up the spill should be disposed of in a trash can outside of the building.

177. **d** Local anesthetics are injected around nerves, not neuromuscular blocking agents.

178. **b** The sequence of muscle relaxation after IV injection is oculomotor, palpebral, facial, tongue and pharynx, jaw and tail, limbs, pelvic, caudal abdominal, cranial abdominal, intercostal, larynx, and diaphragm.

179. **c** Neuromuscular blocking agents interfere with nicotinic neuromuscular transmission by either competing with acetylcholine at the receptor site or by blocking acetylcholine at the receptor site.

180. **b** Local anesthetics prevent nerve cell depolarization, thus stopping the conduction of nerve impulses.

181. **c** Preanesthetic drug administration lowers the amount of anesthetic gas needed to produce anesthesia. Increased age and debilitation such as anemia will also lower the amount of anesthetic gas needed to produce anesthesia.

182. **b** The gas anesthetic solubility coefficient and potency determine the rapidity of onset and recovery.

183. **b** Precision vaporizers limit the concentration of gas vapors from highly volatile anesthetics to lower nontoxic levels. Volatile anesthetics are never administered IV.

184. **d** The longer an animal is under anesthesia, the more volatile anesthetic will be stored in tissues such as fat. The higher the percentage of biotransformation, the longer it takes to eliminate the anesthetic because of the limitations of metabolism. The higher the solubility coefficient, the longer it takes to induce and recover.

185. **d** The anesthetic with the lowest MAC is the most potent.

186. **b** Agent B has a low solubility coefficient combined with a low MAC.

187. **c** *MAC* is minimum alveolar concentration. Agent C has the lowest number under the column labeled *MAC*.

188. **c** Agent C has the highest solubility coefficient, and thus this agent will produce long induction and recovery times.

189. **b** You want to decrease the frequency of ventilating breaths to have carbon dioxide concentration increase in the blood. Increased carbon dioxide will stimulate spontaneous respiration.

190. **c** Increased levels of carbon dioxide in the blood stimulate the respiratory center in the brain.

191. **a** Inspiration is the active phase of respiration. Inspiration/expiration ratio in small animals is 1:2 to 1:4.5.

192. **b** Overinflation of the lungs during artificial ventilation can cause alveolar rupture that results in enlargement or coalition of the alveolar air spaces.

193. **d** Neuromuscular blocking agents do paralyze skeletal muscles, including the diaphragm, provided that the dose is appropriately high. Neuromuscular blocking agents do not provide any sedation or analgesia.

194. **b** Neuromuscular blocking agents paralyze the diaphragm last. Reflexes are absent. Gut motility is not affected, because neuromuscular blocking agents do not paralyze smooth muscles. They work in the periphery at the NMJ, not centrally, to cause muscle relaxation.

195. **a** Neuromuscular blocking agents provide no analgesia.

196. **b** Acetylcholinesterase inhibitors can exacerbate the blockade by depolarizing neuromuscular blocking agents, because additional depolarization results from the increase of acetylcholine in the NMJ. Acetylcholinesterase inhibitors increase the concentration of acetylcholine in the NMJ by preventing the breakdown of acetylcholine.

197. **b** Local anesthetics are not readily absorbed through skin. They should be injected near, not into, the nerve. They are combined with vasoconstrictor drugs to prolong their action at the site of injection by slowing their absorption into the circulation.

198. **c** The term *visceral* means "pertaining to internal organs."

199. **b** *Preemptive* means "preventive."

200. **c** It is the anesthetic gas that the animal is breathing in that is keeping the animal under anesthesia, so turning the anesthetic vaporizer setting off or down is the correct answer.

201. **d** If the endotracheal tube were kinked, the animal would not be getting any anesthetic gas or oxygen and would be hypoxic and possibly too light, not too deep.

202. **d** Animals in shock have poor vascular perfusion. The symptoms of shock include prolonged CRT, pale mucous membranes, tachycardia, and hypotension.

203. **c** The soda lime absorbs carbon dioxide from the exhaust limb of the breathing circuit of the anesthesia machine. If the soda lime were not working, the carbon dioxide would not be removed, and the patient would breathe in more carbon dioxide, thus becoming hypercapnic.

204. **c** If the pressure relief valve is closed, the pressure in the breathing circuit could quickly become dangerously high. Disconnecting and attaching the patient to another anesthesia machine would be preferable.

205. **d** At that blood pressure, the patient is hypotensive. A bolus of IV fluids is the best choice listed.

206. **d** If the patient is having difficulty breathing, the animal may be too deep, so turning down the vaporizer is a good idea. The endotracheal tube could be kinked, so checking that is a good idea. The oxygen tank could be empty, so checking that would be a good idea. The anesthesia machine could be used to ventilate the animal, so disconnecting it from the machine would not be a good idea.

207. **c** A heart rate of 230 beats/min is not normal for a dog. If the animal were too deep or hypothermic, the heart rate would be low.

208. **b** A patient in shock will be hypotensive.

209. **d** If the patient is not breathing, the heart may or may not still be beating. Ventilating breaths will do no good if the endotracheal tube is blocked. Tell the surgeon, because he or she must know.

210. **a**

211. **b** The other choices would increase waste anesthetic gas exposure.

212. **b** Expanding the patient's fluid volume would help increase its blood pressure.

213. **b**

214. **c** Isoflurane undergoes very little biotransformation in the body. Most of it leaves the body via the respiratory system.

215. **b** Once the patient can swallow, it is in less danger of aspirating fluid into the lungs.

216. **d** Prolonged anesthesia does not increase patient safety.

217. **a**

218. **c**

219. **c** Epidural anesthesia blocks sensation and motor control to the rear abdomen, pelvis, tail, pelvic limbs, and perineum.

220. **d** Lidocaine is a local anesthetic drug.

221. **b** Barbiturate drugs have a very alkaline pH.

222. **d** Ketamine is not a barbiturate and thiopental and pentobarbital both cause prolonged recovery times in sight hounds.

223. **a** 97% of sevoflurane is eliminated via respiration.

224. **c** Induction range for halothane is 1% to 4%, and isoflurane, 2% to 6%. Sevoflurane is not a very potent anesthetic.

225. **b** Maintenance range for halothane is 0.5% to 2%, and isoflurane, 1% to 3%. Sevoflurane is a less potent anesthetic than the other two drugs.

226. **a**

227. **b**

228. **d**

229. **c** Yohimbine is an antagonist for xylazine, Dopram is a respiratory stimulant, and naloxone is an opioid antagonist.

230. **d**

231. **a** Lidocaine is a local anesthetic, morphine is an opioid, and yohimbine is a reversal agent for xylazine.

232. **d** Sevoflurane has the lowest blood/gas coefficient (0.68) of the commonly used anesthetic agents in veterinary medicine. This property allows for rapid induction and recovery of the patient. Nitrous oxide is an inhalant analgesic, not an anesthetic.

233. **d** Sevoflurane has a slight depressive effect on the heart, unlike halothane, which has a severe depressive effect.

234. **a**

235. **c**

236. **a** A fentanyl patch should be applied at least 6 hours before the start of surgery in cats and at least 12 hours before surgery in dogs, because there is a delay before therapeutic blood levels are reached.

237. **a**

238. **b**

239. **c** Buprenorphine lasts 6 to 12 hours, morphine and oxymorphone 3 to 4 hours, and butorphanol 1 to 2 hours.

240. **c**

241. **d**

242. **b** Acepromazine is a phenothiazine sedative, diazepam is a benzothiazine tranquilizer, and ketamine is a dissociative anesthetic.

243. **b**

244. **c**

245. **d**

246. **b**

247. **a** Nonrebreathing systems do not use a carbon dioxide absorber.

248. **c**

249. **d**

250. **b**

251. **a** Movement of personnel in the operating room stirs up gases.

252. **c**

253. **d** The color reaction is time limited, and granules that have changed color may revert back to the original color after several hours, although they are saturated with carbon dioxide.

254. **d**

255. **c** The lungs are filled with oxygen by the pressure of gas that enters the airways from the mechanical ventilator; this is in contrast to normal breathing when the chest is under negative pressure.

256. **c**

257. **b**

258. **a** Noncuffed tubes are used in very small patients, such as newborn kittens and puppies, birds, and ferrets, because noncuffed tubes preserve a larger airway.

259. **d**

260. **a** Normal values should be more than 95%; values less than 90% indicate hypoxia; it is impossible to have greater than 100% oxygen saturation of hemoglobin.

261. **a** Probe can be placed on the tongue, lip fold, toe web, ear, skin folds, nasal septum, or vulva.

262. **c**

263. **c** Emergency drugs can be given by the intratracheal route at twice the recommended IV dose. The intracardiac and intraperitoneal routes carry too much risk of damage, and absorption of emergency drugs from an intramuscular injection is too slow.

264. **b** Doxopram stimulates the respiratory center in the brainstem.

265. **c** General anesthesia is usually avoided because of the likelihood of bloat.

266. **b** Of the options given this is the least likely to have an impact on the anesthetic regimen.

267. **d** Younger or smaller animals may require a shorter fast.

268. **d** The rest activate the parasympathetic system.

269. **b** Anticholinergics decrease intestinal peristalsis.

270. **d** The presence or absence of infection cannot be determined from PCV/TP values.

271. **a** Diazepam is a benzodiazepine tranquilizer.

272. **b** Obese animals are actually usually overdosed, because fat is not very metabolically active.

273. **a** Diazepam is a weak sedative.

274. **d** Ketamine generally causes some degree of cardiovascular stimulation rather than depression.

275. **c** Ketamine IV has a shorter duration of effect than by the IM route.

276. **d** Barbiturates suppress the respiratory center that usually responds to increased carbon dioxide.

277. **a** Although it is commonly used in other species, ketamine is approved for use in cats and primates only.

278. **c** Propofol does not provide analgesia, so supplemental analgesics should be given postoperatively.

279. **c** Ketamine causes apneustic respirations, which slow, rather than elevate, the respiratory rate.

280. **d** Transient apnea is more likely if barbiturates are given by IV too quickly. If administered perivascularly, absorption of the drug will actually be slower than normal.

281. **b** They are more potent in their unbound form and thus should be used with caution in hypoproteinemic animals.

282. **a** Intravenous administration is the only route listed that would increase the blood level of the drug quickly and safely enough to induce general anesthesia.

283. **c** Inhalant anesthetics, such as isoflurane or sevoflurane, are generally more expensive to use than injectables.

284. **d** This will minimize the possible negative side effects of barbiturate induction.

285. **d** Passive scavenger systems are ineffective if the hose is longer than 20 feet.

286. **c** Sometimes when the endotracheal tube is in the esophagus, air in the stomach could come out when the chest is pressed.

287. **b** Oxygen cylinders are green, with a full pressure of 2000 psi.

288. **d** This results in a more rapid anesthetic induction than with a drug that is more soluble in body fluids.

289. **b**

290. **c**

291. **b** Colic has been associated with atropine use in horses because of its depressant effect on gut motility.

292. **c**

293. **d** 10% = 10 g/100 ml = 10,000 mg/100 ml = 100 mg/1 ml

294. **d**

295. **c** Nitrous oxide is avoided when trapped gas spaces might be present, because it readily diffuses into these spaces, making the problem worse.

296. **d** Dissociative agents such as ketamine are not a normal part of balanced anesthesia.

297. **b** A high solubility coefficient leads to prolonged inductions, recoveries, and reactions to changes in concentration.

298. **d** Diffusion hypoxia can result when a patient that has been receiving nitrous oxide is allowed to breathe room air immediately after cessation of the nitrous oxide administration. The nitrous oxide diffuses out of the bloodstream into lung alveoli so quickly that it dilutes the oxygen content of the inhaled air, resulting in diffusion hypoxia. This can be prevented by allowing the patient to breathe 100% oxygen for at least 5 minutes after cessation of nitrous oxide administration.

299. **b** Administration of inhalant anesthetics at the MAC level results in lack of response to painful stimuli in about 50% of patients. Surgical anesthesia usually requires administration of 1.5 MAC.

300. **c**

301. **d** These characteristics describe an anesthetic that would produce rapid anesthesia at fairly low concentrations.

302. **c**

303. **c** The pupils generally dilate in stage IV of general anesthesia.

304. **d** Pulse oximeters estimate the percentage of arterial hemoglobin oxygen saturation.

305. **b** However, it is lost as the patient gets deeper.

306. **b** This is the moderate plane of surgical anesthesia. Plane 1 of stage 3 is light surgical anesthesia, and stage 2 is the excitement stage of anesthesia.

307. **c** Jaw tone is not a reflex response.

308. **b** Rather than stage II of anesthesia (excitement), transient apnea or cardiovascular compromise is more likely to be seen with too rapid administration of an anesthetic IV. Stage II is more likely to result from injecting an anesthetic by IV too slowly.

309. **a** A high level of arterial oxygen and a low level of arterial carbon dioxide are safest for an anesthetized patient.

310. **b** Monitoring central venous pressure requires insertion of an intravenous catheter, so the tip is in the cranial vena cava.

311. **b** Doxapram is both a respiratory stimulant and an analeptic agent.

312. **d** Although they may sound as though they are having laryngospasm, because they have sounds on inspiration, it is actually due to the excessive soft tissue in the pharynx.

313. **d**

314. **d** They all have high vapor pressures, thus they require precision vaporizers.

315. **c**

316. **a** The others are components of a circle anesthetic system.

317. **b** Blue is the standard color for medical nitrous oxide cylinders. The pressure in a nitrous oxide cylinder reads 750 psi until all of the liquid is vaporized. The pressure reading then quickly decreases.

318. **c**

319. **b**

320. **a**

321. **b** Cattle should be placed in sternal recumbency to avoid bloat.

322. **d** The intravenous (IV) route is preferable if venous access is already established. If IV is not possible, intratracheal (IT) is less traumatic than intracardiac (IC) drug administration.

323. **a** The potential for the other long-term side effects can be minimized with proper anesthetic techniques, including use of scavenging systems.

324. **b** Cuffed tubes are not necessary in birds.

325. **b**

326. **b** Dopamine is an inotropic agent that increases the force of myocardial contractions.

327. **a** Succinylcholine is a nonreversible type of muscle-paralyzing agent.

328. **b** Geriatric patients have a difficult time coping with the respiratory and cardiovascular depressions associated with xylazine.

329. **b**

330. **d**

331. **c** An airway must be secured as soon as possible in these patients.